Paediatric Kawasaki Disease

Hong Wang
Editor

Paediatric Kawasaki Disease

Clinical Analysis and Cases

PMPH
PEOPLE'S MEDICAL PUBLISHING HOUSE

Springer

Editor
Hong Wang
Department of pediatric cardiology
Shengjing Hospital, China Medical University
Shenyang
China

ISBN 978-981-15-0037-4   ISBN 978-981-15-0038-1 (eBook)
https://doi.org/10.1007/978-981-15-0038-1

Jointly published with People's Medical Publishing House, PR of China
The print edition is not for sale in China (Mainland). Customers from China (Mainland) please order the print book from: People's Medical Publishing House, PR of China.

This Springer imprint is published by the registered company Springer Nature Singapore Pte Ltd.
The registered company address is: 152 Beach Road, #21-01/04 Gateway East, Singapore 189721, Singapore

Foreword

I met Professor Hong Wang for the first time at a pediatric academic conference about three years ago, in which many pediatric cardiologists gathering for annual meeting. By talking I noticed that we are alumna of China Medical University. About one and half years ago, she kindly gave me as a gift her just published book about Kawasaki disease (KD) cases she collected. I was very impressive by these cases. All cases were special and with details clinical features, images, and analysis. I suggested her to publish these valuable cases collection in English, which could spread all over the world and may help medical student, professional, and even the families of their children suffering from this disease. One year later, this idea also confirmed by People's Medical Publishing House. This book was selected with other valuable books to publish in English version by Springer. From then on we worked together to make it possible.

The KD cases collected from more than twenty year ago by Dr Wang. They including 53 KD cases which either typical KD or with complications involved different systems, such as cardiovascular, digestive, nervous, blood, respiratory, urinary, bone and joints, and endocrine systems complications. In this book, each case presented with clinical history, physical examination, laboratory findings, diagnosis, treatment, and discussion, all available images also included. All cases in this book come from the authors' clinical practice. Therefore, some cases might not perform all examinations or lost follow up.

As a non-native English as first language, Dr Wang and her team worked very hard to write up this book. Therefor when you read it might not like a native speaker English in somewhere. However I believe that you will get all information you need from these cases. I hope this book will benefit to all readers.

Yan-min Zhang

Preface by Wang Hong

I still remember 30 years ago, when the first case of Kawasaki Disease (KD) was diagnosed in our hospital, I just graduated and started rotation in the pediatric cardiology ward. The special clinical symptoms, signs and novel name left deep impression on me. After successful diagnosis and cure of a few cases, I felt the diagnosis and treatment of KD was straightforward. However, about 20 years ago, a 6-month infant was brought to our ward on Day 12 of his illness with regular treatment proven unsuccessful, presented not only continuous fever but also successive coronary dilation, facial nerve palsy, sleepiness, aseptic meningitis. During intravascular mannitol treatment, the patient also developed acute heart failure. Although the final prognosis was well, from then on, I began to re-evaluate the KD, and once created a sense of fear. In the following years, I encountered countless special cases one after another, which always made me feel it is the first time I have met the disease. In recent 7 years, a total of three cases in our center with KD or AKD died of chronic heart failure (CHF) for prior misdiagnosis in local hospital. They developed giant coronary artery aneurysms (CAA), coronary thrombosis, and ischemic cardiomyopathy. One of them developed the aortic valve serious damage. Another patient, who survived two and a half years after diagnosed KD, was still struggling with CHF. In China, the relationship between doctors and patients is somewhat sensitive. Furthermore, glucocorticoids application was controversial. Once developed rash during fever, applying glucocorticoids is very common, especially in clinics in rural and/or remote regions. Thus, some atypical clinical symptoms usually delayed the diagnosis of KD and results in severe coronary artery complications. As a pediatric cardiovascular professional doctor, I am very distressed. After KD was first reported more than 50 years ago, there are still patients losing life or being disabled because of the disease. I am obligated to parents and to all pediatric medical coworkers to let known the knowledge of KD. That's why I wrote this book. To accumulate these cases and experience, I would like to thank our distinguished predecessors, Prof. Yong-ji Wang, Prof. Ying-ai Piao, Prof. Ya-nan Zhu, Associate Prof. Shu-chun Hu and Prof. Xian-yi Yu. They laid a solid foundation to help us evolve into an organization that nowadays encountering more than 500 cases of KD every year, and accumulating rich experience in the diagnosis and treatment. At the same time I would also like to thank pediatric related colleagues for their timely consultation and guidance, collaboratively saving the young patients regardless of the acute phases. Thanks to the farsightedness and courage of the hospital leaders in developing electronic medical records (EMRs), which enabled preservation of the precious materials and images, making the book more colorful. In order to be more rigorous, we specially invited Prof. Yang Hou from the department of radiology to mark the images of coronary artery CTA and other radiology images. Associate Professor of cardiac ultrasound Xiao-na Yu for the coronary artery ultrasound images and other ultrasound images, blood chamber attending Xuan Liu, and pathology department attending physician Yun-long Huo responsable in their respective fields. In order to complete this book, naive but all-out, we are using the out of office hours during nights or holidays, lasting for more than 1 year. Admittedly due to the capability limitation and language gap, inevitably there will be errors or mistakes. Hence, I sincerely look forward to the comments and corrections from peer experts.

Hong Wang
Shenyang, China

The original version of the book was revised. The correction to the book can be found at https://doi.org/10.1007/978-981-15-0038-1_17

Contents

Abbreviations

Abbreviations	The full name (Normal value)
ABEP	Auditory brainstem evoked potential
ADV	Adenovirus
AECG	Ambulance Electrocardiogram
AEEG	Ambulance Electroencephalogram
AKD	Atipical Kawasaki disease
ALT	Alanine aminotransfer ase (0–40 U/L)
ANA	Antinuclear antibody
ASA	Acetyl salicylic acid
ASD	Atrial septal defect
ASO	Anti-hemolytic streptococcus O (<200 U/L)
AST	Aspartate aminotransferase (<35 U/L)
CAA	Coronary artery aneurysm
CABG	Coronary artery bypass grafting
CAD	Coronary artery disease
CAL	Coronary artery lesion
CHD	Congenital heart disease
CK	Creatine kinase (<145 IU/L)
CKMB	Creatine kinase-MB isozyme (<24 IU/L)
CKMB-M	Creatine kinase-MB Mass (<6.3 mg/L)
CP	Chlamydia pneumoniae
CRP	C reactive protein (<8 mg/L)
CSF	Cerebrospinal fluid
CT	Computed tomography
CTA	Computed tomographic angiography
CTNI	Cardiac troponin I (<0.04 μg/ml)
D Bil	Conjugated bilirubin (<21mmol/L)
ECG	Electrocardiogram
Echo	Echocardiography
EEG	Electroencephalogram
ESR	Erythrocyte sedimentation rate (M<15mm/h, F<20mm/h)
FDP	fibrinogen degradation product (FDP) (0–5mg/L)
FDS	Fructose Dipllosphate sodium
HS-CTNT	High-sensative Troponin T (<0.014 ng/L)
IKD	Incomplete Kawasaki disease
IL6	Interleukin - 6
INR	International normalized ratio (<1.5)
IVIG	Intravenas immunoglobulin
KD	Kawasaki disease
KDSS	Kawasaki disease shock syndrome
LAD	Left anterior descending
LCA	Left coronary artery

LCX	Left circumflex branch
LM	Left main coronary artery
LV	Left ventricle
MAS	Macrophage activation syndrome
MP	Mycoplasma pneumoniae
MR	Magnetic resonance
MYO	Myoglobinc (<63 mg/L)
NT-pro BNP	N-terminal brain natriuretic peptide precursor (<300 ng/L)
PINF	Parainfluenza
RCA	Right coronary artery
RSV	Respiratory syncytial virus
T Bil	Total bilirubin (3.4–20.5 μmol/L)
TBA	Total bile acid (0.5–10.0 μmol/L)
UND Bil	Non-conjugated bilirubin (3.4–11.9 μmol/L)
VBEP	Visual brainstem evoked potential

Background

1

Hong Wang

Abstract

Since Kawasaki disease (KD) was described by Japanese doctor Tomisaku Kawasaki in 1967, KD has replaced rheumatic heart disease, becoming the leading cause of acquired heart disease in children of the developed countries [1]. Although its etiology is not yet understood, it has been generally recognized as an acute vasculitis happening in children with allergies, mostly less than 5 years old [2]. KD is self-limited. In patients without treatment, the average duration of fever is about 10 days, 20–25% of patients will have coronary artery aneurysms (CAA), and 1–2% of them will have CAA even after treatment. About 10–20% of them develop resistance to IVIG. About 1–2% has recurrence [2]. Because coronary artery injury is the most serious complication, and coronary artery thrombus can lead to coronary heart disease and even sudden death, more and more pediatric cardiologists are engaged in diagnosis, treatment, and follow-up of KD. Therefore, a vast majority of children with KD have a good outcome.

Since Kawasaki disease (KD) was described by Japanese doctor Tomisaku Kawasaki in 1967, KD has replaced rheumatic heart disease, becoming the leading cause of acquired heart disease in children of the developed countries [1]. Although its etiology is not yet understood, it has been generally recognized as an acute vasculitis happening in children with allergies, mostly less than 5 years old [2]. KD is self-limited. In patients without treatment, the average duration of fever is about 10 days, 20–25% of patients will have coronary artery aneurysms (CAA), and 1–2% of them will have CAA even after treatment. About 10–20% of them develop resistance to IVIG. About 1–2% has recurrence [2]. Because coronary artery injury is the most serious complication, and coronary artery thrombus can lead to coronary heart disease and even sudden death, more and more pediatric cardiologists are engaged in diagnosis, treatment, and follow-up of KD. Therefore, a vast majority of children with KD have a good outcome.

However, clinic symptoms of KD vary in a wide range, and multiple systems can be involved. In cases with the cardiovascular system involved alone, KD may be complicated with myocarditis [3–4], in which myocardial inflammation has been reported almost without exception in myocardial biopsies, even in the absence of CAA [5]. Although these children had acute heart failure in the acute phase, as long as they were treated on time, their prognosis are good. Pericardial effusion can also be seen in KD [5]. Although the amount of pericardial effusion is large, long-term and high dose of antibiotics is not required. Once IVIG and oral aspirin are given to patients for treatment, pericardial effusion can be completely absorbed without the sequelae of pericardial adhesion and constrictive pericarditis. Children with KD can develop ischemic cardiomyopathy [6]. In addition, complications also include CRBBB, ABV, arrhythmia [7], and shock [8]. Unlike hereditary cardiomyopathy, it usually recovers with sustained and aggressive treatments. It has been reported that the incidence of CAA in untreated KD children is 20–25% [9]. In our center, total three children were misdiagnosed, and they developed coronary artery thrombus and coronary heart diseases about 6 months later. Within 3 years, they lost their lives. KD accompanied with myocarditis has been reported previously. Analysis of myocardial biopsies from patients at the early disease course suggests it is a nearly universal incidence [10]. In KD patients with CAA, the myocardium damage is very common, even without any symptoms [11]. Thus, we have explanations for the chronic myocardial damage in KD without CAA. Aortic valve regurgitation (AR) is much less common at presentation (1% of patients) [12]. AR in KD is usually associated with aortic root dilation. But in our center, a 3-year-old girl with aortic valve damage died about 2 years later. Patients with severe coronary artery involvement may also develop aneurysms in other medium-sized arteries, with rare occurrences of thrombosis or rupture at these sites [13–14]. However, in our center, a misdiagnosed KD patient had complication of abdominal aorta and iliac aneurysm with increased blood clots, and died at the end.

H. Wang (✉)
Department of Pediatric Cardiology, Shengjing Hospital of China Medical University, Shenyang, China

H. Wang (ed.), *Paediatric Kawasaki Disease*, https://doi.org/10.1007/978-981-15-0038-1_1

For increased permeability of capillaries, hyponatremia and hypoalbuminemia are common due to natrium, liquid, and albumin leaking out of capillaries. Without treatment timely, volume of circulating blood could be insufficient. At last, hypovolemic shock may be developed. In terms of symptoms only, it is somewhat similar to diarrhea disease; both present vomit and/or watery stool. However, the most significant difference between KD and common vial diarrhea is that KD patients usually lose a lot of albumin. Thus, in KD patients, metabolic acidosis is not severe, but the shock is difficult to correct. Furthermore, albumin and immunoglobulin are essential, while bicarbonate is not indispensable. Hypovolemic shock usually happens in patients at acute phase, mostly in patients who have persistent fever along with vomit and diarrhea. While vomiting and diarrhea are common in children with acute KD, persistent fever is common in children with IVIG resistance, but they are less likely to develop shock. It is not clear whether this is related to a decrease in or inhibition of adrenal function, even the hypothalamus is dysfunctional [15]. Of course, it may also be related to syndrome of inappropriate anti-diuretic hormone [16]. Literature only descripted inhibition of adrenal function after treatment using IVIG combined with GC [17]. In our center, children with KD were inadvertently found to have adrenal calcification before treatment, and this calcification can be partially recovered several years later. It is a pity that we did not realize that this might be a complication of KD, and we did not perform the endocrine level test. What is puzzling us is that patients did not have shock, so the inhibition of adrenal function is not the only mechanism causing shock. Even so, once hypovolemic shock happened, patients could be in extreme danger [18]. In addition to this, both hyponatremia and hypoalbuminemia are independent risk factors for coronary artery aneurysms [19]. Therefore, we must be aware of hyponatremia and hypoalbuminemia in KD patients and treat them timely in order for them have a good prognosis.

Coronary artery aneurysms (CAA) or dilatation is the most common complication associated with KD, and the complication may lead to myocardial infarction, ischemic heart disease, or sudden death. In addition, other relatively infrequent heart complications have been noted, especially cardiac arrhythmia which consist of premature contraction, atrioventricular heart block, ventricular tachycardia, and ventricular fibrillation. These complications can be life threatening sometime. It was reported that about 5.5% KD patients may develop arrhythmias, and 5.6% with ST changes. The possible mechanisms of arrhythmia in KD include myocardial ischemia, myocardial interstitial edema, and micro-thrombus formation. Some KD patients with normal or mildly abnormal ECG at acute phase may develop arrhythmia several years later [20]. In our center, there was a 2-year-old boy with IRBBB, QRS 98ms at initial stage. He developed CRBBB 10 years later, QRS 136ms (case 14), but with normal coronary artery, LVED and LVEF. The prevalence of arrhythmia, such as frequented premature ventricular contraction (PVC) and frequented premature atrial contraction (PAC) [7], is higher in adults who had been diagnosed with KD in childhood than those of health adults [6]. Therefore, regular follow-ups should be performed with patients who have a history of KD.

In terms of morbidity, the digestive system ranks at the top among all complications of KD. The most common symptoms include vomiting, diarrhea, and hypoproteinemia [21], followed by abnormal liver function which is significantly associated with IVIG unresponsiveness [22], cholestasis [23–24], cholecystitis [25], pancreatitis [26], intussusception [27], and so on. In our center, a boy presented with fever along with stomachache and vomiting. Physical examination showed right lower abdominal limited peritonitis. Blood test showed significantly increased WBC and CRP. Abdominal CT revealed flatulence and mesenteric lymph node enlargement. He was diagnosed with acute appendicitis, and underwent laparoscopic appendectomy. Postoperative fever continued and was accompanied with congestive rashes, conjunctival congestion, red and dry lips. He was diagnosed with KD and recovered after timely treatment with IVIG and aspirin. Intraoperative findings revealed peritoneal inflammation in right lower abdomen. Pathology examination reported serosal inflammation, which did not support appendicitis. Although the clinic symptoms of KD are very different, with rehydration, albumin supplementation, conventional IVIG, and aspirin treatment, symptoms described above can be recovered, leaving no serious sequelae. Of course, abnormal liver function in children at the acute phase of ASA need to be treated in time, otherwise it will be aggravated and cause liver damage.

Nervous system involvement in KD is common, including irritability, lethargy, convulsions, aseptic meningitis [21], facial paralysis [28], sensorineural hearing loss [29], visual abnormalities [30], and so on. All these findings disappear completely within six months [31]. In our center, we also found bilateral abductor nerve involvement, which recovered at 2 months of illness. None of these complications remained serious after active treatment. Behavioral abnormalities could also be involved, and these behavior sequelae may remain nearly 10 years [32].

KD can also present with blood system complication. At the beginning of KD, blood routine results maybe normal. With the progress of continuous fever and disease itself, peripheral blood routine changed usually 5 days later: WBC, NE percentage, and PLT increased significantly, with worsen anemia. After IVIG and aspirin therapy, body temperatures in most patients were gradually decreased to normal. Without IVIG resistance, WBC and neutrophils gradually recovered, PLT and anemia would return to normal later. However, with IVIG resistance, additional IVIG and GC will form thrombocythemia within a short period of time, leading to hypercoagulability. At this time, except aspirin, dipyridamole is particularly important. About a week after temperature control, PLT begins to decline and returns to normal within 1–2 months. The exception, of course, is that children start off with low platelets, which is often a predictor of CAA [33]. When IVIG resistant occurred, HGB can go down due to persistent fever and the presence of a hepcidin [34]. With the disease under control, blood transfusions are not required in majority of cases. Of course, the secondary macrophage activation syndrome (MAS) is another matter. KD patients with MAS can develop cytopenia (including thrombocytopenia) [35-36]. In our center, these patients usually have leukemia-like reaction. Complication with anemia, infection, and bleeding can all lead to life-threatening conditions [37]. D-Dimer elevation usually indicates hypercoagulability and suggests tissue disintegration, associated with much severe diseases. It has been reported that, in KD patients with complications in blood system, elevated D-Dimer is usually detected in acute phase and is positively correlated with CAA [38]. However, in our center, patients with elevated D-Dimer may present with complications in multiorgans, including cholestatic hepatitis, MAS, aseptic meningitis or shock, but not necessarily CAA. Unlike reported by Masuzawa, there is no statistically significant correlation between D-Dimer elevation and CAA (n=317, t-test, $p > 0.1$, unpublished). In cases with elevated D-Dimers, we would rather concern about multiorgan damages than CAA.

Pulmonary involvement is uncommon and is not part of the conventional diagnostic criteria [39]. However, this does not mean that KD patients with respiratory system complication are less sick. In our center, there were two patients with necrotizing pneumonia and some pleural effusion, which was related to inflammatory hypoproteinemia. Despite at high risks, such as high fever lasting more than half a month, males, CRP >100mg/L, they, unexpectedly, did not develop CAA.

The incidence of KD with arthritis is reported around 16% [40] and 15–45% [41]. Arthritis at early phase usually occur at interphalangeal joint, cervical spine and temporomandibular joints [42]. Once KD is diagnosed, treatment with routine IVIG and aspirin can relieve swelling and redness at joints naturally. But the arthritis at sub-acute phase (around ten days of illness) usually occur at weight-bearing joints, such as hips and knees. If patients still have fever at the same time, differential diagnosis of rheumatism and JIA should be considered. The first choice to treat arthritis in this situation is to use IVIG [43]. If patients have serious joint symptoms accompanied with fever, they may also need to be treated with GCs and oral aspirin. But the course of treatment is short, usually less than one month. Symptom recovery is fast, without relapse or joint deformity or dysfunction. As for KD with bone injury, as far as the author is aware, there has been no relevant report. In our center, a 3 years boy presented at KD sub-acute phase with combined proximal tibial bone lesion. Because there are no relevant reports, and the pharynx brush culture indicated positive hemolytic streptococcus growth, we cannot conclude this change is certainly not pyogenic osteomyelitis. Thus, bone marrow drainage procedure was performed and no pus was found. Patho-histology of bone marrow found majority of lymphocytes and plasma cells, and immunohistology found tumor antigen negative. He recovered after one year. Based on his history, we can confirm that skeletal changes in this patient are a complication of KD.

Among KD patients with complication of kidney injuries, 30%–80% have pyuria, most commonly in patients ≤ 1 year of age, associated with mononuclear cells (not neutrophils). Sterile pyuria originates from the urethra, and as a result there are mild and sub-clinical renal injuries in kidneys, and/or injuries in the bladder due to cystitis [44]. In addition, there are reports of hematuria [45], proteinuria [46], and renal failure [47].

It has been reported that vaccination can induce KD [48], but there is no significant difference between KD patients and normal children [49–50].

The incidence of IVIG resistance in KD children is 10–20% [9]. According to the literature, the treatment mainly include additional IVIG 2 g/kg [51] within 24 hours, glucocorticoid [52], tumor necrosis factor-alfa (TNF-α) inhibition [53], plasma exchange [54], and so on. Before the publication of AHA's 2017 guideline, we had tried lower doses of glucocorticoid. However, no comparative analysis had been done because fewer cases are completed. Overall, the duration of fever was longer and the incidence of coronary artery aneurysms did not increase significantly.

As to atypical KD (AKD), it usually happens in infants and young children [54]. Patients, particularly, <6 months of age and lacking eye or oral mucosal changes, may experience significant delays in diagnosis [55]. In our center, those who received glucocorticoid within three days of onset were more likely to develop atypical KD. They are at substantial risk of developing coronary artery abnormalities and who may have prolonged fever as the sole clinical finding or have subtle or fleeting clinical signs in addition to fever [56].

In this book, we present total 53 complication cases. Because some cases are more severe, with complications in multiple organs, and they are classified as the more severe cases. Among these, there are 15 cases with complication in cardiovascular system, 5 cases in digestive system, 5 cases in nervous system, 1 case in blood system, 3 cases in respiratory system, 2 cases in urinary system, 2 cases in bone and joints, 1 case with adrenal calcification, 3 cases of IVIG resistance, 4 cases of recurrent KD, 4 cases with misdiagnosis of KD, 3 cases of atypical KD, 3 cases with controversial KD, 1 case with vaccination induced KD, and 1 case with myocardial tumor.

These cases were enrolled in last 20 years. While the diagnostic basis for KD has remained largely unchanged for the last 20 years, the criteria for IVIG resistance is somewhat different. All criteria diagnosis are based on AHA Scientific statement-2017 of US [9] and JCS 2008 of Japan [57].

1.1 Diagnosis of Kawasaki disease (KD)

Classic KD is diagnosed with a presence of fever lasting for at least 5 days (the day of fever onset is taken into as the first day of fever) together with at least 4 of the 5 following principal clinical features:

≥4 principal clinical features, particularly when redness and swelling in hands and feet are present, the diagnosis of KD can be made with 4 d of fever. In rare cases, experienced clinicians who have treated many patients with KD may establish the diagnosis with 3 d of fever.

1. Erythema and cracked lips, strawberry tongue, and/or erythema of oral and pharyngeal mucosa
2. Bilateral bulbar conjunctival congestion without exudate
3. Rashes: maculopapular, diffuse erythroderma, or erythema multiforme-like
4. Erythema and edema in hands and feet presented at acute phase and/or periungual desquamation in sub-acute phase
5. Cervical lymphadenopathy (≥1.5 cm diameter), usually unilateral.

Patients who lack full clinical features of classic KD are often evaluated for incomplete (atypical) KD. In most cases, if coronary artery abnormalities are detected, the diagnosis of KD is finalized.

Laboratory tests typically reveal normal or elevated white blood cell count with neutrophil in predominance and elevated acute phase reactants such as C-reactive protein (CRP) and erythrocyte sedimentation rate (ESR) during the acute phase. Low serum sodium and albumin levels, elevated serum liver enzymes, and sterile pyuria can be present. In the second week after fever onset, thrombocytosis is common.

1.2 Diagnosis of Incomplete KD

The diagnosis of incomplete (sometimes referred to as atypical) KD should be considered in any infants or children with prolonged and unexplained fever, fewer than 4 of the principal clinical findings, and supporting laboratory or echocardiographic findings.

1.3 Coronary Artery Abnormalities

Quantitative assessment of luminal dimensions allows for more accurate classification of coronary artery abnormalities. The Japanese guidelines classify coronary arteries by absolute or relative internal lumen diameter [57]. Dilation or small aneurysms are defined as a localized dilation of the internal lumen diameter but <4 mm, or if the child is ≥5 years of age, dilation but with an internal diameter of a segment measuring ≤1.5 times that of an adjacent segment. Medium aneurysms are defined as an internal lumen diameter >4 mm but ≤8 mm, or if the child is ≥5 years of age, an internal diameter of a segment measuring 1.5 to 4 times that of an adjacent segment. Large or giant aneurysms are defined as those with an internal lumen diameter >8 mm, or if the child is >5 years of age, an internal diameter of a segment measuring >4 times that of an adjacent segment. These criteria do not take patients' size into account, which can substantially affect normal coronary artery dimensions, and potentially lead to under-diagnosis and underestimation of the true prevalence of coronary artery dilation pathophysiology and pathology.

For our patients collected the earliest from twenty years ago, the criteria for assessing coronary artery was based on above Japanese standard.

Normalization of dimensions for BSA as *Z* scores (standard deviation units from the mean) based on regression equations allow for standardization as a continuous measure.

A classification scheme based solely on *Z* scores was proposed, which has been adapted and recommended in these guidelines:

Z-Score Classification

1. No involvement: Always <2
2. Dilation only: 2 to <2.5; or if initially <2, a decrease in *Z* score during follow-up ≥1
3. Small aneurysm: ≥2.5 to <5
4. Medium aneurysm: ≥5 to <10, and absolute dimension <8 mm
5. Large or giant aneurysm: ≥10, or absolute dimension ≥8 mm

1.4 IVIG resistance

The diagnostic criteria for IVIG resistance vary from time to time, and it is generally accepted that there is recrudescent or persistent fever at least 36 hours after the end of their IVIG infusion and are termed IVIG resistant [58–60], and the incidence of IVIG resistance is about 10%–20%.

References

1. Shulman ST. IVGG therapy in Kawasaki disease: mechanism(s) of action. Clin Immunol Immunopathol. 1989;53(2 Pt 2):S141–6.
2. Maddox RA, Holman RC, Uehara R, et al. Recurrent Kawasaki disease: USA and Japan. Pediatr Int. 2015;57:1116–20.
3. Aggarwal P, Suri D, Narula N, et al. Symptomatic myocarditis in Kawasaki disease. Indian J Pediatr. 2012;79(6):813–4.
4. De Rosa G, Andreozzi L, Piastra M, et al. Acute myocarditis as a revealing clue of complete Kawasaki disease. Reumatismo. 2018;70(2):115–6.
5. Okada S, Hasegawa S, Suzuki Y, et al. Acute pericardial effusion representing the TNF-α-mediated severe inflammation but not the coronary artery outcome of Kawasaki disease. Scand J Rheumatol. 2015;44(3):247–52.
6. Komaki H, Nakashima T, Minatoguchi S. Radiofrequency catheter ablation for ventricular tachycardia in ischaemic cardiomyopathy due to Kawasaki disease. Cardiol Young. 2018;28(6):890–3.

7. Sumitomo N, Karasawa K, Taniguchi K, et al. Association of sinus node dysfunction, atrioventricular node conduction abnormality and ventricular arrhythmia in patients with Kawasaki disease and coronary involvement. Circ J. 2008;72(2):274–80.
8. Li Y, Zheng Q, Zou L, et al. Kawasaki disease shock syndrome: clinical characteristics and possible use of IL-6, IL-10 and IFN-γ as biomarkers for early recognition. Pediatr Rheumatol Online J. 2019 Jan 5;17(1):1. https://doi.org/10.1186/s12969-018-0303-4.
9. McCrindle BW, Rowley AH, Newburger JW, et al. Diagnosis, Treatment, and Long-Term Management of Kawasaki Disease: A Scientific Statement for Health Professionals From the American Heart Association. Circulation. 2017;135(17):e927–99.
10. Yutani C, Go S, Kamiya T, et al. Cardiac biopsy of Kawasaki disease. Arch Pathol Lab Med. 1981;105(9):470–3.
11. Yonesaka S, Takahashi T, Eto S, et al. Biopsy-proven myocardial sequels in Kawasaki disease with giant coronary aneurysms. Cardiol Young. 2010;20(6):602–9.
12. Printz BF, Sleeper LA, Newburger JW, et al. Noncoronary cardiac abnormalities are associated with coronary artery dilation and with laboratory inflammatory markers in acute Kawasaki disease. J Am Coll Cardiol. 2011;57(1):86–92.
13. Orenstein JM, Shulman ST, Fox LM, et al. Three linked vasculopathic processes characterize Kawasaki disease: a light and transmission electron microscopic study. PLoS One. 2012;7(6):e38998.
14. Hoshino S, Tsuda E, Yamada O. Characteristics and fate of systemic artery aneurysm after Kawasaki disease. J Pediatr. 2015;167(1):108–12.
15. Garrido-García LM, Peña-Juárez RA, Yamazaki-Nakashimada MA. Cardiac manifestations in the acute phase of Kawasaki disease in a third level children's hospital in Mexico City. Arch Cardiol Mex. 2018 Apr 9. pii: S1405-9940(18)30035-1.
16. Mori J, Miura M, Shiro H, et al. Syndrome of inappropriate anti-diuretic hormone in Kawasaki disease. Pediatr Int. 2011;53(3):354–7.
17. Anno T, Kawasaki F, Takai M, et al. Clinical course of pituitary function and image in IgG4-related hypophysitis. Endocrinol Diabetes Metab Case Rep. 2017 Apr 28, 2017. pii: 16-0148.
18. Richards JB, Wilcox SR. Diagnosis and management of shock in the emergency department. Emerg Med Pract. 2014;16(3):1–22.
19. Gámez-González LB, Murata C, Muñoz-Ramírez M, et al. Clinical manifestations associated with Kawasaki disease shock syndrome in Mexican children .Eur J Pediatr. 2013, 172(3):337-42.
20. Goto M, Miyagawa N, Kikunaga K, et al. High incidence of adrenal suppression in children with Kawasaki disease treated with intravenous immunoglobulin plus prednisolone. Endocr J. 2015;62(2):145–51.
21. Zhang Y, Wan H, Du M, et al. Capillary leak syndrome and aseptic meningitis in a patient with Kawasaki disease: A case report. Medicine (Baltimore). 2018;97(23):e10716.
22. Liu L, Yin W, Wang R, et al. The prognostic role of abnormal liver function in IVIG unresponsiveness in Kawasaki disease: a meta-analysis. Inflamm Res. 2016;65(2):161–8.
23. Koca T, Aslan N, Akaslan Kara A, et al. Kawasaki disease in a 9-year old girl presenting with febrile cholestasis: case report and review of literature. Int J Rheum Dis. 2018;21(11):2046–9.
24. Martínez Vázquez JA, Sánchez García C, Rodríguez Muñoz L, et al. Acute kidney injury and cholestasis associated with Kawasaki disease in a 9-year-old: Case report. Reumatol Clin.2017 Dec 15. pii: S1699-258X(17)30282-6.
25. Mayumi T, Okamoto K, Takada T, et al. Tokyo Guidelines 2018: management bundles for acute cholangitis and cholecystitis. J Hepatobiliary Pancreat Sci. 2018;25(1):96–100.
26. Botti M, Costagliola G, Consolini R. Typical Kawasaki Disease Presenting With Pancreatitis and Bilateral Parotid Gland Involvement: A Case Report and Literature Review. Front Pediatr. 2018;6:90. https://doi.org/10.3389/fped.2018.00090.
27. Hussain RN, Ruiz G. Kawasaki disease presenting with intussusception: a case report. Italian Journal of Pediatrics. 2010;36(1):7–9.
28. Stowe RC. Facial nerve palsy, Kawasaki disease, and coronary artery aneurysm. Eur J Paediatr Neurol. 2015;19(5):607–9.
29. Anand S, Yang YC. Optic disc changes in Kawasaki disease. J Pediatr Ophthalmol Strabismus. 2004;41:177–9.
30. Magalhães CM, Magalhães Alves NR, Oliveira KM, et al. Sensorineural hearing loss: an underdiagnosed complication of Kawasaki disease. J Clin Rheumatol. 2010;16(7):322–5.
31. Terasawa K, Ichinose E, Matsuishi T, et al. Neurological complications in Kawasaki disease. Brain Dev. 1983;5(4):371–4.
32. Carlton-Conway D, Ahluwalia R, Henry L, et al. Behaviour sequelae following acute Kawasaki disease. BMC Pediatr. 2005;5(1):14.
33. Newburger JW, Takahashi M, Gerber MA, et al. Diagnosis, treatment, and long-term management of Kawasaki disease: a statement for health professionals from the Committee on Rheumatic Fever, Endocarditis and Kawasaki Disease, Council on Cardiovascular Disease in the Young, American Heart Association Circulation. 2004, 110(17):2747-2771.
34. Huang YH, Kuo HC, Huang FC, et al. Hepcidin-Induced Iron Deficiency Is Related to Transient Anemia and Hypoferremia in Kawasaki Disease Patients. Int J Mol Sci. 2016 May 12, 17(5). pii: E715.
35. García-Pavón S, Yamazaki-Nakashimada MA, Báez M, et al. Kawasaki Disease Complicated With Macrophage Activation Syndrome: A Systematic Review. J Pediatr Hematol Oncol. 2017;39(6):445–51.
36. Dumont B, Jeannoel P, Trapes L, et al. Macrophage activation syndrome and Kawasaki disease: Four new cases. Arch Pediatr. 2017;24(7):640–6.
37. Lerkvaleekul B, Vilaiyuk S. Macrophage activation syndrome: early diagnosis is key. Open Access Rheumatol. 2018 Aug 31;10:117–28.
38. Masuzawa Y, Mori M, Hara T, et al. Elevated D-dimer level is a risk factor for coronary artery lesions accompanying intravenous immunoglobulin-unresponsive Kawasaki disease. Ther Apher Dial. 2015;19(2):171–7.
39. Leahy TR, Cohen E, Allen UD. Incomplete Kawasaki disease associated with complicated Streptococcus progenies pneumonia: A case report. Can J Infect Dis Med Microbiol. 2012;23(3):137–9.
40. Álvarez EP, Rey F, Peña SC, et al. Has joint involvement lessened in Kawasaki disease? Reumatol Clin. 2017;13(3):145–9.
41. Lee KY, Oh JH, Han JW, et al. Arthritis in disease after responding to intravenous immunoglobulin treatment. Eur J Pediatr. 2005;164(7):451–2.
42. Jen M, Brucia LA, Pollock AN, et al. Cervical spine and temporomandibular joint arthritis in a child with Kawasaki disease. Pediatr. 2006;118(5):e1569–71.
43. Rodriguez MM, Wagner-Weiner L. Intravenous Immunoglobulin in Pediatric Rheumatology: When to Use It and What Is the Evidence. Pediatr Ann. 2017;46(1):e19–24.
44. Watanabe T. Pyuria in patients with Kawasaki disease. World J Clin Pediatr. 2015;4(2):25–9.
45. Wang JN, Chiou YY, Chiu NT, et al. Renal scarring sequelae in childhood Kawasaki disease. Pediatr Nephrol. 2006;22(5):684–9.
46. Bonany PJ, Bilkis MD, Gallo G, et al. Acute renal failure in typical Kawasaki disease. Pediatr Nephrol. 2002;17(5):329–31.
47. Gatterre P, Oualha M, Dupic L, et al. Kawasaki disease: an unexpected etiology of shock and multiple organ dysfunction syndrome. Intensive Care Med. 2012;38(5):872–8.
48. Chang A, Islam S. Kawasaki Disease and Vasculitis associated with Immunizations. Pediatr Int. 2018 May 5; https://doi.org/10.1111/ped.13590.
49. Abrams JY, Weintraub ES, Baggs JM, et al. Childhood vaccines and Kawasaki disease, Vaccine Safety Datalink, 1996-2006. Vaccine. 2015;33(2):382–7.

50. Hua W, Izurieta HS, Slade B, et al. Kawasaki Disease After Vaccination: Reports to the Vaccine Adverse Event Reporting System 1990–2007 The Pediatric Infectious Disease Journal. Pediatr Infect Dis J. 2009 Nov;28(11):943–7.
51. Burns JC, Capparelli EV, Brown JA, et al. Intravenous gamma-globulin treatment and retreatment in Kawasaki disease: US/Canadian Kawasaki Syndrome Study Group. Pediatr Infect Dis J. 1998;17(12):1144–8.
52. Kobayashi T, Saji T, Otani T, et al. Efficacy of immunoglobulin plus prednisolone for prevention of coronary artery abnormalities in severe Kawasaki disease (RAISE study): a randomised, open-label, blindedendpoints trial. Lancet. 2012;379(9826):1613–20.
53. Weiss JE, Eberhard BA, Chowdhury D, et al. Infliximab as a novel therapy for refractory Kawasaki disease. J Rheumatol. 2004;31(4):808–10.
54. Singh S, Jindal AK, Pilania RK. Diagnosis of Kawasaki disease. Int J Rheum Dis. 2018;21(1):36–44.
55. Minich LL, Sleeper LA, Atz AM, et al. Delayed diagnosis of Kawasaki disease: what are the risk factors? Pediatrics. 2007;120:e1434–40.
56. Imagawa T, Mori M, Miyamae T, et al. Plasma exchange for refractory Kawasaki disease. Eur J Pediatr. 2004;163(4-5):263–4.
57. JCS Joint Working Group. Guidelines for diagnosis and management of cardiovascular sequelae in Kawasaki disease (JCS 2008): digest version. Circ J. 2010;74(9):1989–2020.
58. Newburger JW, Sleeper LA, McCrindle BW, et al. Randomized trial of pulsed corticosteroid therapy for primary treatment of Kawasaki disease. N Engl J Med. 2007;356(7):663–5.
59. Tremoulet AH, Best BM, Song S, et al. Resistance to intravenous immunoglobulin in children with Kawasaki disease. J Pediatr. 2008;153(1):117–21.
60. Bar-Meir M, Kalisky I, Schwartz A, et al. Prediction of Resistance to Intravenous Immunoglobulin in Children With Kawasaki Disease. J Pediatric Infect Dis Soc. 2018;7(1):25–9.

Cardiovascular System Involvement

2

Hong Wang, Jing Dong, Xiaozhe Cui, Bai Gao, Yali Zhang, Le Sun, Xiaona Yu, Yang Hou, Xuan Liu, Xuexin Yu, Yanqiu Chu, and Yunming Xu

Abstract

Since Kawasaki disease (KD) was described by Japanese doctor Tomisaku Kawasaki in 1967, KD has replaced rheumatic heart disease becomes the leading cause of acquired heart disease in children in the developed world (Shulman, Clin Immunol Immunopathol 53(2 Pt 2):S141–S146, 1989). Although its etiology is not yet understood, it has been generally recognized as an acute vasculitis happening in children with allergies, mostly less than 5 years old (Maddox et al. Pediatr Int. 57:1116–1120, 2015). Because coronary artery injury is the most serious complication, coronary artery thrombus can lead to coronary heart disease and even sudden death. Therefore, more and more pediatric cardiologists are engaged in diagnosis, treatment and follow-up of KD, therefore, the vast majority of children with KD have a good outcome. However, clinic symptoms of KD vary, and multiple systems can be involved. In the case of the cardiovascular system alone KD may complicated with myocarditis (Aggarwal et al. Indian J Pediatr 79(6):813–814, 2012; De Rosa et al. Reumatismo 70(2):115–116, 2018), myocardial damage, pericardial effusion (Okada et al. Scand J Rheumatol. 44(3):247–252, 2015), cardiomyopathy (Komaki et al. Cardiol Young 28(6):890–893, 2018), CRBBB, ABV, arrhythmia (Sumitomo et al. Circ J 72(2):274–280, 2008), even shock (Li et al. Pediatr Rheumatol Online J 17(1):1, 2019) and so on. Coronary artery dilation and aneurysm dilation are more common complications in KD. In my center, total three misdiagnosed children developed CAA and coronary artery thrombus, coronary heart disease and lost their younger lives. KD accompany with myocarditis has been reported previously and reports of myocardial biopsies perform early in the disease course suggested a nearly universal incidence (Yutani et al. Arch Pathol Lab Med 105:470–473, 1981). In those KD patients with CAA, the myocardium damage was very popular although without any symptom (Yonesaka et al. Cardiol Young. 20(6):602–609, 2010). Thus, we can explain the chronic myocardial damage in KD without CAA.

In this chapter, we present 14 cases with cardiovascular complications.

H. Wang (✉) · L. Sun · Y. Chu · X. Yu · Y. Xu · X. Cui
Department of Pediatric Cardiology, Shengjing Hospital of China Medical University, Shenyang, P.R. China

Y. Zhang
Department of PICU, The First Affliated Hospital of Zhengzhou University, Zhengzhou, Henan, P.R. China

Y. Hou
Department of Radiology, Shengjing Hospital of China Medical University, Shenyang, P.R. China

X. Yu
Department of Ultrasound, Shengjing Hospital of China Medical University, Shenyang, P.R. China
e-mail: yuxn@sj-hospital.org

J. Dong
Department of Cardiology Function, Shengjing Hospital of China Medical University, Shenyang, P.R. China
e-mail: dongj@sj-hospital.org

B. Gao
Department of Neurology Function, Shengjing Hospital of China Medical University, Shenyang, P.R. China

X. Liu
Department of Hematology Laboratory, Shengjing Hospital of China Medical University, Shenyang, P.R. China

2.1 Case 1 KD with Acute Myocarditis

A previously healthy and athletic 10-year-old girl had no significant past medical and family history.

She presented on Day 5 of illness with a remittent fever for 5 days, along with sore throat and loss of appetite. On Day 3, rashes developed on the back causing itches. On Day 4 of illness, bilateral conjunctival congestion was present. On Day 4, she received muscle injection of dexamethasone 5 mg and lysine aspirin 0.5 g. Examination revealed fever, 38.9 °C; HR 102 bpm; smooth breath, RR 20 bpm; BP

H. Wang (ed.), *Paediatric Kawasaki Disease*, https://doi.org/10.1007/978-981-15-0038-1_2

100/60 mmHg; warm hands and feet; cervical lymphadenectasis; urticarial rashes all over the body that changed distribution with fever spiking; palm hyperemia; and bilateral conjunctival congestion, no purulent secretion or photaesthesia, obvious pharyngeal congestion, red lips without crack or strawberry tongue; hepatomegaly (liver edge from right costal margin 1 cm and below the xiphoid 2 cm), but otherwise was normal. Blood test at admission identified elevated WBC (Table 2.1). ECG was normal (Fig. 2.1). Cervical ultrasound showed cervical lymphadenectasis, about 1.6 cm × 0.6 cm on the left, 2.1 cm × 0.9 cm on the right. She had met four of five criteria for the Kawasaki disease (KD). She received (i) oral aspirin: 30–50 mg/kg/d, in three divided doses; oral dipyridamole 3–5 mg/kg/d, in three divided doses; (ii) infusion of creatine phosphate sodium 1 g/d and levocarnitine 20 mg/kg/d; (iii) infusion of second-generation antibiotics after blood culture sample was taken; (iv) PPD test to exclude tuberculosis.

Table 2.1 The dynamic changes of lab parameters

Illness	5 days	6 days	10 days	13 days	15 days
WBC ($\times 10^9$/L)	14.5	14			
NE (%)	73.6	75			
HGB (g/L)	128	122			
PLT ($\times 10^9$/L)	256	251			
CRP (mg/L)	86		12.5		5.6
ESR (mm/h)		64			
CTnI (μg/L)	0.053		0.239	0.042	0.029
hs-cTnT (ng/ml)	0.029		0.042	0.009	
NT pro-BNP (ng/ml)	4804		233		

On Day 6, she developed breathlessness with vomiting. Blood test revealed ASO 43.4 IU/ml, ESR 64 (0–20 mm/h), IgE 337.89(<100 IU/ml), TB-Ab weakly positive, MP-IgG 1:40, MP-IgM negative, normal GTP, Cr, and CK-MB. Chest DR was normal. Echo showed LVED 45 mm, LVEF 47.9% (Fig. 2.2a), mild to moderate mitral regurgitation (Fig. 2.2b) along the posterior lobe. Tricuspid regurgitation v = 3.2 m/s estimated pulmonary artery pressure 45 mmHg in systolic, regurgitation of pulmonary artery, v = 2.6 m/s, estimated the pulmonary artery pressure 27 mmHg in diastolic. All chamber sizes of heart were normal. Left ventricular free wall moved weaken. Coronary lumen was clear, LCA 2.9 mm, RCA 2.7–3.1 mm, with neither local widening nor pericardial effusion. HR was elevated. For she had developed myocarditis but without oliguria, she was given (i) IVIG 1 g/kg/d for 2 days; (ii) oral digoxin tablet 0.125 mg, qd, to slow saturation; (iii) controlled liquid and sodium infusion. Total velocity of infusion was less than 3 ml/kg/h. On Day 7, her body temperature regressed to 37.8 °C with a little bleeding nose. She started to cough up blood-stained sputum. Erythromycin ointment was daubed in nasal cavity. Then bleeding settled and blood-stained sputum subsided. Examination showed the hepatomegaly regressed to right costal margin and 1 cm below xiphoid. After PPD 48 h negative, she was infused with

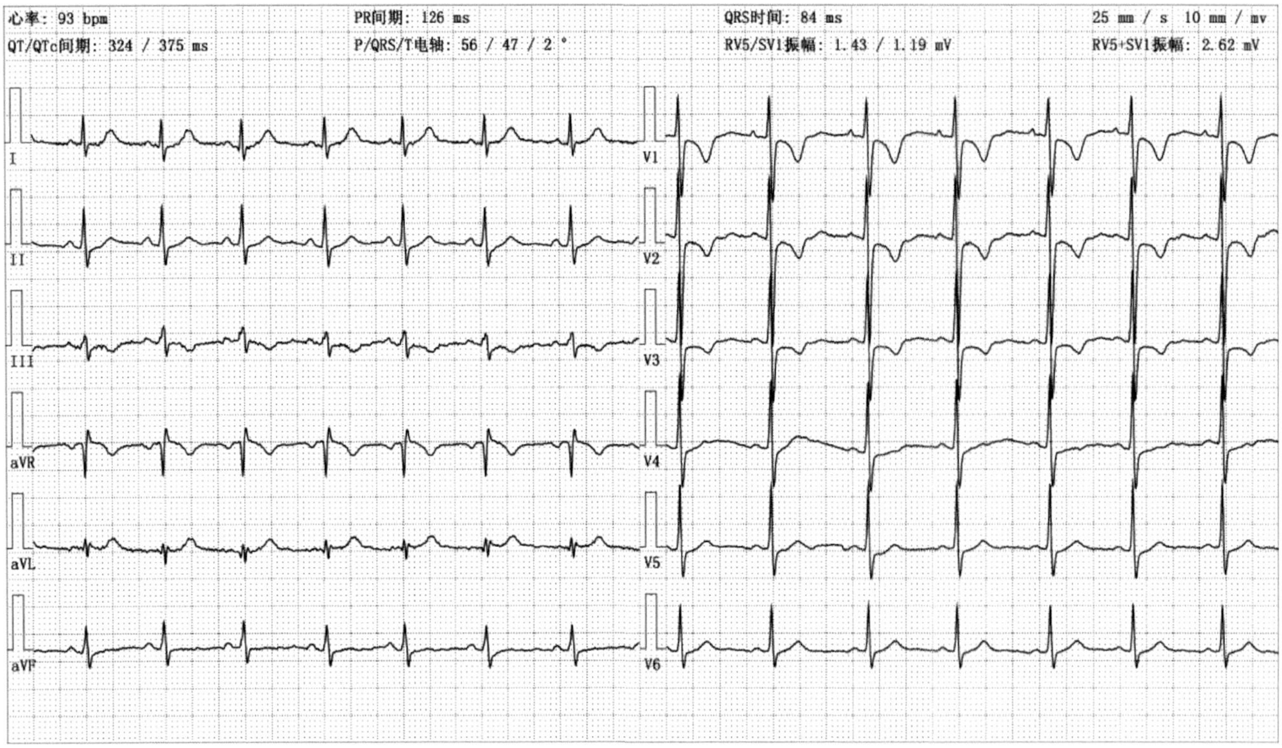

Fig. 2.1 On Day 5 of illness, ECG was normal

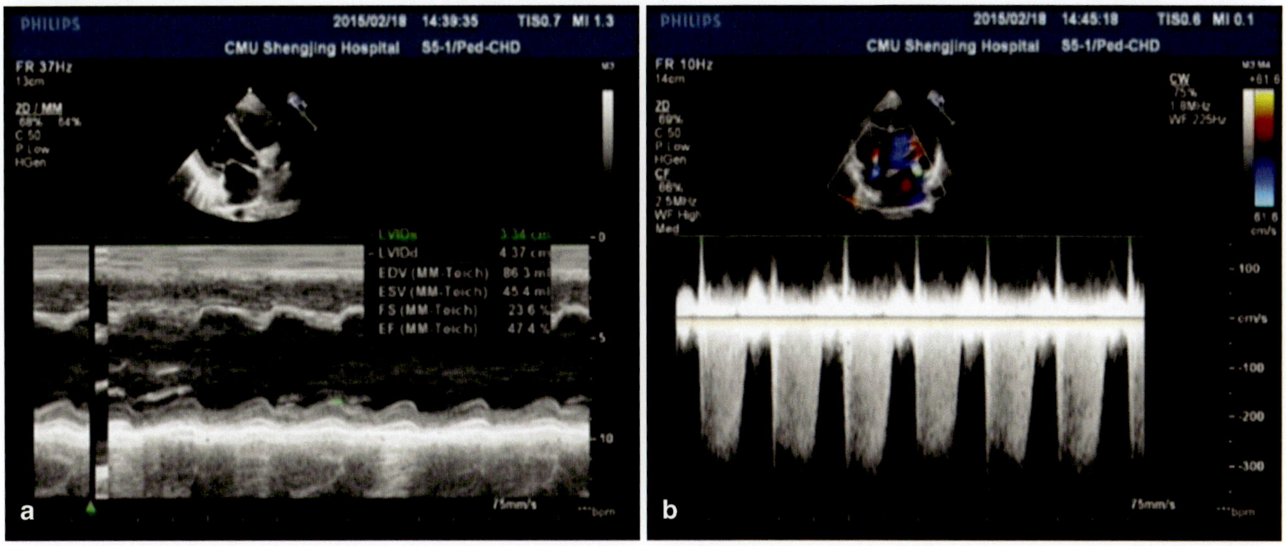

Fig. 2.2 On Day 6 of illness, echocardiography showed the decreased LVEF (47%) (**a**) and moderate mitral valve regurgitation (**b**)

methylprednisolone 2 mg/kg/d. On Day 8, she was afebrile. Rashes and bilateral conjunctival congestion improved. Investigation showed positive PINF. She took Chinese antivirus medicine. Chest CT scan showed pleural effusion upper oblique fissure of right lung (Fig. 2.3). On Day 9, her bilateral conjunctival congestion subsided. Afebrile had been over 48 h. Aspirin was reduced to one dose 3–5 mg/kg/d and antibiotics were stopped. On Day 10, investigation showed both positive MP-IgM and CP-IgM. Blood culture was negative. NT-pro BNP, cTnI, hs-cTnT, and CRP were retested and results were shown in Table 2.1. T wave was still low-flat on LVIW and free wall in ECG (Fig. 2.4a). Echo showed normal LVED (43 mm) and LVEF (67.6%) (Fig. 2.5a). Mitral regurgitation settled (Fig. 2.5b). Pulmonary artery pressure was recovered and coronary artery normal. Methylprednisolone was reduced to 1.5 mg/kg/d. On Day 11 and 12, ECG showed T wave kept low-flat on LVIW and free wall (Fig. 2.4b, Fig. 2.6a). On Day 13, investigation revealed cTnI 0.047 (<0.004 μg/L), hs-cTnT and CRP normal. On Day 14, she had no cough, slept well with good appetite. Examination showed normal BP, HR 80 bpm, no cervical lymphadenopathy, and no skin peeling at finger nails and toe nails. ECG showed sinus arrhythmia, super-ventricular contraction one time, II°II AVB during sleep in the morning (Fig. 2.7).

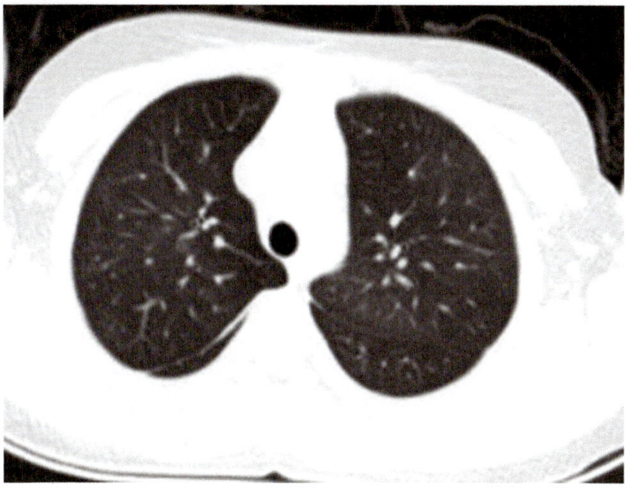

Fig. 2.3 On Day 7 of illness, chest CT scan showed there was a little pleural effusion upper oblique fissure of right lung

On Day 15, blood test revealed normal cTnI and CRP. She was discharged.

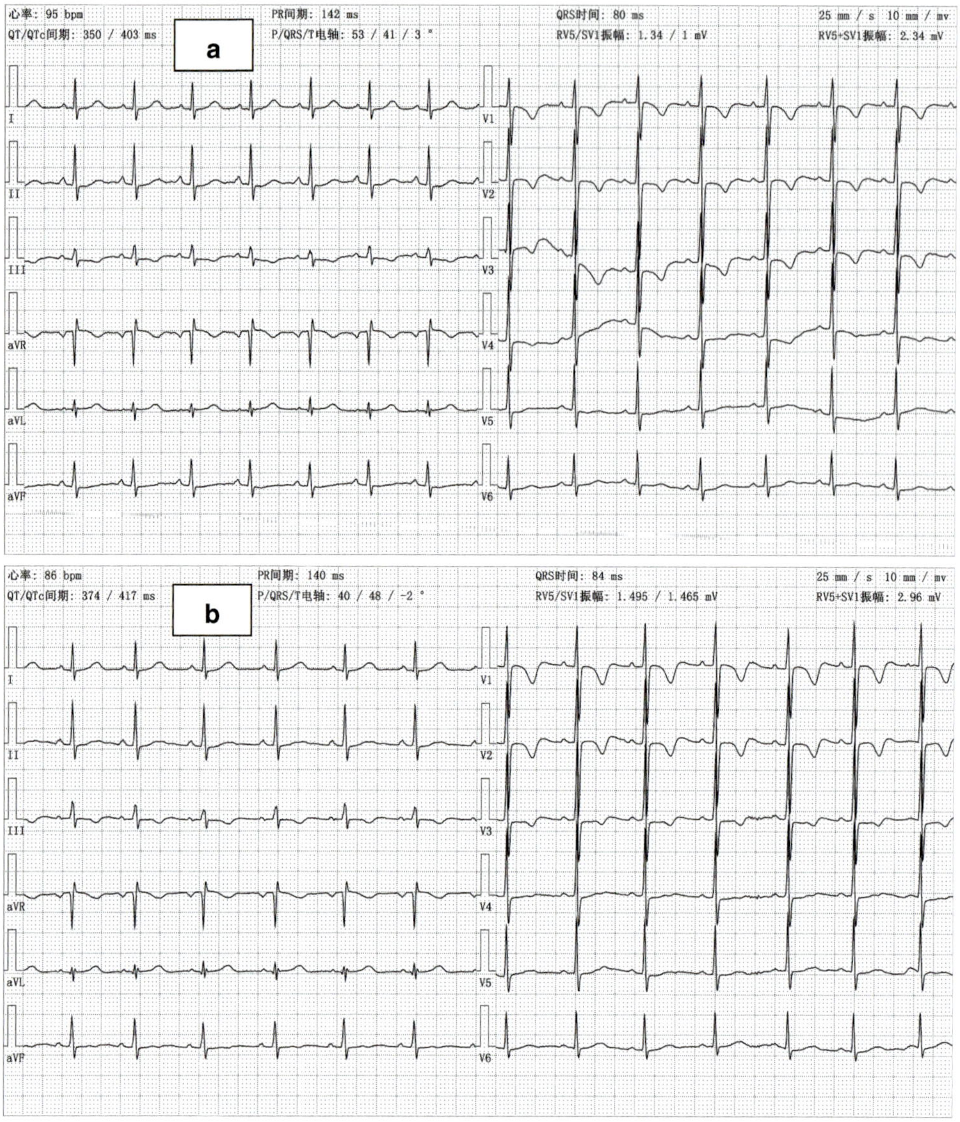

Fig. 2.4 ECG showed T wave low-flat deteriorated on Day 10 (**a**) and 11 (**b**) of illness

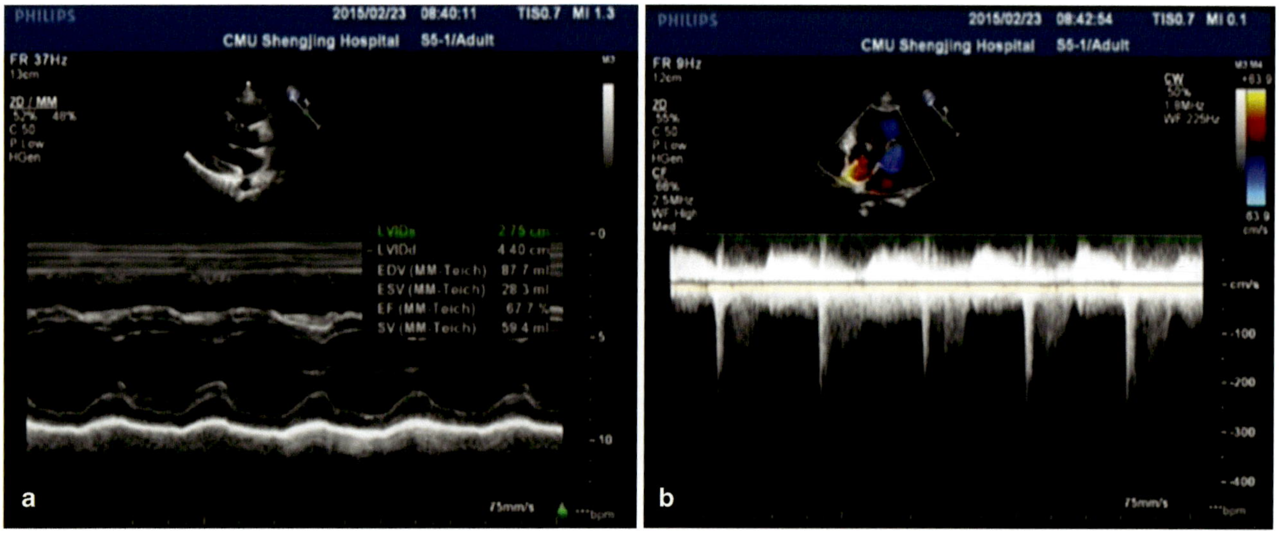

Fig. 2.5 On Day 11 of illness, echocardiography showed normal LVEF (68%) (**a**) and mild mitral valve regurgitation (**b**)

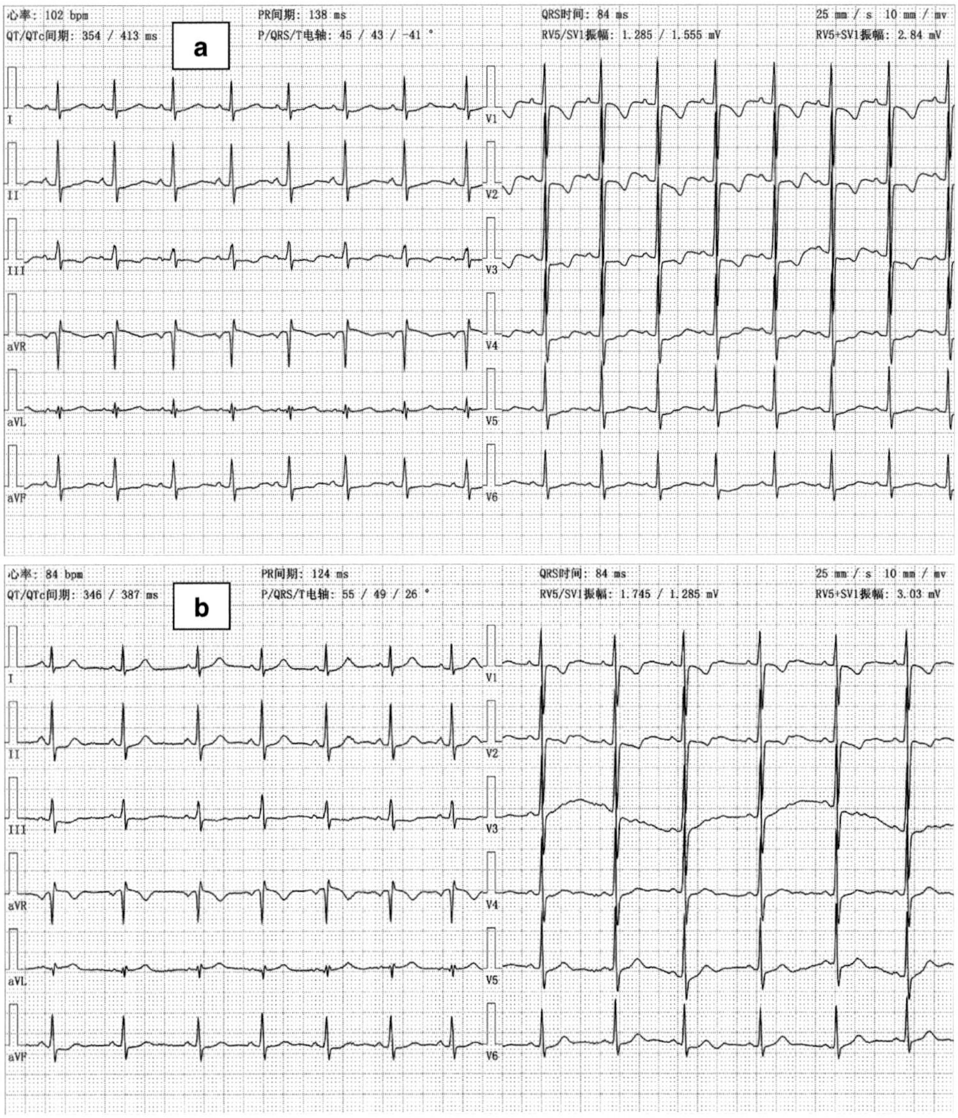

Fig. 2.6 ECG showed T wave low-flat on free side and inferior walls on Day 12 (**a**) and normal on Day 35 (**b**) of illness

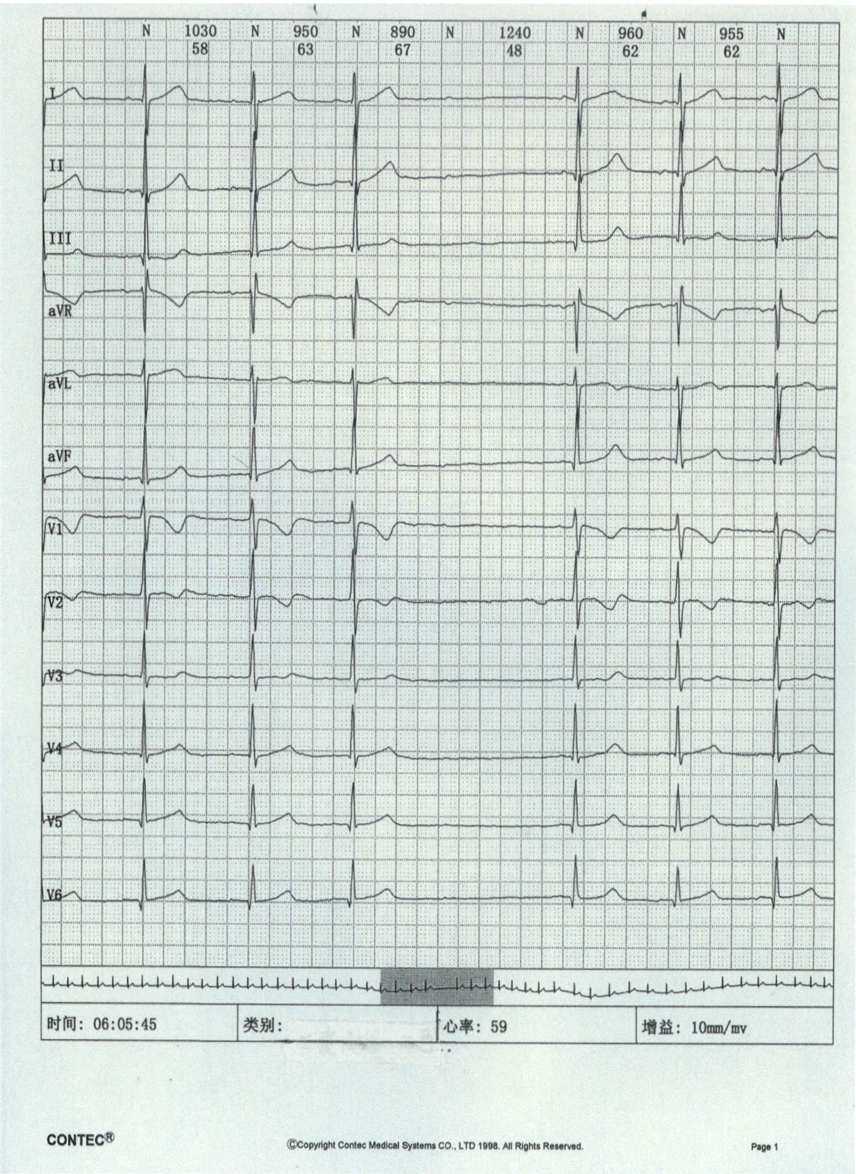

Fig. 2.7 On Day 14 of illness, ECG showed II°II AVB at sleep in the morning

2.1.1 Clinical Course of the Patient

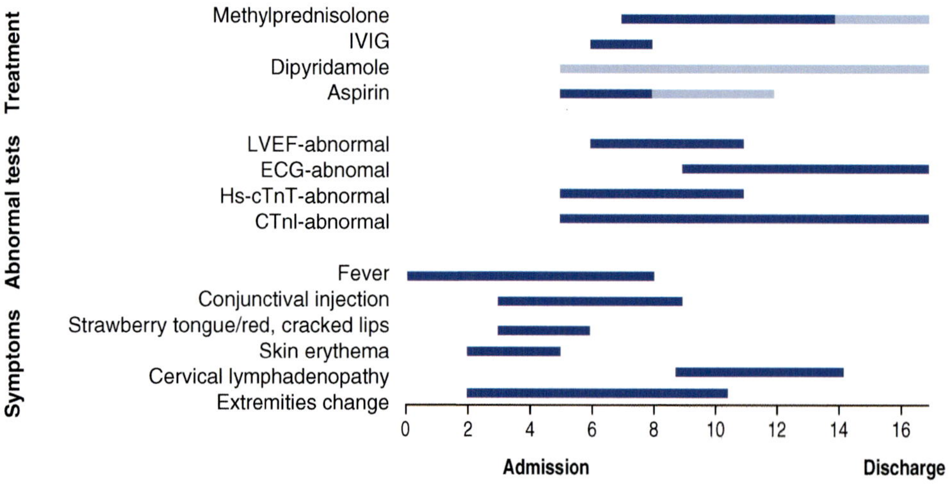

2.1.2 Follow-Up

Since being discharged, she took (i) prednisone 1.0 mg/kg/d, the ratio was morning/night = 2/1. One week later the dose was weaned to 0.5 mg/kg/d, and she only took in the morning for 1 week, then gradually weaned to stop, in total about 1 month; (ii) aspirin and dipyridamole 3–5 mg/kg/d; (iii) FDP and levocarnitine 10 ml, bid; (iv) calcium gluconate, 0.3 g once daily until prednisone withdrawal; (v) digoxin 0.125 mg, once daily for 1 week then stopped.

On Day 35, her ESR settled and ECG was recovered (Fig. 2.6b).

On Day 45, echo showed TI settled.

Two months later, her coronary artery stayed normal (Fig. 2.8). Investigation showed TB-Ab was negative. All medications were stopped.

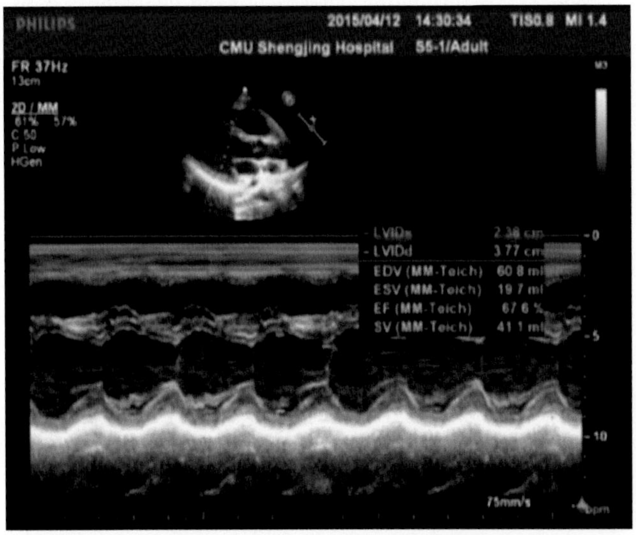

Fig. 2.8 At 2 months of illness, LVEF was normal (68%)

Sixteen months later, her ECG showed: sinus rhythm, 81 bpm, T wave being mild low-flat on the antetheca (Fig. 2.9), while LVED 43 mm and LVEF 64% in echo. Coronary artery was normal. The bicycle exercise-test was denied.

2.1.3 Diagnosis

1. KD
2. Secondary myocarditis
3. Acute heart failure
4. Secondary pulmonary hypertension
5. Mitral regurgitation
6. Tricuspid regurgitation
7. II°II AVB
8. MP infection
9. CP infection
10. PINF infection

2.1.4 Discussion

This girl met criteria of KD [1]. She had continuous high fever over 5 days and not responsive to broad-spectrum antibiotics, along with: (i) polymorphous rashes; (ii) bilateral conjunctival congestion; (iii) palms hyperemia; (iv) cervical lymphadenopathy; significant elevation in CRP and NT pro BNP.

She also met the criteria of myocarditis [2] (i) with KD; (ii) breathless and hepatomegaly; (iii) both increased cTnI and hs-cTnT and elevated NT pro-BNP; (iv) ECG T wave remained low-flat on LVIW over 4 days with dynamic changes; (v) LVEF went down and left ventricular free wall moved weaken. Different diagnosis should be done to acute

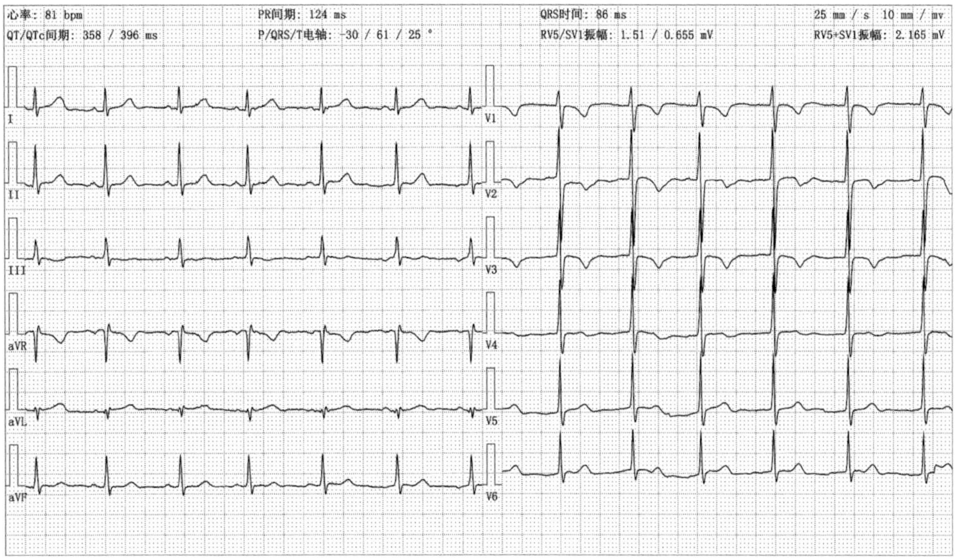

Fig. 2.9 At 16 months of illness, ECG showed T wave mild low-flat on the antetheca (was the similar with beginning of illness)

pharynx conjunctival fever, sepsis, streptococcal infection, and Steven–Johnson syndrome.

Infusion of glucocorticoid (GC) to her was not for IVIG resistance but only for inhibiting myocardium inflammation. The treatment course should last for about 1 month for myocarditis.

Among 2 to 6 years old children, their nasal blood vessels are coarse and crisp. Nose bleeding is common in this age group when the environment is warm and dry or there is an external impact. After taking aspirin and dipyridamole, the bleeding is usually aggravated, such as easily bruised on the shin bone area when touched mildly. If the bleeding gets worse, aspirin and dipyridamole can be stopped for 2–3 days. At the same time, erythromycin ointment is daubed in nasal cavity to soft the blood scab to prevent repeated bleeding.

2.1.5 Case Specific Clinic Features

1. KD with myocarditis was not very common in our center. Before this case, we treated KD only with IVIG and oral aspirin, usually without considering myocardial nutrition management. KD with myocarditis has been reported previously and myocardial biopsies performed at early stage in the disease suggested a nearly universal incidence [3, 4]. In those KD with CAA patients, the myocardium damage was very popular although without any symptoms [5]. In this case, cTnI and hs-cTnT were increased significantly and remained increased on Day 10 of illness. ECG was normal on Day 5, but gradually developed T wave low-flat on Day 9 of illness and kept ST-T abnormal over 4 days and even after NT pro-BNP recovered. T wave settled 1 week later. These dynamic variations were corresponding to the changes of cardiac enzymes. In addition, her echo result showed the LVEF went down and left ventricular moved weakly, which supported myocarditis diagnosis. Therefore, myocardial nutrition supplement should be used.
2. Her ECG changes happened till Day 9 of illness. Therefore, ECG change was not sensitive. ECG abnormalities showed up not only later than cardiac enzymes but also later than events detected in echo. If myocarditis was suspected, ECG should be repeated routinely. Her ECG showed II°II AVB during morning sleep. This was due to vagus nerve effects rather than myocardium damage. Till 16 months of illness, T wave showed low-flat again in her ECG. But it happened on the anterior wall instead of inferior and similar to recording at admission. This also can be noted in healthy children. For KD patients, we should be cautious with myocardial damage. This patient coronary artery remained normal. We suggested her to take exercise test. If the result is positive, the coronary artery CTA should be performed.
3. Generally, to reduce the heart overload, patients with fulminant myocarditis are treated with IVIG 400 mg/kg/d for 5 days. IVIG dose for KD is 1 g/kg/d for 2 days. Although this girl had acute heart failure, her blood pressure was normal, without oliguria. We decided to give her IVIG 1 g/kg/d for 2 days. Infusion of IVIG was controlled at less than 3 ml/kg/h and lasted over 12 h.
4. Her cTnI and hs-cTnT continued to increase on Day 10 of illness while NT pro-BNP had reduced to normal. Her hs-cTnT recovered on Day 14 of illness followed by cTnI 3 days later. This corresponds with the trend of myocarditis recovering reported in literature [6].
5. Her mitral wave was single 1.3 mm at beginning when she was hospitalized, suggesting her left ventricular diastolic function was reduced. This correlated with elevated NT pro-BNP. It is reported that pulmonary artery is widen in KD patients [7]. This girl had pulmonary hypertension, pulmonary valve regurgitation, mitral regurgitation, and tricuspid regurgitation on Day 6 of illness, while both pulmonary hypertension and mitral regurgitation disappeared on Day 12 of illness. About half month later her tricuspid regurgitation also recovered. All above supported these changes were secondary and recovered soon.
6. Myocardium damage may be induced by toxicity from normal dose digoxin. We should not give fast saturation of cedilanid; instead we should give her oral digoxin at half dose (0.125 mg, daily or 0.0625 mg q12h) to slow saturation. Meanwhile, infusion of furosemidum and oral captopril were given to the patient to reduce heart burden. One week later, LVEF recovered, and hepatomegaly regressed. Digoxin was gradually stopped.
7. Once IVIG was not effective, glucocorticoid might be used. Tuberculin test should be done at admission. When her TB-Ab was weakly positive, PPD was performed for 24 h and was negative, chest DR was normal, we deduced that perhaps she had MPI or CPI which is associated with false TB-Ab positive, while her MP-IgM and CP-IgM were negative. It was prudent, chest CT was performed the next day. It showed there was a little pleural effusion, and meanwhile PPD 48 h was still negative. Glucocorticoid was infused. Six days later, both MP-IgM and CP-IgM were positive, which in turn supported our conclusion.

Hong Wang

2.2 Case 2 KD with Shock

A four-year-old girl was previously healthy without any significant past medical history except for some positive antibiotics reaction in skin test.

She presented on Day 5 of illness with fever for 5 days, along with abdominal pain, vomiting 4 to 5 times per day for 3 days. After infused with first-generation cephalosporin for 2 days and third-generation cephalosporin for 3 days in local clinic, her fever did not regress. Congested rash developed on the trunk and it regressed after taking a chlortrimeton on Day 5 of illness. She was admitted in pediatric gastrointestinal ward with BP 80/40 mmHg. Third-generation cephalosporin and liquid were infused. On Day 6, fever did not regress and redden conjunctiva, red and cracked lips, feet and hands developed. After consulting with pediatric cardiologist, she was transferred to pediatric cardiology ward. **Examination** revealed temperature 38 °C, PR104 bpm, RR 23 bpm, BP 64/26 mmHg, cervical lymphadenectasis on the left, bilateral conjunctival congestion, cracked red lips and strawberry tongue, erythema of both palms and feet edema. Others were normal. **Investigation** results are summarized in Table 2.2. Blood gas analysis was normal except for ABE −5.4 mmol/L and sodium 131.6 mmol/L. Cervical ultrasound revealed that the left lymph nodes was enlarged, with the biggest one 1.5 cm × 2.0 cm. Investigation at admission to our ward revealed sodium 129.3 mmol/L. Blood gas analysis was normal; CRP 187 mg/L, PCT 8.47 ng/ml, normal CK, CKMB, CKMB-M, cTnI and cTnT, NT-pro BNP 6454 pg/ml, Liver function ALT 116 U/L, AST 46 U/L, T Bil 74.5μmol/L, D Bil 62.3μmol/L. Amylase and lipase were normal. ASO was negative. ESR was 87 mm/h. Abdomen ultrasound showed abdominal lymphadenopathy. Abdomen CT scan showed there were a great deal of gas and liquid in intestine (Fig. 2.10a), and multiple lymphadenectasis behind it (Fig. 2.10b). The appen-

Table 2.2 The dynamic changes of laboratory parameters

Day of illness	2 days	5 days	6 days	7 days	8 days	10 days	11 days	14 days
WBC ($\times 10^9$/L)	24.9	19		15.32	26.2	16	12.9	
NE (%)	77.1	85.1		93.8	93	58.5	49.7	
HGB (g/L)	125	124		110	101	96	75	
PLT ($\times 10^9$/L)	300	366		309	251	358	384	
CRP (mg/L)	17	61	187		189	93.2		
NT-pro BNP (pg/ml)			6454		26025			625.3
ALT (U/L)			116		48		12	11
ALB (g/L)			36	26	23.4		24.5	39.6
T Bile (μmol/L)			74.5		21.3			
D-D (μg/L)			63.9	915	18.4			

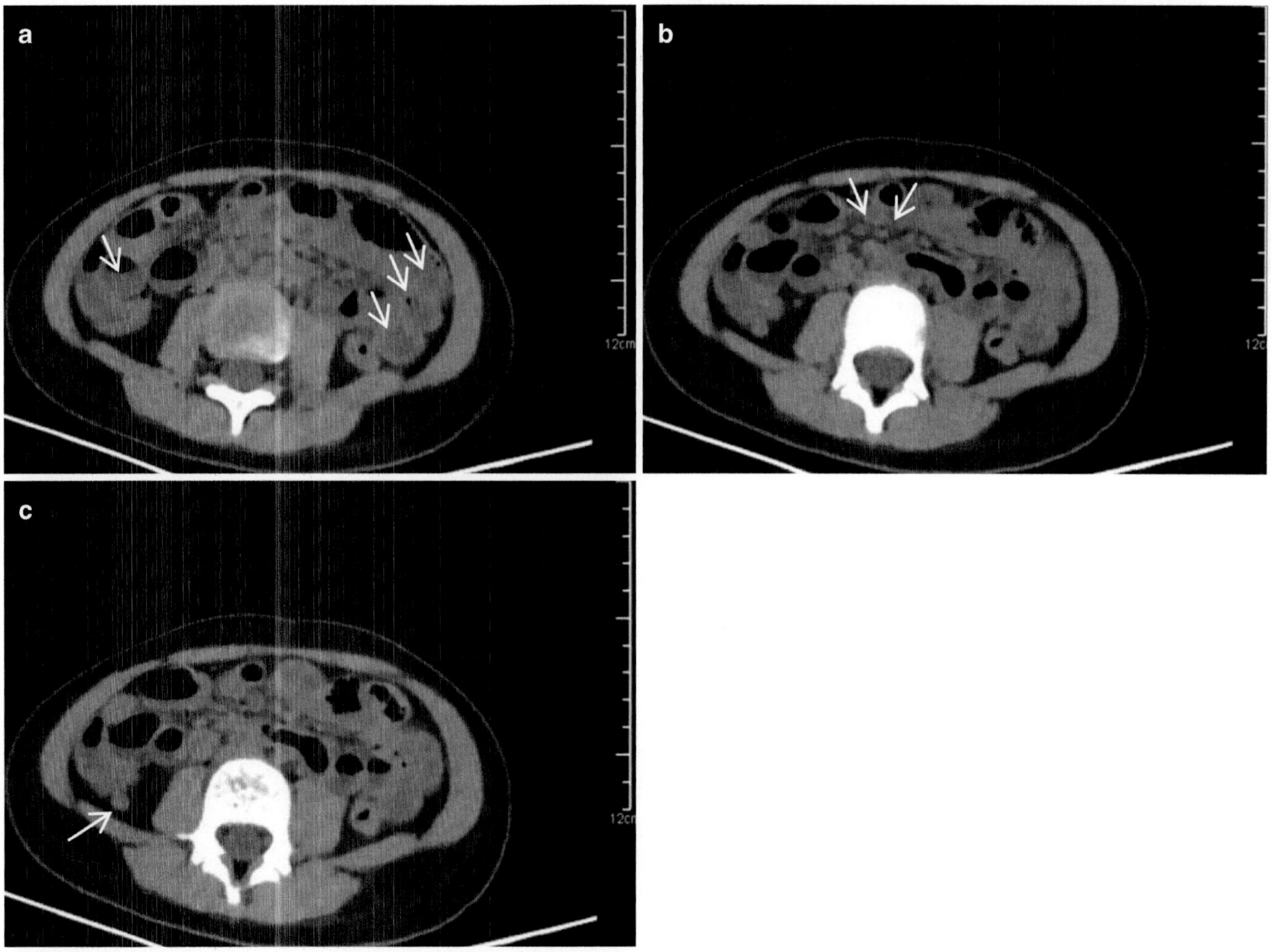

Fig. 2.10 On Day 5 of illness, abdominal CT showed there was much gas and liquid in intestine (**a**), retroperitoneal lymphadenectasis (**b**), the appendix was thickness (**c**)

dix was slightly thicker (Fig. 2.10c). Chest CT scan showed a little inflammation in the lower lobe of both lungs with thickening of the right oblique fissure (Fig. 2.11). There were multiple slightly larger lymph nodes in the mesentery and retroperitoneum. EEG showed multiple episodes of 4–6 Hz θ wave (Fig. 2.12). Head MRI showed bilateral maxillary sinusitis (Fig. 2.13a) and FLAIR showed high signal in left frontal lobe spot-shaped (Fig. 2.13b). ECG showed sinus tachycardia and I degree AVB (Fig. 2.14). The patient met 6 criteria of KD. She was treated with IVIG 1 g/kg/d, aspirin (oral route) 30–50 mg/kg/d, and dipyridamole 3-5 mg/kg/d, both in three divided doses per day; infused with magnesium isoglycyrrhizinate, third-generation cephalosporin, oxiracetam, creatine phosphate sodium, levocarnitine and NS. At midnight, her BP continued to go down to 73/38 mmHg, temperature was 38.6 °C, HR fluctuated between 150 and 170 bpm, the circulation of the extremities was poor. Blood gas analysis results: pH 7.470, $PaCO_2$ 28.1 mmHg, BE −2.2 mmol/L, potassium 3.55 mmol/L, sodium 126.8 mmol/L; DIC parameters: PT 17.3, APTT 38 s, D-dimers 915 μg/L. After infused with 300 ml 1:1 liquid (glucose: NS was 1:1) and 0.2 percent K^+, her BP was 65/35 mmHg. Her HR was fluctuated between 160 and 170 bpm. She was irritability and her peripheral circulation got worse. CRT prolonged to 5 s. She was transferred to PICU. Femoral vein puncture was performed to monitor the central venous pressure, and it was 5 cm H_2O, suggesting that the effective circulating blood volume was insufficient. Treatment: (i) IVIG 1 g/kg/d; (ii) infusion of albumin 20 g; (iii) infusion of 1:1 liquid (glucose: NS) at the speed of 200 ml/h; (iv) infusion of dopamine 5 μg/kg/min and dobutamine 2.5 μg/kg/min to improve the peripheral circulation. Meanwhile procedures were set up to focus on pneumonedema and monitor the amount of urine and the central venous pressure.

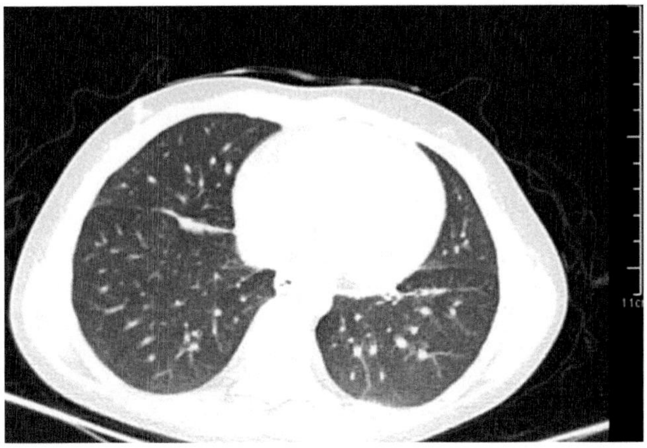

Fig. 2.11 On Day 5 of illness, a little inflammation in the lower lobe of both lungs with thickening of the right oblique fissure

On Day 7, her mental stage was improved but slightly irritability. PR was148 bpm, RR was 32 bpm, and BP was 106/68 mmHg. Laboratory findings include WBC 15.32 × 10^9/L, NE% 93.8%, RBC 4.1 × 10^{12}/L, HGB 110 g/L, PLT 309 × 10^9/L, Protein 45.2 g/L, ALB 23.4 g/L, A/G 1.1:1, ALT 48 U/L, AST 16 U/L, T Bil 21.3 μmol/L, UNDBI 18.4 μmol/L, PCT 7.68 ng/ml, NT-pro BNP 26025 pg/ml, MP-IgM slightly positive, and HSV (I + II)-IgM positive. Venous blood gas analysis showed: pH 7.50, BE −4.4 mmol/L, $PaCO_2$ 33 mmHg, PaO_2 44 mmHg, K^+2.9 mmol/L, Na^+125 mmol/L, glucose 9.3 mmol/L, and lactic acid 1.6 mmol/L. She was treated with (i) infusion of

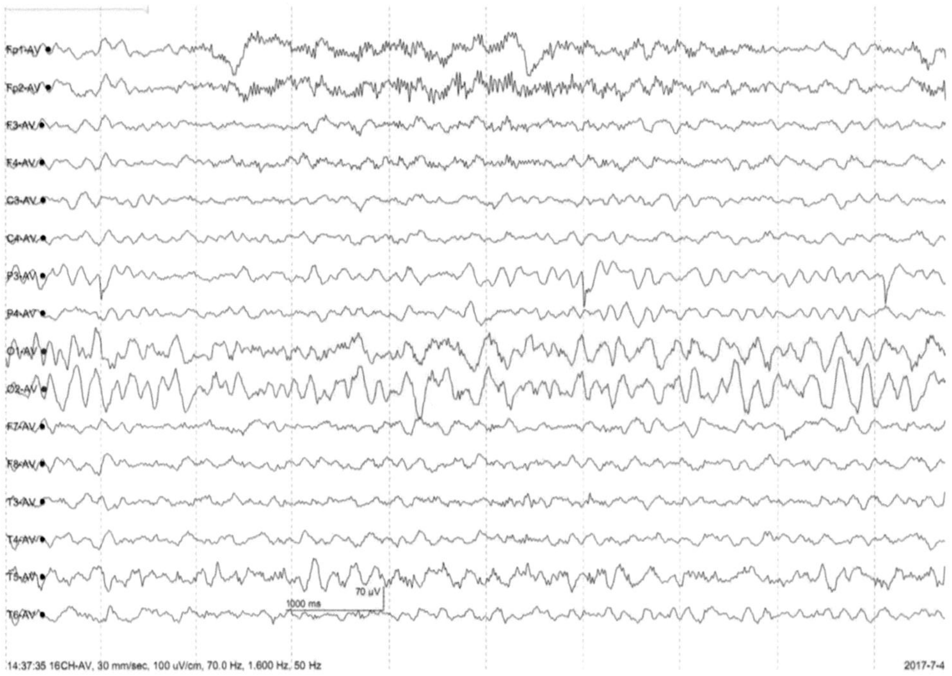

Fig. 2.12 On Day 5 of illness, EEG showed there were more 4–6 Hz slow waves at bilateral occipital brain

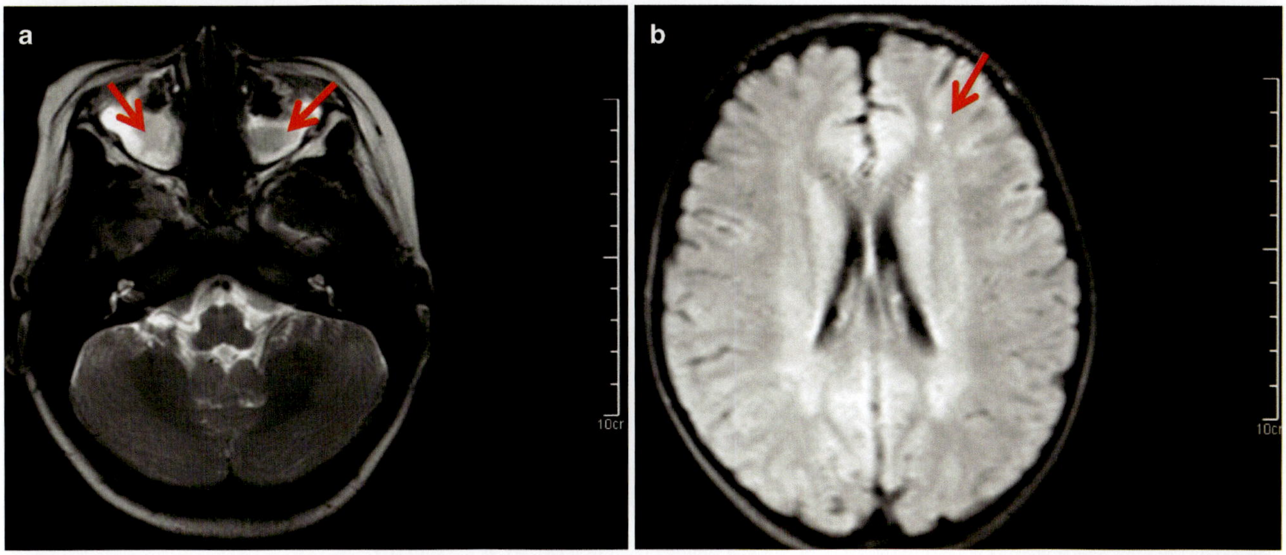

Fig. 2.13 On Day 6 of illness, head MR showed bilateral maxillary sinusitis (**a**), FLAIR showed high signal in left frontal lobe spot-shaped (**b**)

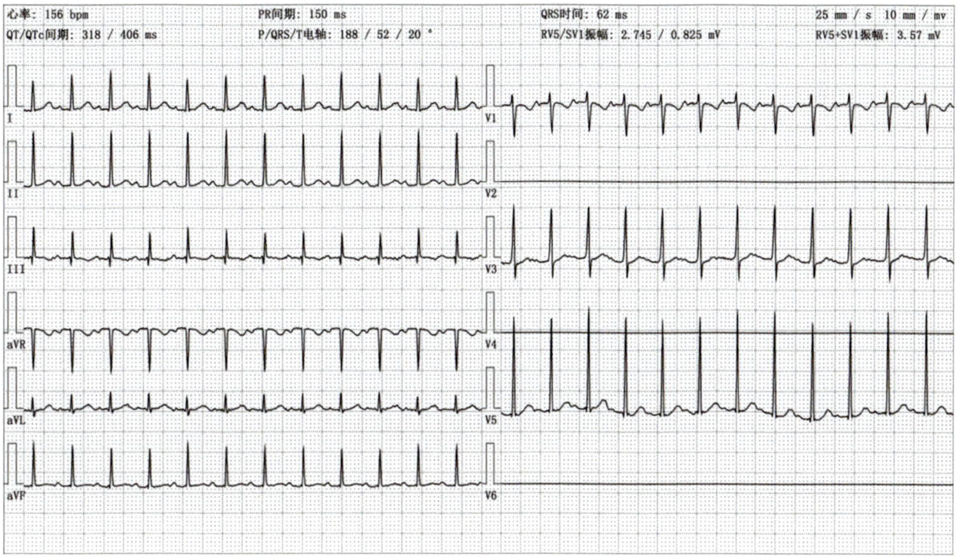

Fig. 2.14 On Day 6 of illness, ECG showed sinus tachycardia and I°AVB (PR 150 ms)

albumin 20 g, IVIG 1 g/kg/d, and 1:1 solution (glucose: NS), supplement sodium and potassium ions. On Day 8, the child had fever again up to 38.9 °C. After oral ibuprofen, the temperature went down to normal. Percutaneous oxygen saturation (SpO_2) remained normal without oxygen supplied. She had abdominal pain around umbilicus occasionally without cough, vomit, or diarrhea. Pediatric surgeon suggested to continue anti-inflammation. If necessary, enema and hot compress should be performed. When her BP was around 90/50 mmHg, we stopped dobutamine infusion. Bilateral conjunctival congestion, cracked red lips and strawberry tongue were not regressed. The circulation of extremities was improved to CRT 3 s. Bilateral Babinski signs were positive. Kernig and Brudzinski signs were negative. Echo showed that LCA (Fig. 2.15a), RCA (Fig. 2.15b), LVED and LVEF (Fig. 2.16a) were all normal. On Day 11, the child had mild fever, and the fever regressed soon by itself. BP was 102/52 mmHg. Repeated CBC showed: WBC 12.9 × 10^9/L, NE 49.7%, RBC 2.80 × 10^{12}/L, HGB 75 g/L, PLT 384 × 10^9/L, CRP 24.8 mg/L, and PCT 1.90 ng/ml. Blood gas analysis and 24-hour urinary protein test were normal. Urinary bacterial and stool culture tests came back as negative.

On Day 12, she was afebrile and everything went well. BP was 117/77 mmHg, CVP was recovered to 10 cm H_2O (Table 2.3). On Day 13, she was transferred back to pediatric cardiology ward. She was afebrile but with occasional headache. On examination she was well except for anemia. She took iron protein succinic acid and vitamin C orally. Retest

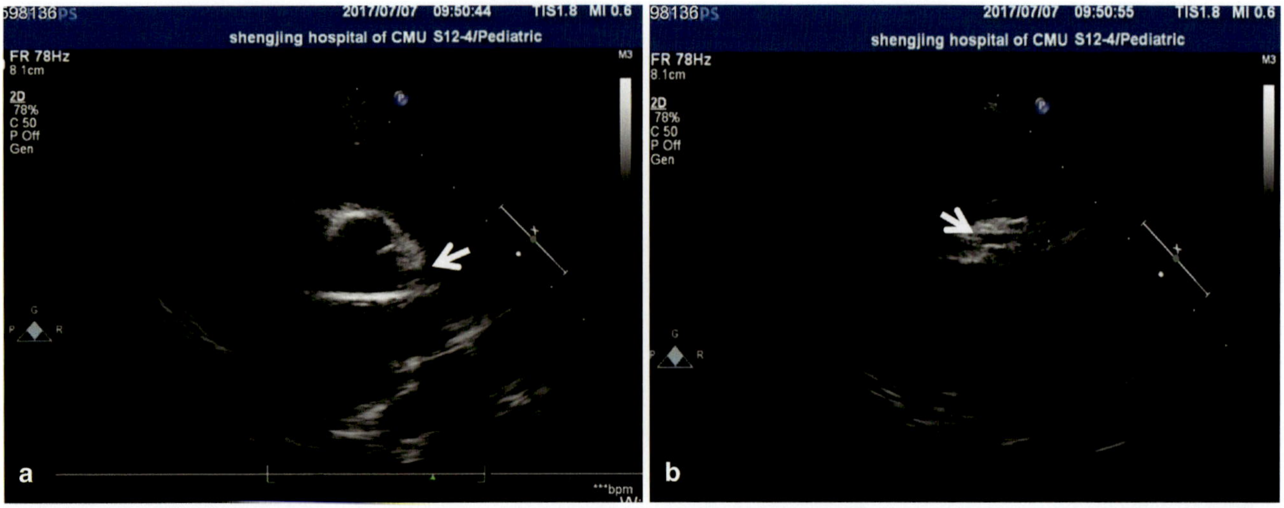

Fig. 2.15 On Day 8 of illness, echocardiography showed LCA diameter 2.5 mm (**a**), RCA 2.3 mm (**b**)

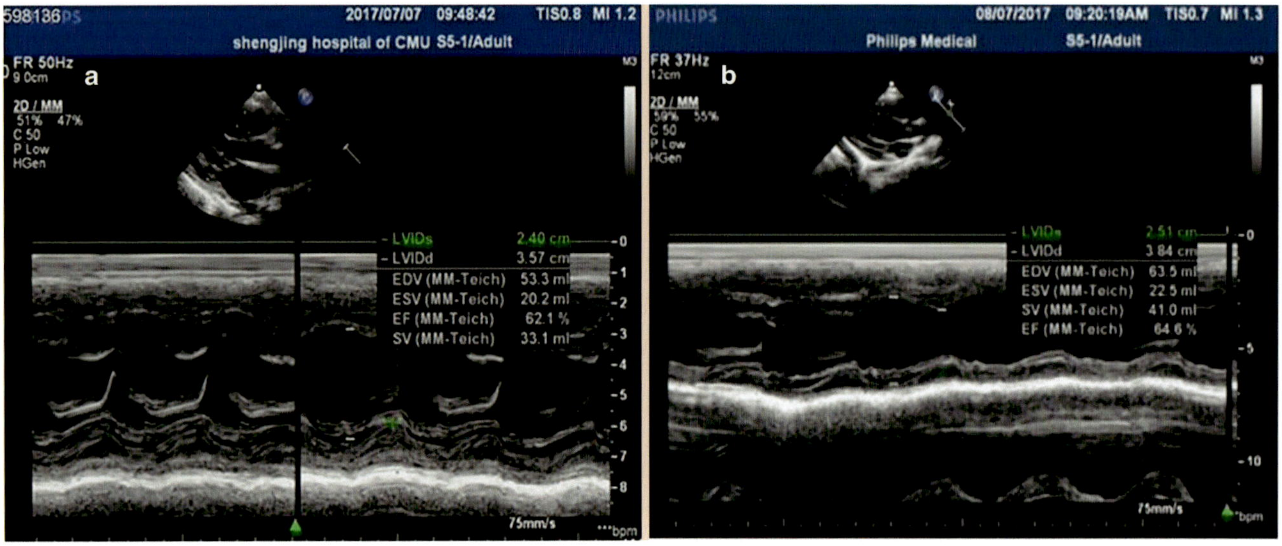

Fig. 2.16 Echocardiography showed LVEF were normal both on Day 8 (**a**) and one month (**b**) of illness

blood routine (see Table 2.2). Retest liver function revealed albumin 24.5 g/L. EEG showed much more 5–6 Hz θ waves (Fig. 2.17). Medication: albumin 20 g was infused and aspirin was reduced to one dose 66 mg/d. On Day 14, investigation revealed NT-pro BNP 625.3 pg/ml; albumin 39.6 g/L. ECG showed almost normal (Fig. 2.18). On Day 15, lymphadenectasis was regressed. Echo showed normal. There was mild regurgitation in mitral and triple valves. Deproteinized calf blood serum was infused to improve cranial nerve function. On Day 20, there was no obvious abnormality in the examination. EEG result was almost normal (a little 5-6 Hz θ wave left) (Fig. 2.19a). She was discharged.

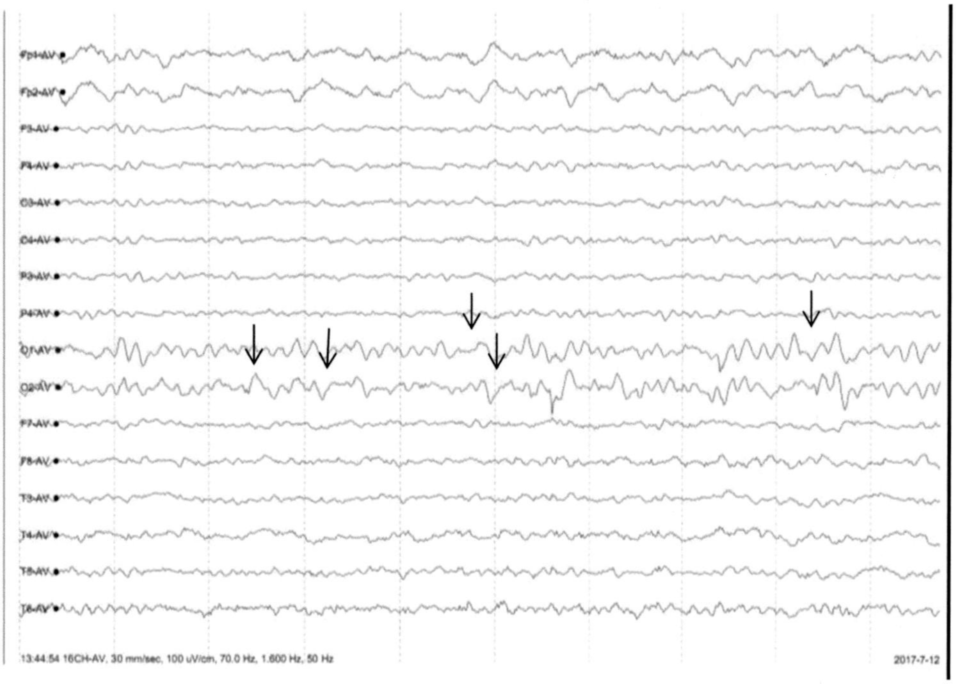

Fig. 2.17 On Day 13 of illness, EEG showed there were more 5–6 Hz slow waves in her bilateral occipital brain

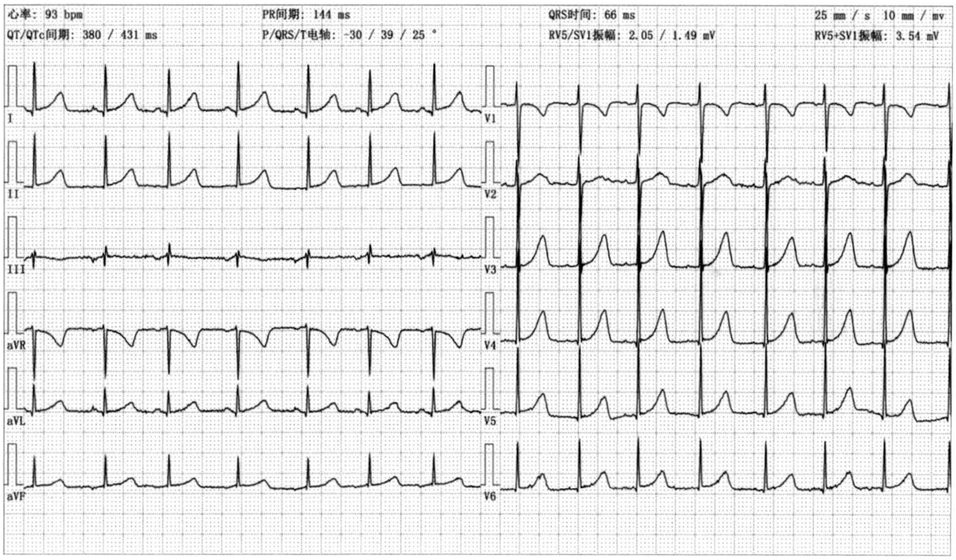

Fig. 2.18 On Day 14 of illness, ECG showed almost normal

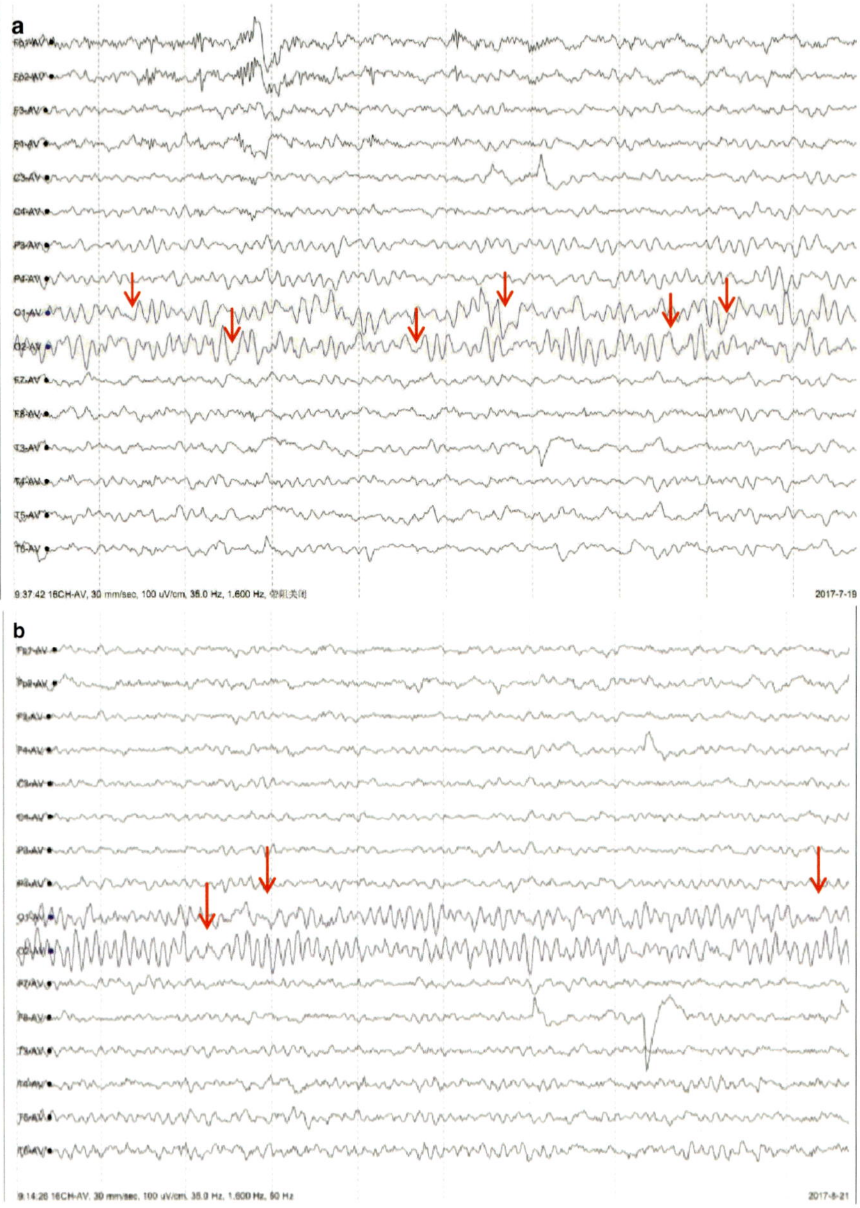

Fig. 2.19 At bilateral occipital brain, EEG showed there were more 8 Hz α waves and mixed with 5-6 Hz slow waves on Day 20 of illness (**a**), and recovered to most 8–9 Hz α waves and mixed with a little bit 5–6 Hz slow waves on Day 53 of illness (**b**)

2.2.1 Clinical Course of Patient

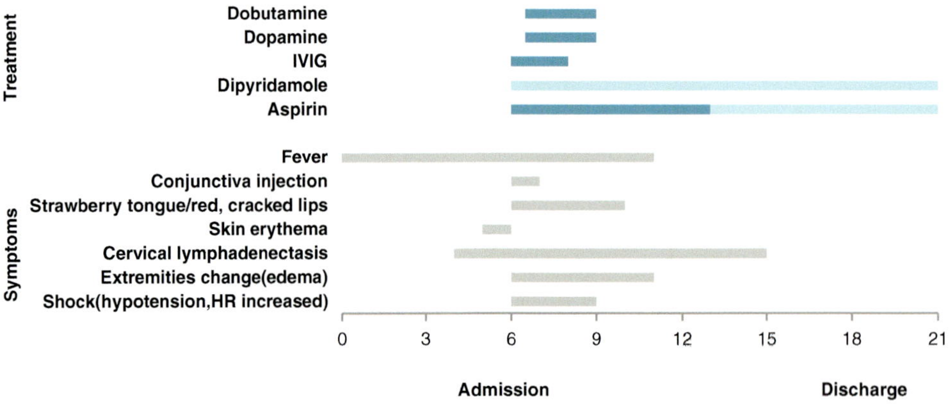

2.2.2 Follow-Up

At 1 month of illness, ECG and coronary and LVEF (Fig. 2.16b) were normal. EEG showed most 8–9 Hz α wave and mixed with a little bit 5–6 Hz slow waves in her bilateral occipital brain (Fig. 2.19b). ECG and echo were performed at 1.5 months, 2 months (Fig. 2.20a) and 6 months (Fig. 2.20b) all were normal. Medications were stopped at 2 months of illness.

2.2.3 Diagnosis

1. KD
2. Hypovolemic shock
3. Hypoproteinemia
4. MP infection
5. Herpes simplex virus infection
6. Aseptic meningitis cannot exclude
7. Moderate anemia
8. Liver dysfunction

2.2.4 Discussion

By now, the etiology of KD is not fully understood. Generally believed it is immune small vasculitis caused by a certain pathogen infection. The clinic symptoms are very different. Multiple systems can be involved. For increasing permeability of capillaries, natrium, liquid, and albumin flow out of capillaries. Hyponatremia and hypoalbuminemia are common. If without treatment timely, amount of circulation blood volume could be insufficient. At last, hypovolemic shock may be developed. If only from symptom, it is somewhat similar to diarrhea disease, both with vomit and/or watery stool. However, the most significant difference between patients with common viral diarrhea and patients with KD is that KD patients usually lose large amount of albumin. Thus, metabolic acidosis is not severe, but the shock is difficult to correct. Furthermore, albumin and immunoglobulin are essential while bicarbonate is not indispensable. Hypovolemic shock usually happens in acute phase, mostly in patients with persistent fever along with vomit and diarrhea. Once hypovolemic shock happens, the patient could be in danger [8]. Meanwhile, both hyponatremia and hypoalbuminemia are independent risk factors for coronary artery aneurysms [9]. Therefore, we must pay attention to hyponatremia and hypoalbuminemia in KD patients and treat them timely in order to have a good prognosis.

The patient met the criteria of KD. She had prolonged fever for 6 days and was not responding to antibiotics, along with (i) skin rashes; (ii) cervical lymphadenectasis over 1.5 cm; (iii) bilateral conjunctiva congestion; (iv) cracked red lips with strawberry tongue; (v) erythema of both palms and edema of the feet. In addition, she also met the criteria of hypovolemic shock [8]: (i) the blood pressure decreased, with the lowest at 65/35 mmHg [systolic blood pressure decreased more than 20% from baseline, and the

Table 2.3 The dynamic changes of venous blood gas analysis and BP

Day of illness	5 days	6 days	7 days	8 days	10 days
pH	7.425	7.454,	7.47	7.5	7.53
BE	−5.4	−2.8	−2.2	−4.4	8.4
K^+(mmol/L)	3.82	3.87	3.55	2.9	3.5
Na^+(mmol/L)	131.6	129.3	126.8	125	136
SBP(mmHg)	80	64	73–65	65	99
DBP(mmHg)	40	26	38–35	35	61

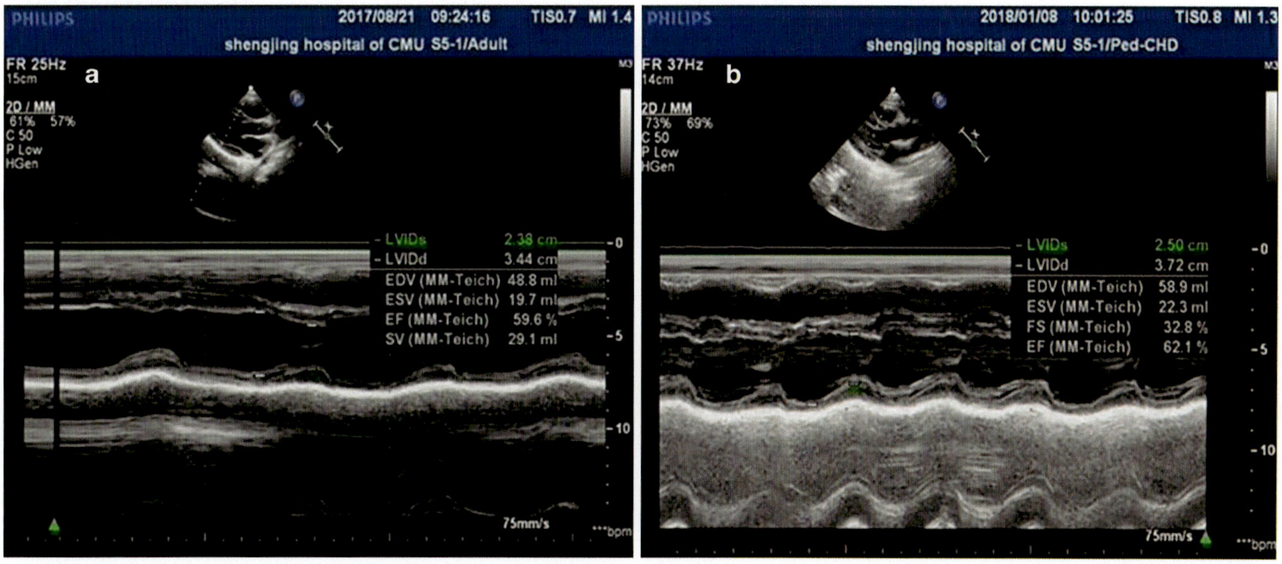

Fig. 2.20 Echocardiography showed her LVEF were normal both at 2 months (**a**) and 6 months (**b**)

average blood pressure (age × 2 + 80 mmHg) decreased by more than 20%]; (ii) the HR increased to 160 bpm; (iii) irritability, cold extremities, CRT 5 s; (iv) blood sodium decreased obviously. Urine was less. The minimum CVP was reduced to 5cmH_2O; (v) the shock was quickly corrected after infusion of NS, albumin, IVIG and increasing BP medicine.

In recent years, experts found some children with KD accompanied with hemodynamic changes, which is called Kawasaki disease shock syndrome (KDSS) [9]. Children with KDSS are in much more danger, like this girl. Currently, the accepted treatment of KDSS is to infuse a large dose of immunoglobulin, albumin appropriate liquid infusion, vasoactive drugs (dobutamine, dopamine, adrenaline, etc.) as well as anti-inflammatory. It is crucial to maintain effective circulating blood volume when a shock develops. As for this case, the patient presented tachycardia and hypotension. We immediately gave IVIG and infuse solution to increase colloid osmotic pressure and crystalloid osmotic pressure. Then dopamine and dobutamine were infused to improve the peripheral circulation and increase blood pressure. Fortunately, she survived from KDSS.

2.2.5 Case Specific Clinic Features

1. A study [10] showed that the level of NT-pro BNP in children with KDSS was significantly higher about eight times than that only with KD. Her NT-pro BNP was 26,025 pg/ml before being transferred to PICU, 79 times as high as normal. It coincides with the literature.
2. It has been reported [11] the inflammation in children with KD accompanied with cervical lymphadenectasis was more severe. Both cervical and abdominal lymphadenectasis, the circulation, nervous, blood and digestive system were involved in this case. Obviously, her inflammation was extremely severe.
3. She had abdominal pain at the beginning of the disease. Ming-Ming Zhang et al. [12] found that some children with KDSS have severe gastrointestinal symptoms in China. One study of Mexican [9] showed that 91% of KDSS patients have gastrointestinal manifestations. With the application of IVIG, abdominal pain was relieved, which indicated that it may be abdominal vasculitis, hypoproteinemia, intestinal wall edema. Several patients had complications such as intussusception, cholecystitis, and pancreatitis (See cases of digestive system involvement).
4. II °AVB may be caused by the injury of myocardial conduction system, and also may be associated with the ion disorder. The ECG of follow-up showed the damage was reversible (see case 11).
5. She was lethargy, lassitude and EEG showed much slow wave. It may be the symptom of aseptic meningitis, or brain edema caused by hyponatremia, and/or may be even caused by IVIG [13]. Unfortunately, the patient did not have lumbar puncture. If CSF showed evidence of pleocytosis, aseptic meningitis could be diagnosed.
6. This girl was consistent with report that KD shock syndrome was more often seen in female and had larger proportions of higher CRP, lower HGB and PLT [14]. But she was inconsistent with the literature reports that KD with shock has higher risk of IVIG resistance, CAA, and prolonged myocardial dysfunction [15]. This patient did not have these complications and survived without sequelae.

Xiao-zhe Cui

2.3 Case 3 KD with Chronic Myocardial Damage

A three-year-old boy was presented with an unremarkable past, personal, allergy, and family history.

He presented on Day 6 of illness with continuous fever for 6 days, along with rashes for 5 days, red conjunctiva, edema in hands and feet for 6 h. On the second day of illness, a lot of rashes with itching developed from his instep, spread to all over the body and gradually merged together. He was admitted to a local infectious disease hospital as "scarlet fever" and treated with second-generation cephalosporin for 3 days. The rashes regressed, but he developed remittent fever up to 39.0 °C. On the morning when he was admitted, hard swelling developed in his hands and feet, and conjunctival hyperemia was present in both eyes. He was admitted to our pediatric cardiology ward as atypical KD. Examination revealed a stable mental stage, fever (38.8 °C), HR 129 bpm, RR 24 bpm, and weight 14 kg. He had red rashes all over skin, along with bilateral conjunctival hyperemia, red lips, and strawberry tongue. Hands and feet were hard swollen, more significant on his left foot. Others were normal. CBC on Day 3 at the local hospital showed: WBC 10.6 × 10^9/L, NE 77.6%, HGB 113 g/L, PLT 306 × 10^9/L. When admitted at our ward, CBC was repeated and showed: WBC 10.8 × 10^9/L, NE 51.2%, HGB109g/L, PLT 409 × 10^9/L, CRP 32.9 mg/L and NT pro-BNP 521.5 pg/ml. Cervical ultrasound showed lymphadenectasis; the larger one was 1.2 cm × 0.8 cm on the left, and 1.2 cm × 0.5 cm on the right. He had met the diagnostic criteria for KD. He received (i) aspirin (oral route), 30-50 mg/kg/d, in 3 divided doses; dipyridamole (oral route) 3-5 mg/kg/d, in 3 divided doses; (ii) creatine phosphate sodium 1 g/d and levocarnitine 20 mg/kg/d infusion; (iii) IVIG 1 g/kg/d for 2 days.

On Day 7, lab tests for liver function, myocardial enzyme, renal function, hs-cTnT, CK-MB mass, MYO, immunoglobulin, and ASO revealed that they were all normal. Lab test showed ESR 20 mm/h, cTnI 0.136 μg/L($\leq$0.04 μg/L), IgE 54.59 (1.31–165.3 IU/ml), and MP-IgG 1:320. TB antibody and measles virus antibody were negative. ADV and PINF virus antibodies were positive. ECG and chest CT were normal. He was infused with azithromycin 10 mg/kg/d for 3 days. On Day 8, his fever reduced, and red conjunctiva regressed. Echo showed normal LCA, RCA (Fig. 2.20a, b), and LVEF (Fig. 2.21). On Day 9, after 48 h afebrile, the dosage of aspirin was reduced to 3–5 mg/kg/d. On Day 11, red lips, swollen hands and feet subsided, and peeling skin occurred around fingernails.

On Day 13, peeling skin was also found around toe nails. Blood test revealed WBC 4.2 × 10^9/L, NE 28.5%, HGB 98 g/L, PLT 465 × 10^9/L, cTnI 0.054 μg/L. ALT, AST, and NT pro-BNP were normal. Repeated echo showed normal results. He was discharged.

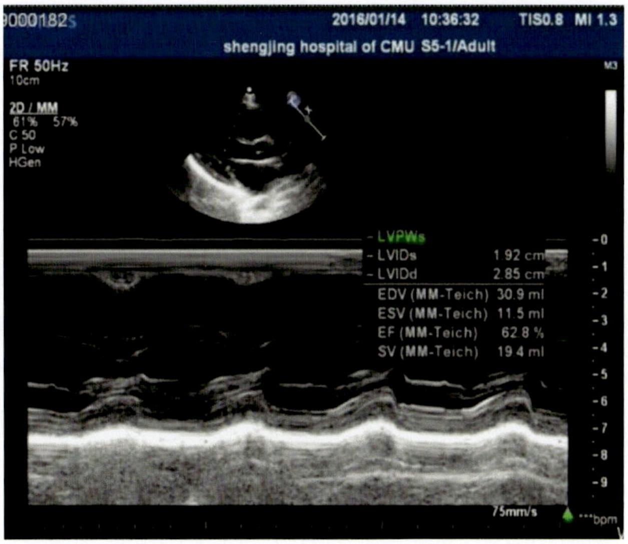

Fig. 2.21 On Day 8 of illness, echo showed normal LVEF

2.3.1 Clinical Course of the Patient

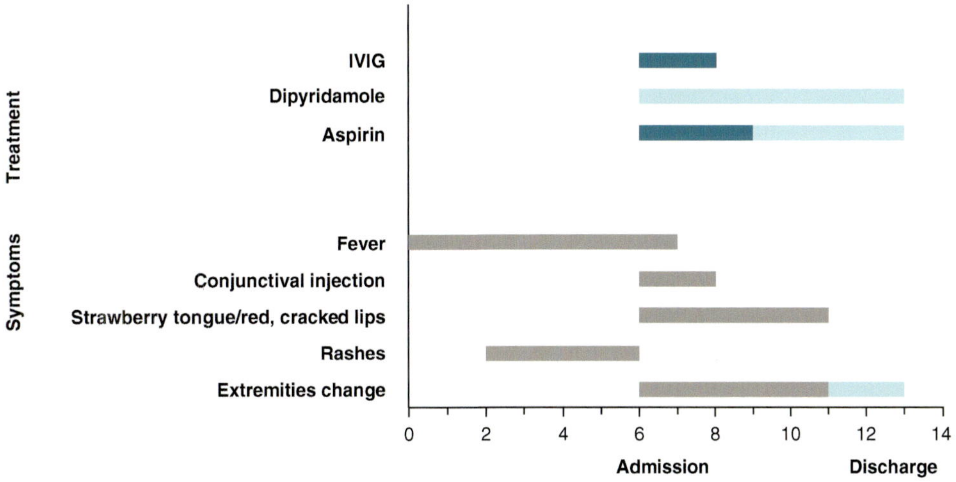

2.3.2 Follow-Up

He was followed up at the clinic over 2 years since discharge. Echo was performed at 3, 4, and 8 weeks of illness, respectively. Coronary artery, LVED, and LVEF remained normal. Aspirin and dipyridamole were discontinued at 2 months. Nevertheless, his cTnI stayed at high level (Fig. 2.22) for 10 months, whereas ECG was normal. Fructose sodium diphosphate oral solution was discontinued at the end of 3 months of illness. He continued to take levocarnitine (oral) for 10 months until cTnI reduced. Unfortunately, at 16 months of illness, his cTnI rose again and stayed high to 48 months of illness. Both ECG (Fig. 2.23) and echo were normal.

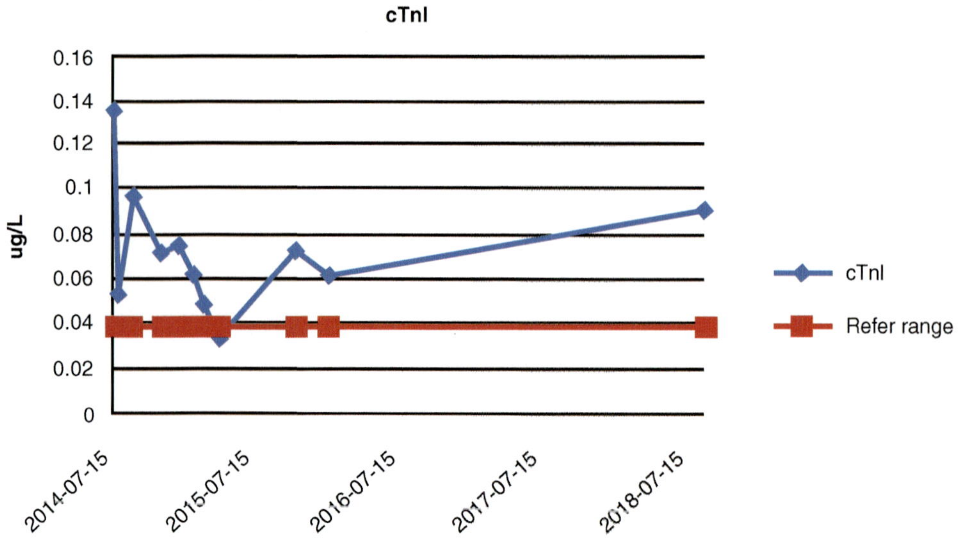

Fig. 2.22 His cTnI kept elevated for 4 years

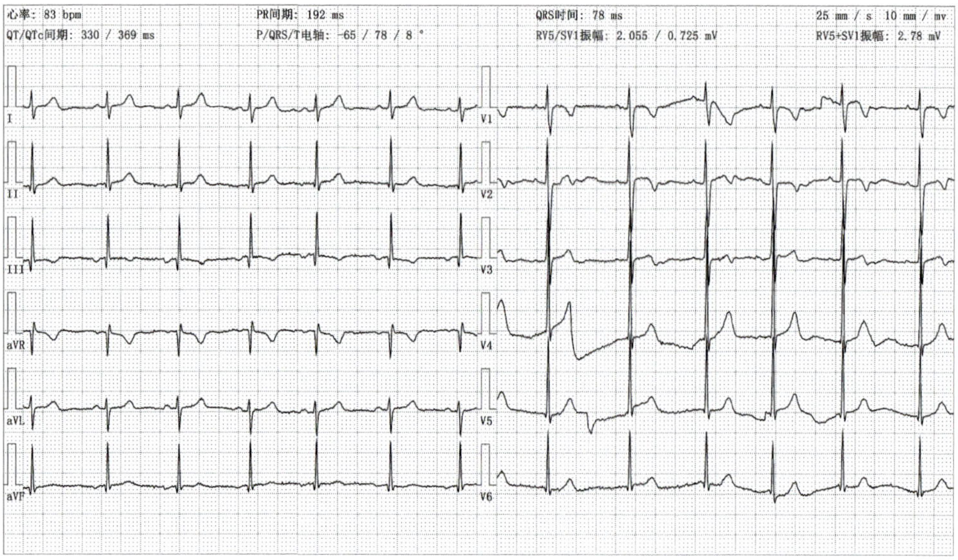

Fig. 2.23 At 4 years of illness, his ECG was normal

2.3.3 Diagnosis

1. KD
2. Myocardial injury
3. MP infection
4. Viral infection (ADV, PINF virus)
5. Mild anemia

2.3.4 Discussion

The patient met the criteria of KD. He had persistent fever over 5 days and did not respond to broad-spectrum antibiotics, along with: (i) congestive rash; (ii) bilateral conjunctival congestion; (iii) red lips and strawberry tongue; (iv) swollen hands and feet, skin peeling around toenails in late period. Differential diagnosis should be looked into for possible streptococcus infection and pharyngeal conjunctival fever.

2.3.5 Case Specific Clinical Features

1. KD is a systemic vasculitis with unknown etiology, which can result in small and medium arterial diseases. Some literatures report that it may be related to infection of microorganisms such as bacteria super-antigen or viruses. Some reports suggest that EB virus infection may be involved in the pathogenesis of KD, while herpes simplex virus, coronavirus OC 43/229E and NL63, respiratory syncytial virus A and B, and PINF virus 1 and 4 are not significantly associated with KD [16]. Furthermore, some studies have found that MP infection may also relate to

KD. The duration of disease in children with MP infection in KD is prolonged, usually combined with other organ damages [17].
2. CTnI is a structural protein in myocardium and has a high content in myocardium. CTnI is released into blood during myocardial injury and serves as a specific marker for myocardial injury. Mycoplasma and viral infection can result in myocardial damages. This patient's MP IGG antibody was positive (1:320). ASV and PINF virus antibodies were positive. Though ECG and echo were normal, elevated cTnI last for 10 months which might be associated with KD [18]. However, the re-increase of cTnI in the later period indicates that KD can cause prolonged myocardial injury. It is commonly noted that transient increases of CK, CK-MB, CK-MB mass, and hs-cTnT occur in patients with myocarditis. They recover usually in 2 weeks [19]. Based on a lack of reproducibility of myocardial cell, persistently elevated cTnI suggests worse prognosis.
3. Conjunctival hyperemia in KD is mostly transient. There is no purulent secretion. It is often not necessary to apply antibiotics locally. The condition rapidly resolved with IVIG treatment. As soon as fever subsided, the conjunctivitis disappeared. The mechanism may be related to the increased IgE in these patients [20]. IgE level reaches its peak at 1–2 weeks after diagnosed with KD, and disappears after one or 2 months. Some reports showed that children with KD and elevated IgE and IL_5 may develop allergic dermatitis [21].
4. In our ward, the chronic injury of the myocardium has been seen in 3 cases of inflammatory cardiomyopathy. All of them died within 6 months [6]. It is the first time for us to see a long-term cTnI elevation along with a normal hs-cTnT in KD patients. The pathogen was re-checked. Virus antibodies were negative at late phase. Both coronary artery and ECG were normal. Thus, this patient had not yet reached the criteria of inflammatory cardiomyopathy. Sustained myocardial damages can result in worse prognosis in long run.

Ya-li Zhang

2.4 Case 4 KD with Large Pericardial Effusion

A previously healthy 7-month-old girl was with an unremarkable past and family history. She always had cyanosis around the mouth after crying.

She presented on Day 20 of illness with a prolonged fever lasting for 20 days, along with rashes for 2 days, redden conjunctiva and lips for 7 days, cough and hoarse voice for 5 days. She was infused with second-generation cephalosporin for 4 days at a local clinic and then took amoxicillin (oral route) at home. Fever did not regress and trunk rashes, bilateral conjunctivitis, and red and cracked lips developed on Day 4 of illness. Two days later the rashes were subsided. But fever was persistent at around 39 °C. Cough developed along with hoarse voice 2 days after illness. The conjunctiva and lips symptoms had gradually improved 1 week after onset. Cough improved without wheeze. She was admitted in a local hospital and infused with IVIG 2.5 g for 1 day on Day 18 of illness. But fever did not subside. She was transferred to our pediatric respiratory ward on Day 19 of illness. After consulting pediatric cardiologist, she was transferred to the cardiology ward as a KD patient on Day 20 of illness. Since onset, she had watery diarrhea for 5 days, 4–5 times a day. Examination found: body temperature 38.2 °C, PR 140 bpm, RR 36 bpm, and weight 6 kg. Her mental stage was stable. She had cervical lymphadenectasis about 2 cm. Auscultation found blisters at the bottom of her right lung. HR was 140 bpm, with 2/6 level of systolic murmurs on the second costal by the left side of sternum. Liver was enlarged 2.5 cm below right costal margin. Spleen was enlarged 1.0 cm below left costal margin. Peeling skin was found around fingernails. Others were normal. Echo revealed: a second atrial septal defect (ASD) 10 mm and slight pulmonary valve stenosis (Fig. 2.24a); LCA aneurysm like dilated diameter about 7.2 mm, RCA aneurysm like dilated diameter about 7.5 mm (Fig. 2.24b); massive hydro-pericardium (Fig. 2.24c); and LVED 19 mm. She had met the criteria of KD, complicated with bilateral CAA and massive hydro-pericardium. CHD of ASD. She was treated with (i) aspirin (oral) 30–50 mg/kg/d and dipyridamole (oral) 3–5 mg/kg/d, in three divided doses; (ii) IVIG 2 g/kg/d in 24 h; (iii) infused with dexamethasone 0.2 mg/kg/d for 4 days; (iv) digoxin (oral route) 0.01 mg/kg per day; (v) furosemidum 1 mg/kg/d every day and spironolactone in 1 mg/kg per day for 4 days in 1 week; captopril 0.6 mg/kg/d, in 2 divided doses, all oral route; (vi) montmorillonite powder to control diarrhea, and live combined bifidobacterium to regulate the intestinal flora; oral route; vii) intramuscular injection of vitamin K_1 5 mg/d for 3 days to prevent delayed vitamin K deficiency; viii) infused with ceftezole.

On Day 21, fever subsided. Blood test revealed that WBC, PLT, CRP, ESR, BNP were elevated (Table 2.4); cTnI, MP-Ab, EBV, and TORCH were normal. The ECG showed sinus tachycardia, myocardial damage (T wave was low and flatter at left ventricular inferior wall and lateral wall) (ECG strip was failed to save as file). On day 27, peeling skin occurred at ends around fingernails and toenails. Investigation revealed that WBC, PLT, ESR remained elevated (Table 2.4). CRP was normal. Repeated echo showed LVED 22.3 mm. LM and LAD aneurism dilated stayed unchanged about 7.5 mm. The RCA aneurism continually dilated to 8.3–10.5 mm. Hydro-pericardium diminished to mild. Her parents refused to give her oral warfarin. She was discharged next day.

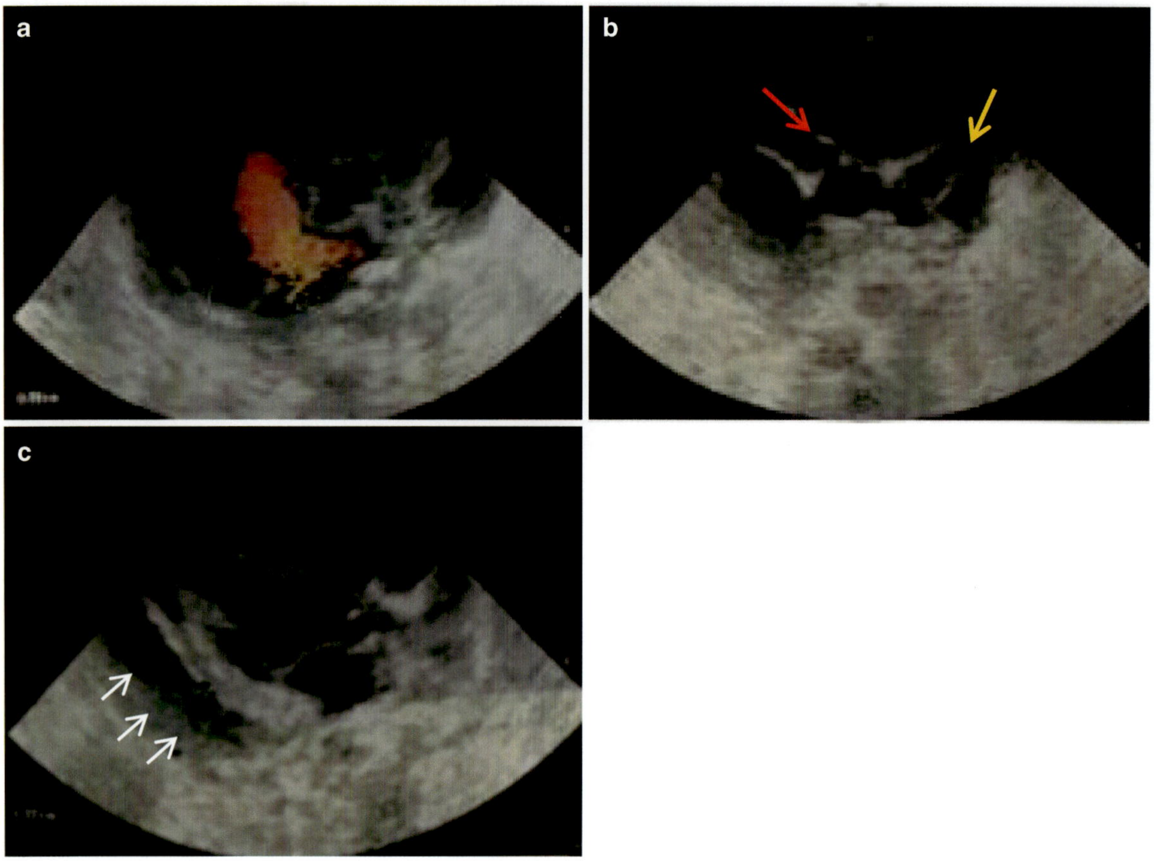

Fig. 2.24 On Day 20 of illness, echocardiography revealed secondary atrial septal defect 10 mm (**a**), *red shunt from left to right*. LCA dilated up to 7.2 mm (**b**), *red arrow*, RCA dilated up to 7.5 mm (**b**), *orange arrow*. 14 mm large amount of pericardial effusion behind the posterior wall of the left ventricle (**c**)

Table 2.4 The dynamic changes of lab parameters

Time of illness	21 days	27 days	32 months	57 months	86 months	110 months
WBC ($\times10^9$/L)	9	16.9	10	7.4		10
HGB (g/L)	73	85	124	123		133
PLT($\times10^9$/L)	481	730	230	351		230
CRP (mg/L)	15.3	5.78	N	N		
ESR (mm/h)	21	21	N	N		
BNP (pg/ml)	284.59		N		N	

N normal

2.4.1 Clinical Course of the Patient

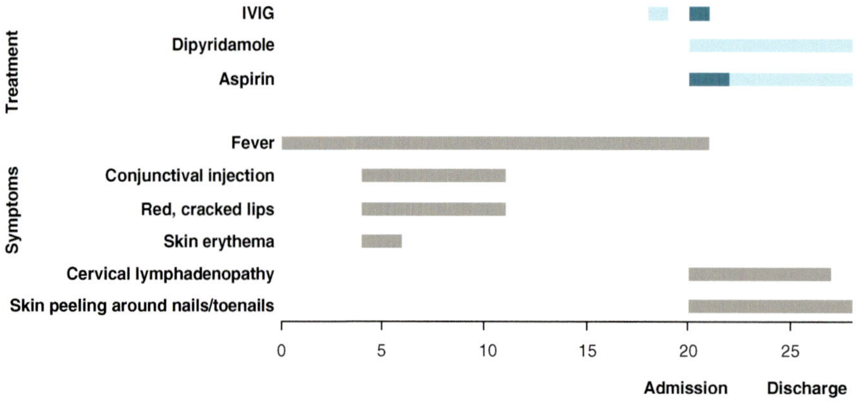

2.4.2 Follow-Up

She was taking oral aspirin and dipyridamole after discharge and was followed up with us as an out-patient. In the follow-up, 2D echo was performed as scheduled. (Tables 2.4 and 2.5) (Figs. 2.26, 2.27, 2.28, 2.29, 2.30, 2.31, 2.32, 2.33, 2.34, and 2.35).

At nearly 5 years of illness, repeated echo showed no pericardial effusion (Fig. 2.25). LM was filled with a strong echo reflex size of 6.8 mm × 1.5 mm (Fig. 2.26a). The RCA regressed to 4.5 mm (Fig. 2.26b). Coronary artery CTA showed that LM aneurism dilated to 12.5 mm (Fig. 2.27a), proximal segment of RCA dilated slightly (Fig. 2.27b, left arrow) with calcification (Fig. 2.27b, right arrow), the coronary lumen was irregular. Coronary artery CTA showed no stenosis (Fig. 2.27c).

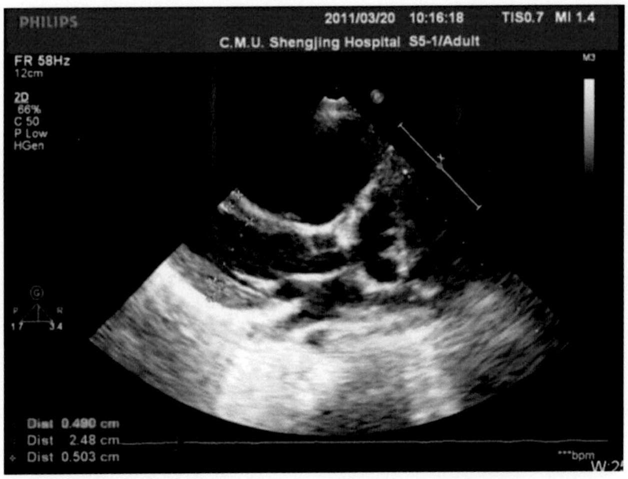

Fig. 2.25 At nearly 5 years of illness, echocardiography showed the pericardial effusion was absorbed

At nearly 5.5 years of illness, the child was admitted to the department of cardiology of our hospital for the treatment of ASD occlusion. The procedure went well.

At nearly 6 years of illness, the CTA showed both LM and RCA calcification, and the child took warfarin 0.1 mg/kg/d orally, and DIC was monitored to keep her INR in 2-3.

At nearly 7 years of illness, echo showed that LCA dilated to 10.3 mm (Fig. 2.28a) with thrombus inside of it (Fig. 2.28b). RCA dilated to 3.5–4.2 mm without thrombus, and its inner intima was not smooth (Fig. 2.28c). Coronary artery CTA showed that LCA aneurism dilated to 16 mm × 12 mm, LDA and LCX all originated from the aneurism (Fig. 2.29a); there were calcifications (Fig. 2.29b, upper arrow) on the wall of RCA with thrombus (Fig. 2.29b, lower arrow) in it.

At nearly 9 years of illness, echo showed the proximal segment of LCA dilated to 8.5 mm without thrombus (Fig. 2.30a).

At nearly 10 years of illness, echo showed the opening of the LCA dilated to 10 mm (Fig. 2.30b). There was no echo reflex in the wall, without thrombus; the RCA dilated to 6 mm, its inner intima was not smooth, and the coronary lumen was irregular. ECG was normal (Fig. 2.31).

At nearly 11 years of illness, echo showed LCA dilated to 10 mm (Fig. 2.32a), RCA dilated to 4.5 mm, inner intima was not smooth (Fig. 2.32b), LVEF was 0.52 (Fig. 2.32c), while the position of interatrial septal plug was normal, without additional echocardiography findings on it (Fig. 2.32d).

At nearly 12 years of illness, echocardiography showed LCA dilated to 4.2–8.2 mm (Fig. 2.33a), RCA 4.6 mm (Fig. 2.33b). ECG was almost normal (Fig. 2.34). Coronary artery CTA showed LAD aneurism dilated to 20 mm × 12.2 mm (Fig. 2.35a), LDA and LCX all originated from the aneurism; the RCA dilated to 4.5 mm (Fig. 2.35b). There were calcifications on aneurysm of LCA (Fig. 2.35c) and RCA (Fig. 2.35d).

Table 2.5 The dynamic changes of coronary artery

Time		20 day	27 day	57 month	73 month	85 month	98 month	110 month	122 month	134 month	146 month
ECHO	LAD (mm)	7.2	7.5	11.4		10.3	13 × 10	8.5	10	10.3	4.2–8.2
	RCA (mm)	7.5	8.3–10.5	4.5		3.5–4.2	4.2	3.8–4.4	6	4.4	4.6
	PE	Massive	Mild	No	No	No	No	No	No	No	No
	Thrombus			LCA		LCA/ RCA					
CTA	LAD (mm)	12.5		12 × 16					12.2 × 20	12.5	
	RCA (mm)										
	Calcification		LCA	RCA	RCA	RCA			LCA		LCA/RCA

PE Pericardial effusion

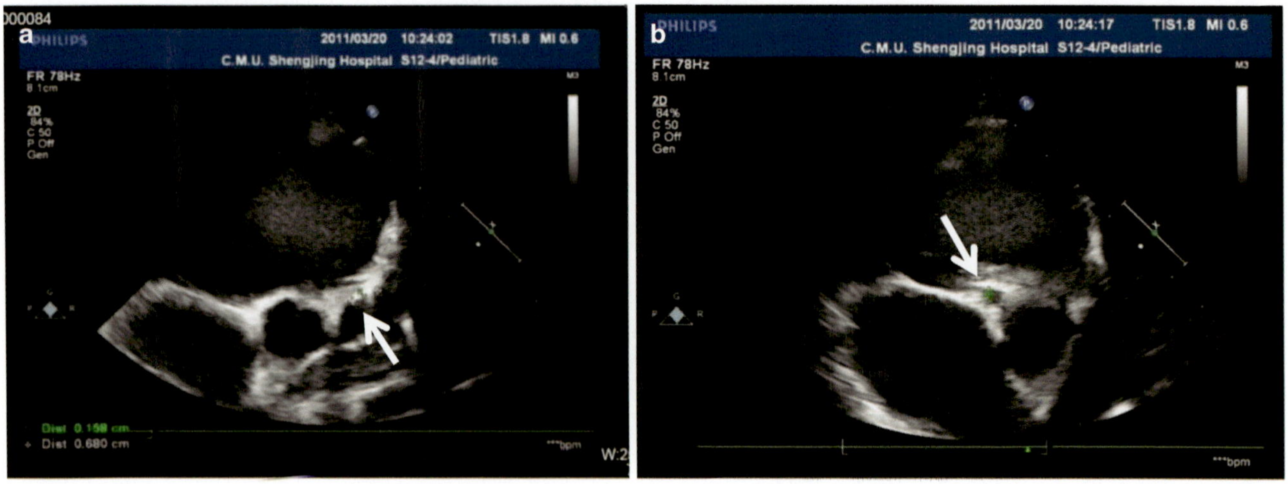

Fig. 2.26 At nearly 5 years of illness, echocardiography showed LM dilated up to 11.4 mm with 6.8 mm × 1.5 mm thrombus inside (**a**), while RCA was returned to 4.5 mm (**b**)

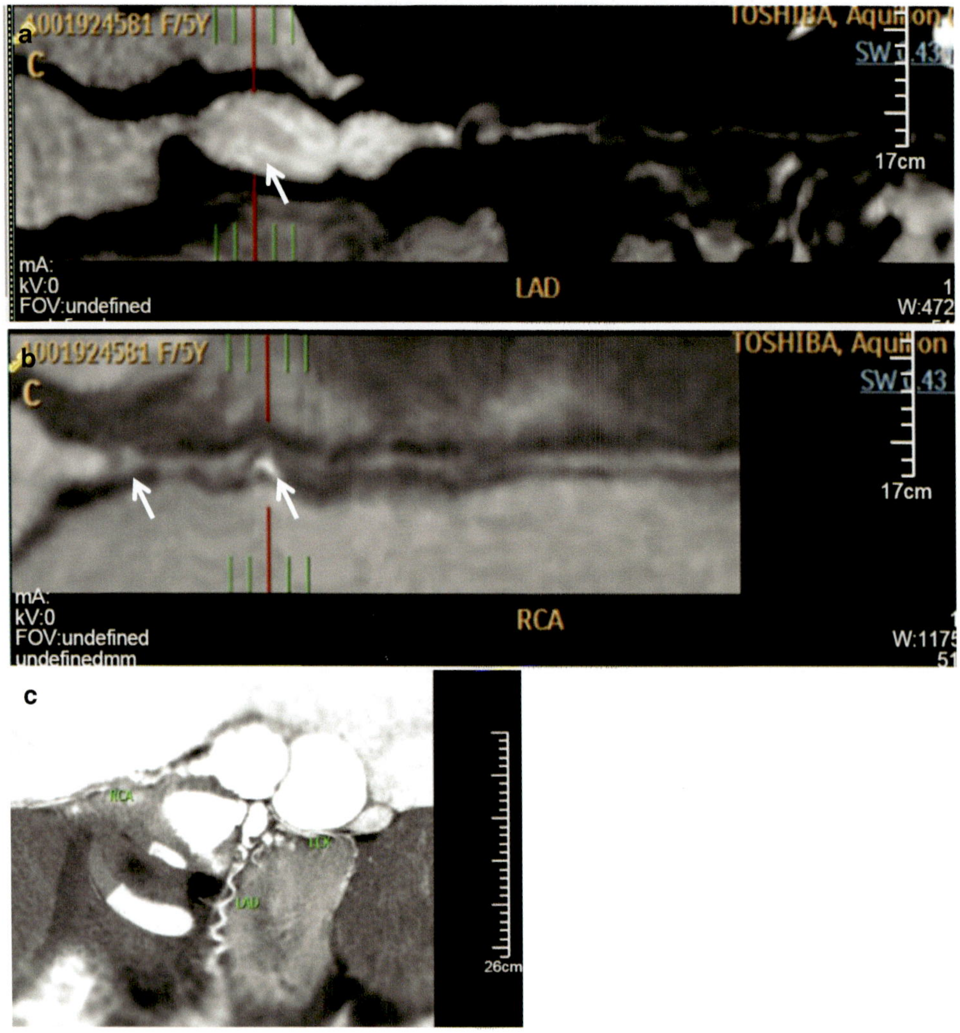

Fig. 2.27 Fig. 2.27 At nearly 5 years of illness, coronary artery CTA showed Two aneurysms in the LM and the proximal segment of LAD (**a**-white arrow), proximal segment of RCA dilated slightly (**b**-left arrow) with calcification (**b**-right arrow), Multiple stenosis in the proximal and middle segments of the RCA. 2D-map reconstruction of coronary CTA showed LAD aneurysm, RCA dilated

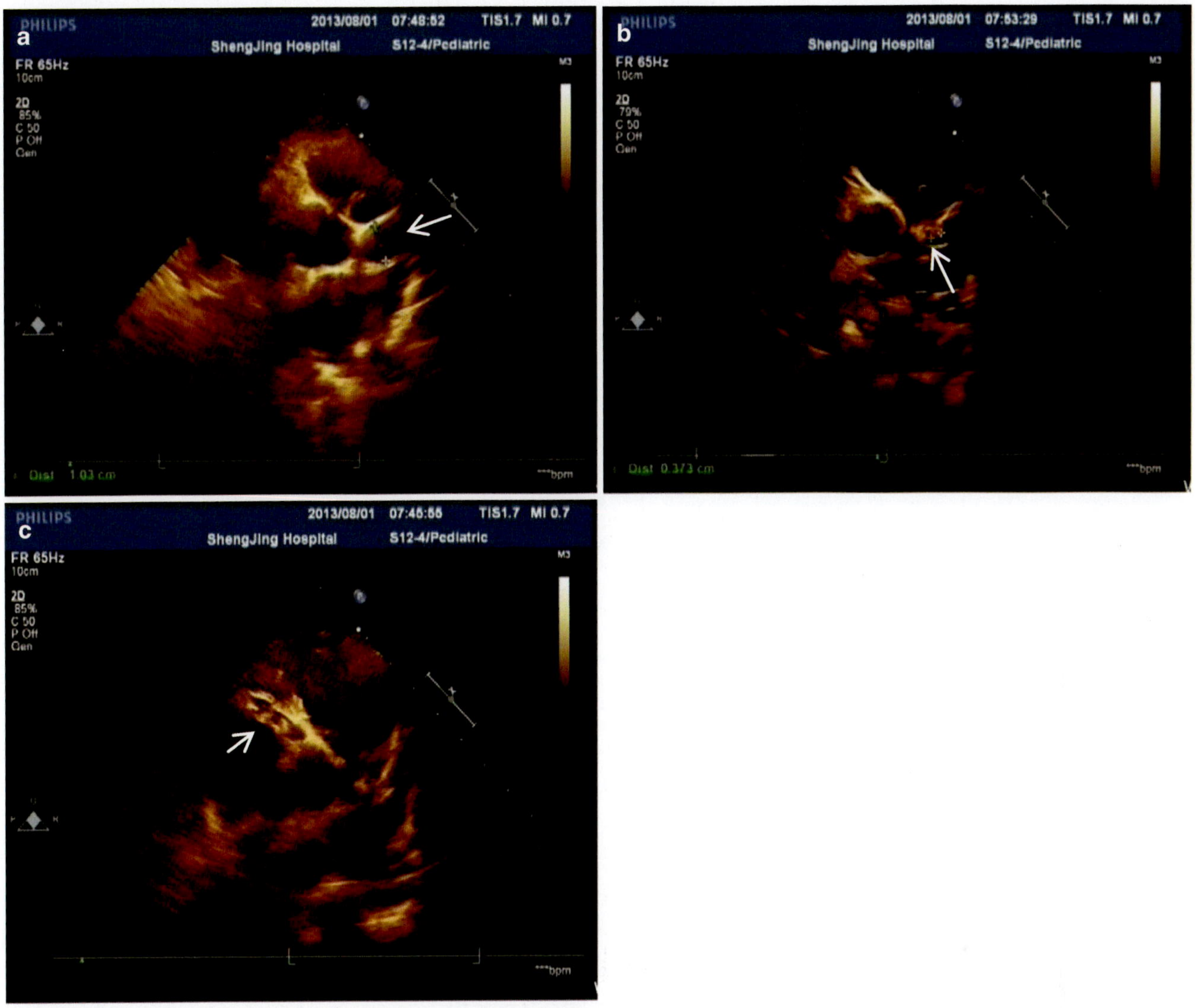

Fig. 2.28 AT nearly 7 years of illness, echocardiography showed LCA dilated up to 10.3 mm (**a**) with a thrombus inside (**b**). RCA dilated to 3.5–4.2 mm with rough wall (**c**) but no thrombus

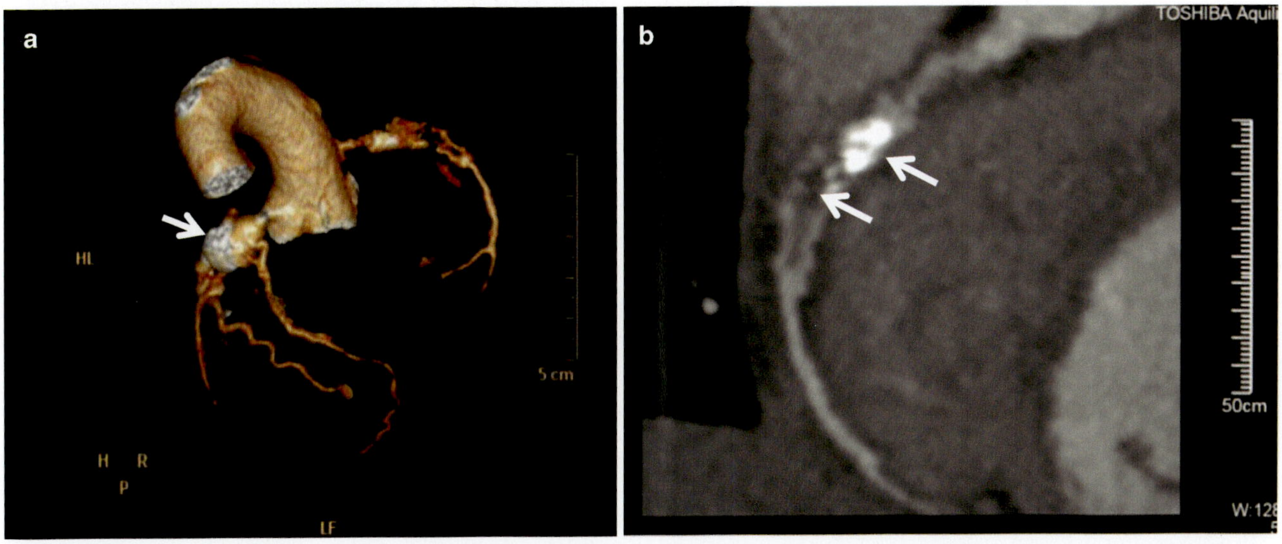

Fig. 2.29 At 86 months of illness, coronary artery CTA showed LCA aneurism dilated to 16 mm × 12 mm, LDA and LCX all originated from the aneurism (**a**); there were calcifications (**b**-upper arrow) on the wall of RCA and thrombus (**b**-lower arrow) inner aneurysm of RCA

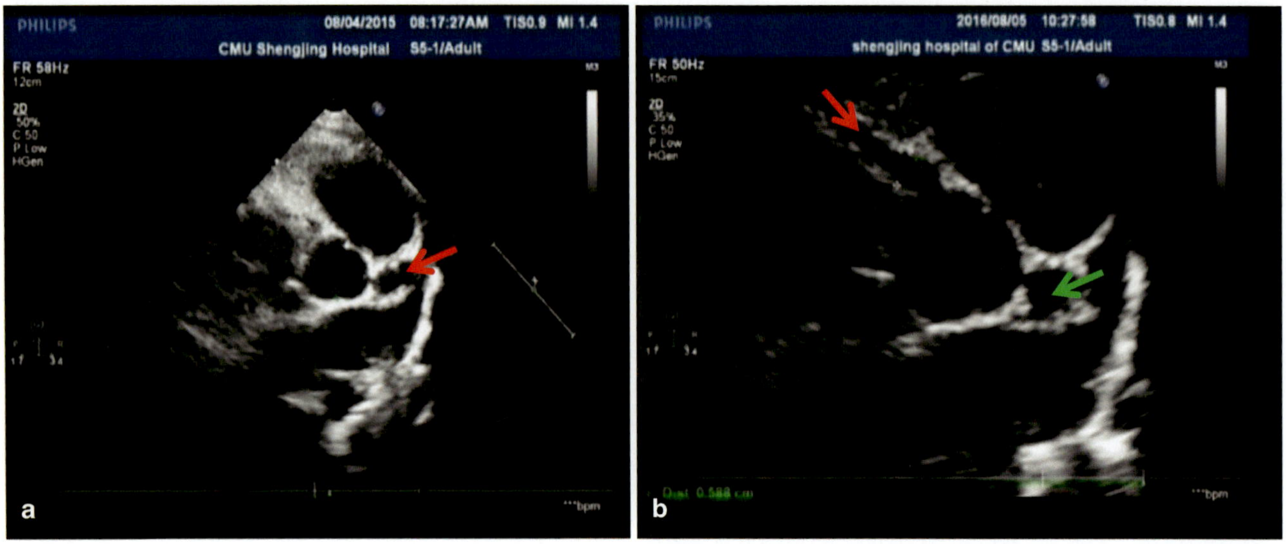

Fig. 2.30 After about 9 years of illness, echocardiography showed LCA dilated up to 8.5 mm (**a**, red arrow). After about 10 years, LCA dilated up to 10 mm (**b**, green arrow), RCA dilated to 6 mm (**b**, red arrow)

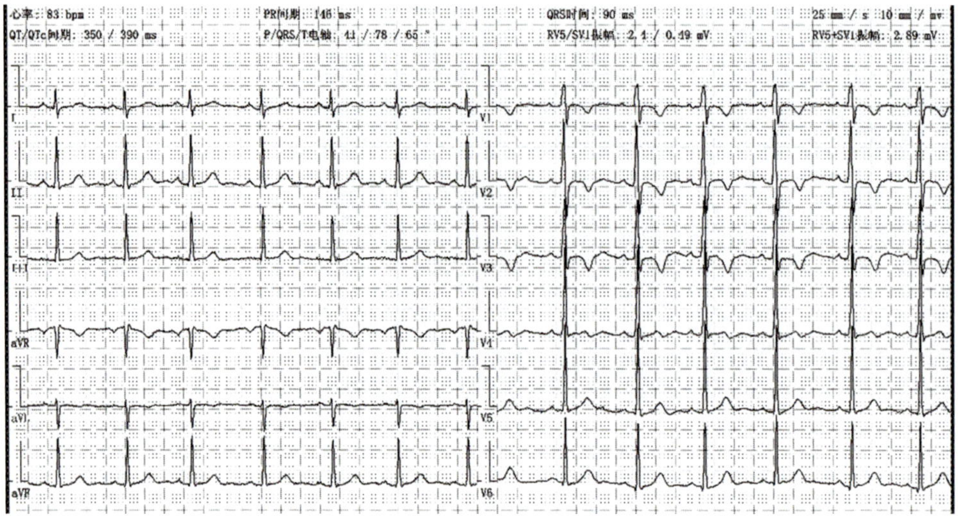

Fig. 2.31 At about 10 years of illness, ECG showed sinus rhythm, basically normal ECG

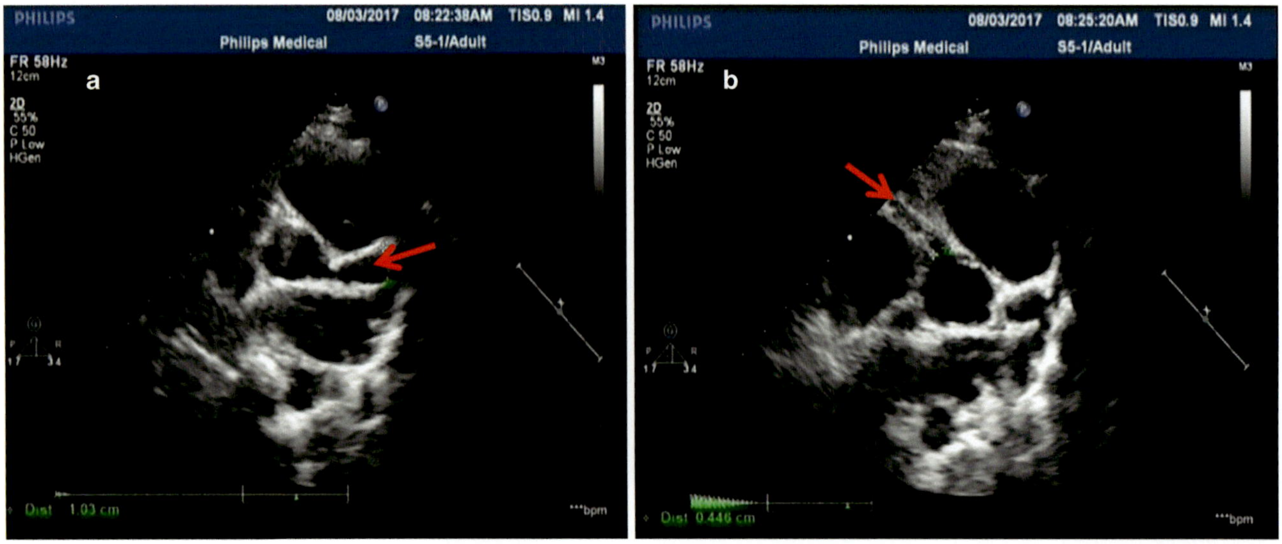

Fig. 2.32 After about 11 years, echocardiography showed LCA dilated to 10 mm (**a**), RCA dilated to 4.5 mm with rough wall (**b**), LVEF was 52% (**c**), the position of ASD occlusion device was normal, no additional echogenicity on it (**d**)

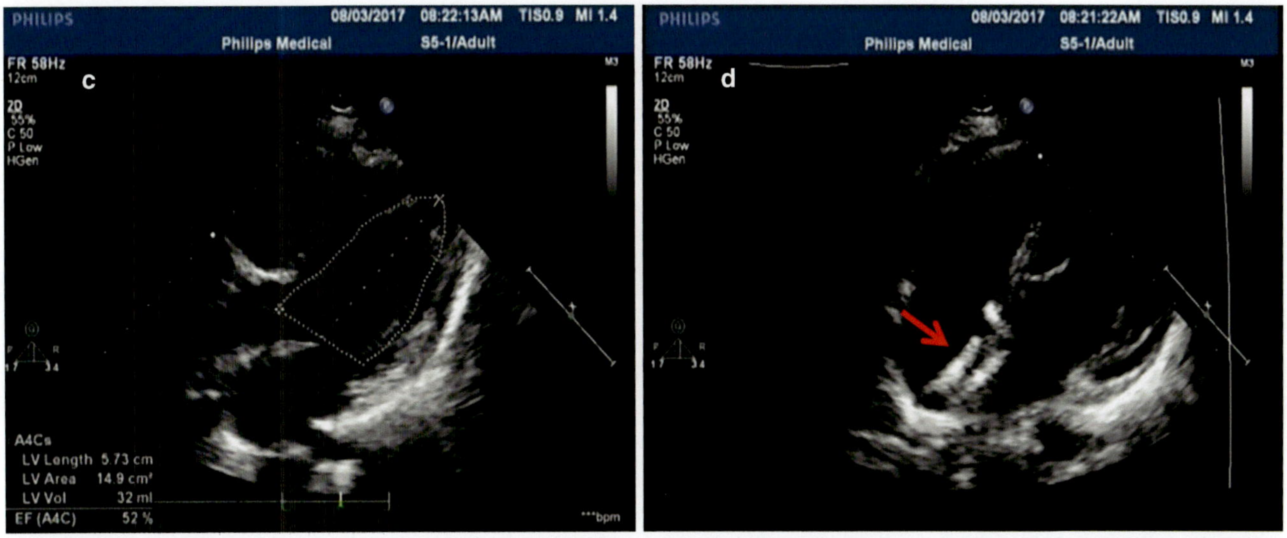

Fig. 2.32 (continued)

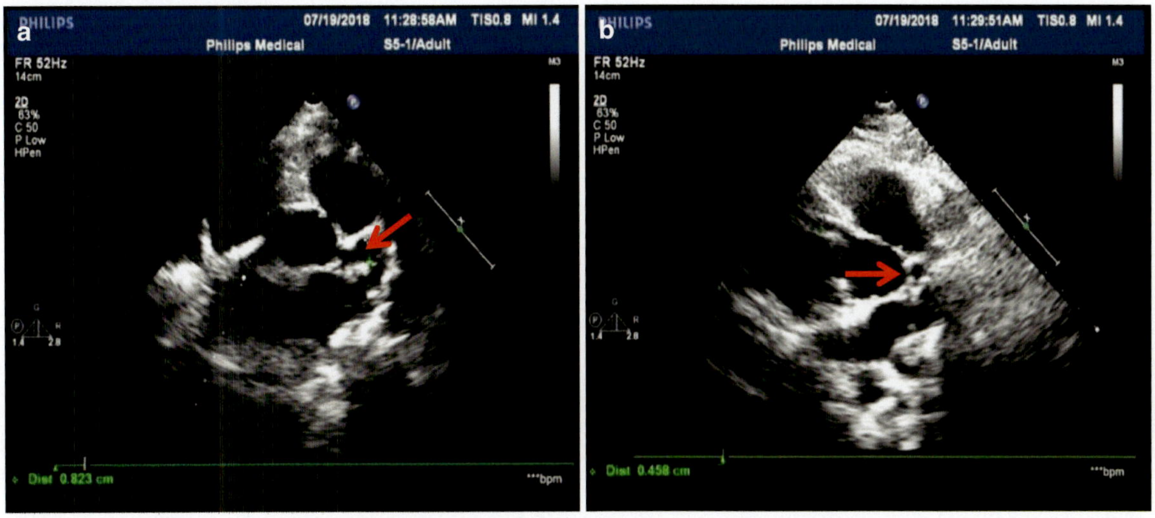

Fig. 2.33 After about 12 years, echocardiography showed LCA dilated to 4.2–8.2 mm (**a**), RCA 4.6 mm (**b**)

Fig. 2.34 At 12 years of illness, ECG was almost normal

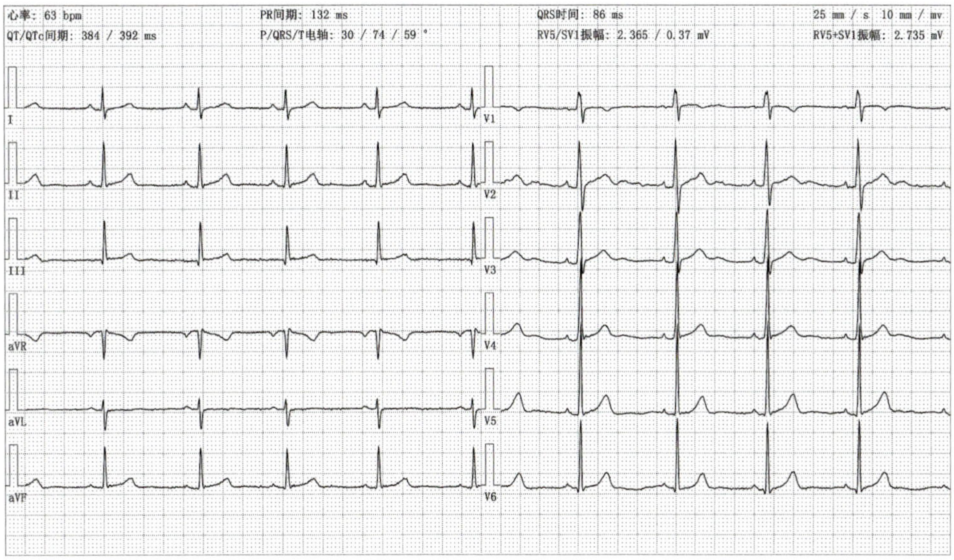

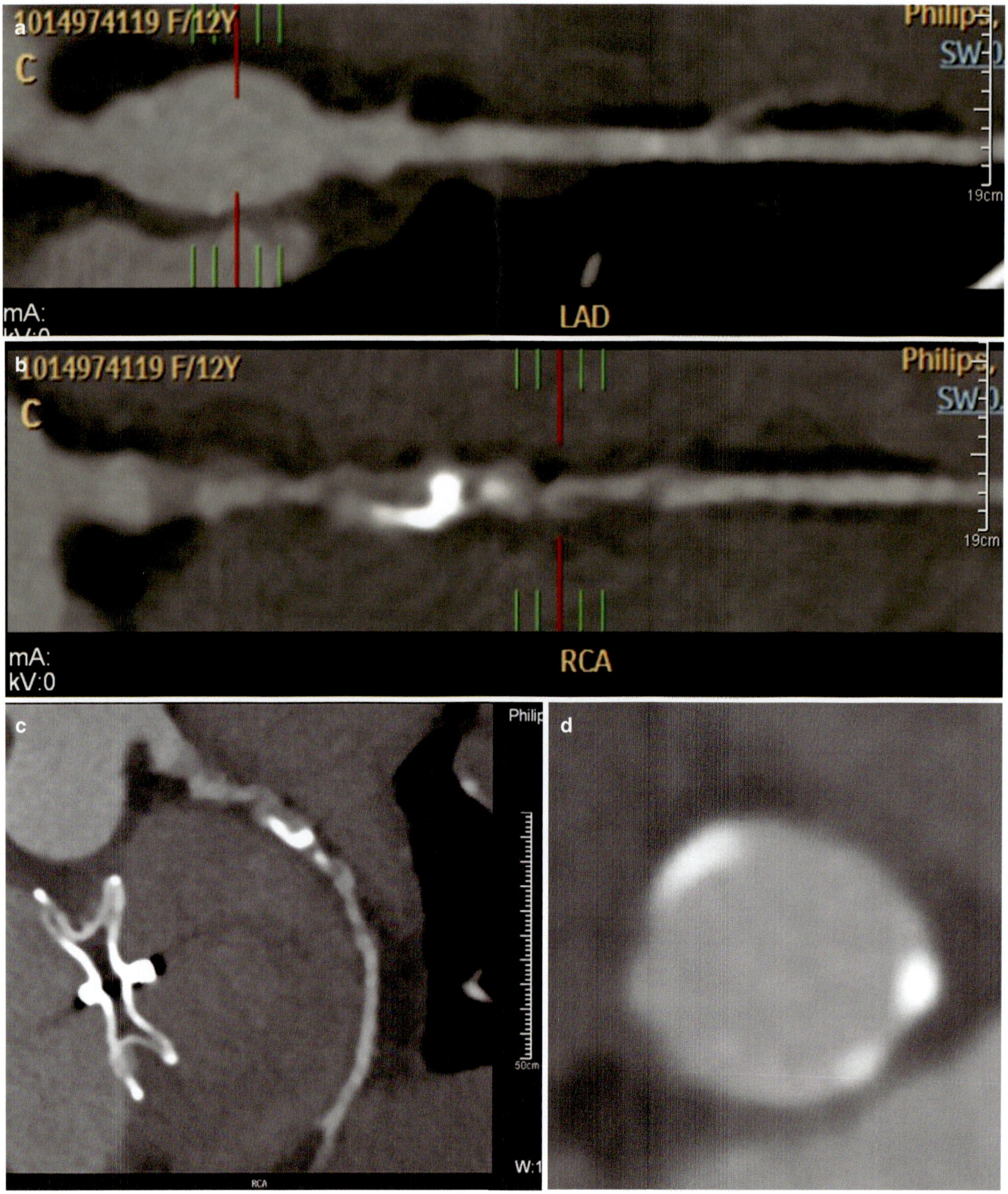

Fig. 2.35 At 12 years of illness, coronary artery CTA showed LAD aneurism dilated to 20 mm × 12.2 mm (**a**), LDA and LCX all originated from the aneurism; the RCA dilated to 4.5 mm (**b**), there were calcifications on aneurysm of LCA (**c**) and RCA (**d**)

2.4.3 Diagnosis

1. KD
2. Bilateral CAA
3. Massive hydro-pericardium
4. Coronary artery calcification
5. After the closure of ASD.

2.4.4 Discussion

She met the criteria of KD. Thus she had persistent fever for more than 5 days with (i) skin rashes; (ii) red conjunctiva; (iii) red and cracked lips; (iv) peeling skin around fingernails; (v) cervical lymphadenectasis; (vi) bilateral CAA shown in echocardiography.

The best time for giving IVIG should be within 10 days of the onset since fever. If some atypical patients were not diagnosed less than 10 days, but within 14 days, there were still high fever, and the laboratory index still increased, the IVIG should be given, too. If the course of disease had exceeded 10 days, in the absence of fever, or significant elevation of inflammatory markers, or coronary artery abnormality, IVIG was unnecessary, but only aspirin and dipyridamole treatment. The prevalence of coronary abnormalities was related to the total dose of IVIG and was independent of dose of aspirin. 2 g/kg IVIG in 24 h provides maximum protection against development of coronary abnormalities after KD [22].

ECG was not sensitive to myocardial ischemia in KD. There was no significant change in the ECG when the patient had coronary artery thrombosis or the distal coronary artery had poor supply. It may be due to short ischemia time or the establishment of collateral circulation. Clinically, it was more common after the occurrence of ischemic cardiomyopathy and chronic cardiac dysfunction.

2.4.5 Case Specific Clinical Features

1. This child had been feverish for more than 20 days when she was admitted to our hospital. Other symptoms were not obvious except peeling skin around fingernails. She was suffering from pneumonia with a large amount of pericardial effusion. LVED was normal. We speculated that this pericardial effusion was caused by vasculitis of KD other than heart failure or purulent pericarditis. Therefore, antibiotics and corticosteroids were added after IVIG, rather than single corticosteroids at initial treatment, which may aggravate the coronary artery injury. After 1 week treatment, pericardial effusion diminished to mild. Infusion of antibiotics was stopped without resulting in constrictive pericarditis. Thus, it supports our speculation.
2. The method of estimating the amount of pericardial effusion as followed [23]:

Echocardiography-free space		Microscale	Small	Medium	Large
Behind LVPW	(cm)	0.2–0.3	0.5	1.0–2.0	>2.0
	(ml)	30–50	50–200	200–500	> 500
	Location	Atrioventricular groove			
Before AWRV	(cm)			0.5–1.0	>1.5
	(ml)			200–500	>500

In this case, echocardiography revealed massive hydropericardium: about 14 mm behind the posterior wall of the left ventricle; the lateral wall of the left ventricle was 15 mm, it was about 8 mm in front of the anterior wall of the left ventricle; at the bottom of the xiphoid, it was about 10 mm. The patient did not have symptoms such as chest tightness, shortness of breath, discomfort in the anterior cardiac region. After 1 week of treatment, there was only a small amount of hydropericardium left. The pericardial drainage was not performed.

3. The efficacy of glucocorticoids in treating KD was still controversial. In 1997, Kato's research suggested that steroids might aggravate coronary artery disease [24]. Kobayashi T found that the addition of prednisolone to the standard regimen of IVIG improves coronary artery outcomes in patients with severe KD in Japan [25]. Athappan G considered that the inclusion of corticosteroids in regimens for the initial treatment of KD decreased rates of re-treatment with IVIG. However, the addition of corticosteroids to standard therapy did not decrease the incidence of CAA or adverse events [26]. At present, the usefulness of steroids in the initial treatment of KD is not well established, because these studies did not compare with those using glucocorticoid alone. Currently, because glucocorticoid is potentially dangerous to the prognosis of KD, the role of glucocorticoids in the treatment of KD is an adjuvant treatment and replacement of IVIG. If IVIG is unavailable, steroids are a logical primary treatment, especially for patients with severe myocarditis and cardiac dysfunction, hydropericardium, IVIG non-responsive cases, or patients with uncontrollable symptomes after repeated use of IVIG [27, 28].
4. The thrombus in the coronary artery was usually relatively stable after half a year and tended to be calcificated. Therefore, the child could still have the opportunity to go through atrial septal occlusion procedure.

Le Sun

2.5 Case 5 KD with ECG ST-T Changes

A previously healthy 5-years-old boy presented with unremarkable antenatal and family history.

He presented on Day 5 of illness with a prolonged fever for 5 days, along with cervical lymphadenopathy for 5 days and red conjunctiva for 3 days. He was treated with erythromycin for 4 days at a local hospital. Fever didn't subside, cervical lymphadenopathy improved and he developed red conjunctiva 3 days ago. He was then transferred to our clinic and infused with third-generation antibiotics for 2 days. Fever was unresponsive to the treatment, and the patient lost appetite. He was then admitted in our pediatric cardiology ward. Examination found: fever (37.5 °C), PR 120 bpm, RR 27 bpm, weight 37 kg. His mental stage was well, with conjunctival hyperemia, red lips, strawberry tongue, conjested pharynx and cervical lymphadenopathy. Skin around the anus was red and started to peel off. Blood test revealed: WBC 18.2×10^9/L, NE 80.4%, HGB 107 g/L, PLT 390×10^9/L, CRP 318 mg/l, ESR 55 mm/h, and NT-pro BNP 1792 pg/ml. ECG presented a low T wave, and the ST segment slightly moved downwards (Fig. 2.36). He had met the criteria for IKD, and was treated with (i) aspirin 30–50 mg/kg/d and dipyridamole 3–5 mg/kg/d, in three divided doses; oral route (ii) IVIG 1 g/kg/d for 2 days; (iii) infusion of therapeutic nutritions for myocardium.

On Day 7, red conjunctiva and red lips recovered, and investigation revealed ALB 28.4 g/L. He was infused with albumin 1 g/kg/d for 2 days. ECG was normal (Fig. 2.37). On Day 9, he was afebrile over 48 h, there was peeling skin around fingernails. Aspirin was reduced to 3–5 mg/kg/d. On Day 11, investigation revealed: WBC 11.1×10^9/L, NE 57.1%, HGB 104g/L, PLT 613×10^9/L. CRP 15.40 mg/L, ESR 31 mm/h, ALB 45.0 g/L, NT-pro BNP 225.2 pg/ml. Echocardiography showed LCA was 2.9–3.4 mm (Fig. 2.38a), RCA was about 4.5–5.8 mm (Fig. 2.38b). He had right CAA.

On Day 12, everything went well and he was discharged.

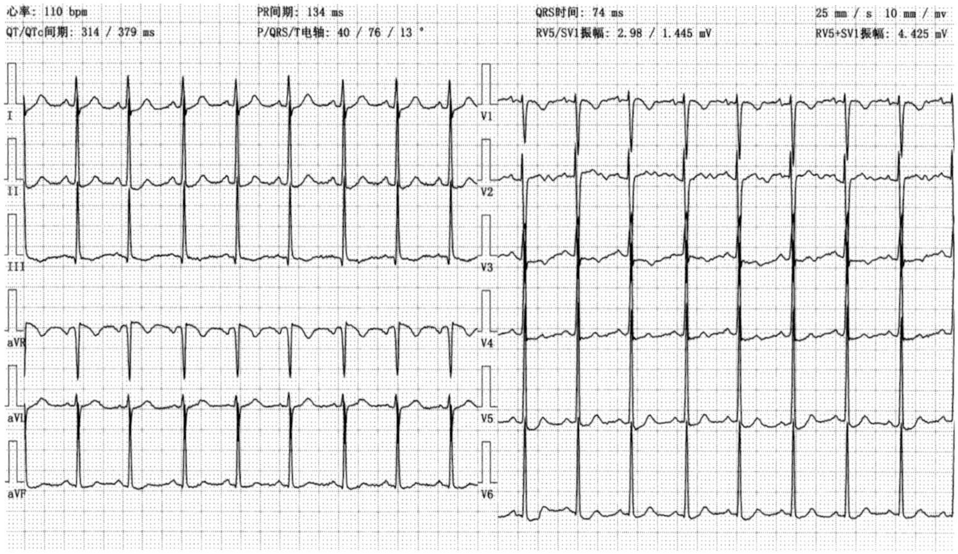

Fig. 2.36 On Day 6 of illness, ECG showed a low T wave, and the ST segment moved down a little bit

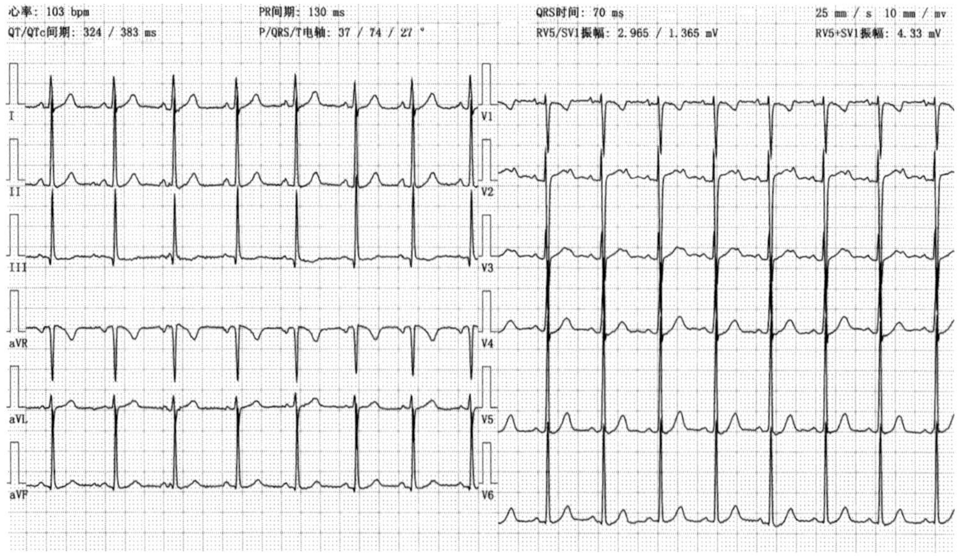

Fig. 2.37 On Day 7 of illness, ECG was normal

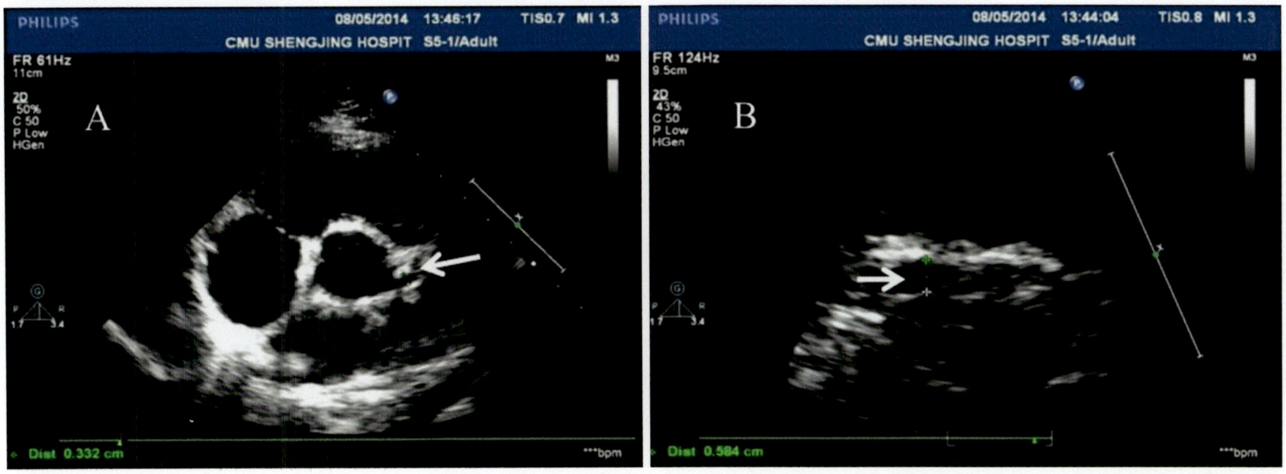

Fig. 2.38 On Day 11 of illness, echocardiography showed LCA diameter 3.3 mm (**a**). RCA 5.8 mm (**b**)

2.5.1 Clinical Course of the Patient

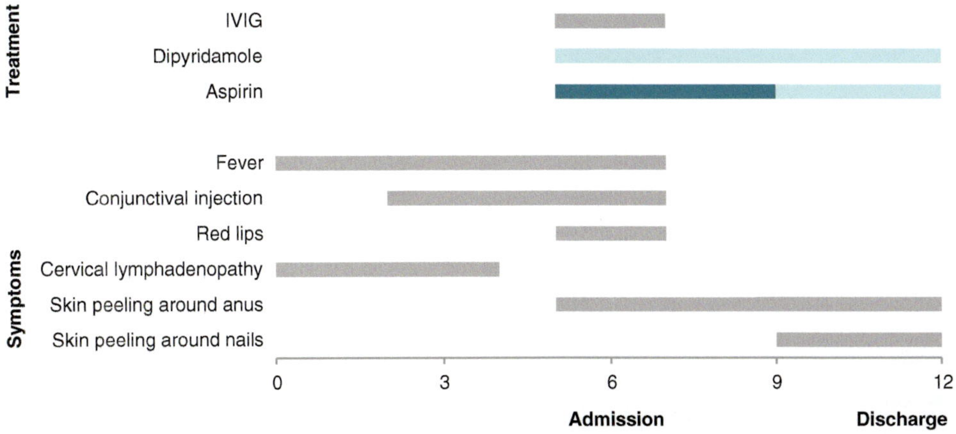

2.5.2 Follow Up

He was followed up since discharge and oral aspirin and dipyridamole, echocardiography was performed on Day 17, LCA 2.9–3.4 mm, RCA 4.4–5.3 mm. On Day 24, LCA was normal and RCA wasn't regress.

At 1 month, echocardiography showed RCA was 5.5 mm (Fig. 2.39).

At 2 months, echocardiography showed RCA was 4.4–5.9 mm (Fig. 2.40).

At 6 months, echocardiography showed RCA was 3.1 mm (Fig. 2.41).

At 7 months, echocardiography result was normal (Fig. 2.42).

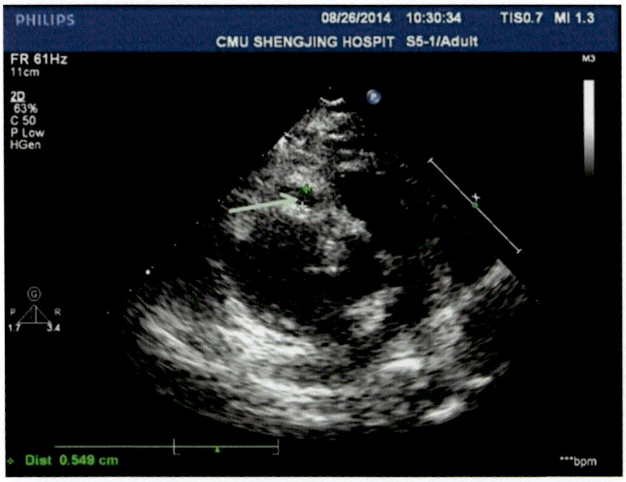

Fig. 2.39 At 1 month of illness, echocardiography showed RCA diameter 5.5 mm without thrombus inside

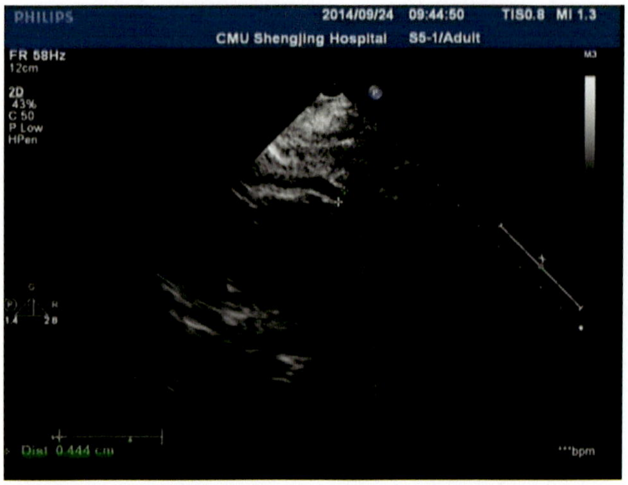

Fig. 2.40 At 2 months of illness, echocardiography showed RCA diameter 4.4–5.9 mm

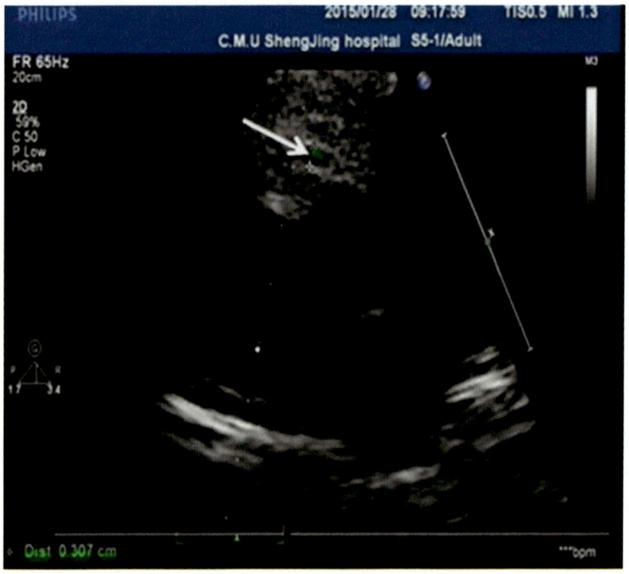

Fig. 2.41 At 6 months of illness, echocardiography showed RCA diameter 3.1 mm

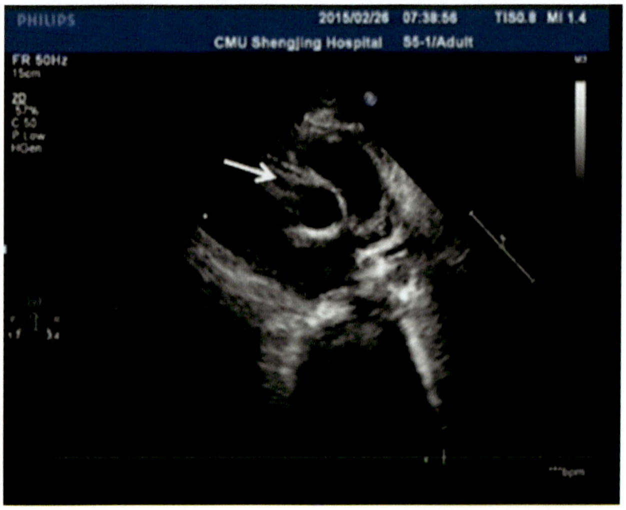

Fig. 2.42 At 7 months of illness, echocardiography showed the normal RCA (2.3 mm)

2.5.3 Diagnosis

1. KD
2. Right CAA
3. Hypoproteinemia
4. Thrombocythemia.

2.5.4 Discussion

He had met the criteria of KD. He had persistent fever for more than 5 days along with (i) cervicallymphadenopathy; (ii) non-purulent conjunctivitis; (iii) red lips and strawberry tongue; (iv) peeling skin around fingernails; (v) CAA at RCA; (vi) additional: WBC > 15 × 10^9/L, PLT 390 × 10^9/L, CRP > 30 mg/L, ESR > 40 mm/h, NT-pro BNP 1792 pg/ml.

2.5.5 Case Specific Clinical Features

1. KD is a self-limited disease, most time with good prognosis. Approximately 15% of KD children have CAL complication, even when treated with high-dose of IVIG [29]. This child developed CAA although he received standard and timely treatment. There are reports describing that the risk factors for developing CAA include: (i) boy; (ii) Age < 6 months or > 3 years old; (iii) persistent fever for more than 2 weeks or repeated fever; (iv) cardiomegaly, arrhythmia; (v) laboratory examination: HGB < 80 g/L, without recovery; WBC > 16–30 × 10^9/L; PLT > 1000 × 10^9/L. ESR>100 mm/h, or not reduced for more than 5 weeks; (vi) recurrent cases [29]. In Tohru Kobayashi's article [30], cutoff points and scorepoints for each variable were as follows:

	Points
Sodium≤133 mmol/L	2
Days of illness at initial treatment≤4	2
AST ≥ 100 IU/L	2
NE ≥ 80%	2
CRP ≥ 10 mg/dL	1
Age ≤ 12 months	1
PLT ≤ 30.0 × 10^4/mm^3	1

In the high-risk group (scores≥4), the occurrence of IVIG resistance was 43%, whereas it was only 5% in the low-risk group (scores 0 to 3). Similarly, the occurrence of coronary artery abnormalities was 16% in the high-risk group, while it was only 1% in the low-risk one. Especially in patients with very high scores (score ≥ 7), the occurrence of IVIG resistance and coronary artery abnormalities was extremely high (75% and 36%, respectively). But this boy was exceptional. His NE was 80.4%, 2 points; CRP was 318 mg/L, 1 point. The total score was only 3 points.

2. In this case, CRP and NT-pro BNP were significantly high. The ECG showed a low T wave, and the ST segment moved downwards a little bit. These suggested that there was myocardial damage. These were all associated with the development of CAA in children.
3. His RCA aneurysm was regressed to normal 7 months later. We advised to have a coronary artery CTA, which could identify narrownessand calcification [31]. But they refused to take the test.

Le Sun

2.6 Case 6 KD with Coronary Artery Calcification

A previously healthy 3-year-old boy was with an unremarkable antenatal and family history.

He presented on Day 8 of illness with a fever lasting for 8 days, along with red conjunctiva for 5 days, rash for 3 days. On Day 3, he developed bilateral conjunctivitis and red lips. He was infused with fosfomycin and ribavirin for 5 days at a local clinic. His fever did not regress and stayed up to 38.8 °C. Rashes developed on the trunk on Day 5. After intramuscular injection of dexamethasone, the interval of fever prolonged. He was infused with azithromycin for 2 days and third-generation cephalosporin for 1 day. The day before admission, he had spikes of high fever up to 39 °C. He was admitted in our pediatric cardiology ward. Examination found his mental state was stable, with normal vital signs (axillary temperature 36.6 °C, PR100 bpm, RR 20 bpm, BP 90/65 mmHg). His weight was 16 kg. He had red and cracked lips, along with strawberry tongue. A lot of rashes were on the trunk, without cervical lymphadenopathy. Lungs, heart, and abdomen were normal by examination. Skin was peeling around anus. Neurological system was normal. He had met the criteria for IKD, and was treated with (i) oral aspirin 30–50 mg/kg/d and dipyridamole 3–5 mg/kg/d, in 3 divided doses; (ii) IVIG 2 g/kg/d in 24 h; (iii) infused with ceftezole for anti-infective therapy after blood sample taken for culturing; (iv) nutritional myocardium. On the day of admission, fever was up to 39.4 °C, aspirin IM resulted in fever regress-

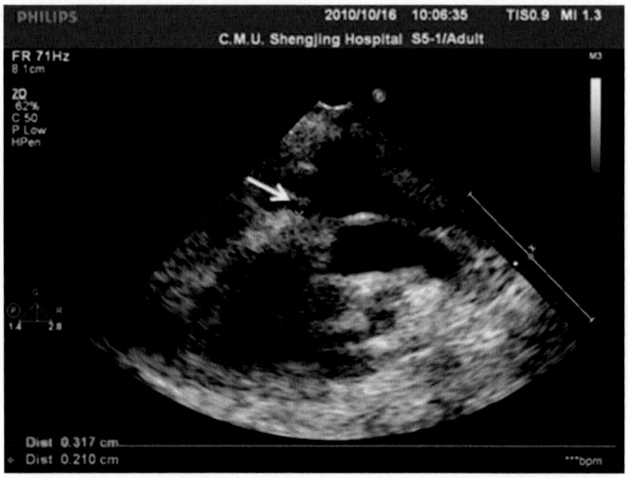

Fig. 2.43 On Day 11 of illness, RCA dilated to 2.1–3.2 mm

ing to 38.7 °C.10 min oral admission of nimesulide 25 mg later, he had a hoarse voice without dyspnea, along with large sheet of rash on the trunk and swollen lips and feet edema. After intramuscular injection of 3 mg dexamethasone, all the symptoms were improved except the swollen feet.

On Day 9, his fever subsided. There were still red rashes on the trunk. The palms of the hands and feet were a little red without skin peeling around fingernails and toenails. Skin peeling was still around the anus. Blood work showed WBC 18.3 × 10^9/L, NE 86.7%, HGB 115 g/L, PLT 378 × 10^9/L. ASO 87.0 IU/ml. CRP 123 mg/L. ESR 50 mm/h. TP 72.9 g/L, ALB 31.1 g/L, BNP 29.7 pg/ml, and cTnI 1.1μg/L. CK, CK-MB, and CKMB mass were normal. On Day 10, the patient was afebrile. His rash faded. Lips and tongue subsided. The palms of the hands and feet were still a little red. Skin around the anus was still peeling. On Day 11, skin peelings were around fingernails, toenails, and anus. Echocardiography showed LVED 30.5 mm, LVEF 69%, and LM 2.9 mm. RCA dilated to 2.1–3.2 mm (Fig. 2.43). He had met the criteria for KD and he was afebrile over 48 h. Aspirin dose was reduced to 3–5 mg/kg/d.

On Day 13, blood test results showed WBC 9.7 × 10^9/L, NE 37.2%, HGB 114 g/L, PLT 382 × 10^9/L. CRP 5.89 mg/L, ESR 65 mm/h, TP 84.5 g/L, and ALB 35.5 g/L. Everything was in normal range and he was discharged.

2.6.1 Clinical Course of the Patient

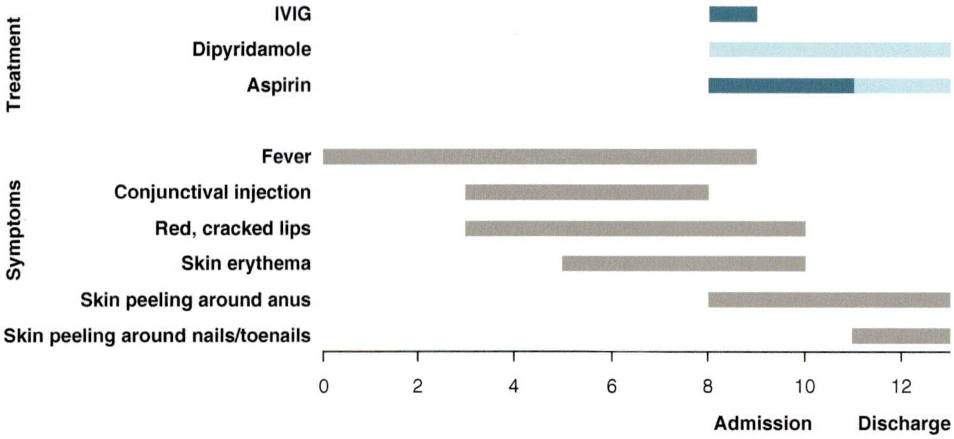

2.6.2 Follow-Up

He was followed up since discharge and used oral aspirin. Echocardiography was performed on routine schedule.

At 3 weeks of illness, echocardiography showed LM dilated to 3.3–5.5 mm (Fig. 2.44a). RCA dilated to 2.8–4.9 mm (Fig. 2.44b).

At 1 month of illness, echocardiography showed LM dilated to 3.6 mm, LCX dilated to 4.5 mm (Fig. 2.45a), and LAD dilated to 4.5 mm. The proximal segment of RCA was about 2.8 mm. The far-end of RCA dilated to 5 mm (Fig. 2.45b).

At 5 months of illness, LM regressed to 3.1 mm, LCX 4.2 mm, LAD 4.5 mm. The proximal segment of RCA was

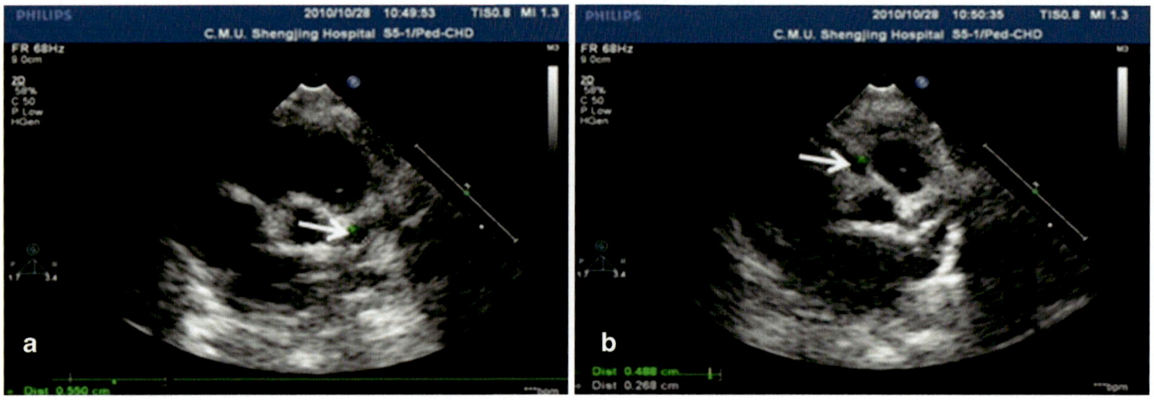

Fig. 2.44 At 3 week of illness, LM dilated to 3.3–5.5 mm (**a**), RCA dilated to 2.8–4.9 mm (**b**)

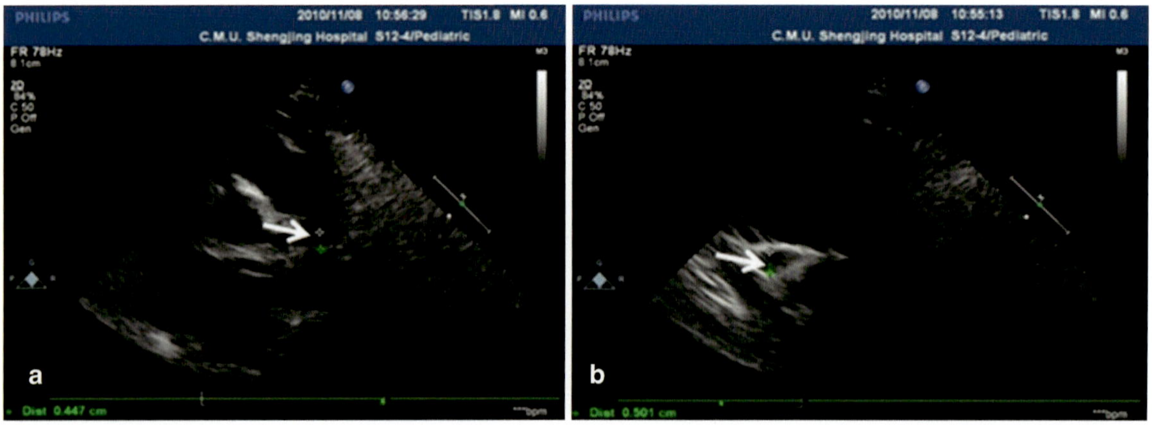

Fig. 2.45 At 1 month of illness, LCX dilated to 4.5 mm (**a**), the distal segment of RCA dilated to 5 mm (**b**)

about 2.4 mm; the far-end of RCA dilated to 6.1 mm (Fig. 2.46).

At 8 months of illness, examination revealed INR 1.0. Echocardiography showed the proximal segment of LAD dilated to 6.8 mm (Fig. 2.47a), the proximal segment of RCA was about 2.7 mm, 16 mm away from opening, dilated to 6.1 mm (Fig. 2.47b). Coronary artery CTA showed dilated left and right main coronary arteries. The proximal segment of LAD dilated (Fig. 2.48). Aneurysm dilated to 8.6 mm and identified thrombus inner the proximal and mid-segment of RCA (Fig. 2.49). The constriction and dilatation alternately existed like a string of beads (Fig. 2.50), and the wall of mi-segment thickened with thrombus. He had right giant CAA and RCA thrombosis, and was treated with oral warfarin 0.1 mg/kg/d, and DIC was monitored to keep his INR between 1.5 and 2.5.

At 22 months of illness, blood work results came back showing WBC 5.8 × 10^9/L, NE 48.8%, HGB122g/L, PLT 235 × 10^9/L; PT 16.2s, INR 1.2 and APTT 44 s. Follow-up echocardiography showed LVED 34.6 mm, LVEF 62%, LM 2.9 mm, LCX 2.5 mm. LAD aneurysm dilated to 5.7–7.1 mm without thrombosis. The proximal segment of RCA was about 2.7 mm, 16 mm later. RCA aneurysm dilated to 8.4 mm without thrombosis, and its intima was not smooth. The distal segment of RCA was not clear. Left ventricular systolic function was normal. Coronary artery CTA showed no calcified plaques in the LAD or RCA. The proximal segment of LAD dilated to 7 mm (Fig. 2.51). The distal segment of RCA showed segmental dilation about 8 mm. There were no calcified plaques at the proximal segment of LCX (Fig. 2.52).

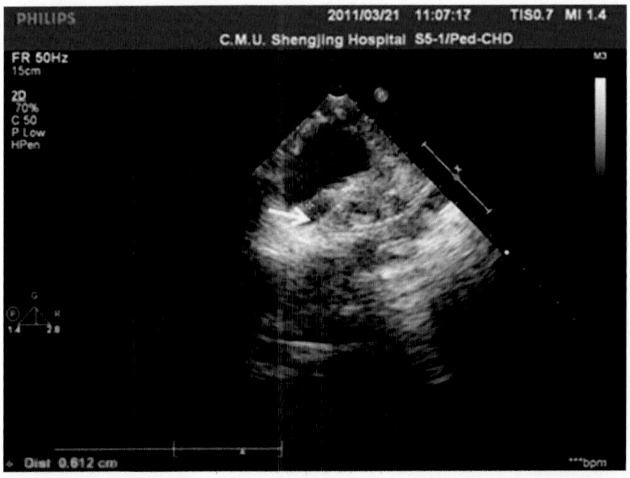

Fig. 2.46 At 5 months of illness, the distal segment of RCA dilated to 6.1 mm

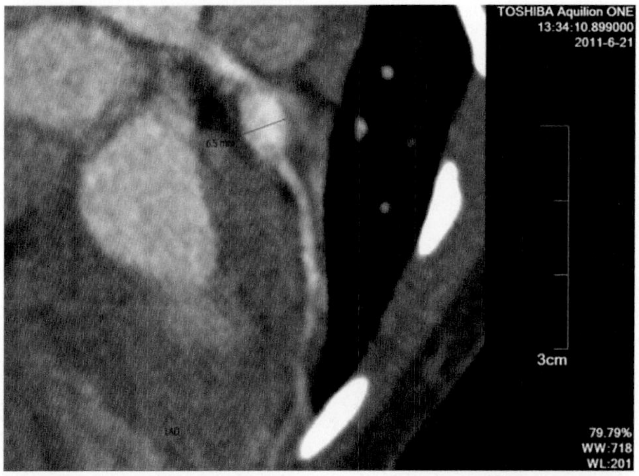

Fig. 2.48 At 8 months of illness, coronary artery CTA showed the proximal segment of LAD diameter was 6.5 mm

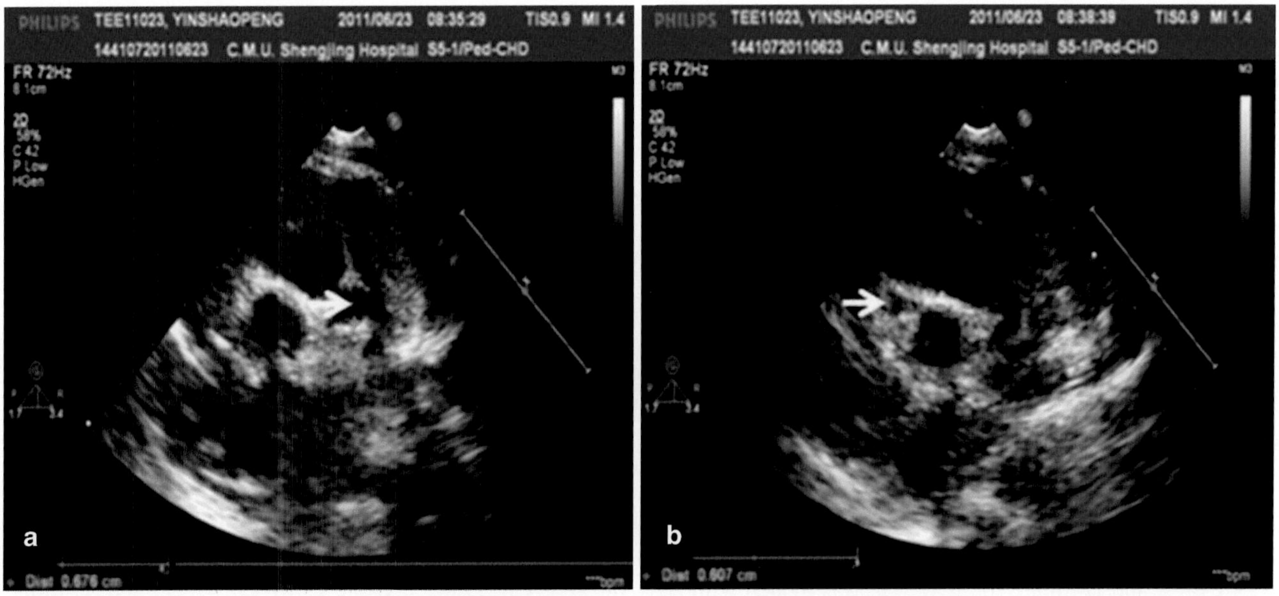

Fig. 2.47 At 8 months of illness, LAD dilated to 6.8 mm (**a**), the distal segment of RCA dilated to 6.1 mm (**b**)

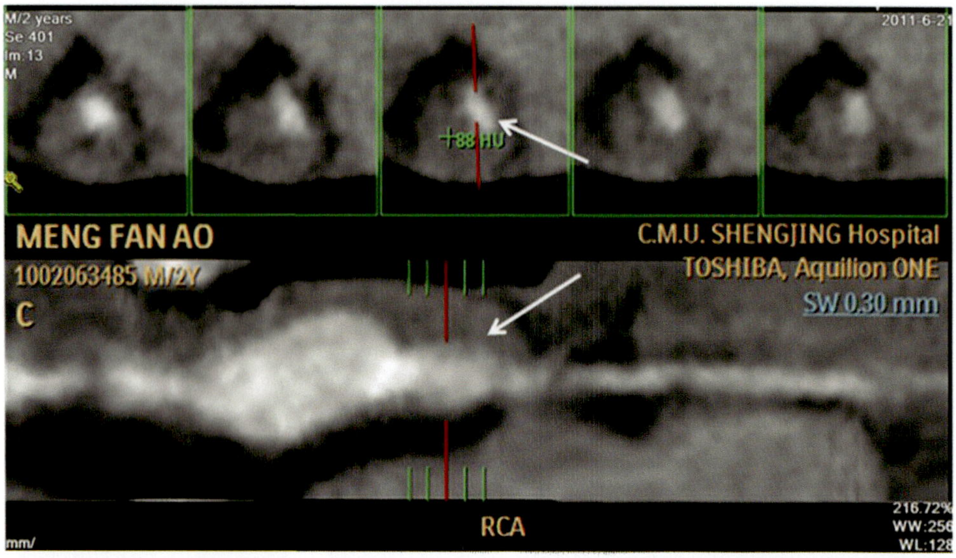

Fig. 2.49 At 8 months of illness, coronary artery CTA showed that aneurysm dilated to 8.6 mm at the near and middle segment of the RCA with thrombus in it (longitudinal and horizontal surface)

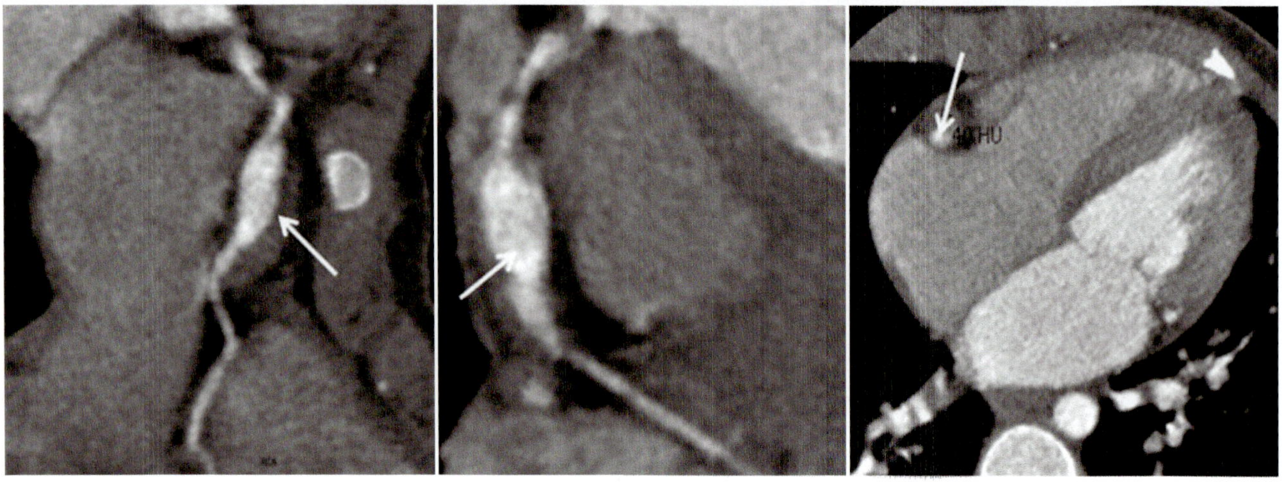

Fig. 2.50 At 8 months of illness, coronary artery CTA showed RCA aneurysm dilated to 8.6 mm at the middle segment with thrombus in it (longitudinal surface), the constriction and dilatation alternately existed like a string of beads

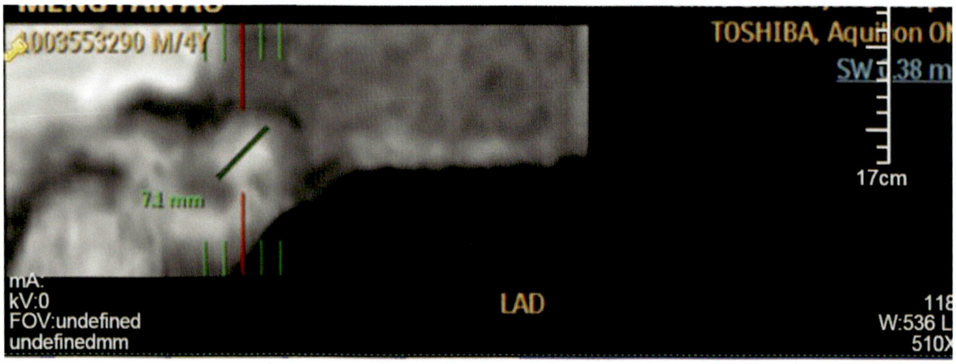

Fig. 2.51 At 22 months of illness, coronary artery CTA showed LAD dilated to 7 mm

At about 3 years of illness, blood work showed CKMB mass 6.7 μg/L; cTnI, NT-pro BNP, hs-cTnT, normal cTnI, NT-pro BNP, hs-cTnT, CK, and CKMB. PT 16.2s, INR 1.5, APTT 45 s, and D-dimer 100 μg/L. He was treated with (i) oral warfarin 0.1 mg/kg/d and DIC was monitored; (ii) oral aspirin 3–5 mg/kg/d; (iii) nutritional myocardial therapy. Four days after eating a lollipop, a purple petechiae about 2 cm in diameter was seen on his mandible. Blood test showed PT 17.0s, INR 1.5, APTT 43 s, and D-dimer 34 μg/L. Scheduled echocardiography showed LVED

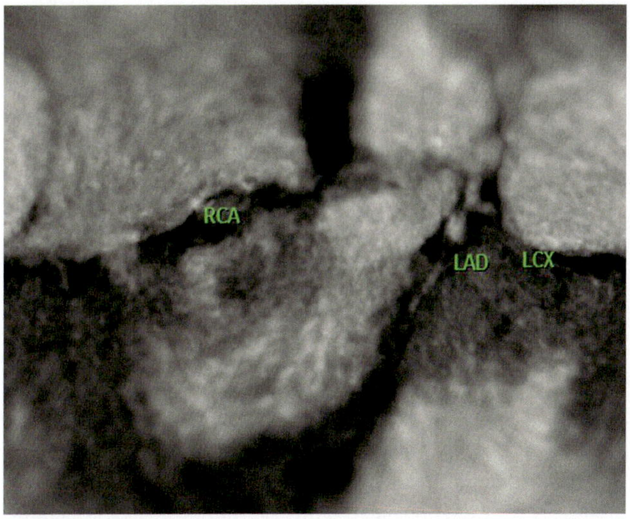

Fig. 2.52 At 22 months of illness, coronary artery CTA showed that there were no calcified plaques in the LAD or RCA. The distal segment of RCA showed segmental dilation, the diameter to 8 mm, the proximal LAD dilated to 7 mm, there were no calcified plaques at the proximal segment of LCX

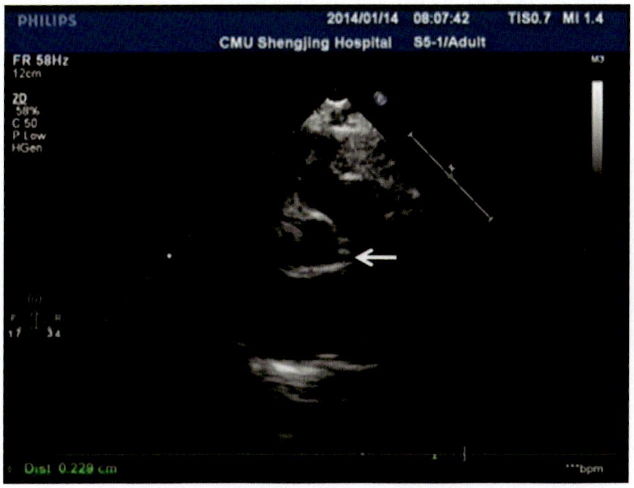

Fig. 2.53 At about 3 years of illness, echo showed LM diameter 2.3 mm

38 mm, LVEF 63%, and normal LCA and RCA (Fig. 2.53). Left ventricular systolic function was normal. Coronary artery CTA showed that there were calcified plaques in the LAD and RCA. LM dilated to 3.5 mm. The proximal segment of LAD aneurysm dilated to 6.7 mm × 5.0 mm with calcification. The proximal segment of LCX was 2.8 mm. The proximal segment of RCA was 3.0 mm. The mid-segment of RCA dilated to 9.7 mm, and 22 cm in length with calcifications and thrombosis (Fig. 2.54).

Since last examination, he has not been followed up in our hospital.

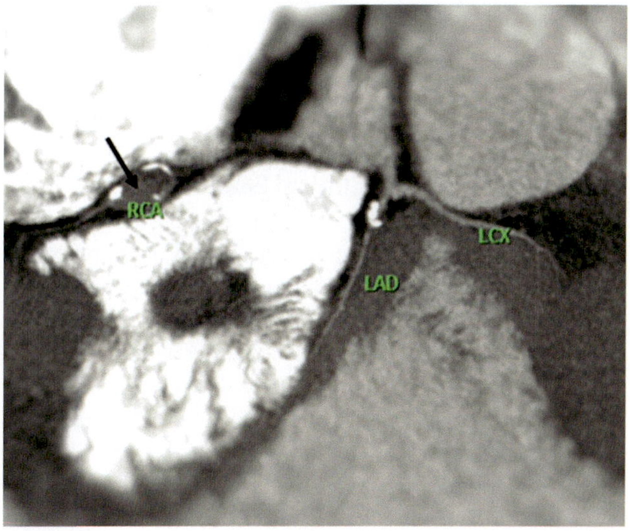

Fig. 2.54 At about 3 years of illness, the proximal segment of LAD aneurysm dilated to 6.7 mm × 5.0 mm and the wall had calcification. The proximal segment of LCX was 2.8 mm. The proximal segment of RCA was 3.0 mm. The middle segment of RCA dilated to 9.7 mm, and 22 cm in length with calcifications and thrombosis (black arrow)

2.6.3 Diagnosis

1. KD
2. Right giant CAA
3. RCA thrombosis
4. Myocardial damage

2.6.4 Discussion

This patient met the criteria of KD for he had prolonged fever over 5 days, along with (i) rashes on the trunk; (ii) non-purulent conjunctivitis; (iii) red, cracked lips, and strawberry tongue; (iv) skin peeling around fingernails, toenails, and anus; (v) echocardiography showed both dilated LCA and RCA. Additional: WBC 18.3 × 10^9/L, NE 86.7%, CRP 123 mg/L, and ESR 50 mm/h.

Differential diagnosis with streptococcus infection should be considered.

The most common antithrombotic regimen for patients with giant CAA is to admit low-dose aspirin together with warfarin [27]. Application of warfarin has no significant effect on the regress of giant CAA. However, retrospective studies show that combination therapy using warfarin and aspirin was associated with a decreased risk of myocardial infarction. No major bleeding events occurred in KD patients with CAA when combination of aspirin and warfarin was administered [32]. Warfarin had anticoagulant and antiplatelet effects and it was convenient and effective. However, it could be affected by many factors, such as drugs, food, and the individual difference. Therefore, the INR needed to be monitored.

2.6.5 Case Specific Clinical Features

1. At 8 months of illness, coronary artery CTA showed the constriction and dilatation alternately existed like a string of beads on the proximal and middle segment of RCA. The wall of middle segment thickened. At about 3 years of illness, follow-up echocardiography showed that there was no dilation in the LCA or RCA. However coronary artery CTA showed both dilated LCA and RCA with calcification. Coronary artery CTA has an advantage for evaluating CAL, especially the mid-distal segment, morphology change, the stenosis, and/or calcification [31]. As to dilatation on the proximal and middle segment of RCA could not be found in echocardiography, the patient should have coronary artery CTA test done before aspirin withdrawal if suspected of CAA.
2. This patient was followed up for more than 3 years. The CAL gradually developed into giant CAA with thrombosis and calcifications. Giant CAA had difficulties to regress to normal and also had risks of calcifications or thrombosis. Long-term prognosis requires further follow-up and observation. Patients with KD accompany with CAL show more evidence of coronary calcifications. Detection of coronary artery calcifications may be useful for risk stratification in the long-term management for patients with KD [34].

Le Sun

2.7 Case 7 KD with Chronic Coronary Artery Thrombus and Calcification

A previous healthy 2-year-old girl was presented with no remarkable past medical history and family history.

She presented at 13 months of illness with KD. Thirteen months before she presented with continuous fever for 12 days, along with rash, bilateral conjunctivitis, hands and feet edema for 8 days. In Beijing An Zhen hospital she was diagnosed with KD and CAA. After discharge, she was taking (oral) aspirin and dipyridamole. 5 months after the onset of illness, the patient was scheduled the first follow-up with us at our out-patient center. Echocardiography showed LM was 2.4–3.2 mm (Fig. 2.55a, red arrow), and LAD was 3.6–4.2 mm (Fig. 2.55a, green arrow). RCA was intermittently dilated, proximal to 2.8–4.2 mm, and middle section was dilated to

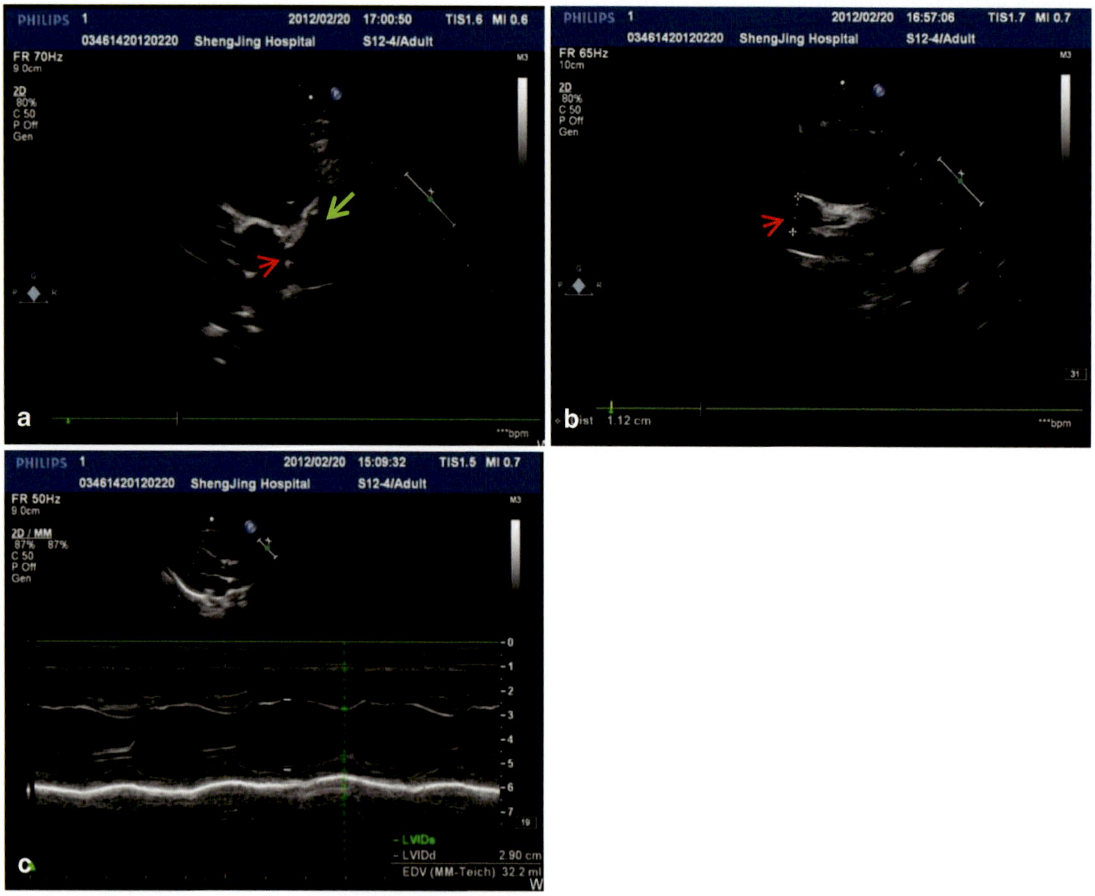

Fig. 2.55 At 8 months of illness, echocardiography showed LM diameter 3.2 mm (**a**, red arrow), LAD 4.2 mm (**a**, green arrow). 11.2 mm tumor-like expansion at distal segment of RCA (**b**). LVEDD was normal (**c**)

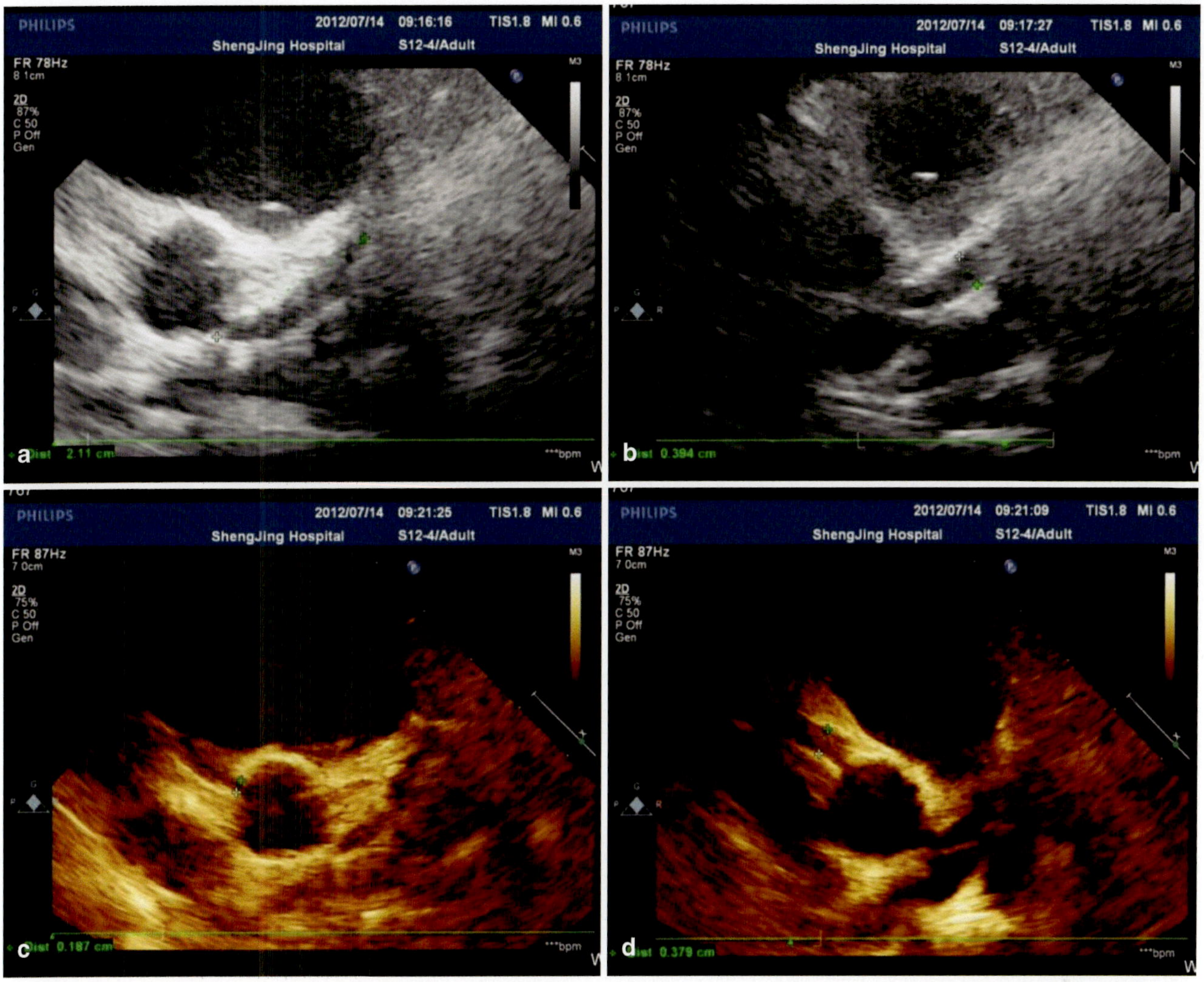

Fig. 2.56 At 13 months of illness, echocardiography showed LAM 3.3 mm, LCA was displayed 7.1 mm in length (**a**), LAD was dilated to 4.2 mm (**b**). RCA was irregularly dilated from 4.2 mm (**c**) to 11.2 mm (**d**), without thrombus in it

9.9–11.2 mm (Fig. 2.55b). LVED (29 mm) was normal (Fig. 2.55c), LVEF 54%. Her RCA had two aneurysms. We recommended coronary CTA test, but her parents turned it down due to financial concerns. Blood test revealed normal CBC and DIC. We prescribed warfarin, aspirin and dipyridamole for her to take orally. At 7 months after the illness, she was follow-up at out-patient center again. Blood test revealed almost normal CBC (WBC 11.2 × 10^9/L, NE 43.7%, RBC 4.3 × 10^{12}/L, HGB 123 g/L, PLT 670 × 10^9/L). DIC: PT 27.9s, PTA 27%, INR 1.9, PTR 2.2. She had been taking aspirin and dipyridamole orally, but stopped taking warfarin, for couldn't monitor DIC and without any discomfort. At 13 months of illness, she was admitted to our hospital for CTA. Physical examination didn't find any abnormal signs. Investigation CBC revealed WBC 6.7 × 10^9/L, NE 1.25 × 10^9/L, RBC 4.0 × 10^{12}/L, HGB 114 g/L, PLT 283 × 10^9/L. Normal NT-pro BNP, DIC, Liver and kidney function. hs-cTnT 0.018 ng/ml (<0.014 ng/ml). ECG was normal. Echo showed that LM was 3.3 mm, and the length of LCA was 7.1 mm (Fig. 2.56a). LAD was dilated to 4.2 mm (Fig. 2.56b). RCA was with interval aneurysm dilation. Proximal section was 4.2 mm (Fig. 2.56c) and middle section was dilated to 9.9–11.2 mm (Fig. 2.56c), without thrombus in it. LVED was normal. In addition to continue taking oral aspirin and dipyridamole, she took warfarin orally again at a dose of 0.1 mg/kg/d, QD. She was also prescribed to take oral FDP and levocarnitine.

On Day 5 of admission, hs-cTnT and CRP were retested and they were normal. DIC revealed PT 15.3s, INR 1.2. Coronary artery CTA showed the atrioventricular size of the heart was basically normal. The proximal segment of the LCA was slightly dilated to 4 mm and the distal end was not clear to define. The proximal segment of the RCA was slightly dilated to 4.6 mm. The middle section was highly expanded with a diameter of about 12 mm (Fig. 2.57), and the shape of the far end section was almost normal. On Day 7, DIC was repeated and it was normal. Warfarin was increased to 0.12 mg/kg/d.

On Day 8 of admission, DIC revealed PT 27.9 s, PTA 27%, INR1.2, PTR 2.2. The patient was discharged. She lived in a remote rural area in inner Mongolia. There is no hospital nearby for her to take DIC for monitoring purpose.

2.7.1 Follow-Up

She followed up with us at 24, 32, 34, 46, and 58 months. Lab tests and echocardiography were shown in Tables 2.6 and 2.7. Investigation revealed normal CK, CKMB, CKMB-M, cTnI, hs-cTnT, ALT, BUN, Cr, and NT pro-BNP. ECG was normal. RCA was permanently with aneurysmal dilation (Figs. 2.58, 2.59, 2.61, 2.62, 2.64 and 2.65) and with deterioration at 32 and 58 months.

At 25 months of illness, echocardiography showed LAM about 2.0 mm (Fig. 2.58a). RCA had similar aneurysm dilation, 3.9 mm (Fig. 2.58b) and 12.3 mm (Fig. 2.58c).

At 32 months, she presented again with nose bleeding for 2 months. She took aspirin and warfarin (oral route) since discharge. Two months ago, her PLT count was 37 × 10^9/L and normal WBC and HGB with nose bleeding. She stopped taking warfarin for 1 week, then resumed at a dose of 0.1 mg/kg/d. One week later retested DIC and INR still 1.5, then she went back to our hospital. Examination did not find any abnormal symptoms and signs. Blood test revealed WBC 7.6 × 10^9/L, NE 31.5%, RBC 3.9 × 10^{12}/L, HGB 110 g/L, PLT 16 × 10^9/L. Routine DIC showed INR 1.1, APTT almost normal, FIB 1.6 (NR 2–4)g/L. MP-IgG 1:160. EBV-IgG both NA (297) and VCA (205) positive, while EA negative. PINF-IgM was positive. She was suspected to have acute immune thrombocytopenia, with MP and PINF infection. She was treated with IVIG 500 mg/kg/d for 4 days and was warned not touching sharp objects and not getting over excited. Bone marrow puncture was performed and aspirin and warfarin were temporarily stopped. Echocardiography showed that RCA was discontinuously dilated from 3.1 mm (Fig. 2.59a) at proximal to about 10.3 mm at middle-section with aneurysmal dilatation (Fig. 2.59b). LCA was 3.0 mm (Fig. 2.59c). LVED and LVEF were normal. Azithromycin (10 mg/kg/d) was infused for

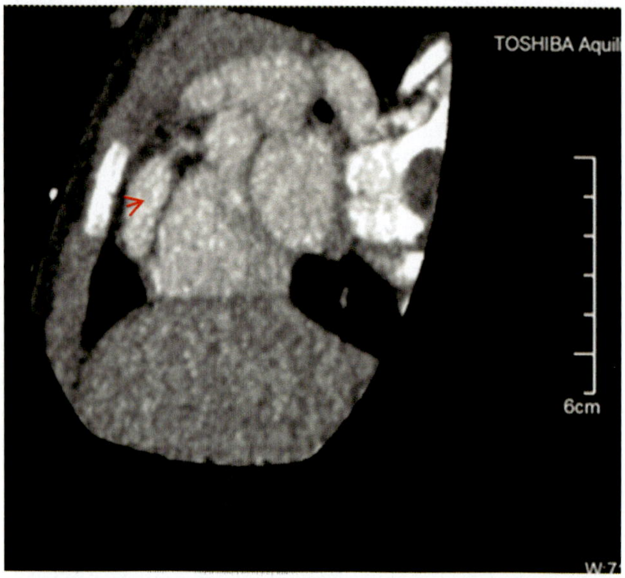

Fig. 2.57 At 13 months of illness, coronary artery CTA showed the proximal segment of the RCA was slightly dilated to 4.6 mm. The middle section was highly expanded with a diameter of about 12 mm

Table 2.6 The dynamic changes of lab parameters and treatment

Time of illness	5months	5months + 7days	7months	13months	24months	32months	34months	46months	58months
WBC (×10^9/L)	6.7		11.2	6.7	7.1	7.6	6.5	9	6.5
HGB (g/L)	118.5		123	114	111	112	133	124	133
PLT (×10^9/L)	363.2		670	283	292	16–101	288	287	297
INR	1	1.1	1.9	1.3–2.5	1.3	1.3–1.1	1.1	1.4	1.4
Aspirin (mg/kg/d)	3	3	3	3	3	3–0	3	3	3
Persantine (mg/kg/d)	3	3	3	3	3	3–0	3	3	3
Warfarin (mg/kg/d)	0.1	0.12	0.12	0.12	0.1–0.012	0.12–0.08	0.08–0.09	0.09	0.09

Table 2.7 The dynamic changes of coronary artery

Time of illness		5months	13months	24months	32months	34months	46months	58months
Echo	LCA (mm)	2.4–3.3	2.2–3.7	2.3	3.3	3.3	3.1	2.9
	LAD (mm)	3.6–4.2	3.9	2.1				
	RCA-1 (mm)	2.8–4.2	3.5–3.8	2.8	2.3	2.5	3.3	3.8
	RCA-2 (mm)	9.9–11.2	9.8–10.9	12.6 × 23.4	10.1	11	11	11
	Thrombus	N	N	N	N	N	N	N
CTA	LCA (mm)		4			2.9		3
	LAD (mm)		Unclearly			2.8		3
	RCA-1 (mm)		4.6			3.2		2.9–3.8
	RCA-2 (mm)		12			12.1 × 27.2		11.1 × 28.1
	Thrombus		N			N		Positive/ calcification

RCA-1 proximal of RCA, *RCA-2* distal of RCA, *N* negative

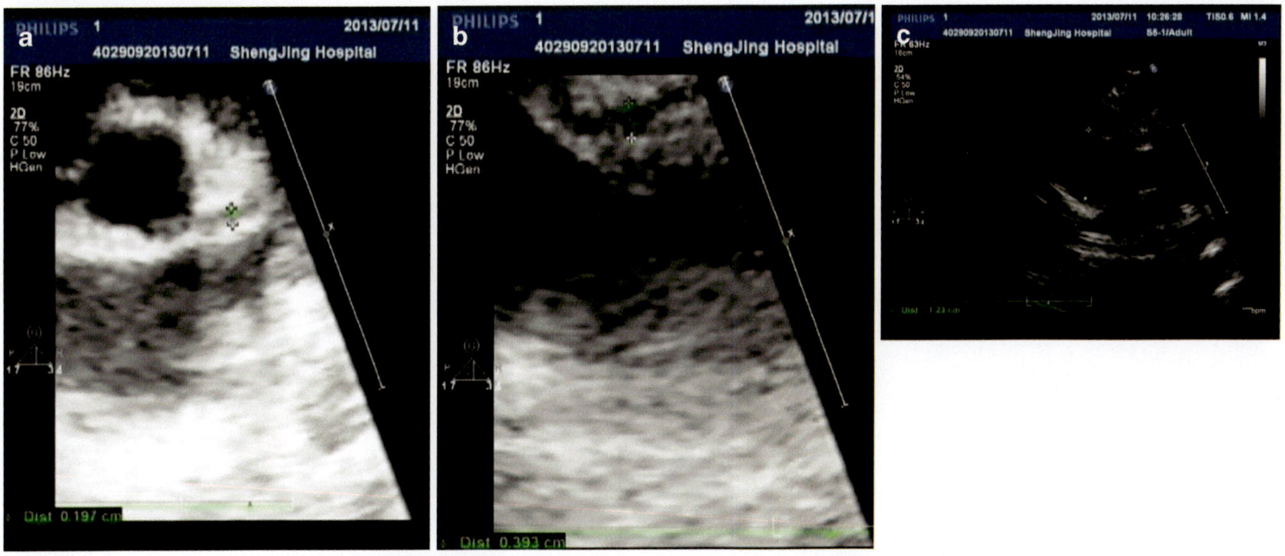

Fig. 2.58 At 25 months after illness, echocardiography showed LM diameter 2.0 mm (**a**). RCA diameter 3.9 mm (**b**) to 12.3 mm (**c**)

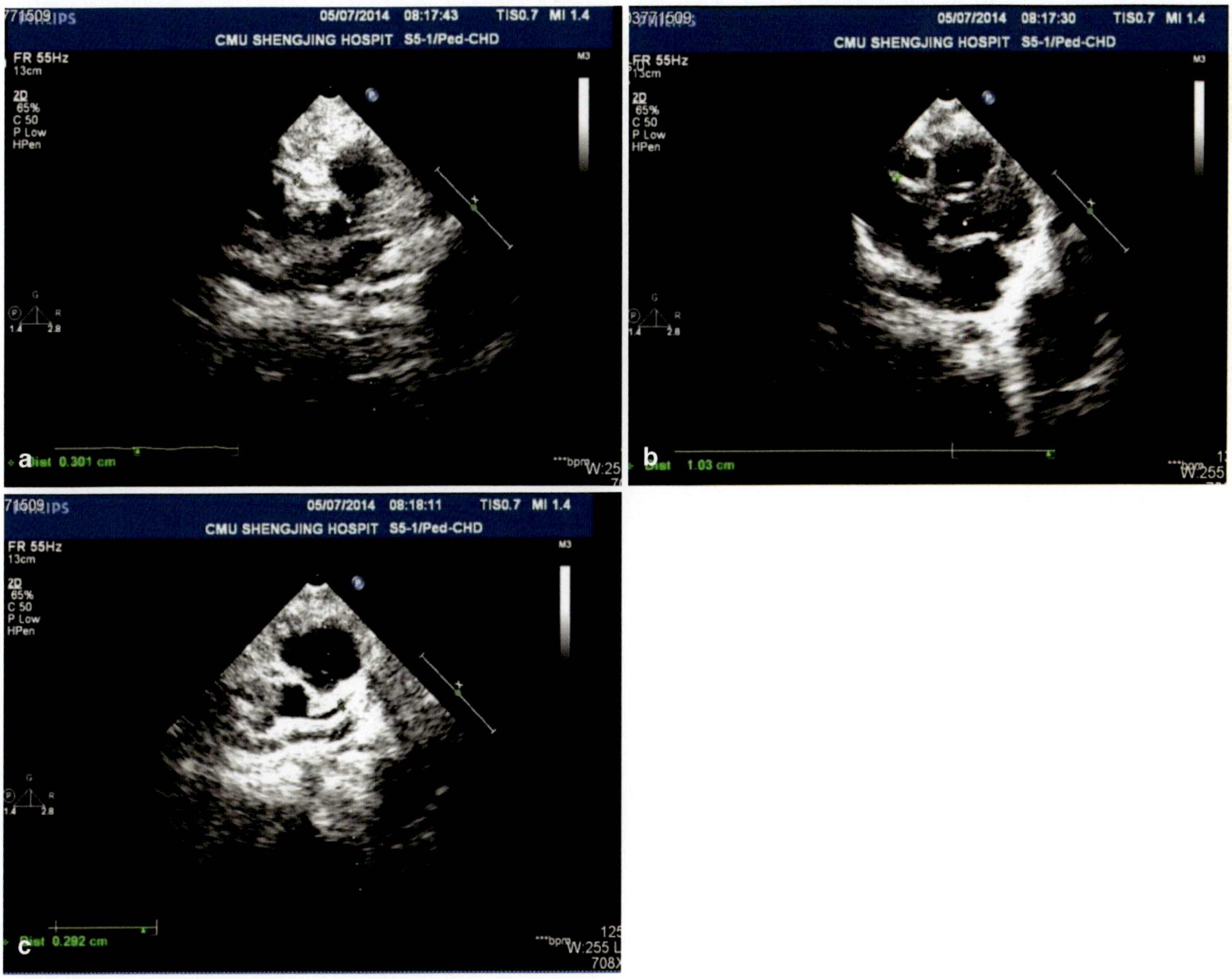

Fig. 2.59 At 32 months of illness, echocardography showed an interval dilation in RCA, proximal 3.1 mm (**a**) and middle section was dilated to 10.3 mm (**b**). LCA was normal (**c**)

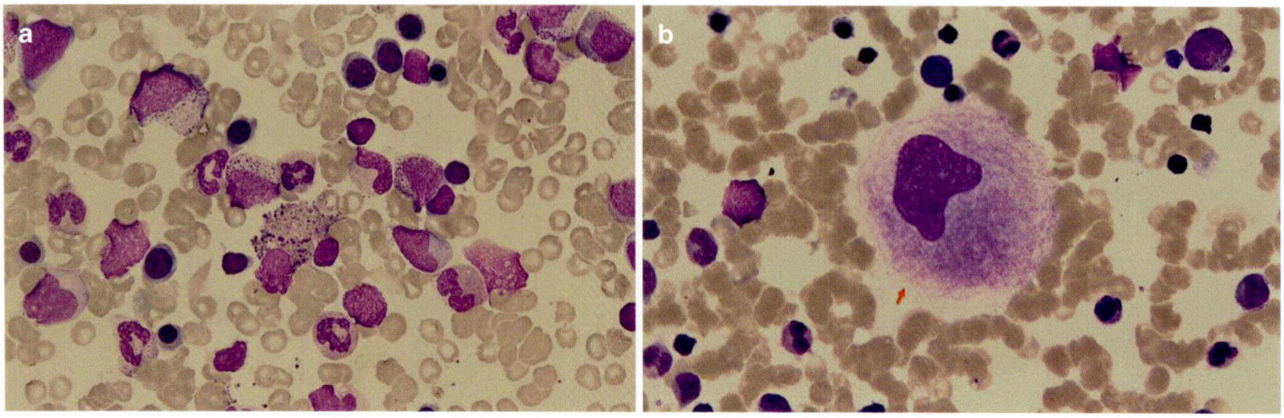

Fig. 2.60 At 32 months of illness, bone marrow smear: Wright-Giemsa ×1000 showed cellular marrow with low myeloid-to-erythroid ratio (**a**), cellular morphology revealed normal. Platelets were absent (**b**)

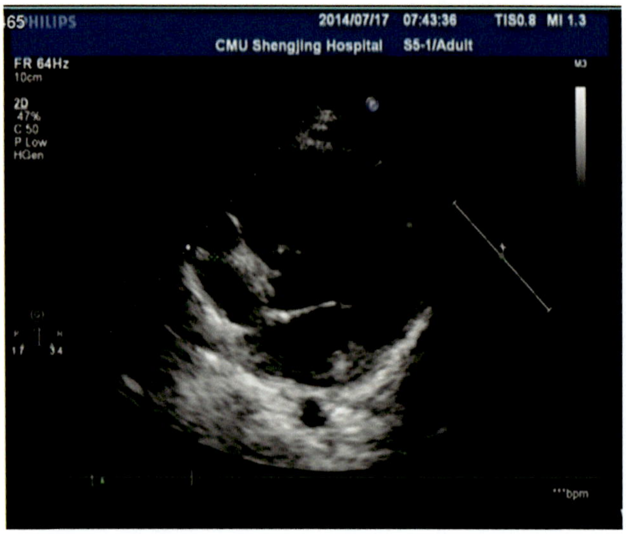

Fig. 2.61 At 34 months of illness, echo showed her RCA was 11 mm

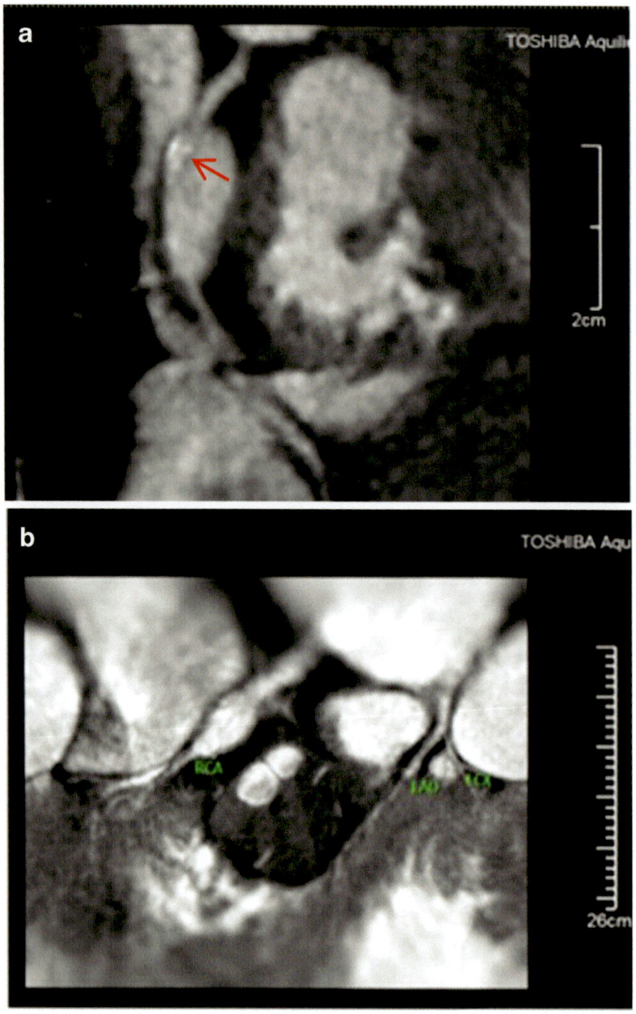

Fig. 2.62 At 34 months of illness, coronary artery CTA showed her RCA middle section aneurysmal dilation 12 mm and the wall with calcification (**a**-red arrow) and far-end, LCX and LAD were normal (**b**)

3 days. Three days later, she stopped bleeding. Investigation revealed PLT up to 101 × 10^9/L. Marrow showed hyperplasia, obviously active, the ratio of akaryocyte to karyote was 1000 to 64, the percentage of granulocyte and erythrocyte were 48.8 and 27.2, the ratio of granulocyte to erythrocyte was 1.79 to 1. Granulocyte was hyperplasia active and the ratio was nearly normal. Some granulocytes had different granules and they were not in balance. Eosinophil was 2.8%. Erythrocyte was also active, mainly in middle and late erythrocyte. Cellular marrow was with low myeloid-to-erythroid ratio (1.79 to 1) (Fig. 2.60a). Cellular morphology was normal. After scanning all slices 123 megakaryocytes had been found, without producing PLT at the ratio of one in three slices. It showed the function of platelet production was low. Platelets were absent (Fig. 2.60b). Routine blood work indicated the granulocyte

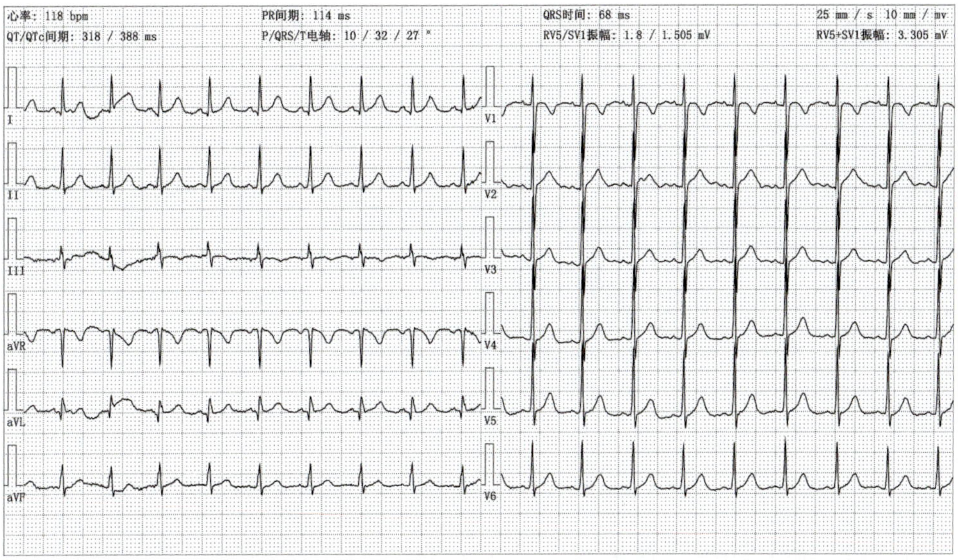

Fig. 2.63 At 46 months of illness, ECG was normal

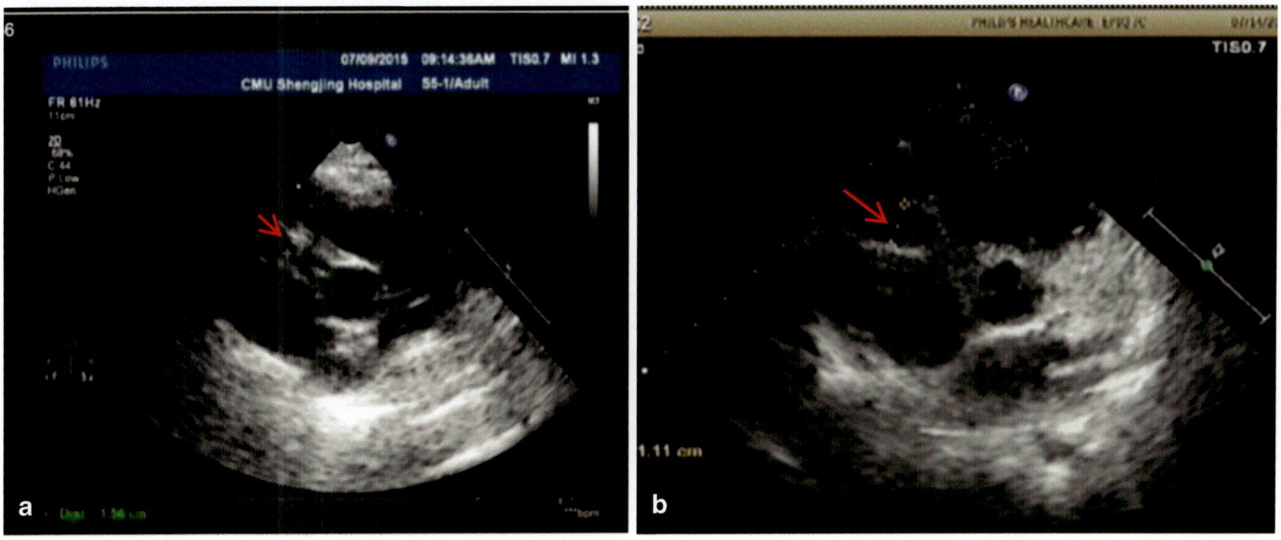

Fig. 2.64 Echo showed RCA aneurysmal dilation stay 11 mm unchanged at 46 months (**a**), and at 58 months (**b**) of illness

nucleus moved to the left. There was grain in mature granulocyte. NPA score was a little high. Consulted with hematologist, hematologist suggested that MP-IgG and PINF IgM were positive. PLT 16 × 10^9/L, marrow showed megakaryocyte active without producing PLT one. After treatment for 3 days, PLT had improved up to 101 × 10^9/L. Now PLT was in a safe range and IVIG was stopped. The patient did not have fever and bleeding. The patient was prescribed with leucogen tablet and was discharged. Then the patient took azithromycin orally for 3 days, followed by aspirin 10 days later and warfarin 1 month later if PLT stayed normal. The patient was advised not be vaccinated within 3 months. Follow-up appoints were scheduled at outpatient clinic.

At 34 months of illness, echocardiography and coronary artery CTA were performed. ECG and echocardiography results were shown in Fig. 2.61 to Fig. 2.64a following up at 46 months of illness.

At 58 months of illness, she came back to the hospital for coronary artery CTA. Echocardiography showed normal LVED and LVEF, LCA 2.9 mm, RCA distal 11 mm, without thrombus (Fig. 2.64b). On the following days, her coronary artery CTA showed proximal RCA was mildly wide, aneurysmal dilation was in middle section about 11.1 mm × 28.1 mm, with a small soft tissue density filling defect (Fig. 2.65), and the distal section was normal.

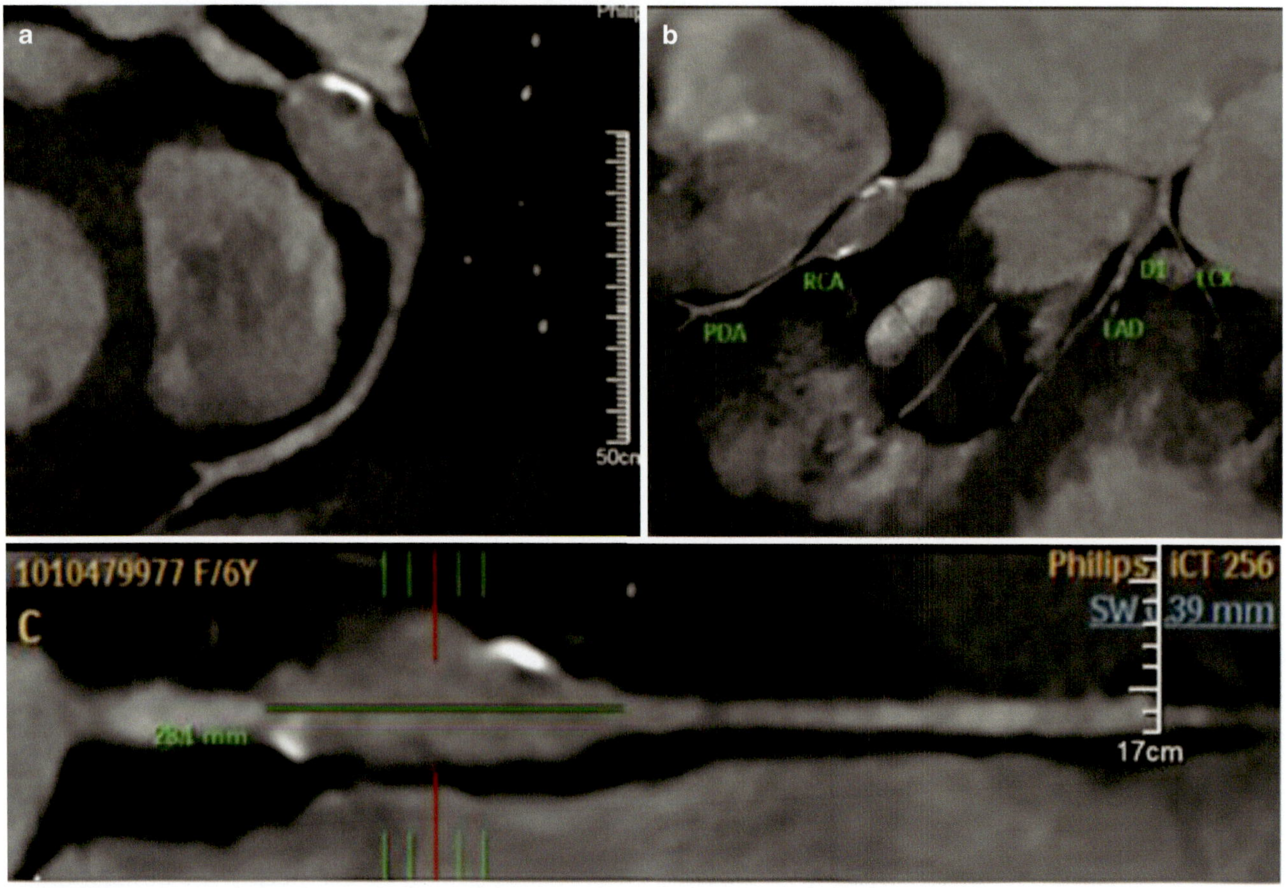

Fig. 2.65 At 58 months of illness, coronary artery CTA showed RCA middle section aneurysmal dilated 11.1 mm (**a**) and the length was 28.1 mm (**c**), there was some calcification on the wall, the distal section was normal (**b** and **c**)

2.7.2 Diagnosis

1. KD recovery stage
2. Giant RCAA
3. Acute immune thrombocytopenia
4. Myocardium damage.

2.7.3 Discussion

This disease often reoccurred, and blood routine test should be repeated dynamically. Once PLT down to 30×10^9/L, IVIG should be admitted again together with glucocorticoid if patients do not have glucocorticoid contraindication.

This girl had met the criteria for KD. She had continuous fever over 5 days and did not response to antibiotics, along with (i) red lips; (ii) bilateral conjunctival congestion; (iii) edema in feet and hands. (iv) RCA with dilatation, calcification, and thrombus.

Differential diagnosis of pharyngo-conjunctival fever and infant nodular polyarteritis nodosa should be considered.

2.7.4 Case Specific Clinical Features

1. We did not have knowledge of her cTnI value tested in An Zhen hospital. At 13 months of illness, her cTnI was increased. Some literature reports the myocardium damage can last for several months even for several years, especially in CAA patients [35]. This damage also can be seen for over 1 year without CAA (see case 3). Therefore we could not conclude the source (CAA or recent infection) causing her increased cTnI.
2. Though she orally took aspirin, warfarin and dipyridamole regularly, her CAA still progressed 4 years after onset of the disease, which is not in agreement with literature report [36]. If there was calcification with non-dilatable lesions, rotation atherectomy can be applied when patients grew up [37]. The prognosis is very different for each patient.

3. At 5 year of illness, repeated echocardiography only suggested RCAA, but coronary artery CTA showed there was thrombus in RCAA with calcification. We consulted with the same ultrasound doctor to review the imaging, but he could not find thrombus at the distal ends of the aneurysm of RCA. Thus, echocardiography has its limitations on middle or far-end CAA. Coronary CTA can find some abnormities, whereas ultrasound cannot [31].
4. Both giant CAA and thrombus in coronary artery need to be treated with warfarin. Meanwhile, aspirin is used for antivasculitis, and together with dipyridamole to prevent PLT aggregation. Thrombocytopenia is very dangerous. All these medications do not have side effects of suppressing bone marrow. Therefore we need to identify other reasons in this patient. In the absence of fever, lymphadenectasis or hepatosplenomegaly, leukemia was not concerned. We also excluded aplastic anemia based on her bone marrow results. The duration of MPI and PINF infection were consistent with that of thrombocytopenia. Thus, the diagnosis of acute immune thrombocytopenia was established. With IVIG treatment, platelets returned to normal, which in turn supports this diagnosis.
5. When she started to take warfarin, we recommended her stay in the hospital to have DIC monitored, which would help doctors adjust dose to keep the INR between 2.0 and 2.5 [27]. But her family lived far away from our hospital (the edge of Inner Mongolia, over 1000 km away), and her parents insisted on going home. Once they were back to home, they found a near hospital where DIC could be performed. Since that hospital was over 100 km away from her family, without a private car, the patient could only have DIC test once every 3 months, especially after she suffered from acute immune thrombocytopenia. Local pediatricians refused to add warfarin in her medications for they were concerned about bleeding. Later, during the follow-up appointments at our clinics, her parents refused to increase the dose of warfarin for being concerned about bleeding. INR almost did not meet criteria of thrombolysis and perhaps this is the reason she had thrombosis.

Hong Wang

2.8 Case 8 KD with Dilated Cardiomyopathy

A previous healthy 4-year-old male was with a significant past medical history of MP pneumonia and an unremarkable antenatal, family history.

He presented on Day 6 of illness with a 6-day history of high fever (39 °C, with shivering) along with cervical lymphadenectasis. On Day 4, rashes developed all over his body. One day later, rashes regressed but bilateral conjunctival congestion developed. In local clinic, second-generation cephalosporin, ribavirin, and dexamethasone were infused for 2 days, but all turned out to be ineffective. Thus, he was admitted to our pediatric cardiology ward. Since the onset of illness, he had a little bit cough and watery stool 2–3 times daily, along with vomit occasionally. **Examination** revealed mild fever (37.4 °C), weight 20 kg, height 105 cm, bilateral conjunctivitis, red fissuring lips, strawberry tongue, and labial angular ulcer. Cervical lymphadenectasis was about 2.0 cm. The liver was enlarged 5 cm below the right costal margin, the quality was medium hard. The skin around crissum peeled, without rash on the body. Others were normal. Admission blood tests revealed WBC 37.1 × 10^9/L, NE 92.3%, HGB 105 g/L, PLT 387 × 10^9/L. NT-pro BNP 45674 pg/ml. hs-cTnT<0.003 ng/ml. CRP 92.4 mg/L. Cervical ultrasound revealed bilateral lymphadenectasis, 1.7 cm × 1.5 cm on the left. He had met the criteria of KD with 4 out of 5. He was treated with (i) IVIG 1 g/kg/d for 2 days; (ii) oral aspirin 30–50 mg/kg/d, dipyridamole 3–5 mg/kg/d both divided into 2–3 times doses; (iii) infusion with first-generation cephalosporin.

On Day 7, investigations revealed ESR 52 mm/h. ALT 80 U/L, ALB 28 g/L, γ-GT 167 U/L, D Bil 12.0 μmol/L. MP-IgM, CP-IgM, and RSV-IgA were positive, MP-IgG 1:320. Abdominal ultrasound showed swollen liver, with upper border at the 6 right rib; 4.3 cm below the right costal margin; the surface was smooth. He was treated with (1) polyphosphatidyl choline 5 ml/d; (2) albumin 1 g/kg/d for 2 days; (3) azithromycin 10 mg/kg/d for 3 days. On Day 8, he was still febrile (up to 38.7 °C) 36 h after IVIG. Meanwhile, moderate middle-to-small rales could be heard on bilateral lower lungs. Chest CT revealed mild inflammation on bilateral lower lobes. On Day 10, his fever reduced and bilateral rales stayed unchanged. Retested blood work revealed WBC 15.5 × 10^9/L, NE 52.1%, HGB 94 g/L, PLT 661 × 10^9/L. CRP 72.2 mg/L. ESR 60 mm/h showed dilation of LCA 4.2–4.5 mm, LVED 35.9 mm, EF 61%. On Day 11, he had been afebrile for 36 h, skin around his fingernails desquamated, and the rales were rarely heard. Thus we tapered off aspirin.

On Day 16, all the symptoms were settled. Physical examination did not find significant abnormalities. Re-tested blood work revealed WBC 7.2 × 10^9/L, NE 34.5%, HGB105g/L, PLT 886 × 10^9/L. CRP 3.82 mg/L. NT-pro BNP 41.49 pg/ml. ALT 12 U/L, γ-GT 45 U/L, ALB 38.3 g/L. Echocardiography revealed LCA 3.8 mm (Fig. 2.66a), LVED 38 mm (Fig. 2.66b), EF 53%. For his LVED was significantly increased, cedilanid was injected to fast saturation. The next day, he continued to take oral digoxin and he was discharged.

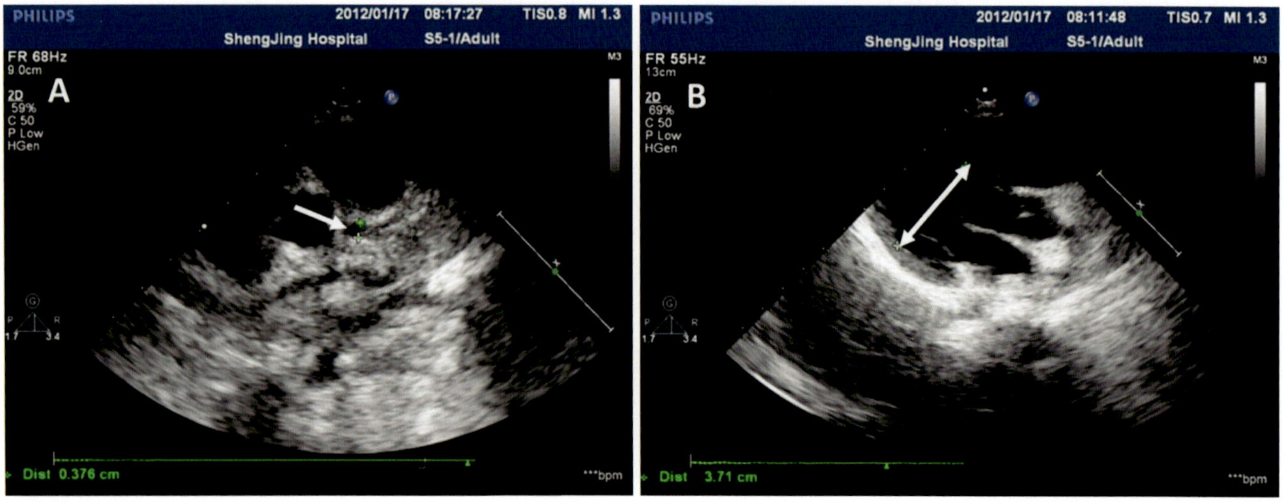

Fig. 2.66 On Day 16 of illness, echo showed LCA 3.8 mm (**a**), LVED 38 mm (**b**)

2.8.1 Clinical Course of this Patient

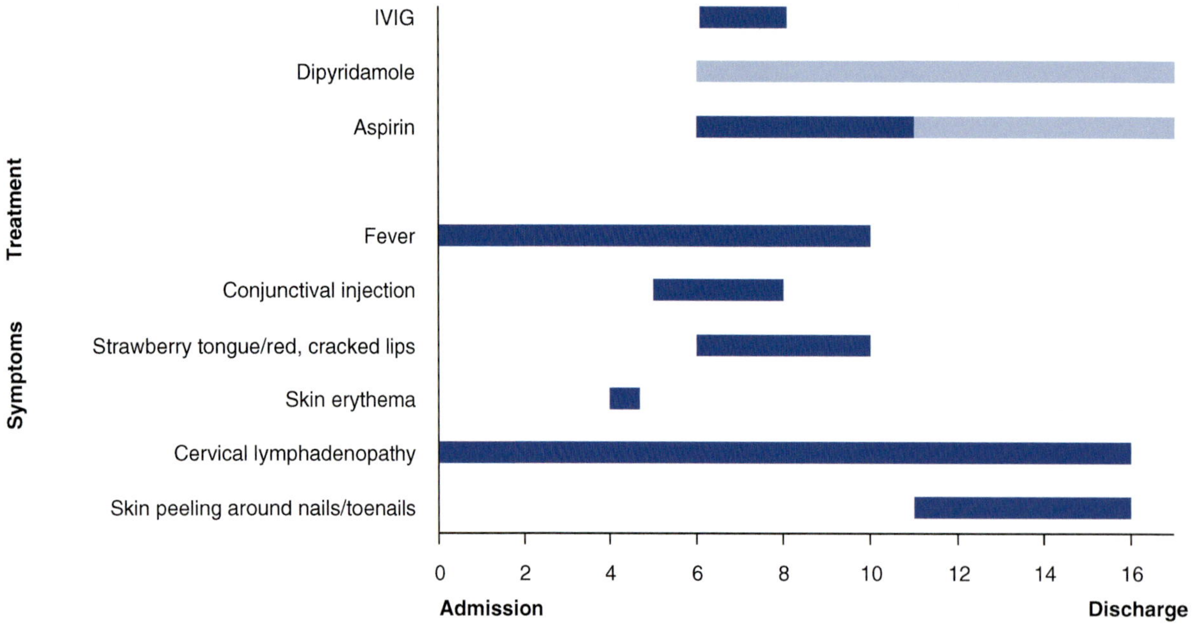

2.8.2 Follow-Up

After being discharged, he was on digoxin 0.125 mg, once a day, aspirin, dipyridamole, and CoQ10 10 mg, in three divided dose. Echocardiography was performed regularly, the data of echocardiography were listed in Table 2.8 (Fig. 2.67a, b).

One month later, routine blood work revealed WBC 14.37 × 10^9/L, HGB 119.2 g/L, PLT 465.4 × 10^9/L.

Seven months later, coronary artery CTA was performed, and revealed LCA 3.9 mm (Fig. 2.68a). LAD 2.2 mm, LCX 1.8 mm, RCA 2.5 mm (Fig. 2.68b). All the branches were in normal distribution and shape, without stenosis or aneurysm dilation (Fig. 2.69a, b). For the larger left ventricle, oral captopril was prescribed, 1 mg/kg/d, in divided 2 doses.

Table 2.8 The dynamic changes of echo parameters

Time of illness	11days	17days	1months	2months	7months	3.5years
LCA (mm)	4.2–4.5	3.8	3.2–3.4	3.4	3.5	3.5
LVED (mm)	35.9	38	33.6	40	43	47
LVEF (%)	61	53	58	59	67	59

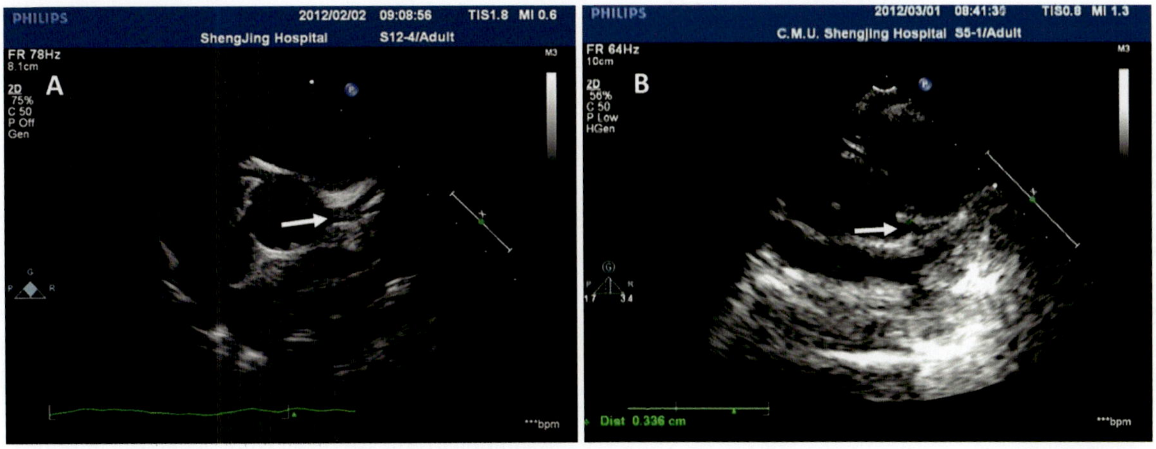

Fig. 2.67 Echocardiography showed LCA diameter 3.2–3.4 mm at one month (**a**) and 3.4 mm at 2 months (**b**)

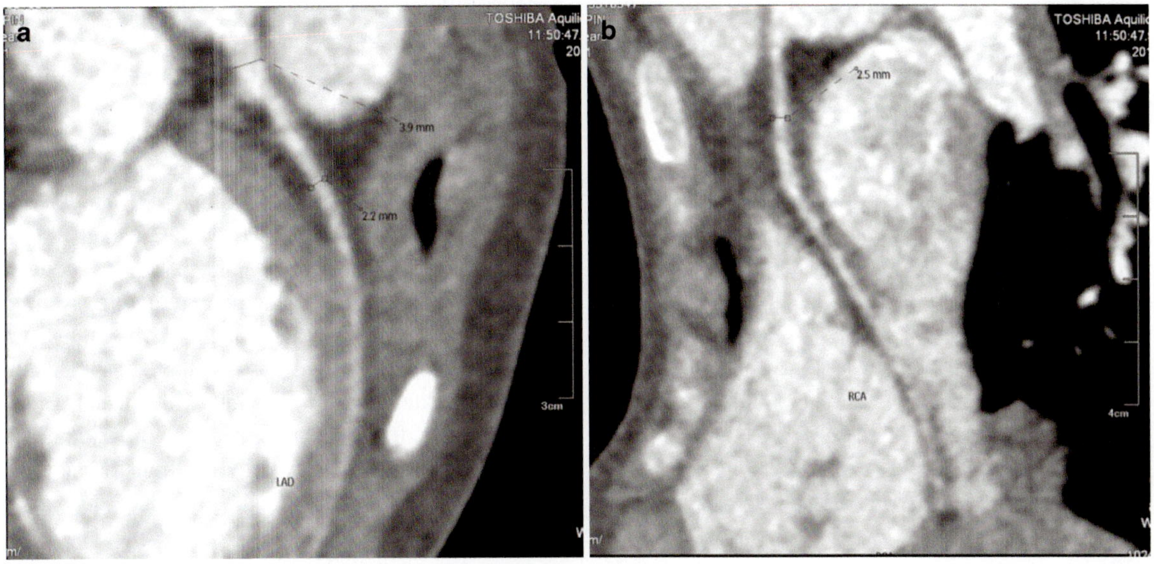

Fig. 2.68 At 7 months of illness, coronary artery CTA showed LMA 3.9 mm, proximal LAD 2.2 mm (**a**), RCA 2.5 mm (**b**)

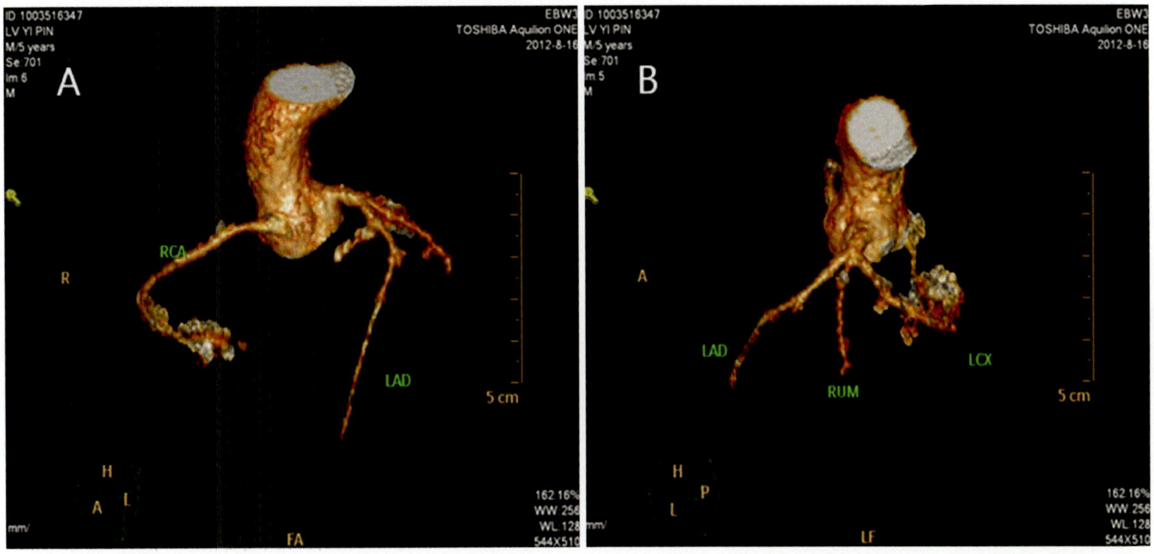

Fig. 2.69 On 7 months of illness, coronary artery CTA showed LM mild dilatation (**a**), while proximal and RCA were normal (**b**)

2.8.3 Diagnosis

1. KD
2. Left CAA
3. Left ventricular dilation
4. Liver dysfunction
5. Hypoalbuminemia
6. Acute bronchopneumonia
7. CP infection
8. RSV infection
9. MP infection
10. Thrombocytosis.

2.8.4 Discussion

The diagnosis of KD was definitive, the high fever was accompanied (i) rashes all over the body; (ii) bilateral conjunctivitis, without purulent excretion; (iii) cervical lymphadenopathy; (iv) cracked red lips and strawberry tongue; additional WBC 37.1 × 10^9/L, NE 92.3%. NT-pro BNP 45674 pg/ml. CRP 92.4 mg/l. ESR 52 mm/h.

In regard of pneumonia, azithromycin was applied instead of another 2 g/kg of IVIG. 36 h after the first IVIG infusion, the patient still had persistent high fever without other symptoms of KD. We considered it was associated with pneumonia. Therefore we treated the patient with azithromycin instead of second round of IVIG after a resistance to the first IVIG.

2.8.5 The Special Features of the Patient

1. The dilation of LCA was identified on Day 11 after illness, which gradually regressed to 3.5 mm. However, with the detection of slight dilation of left ventricle (LVED 38 mm, normally 31.5 ± 1.6 mm) according to his standard weight and height, we had to take dilated cardiomyopathy into account. Cedilanid and subsequent digoxin were applied as cardiac inotropes. The LVED was 33.6 mm after 1 month, reached 40.7 mm after 2 months. On account of the continuous increase (43 mm 6 months later), captopril was added for treatment. Echocardiography 3.5 years afterwards revealed LVED 47 mm (normally 38.6 ± 2.6 mm), LCA 3.5 mm, LVEF 59%. This increasing trend suggested complications of dilated cardiomyopathy and cardiac insufficiency, besides the aneurysm and thrombosis. Clinicians should be aware of the above complications to ensure treating the patient timely.
2. Acute coronary artery injury would appear in 15%–25% untreated KD patients. Once treated with IVIG within 10 days, this incidence will fall down to less than 5% [38]. Risk factors of coronary artery injury include male, atypical KD, long fever duration, lagged initial IVIG infusion, ALB<35 g/L, serum $Na^+ \leq 133$ mmol/L, CRP>100 mg/L, IVIG resistance and adoption of GC [39]. GC was independent risk factor for formation of aneurism and giant aneurysm [40]. The risk factors of aneurysm include age (<1 year old), NE ≥ 80%, CRP>100 mg/L, PLT<300 × 10^9/L, serum Na + ≤133 mmol/L, ALT≥100 U/L and initial IVIG infusion within 4 days [41]. He was treated with IVIG on 7–8 days after fever onset as soon as KD was diagnosed, in addition to oral aspirin and dipyridamole. Unfortunately, he still developed CAA, which may be related to infusion of GC at early stage.
3. According to above criteria, except for his NE over 80%, perhaps infusion with dexamethasone within 3 days of initial fever onset was the key for treating his CAA and enlarged LV, though he was diagnosed and treated timely.
4. The immunoreaction of KD could last for many years. Coronary artery injury may develop into chronic dilation of left ventricle, and heart failure [42]. However, severe cardiac insufficiency caused by KD usually happens in cases of misdiagnosis. Regularly performed echocardiography is needed to evaluate heart structure, systolic function, and coronary artery changes. Even lesions were absent when the patient was discharged. As to giant CAA, anticoagulant therapy was vital, which usually comprised of warfarin, low-dosage aspirin, and dipyridamole.
5. Accounting for the limitation of transthoracic echocardiography, after the acute stage of KD, coronary artery enhanced CT was necessary for the patients with aneurysm if permitted. The CTA could demonstrate distribution of coronary artery, also the location, shape, and quality of the lesions multi-dimensionally. CTA was in accordance with echocardiography in proximal lesions, and better in distal lesions [31]. Thus it is advised that once the coronary artery dilated, CTA would be supplemental exam to echocardiography, in case the distal coronary artery was misdiagnosed.
6. According to the KD criteria, if antibiotics were standardly administrated but ineffective in the initial 3 days, blood bacteria culture was recommended. IVIG may replace antibiotics after 5 days of illness. The adoption of antibiotics was depending on the microorganism test and blood bacteria culture. In this case, the cephalosporin was infused for the presence of pneumonia.

Xue-xin Yu

2.9 Case 9 KD with CAA After Cease Medicine-1

A 5-month-old boy presented with a significant past medicine history of eczema, allergy to cephalosporin and milk. Therefore, he was not on vaccination schedule for allergy condition. His family history was non-remarkable.

He presented on Day 4 of illness, with cough and fever for 4 days, along with rash for 3 days. Four days ago, after contacting his old sister who had herpangina, he had fever up to 38.9 °C. Fever presented twice per day, along with cough and sputum. He took first-generation cephalosporin orally at home, fever did not regress and urticarial rash developed around his nose and eyes. He was sent to clinic and infused with third-generation cephalosporin. After infusion, urticarial rash developed all over the body. Dexamethasone 5 mg was intramuscularly injected. He went home and took erythromycin orally for 2 days. His fever sustained at 39 °C without regression. He was then admitted to respiratory ward. His mental state was mildly irritable and he lost appetite, but he had normal sleep and normal stools. Examination showed fever (T 38.7 °C), PR 118 bpm, RR 32 bpm. WT 7.5 kg. His common state was generally normal. Urticaria could be seen all over body without hemorrhagic spot. Lips were red without strikingly cracked. Slight wheeze could be heard on bilateral lungs by auscultation. Others were normal. CBC on Day 2 revealed WBC 16.4 × 10^9/L, NE 12.7 × 10^9/L, HGB 108 g/L, PLT 455 × 10^9/L. On Day 3, urine routine revealed WBC 16.0/HP. On Day 4, he was crying at night. Abdominal ultrasound was performed and result was normal. His stool was gelee-like and occult blood was positive. He was treated with (i) infusion of erythromycin; (ii) compound glycyrrhizin; (iii) vitamin C; (iv) dexamethasone 3 mg; (v) oral chlortrimeton to release allergy.

On Day 5, he was afebrile and not crying, but cough aggravated. Mucosolvan was infused. CBC revealed WBC 17.0 × 10^9/L, NE 50.0%, HGB 101 g/L, PLT 422 × 10^9/L. Stool occult blood was positive. PCT 0.267 ng/ml. CRP 78.2 mg/L. Liver function was normal except ALB 34.5 g/L. CK was normal, CKMB 37.7 U/L. Chest DR was almost normal. Mild anemia was considered physiological anemia. His parents were advised to pay attention to adding complementary foods. He was treated with oral erythromycin. On Day 6, he was afebrile. Lips redness improved, rashes disappeared. Investigation showed stool occult blood was negative. CBC revealed WBC 20.4 × 10^9/L, NE 43.9%, PLT 634 × 10^9/L. CRP 18.8 mg/L. On Day 10, he was still afebrile, with a mild cough. Rash had disappeared. Skin peeled off around his fingernails. Investigation revealed WBC 13.8 × 10^9/L, NE 56.6%, HGB 91 g/L, PLT 469 × 10^9/L. CRP 22.8 mg/L. Blood culture reports staphylococcus haemolyticus growth on two bottles. For he had (i) sepsis (staphylococcus haemolyticus); (ii) KD was suspected. He was treated with (i) continual oral erythromycin; (ii) test PCT and redo the blood culture; (iii) echocardiography test. On Day 11, echocardiography showed LCA was dilated to 2.8–3.8 mm (Fig. 2.70a), RCA was dilated 2.8–3.4 mm (Fig. 2.70b). ASD 2 mm. Consulted pediatric cardiology: by talking to his mother. On Day 2, his bilateral conjunctiva was congested, with strikingly red lips. He had met all criteria for KD and was transferred to cardiology ward. Retested CBC revealed WBC16.5 × 10^9/L, NE 51.7%,

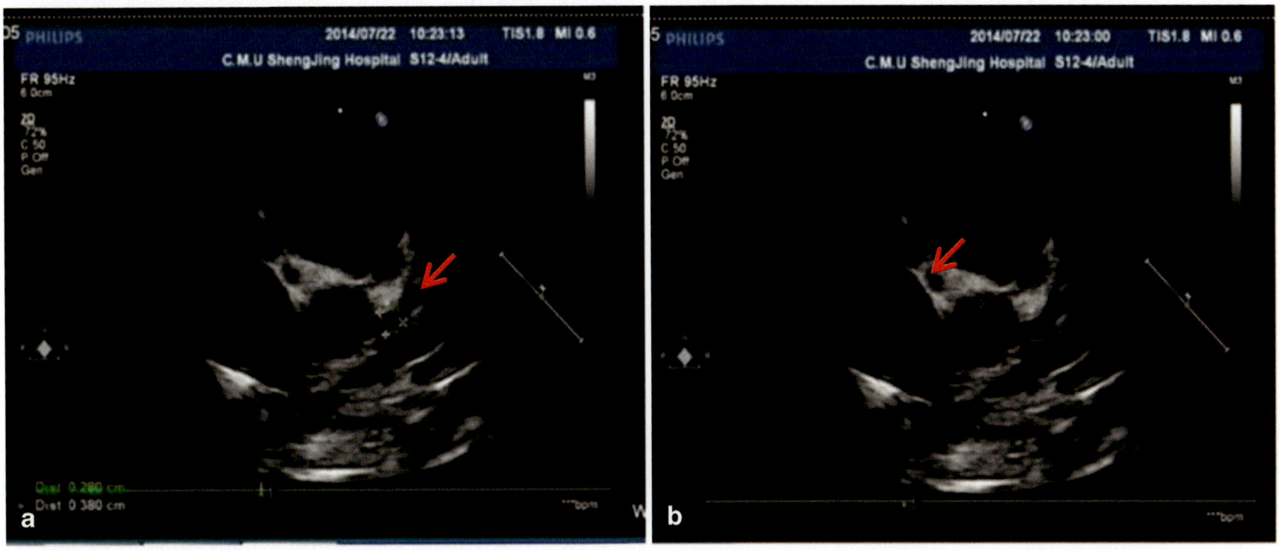

Fig. 2.70 On Day 11 of illness, echocardiography showed LCA dilated to 2.8–3.8 mm (**a**), RCA dilated to 2.8–3.4 mm (**b**)

RBC 4.0×10^{12}/L, HGB 93b/L, PLT 535×10^{9}/L. cTnI, MYO, CKMB-M and hs-cTnT were normal. NT pro-BNP 314.9 pg/ml. He was treated with (i) test HIV + TPPA+RPR; (ii) IVIG 2 g/kg, infused over 12 h and mannitol (20%) and furosemidum were infused after IVIG 1 g/kg infused; (iii) oral aspirin and dipyridamole in 3–5 mg/kg/d; (iv) oral erythromycin.

On Day 13–14, he had mild fever. Examination revealed no additional signs. On Day 15, he was afebrile. Examination found skin peeling off like a cap around fingernails (Fig. 2.71). On Day 17, he was still afebrile. Investigation revealed WBC 4.9×10^{9}/L, NE 12.9%, RBC 3.4×10^{12}/L, HGB 80 g/L, PLT 591×10^{9}/L. CRP and NT-pro BNP were normal; Second blood culture was negative. For he had granulocytopenia and anemia, he was treated with oral traditional Chinese medicine, ferralia, and vitamin C. On Day 19, CBC revealed WBC 5.3×10^{9}/L, NE 0.43×10^{9}/L, RBC 3.6×10^{12}/L, HGB 86 g/L, PLT 560×10^{9}/L. He was treated with rhG-CSF 60 μg hypodermic injection. On Day 20, CBC revealed WBC 12.1×10^{9}/L, NE 5.36×10^{9}/L, RBC 3.8×10^{12}/L, HGB 94 g/L, PLT 373×10^{9}/L. He was discharged.

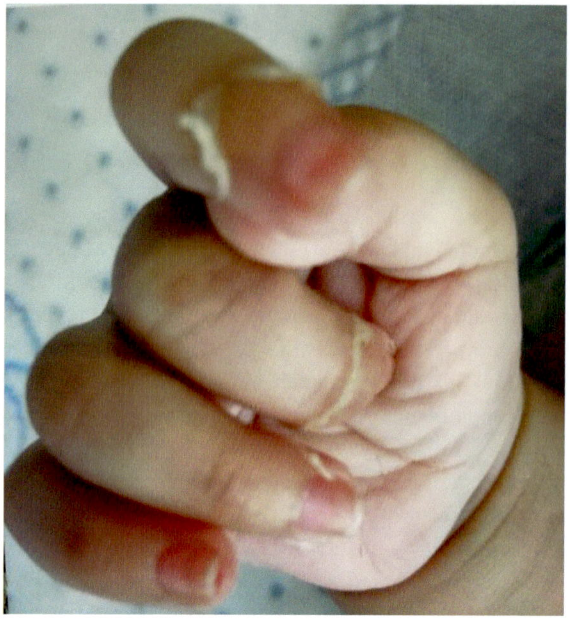

Fig. 2.71 On Day 15, skin peeling off like a cap around fingernails

2.9.1 Clinical Course of the Patient

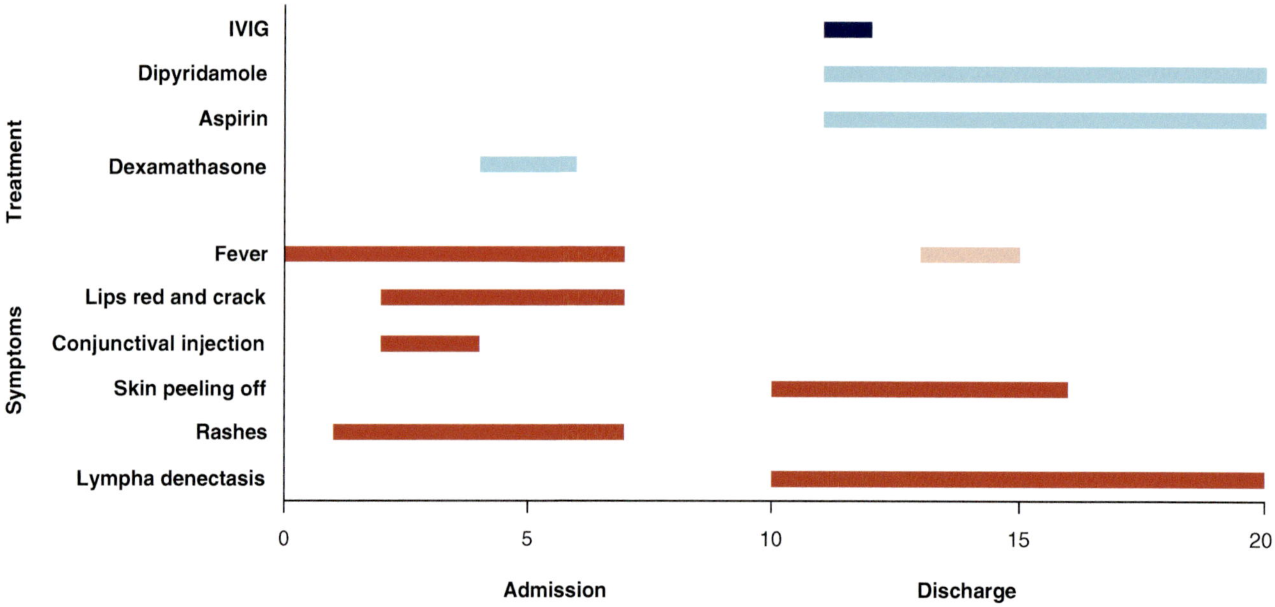

2.9.2 Follow-Up

After discharged, he was taking (i) oral aspirin and dipyridamole; (ii) ferralia and vitamin was performed on Day 26 of illness, both LCA (Fig. 2.72a) and RCA (Fig. 2.72b) were normal.

Echocardiography was performed at 3 months of illness, both LCA (Fig. 2.73a) and RCA (Fig. 2.73b) were normal. All medications were stopped.

Echocardiography was performed at 6 months of illness, anomalous origin of the LCA, the inner diameter of the posterior coronary artery dilatation about 3.3 mm (Fig. 2.74a). We

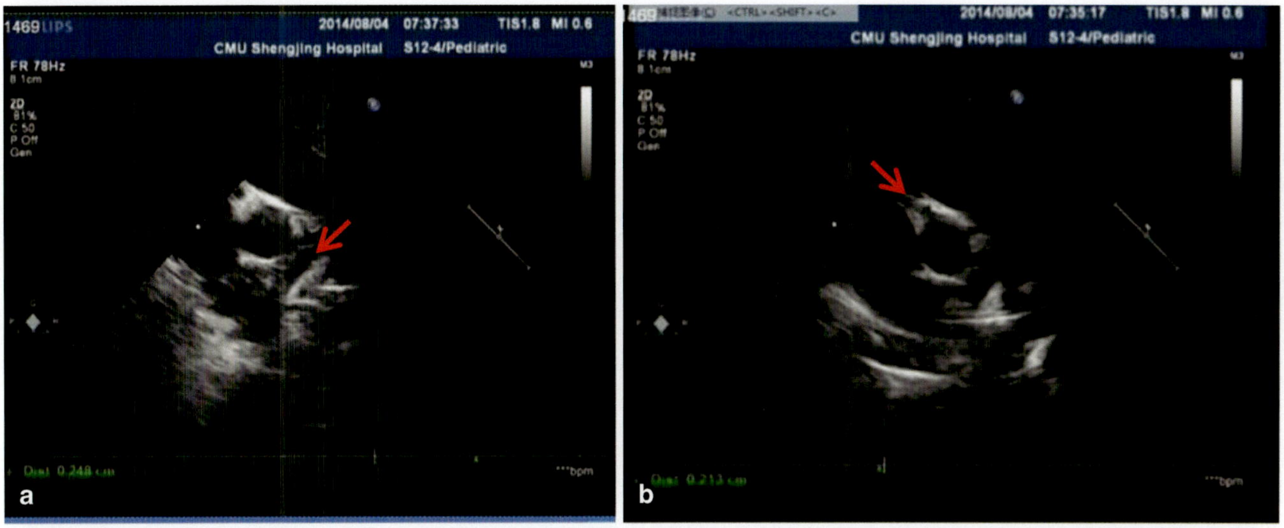

Fig. 2.72 On Day 26 of illness, echo showed normal LCA (**a**) and RCA (**b**)

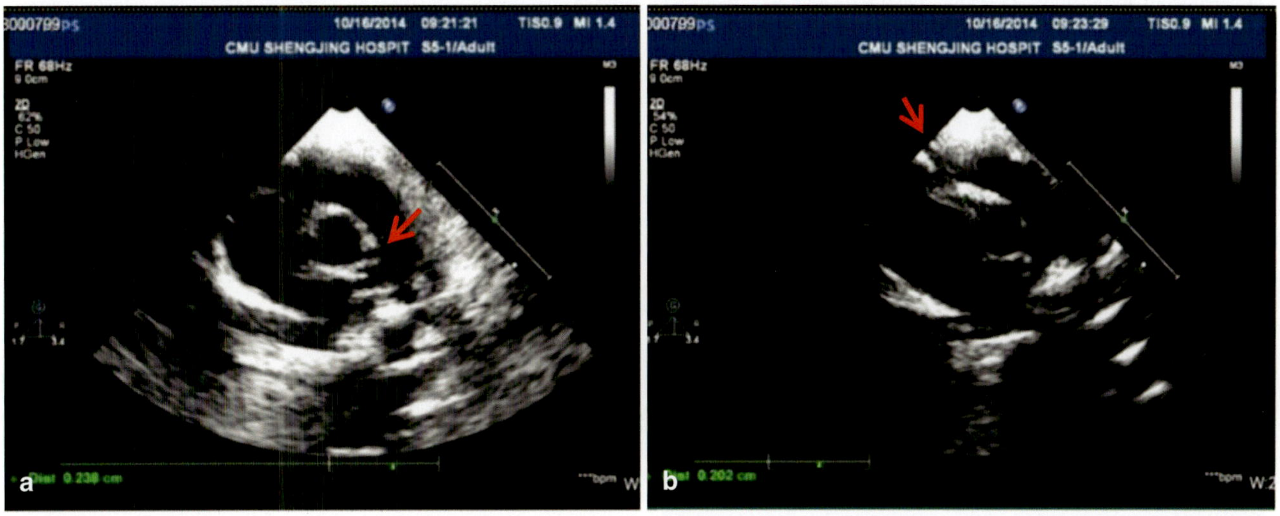

Fig. 2.73 At 3 months of illness, echo showed normal LCA (**a**) and RCA (**b**)

recommended coronary artery CTA to his parents, but they refused for he was too young. Then he went to Beijing, had echocardiography done in both An Zhen Hospital and Beijing Children Hospital, and results showed coronary were normal.

Echocardiography was performed at 10 months showed anomalous origin of the LCA, the inner diameter of the posterior coronary artery dilated to 4.1 mm (Fig. 2.74b). Coronary artery CTA was recommended but was rejected again by his parents. He resumed oral aspirin.

Echocardiography was performed at 13 months, anomalous origin of the LCA, the inner diameter of the posterior coronary artery dilated to 4.1 mm (Fig. 2.75). Thus, he was admitted again for coronary artery CTA. Blood test revealed WBC 6.2×10^9/L, NE 37.5%, HGB 127 g/L, PLT 282×10^9/L. NT-pro BNP, hs-cTnT, MYO, cTnI, ALT and DIC were normal; AST 45 U/L, CK 231 U/L, CKMB 52 U/L, CKMB-M 7.5 μg/L were elevated. Coronary artery CTA failed for rapid HR and RR, with more false images on aortic roots. Right coronary was dominant, the inner diameters of LCA, LAD near-section, and RCA were normal. Others section were indistinct, LM 2.8 mm, RCA 2.9 mm (images were blur and cannot be saved). For he was too young to perform CTA again in short period, he was on oral aspirin and was discharged.

At 15 months, echocardiography performed in Beijing Children Hospital showed LCA dilated to 3.4 mm.

At 18 months, echocardiography performed in our hospital showed LCA dilated to 3.1 mm (Table 2.9). Continued to take oral aspirin.

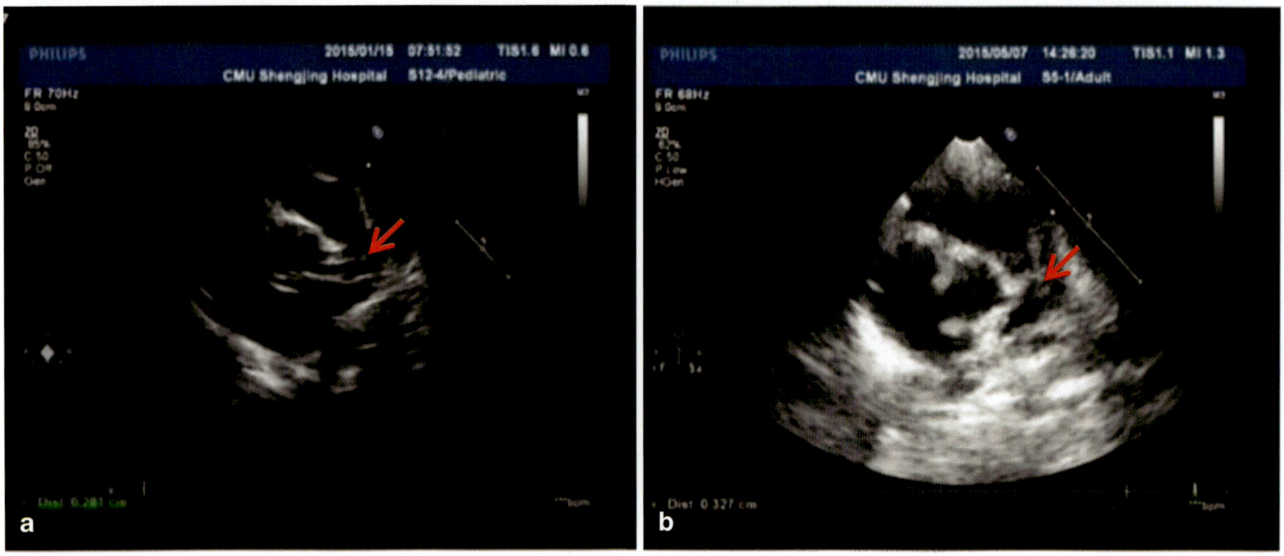

Fig. 2.74 Echocardiography showed two LCA (anterior and posterior) originated from aortic sinus, located at 3 and 4 o'clock with diameter 2.4 mm and 2.8 mm, respectively. The posterior LCA was slightly dilated to 3.5 mm (**a**) at 6 months and 3.3 mm at 10 months (**b**) of illness

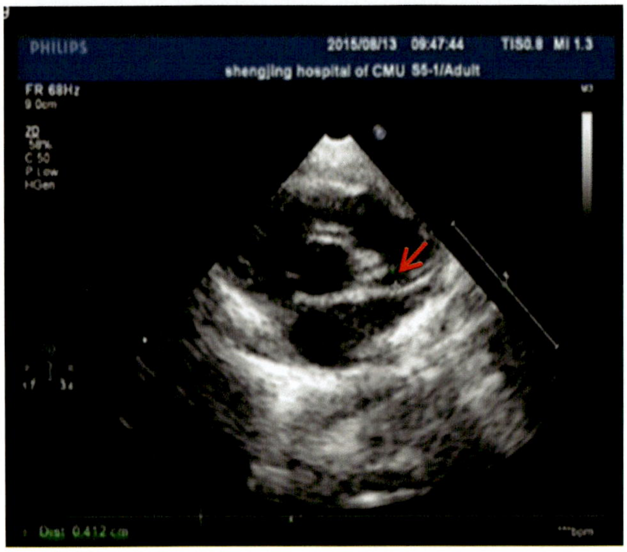

Fig. 2.75 At 13 months of illness, echocardiography showed two LCA, posterior LCA diameter was 3.0 mm, then slightly dilated to 4.1 mm

2.9.3 Diagnosis

1. KD, bilateral coronary artery dilatation
2. Acute capillary bronchitis
3. Septicemia (Staphylococcus Haemolyticus)
4. Moderate microcytic anemia
5. Agranulocytosis (Table 2.9)

2.9.4 Discussiom

He had met all criteria for KD, his fever last over 5 days and failed to respond to antibiotics. Fever regressed after dexamethasone 5 mg injection on Day 4, 3 mg on Day 5. He had (i) rashes all over body; (ii) bilateral conjunctive congest; (iii) strikingly red lips at beginning of fever; (iv) skin peeled off around fingernails on Day 10 of illness; (v) LCA dilated to 4.1 mm.

Differential diagnosis for suppurative meningitis should be considered.

Table 2.9 The dynamic changes of coronary artery

Time of illness		11days	26days	4months	6months	10months	13months	18months
Echo	LCA(mm)	2.8–3.8	N	N	3.5	3.3	4.1	3.1
	RCA(mm)	2.8–3.4	N	N	N	N	N	N
CTA	LCA(mm)					2.8		
	RCA(mm)					2.9		
Aspirin		√	√	√	–	√	√	√

N normal

2.9.5 Case Special Clinical Features

1. Coronary artery dilatation up to 6 weeks of illness [43]. As to the time of stopping medication, there are different opinions. Some physicians recommend aspirin be continued until coronary artery normal [44]. It was also suggested that once coronary artery lesion occurred, aspirin should be taken orally for extra 3 months after coronary artery regressed to normal. This boy took aspirin for total 4 months (after 3 months his coronary artery was normal). Although aspirin could not lower the frequency of development coronary artery abnormalities [46], his coronary artery dilated again 2 months later and then there is the trend of continuing to broaden. Maybe he belongs to KD patients whose vascular inflammation can last for a long time or even permanent coronary artery aneurysms [47].
2. Echocardiography and coronary CTA are common methods to evaluate coronary artery, and theoretically the later one should be superior, particularly along with coronary artery stenosis or calcification [31]. But to perform CTA HR must be less than 90 bpm and be absolutely calm during the performing time. To prevent vomit or aspiration after infused with the contrast agent, the child fasted over 4 h. It is difficult to stay calm when the child is hungry. Thus, sometime coronary artery CTA was unsatisfactory in some babies.
3. When LCA abnormally originated from RCA, if it is not between the aorta and the pulmonary artery, it usually does not cause myocardial ischemia; if it is between the aorta and pulmonary artery, it does not cause myocardial ischemia either unless strenuous exercise occurs. This anomaly is not related to KD or coronary artery dilatation.
4. IgE may be increased significantly in KD in initial 1–2 weeks and go down after 1–2 month [20]. Therefore, the rash at the beginning may be related to it. But most of them had a history of using antibiotics. Pediatricians may first suspect that rash was allergic reaction to medication and treat patients with glucocorticoid. This boy was infused with dexamethasone twice, consequently, its anti-allege effect was obvious. But if infused with glucocorticoid before Day 5, especially before Day 3 of illness, it may mask the early symptoms of KD. If single glucocorticoid infused in early stage of KD, it may promote coronary artery thrombosis and result in coronary artery aneurysm [44, 39]. This boy with the symptoms of conjunctival congestion, red and cracked lips are all happened at home, both parents and pediatrician focused on rashes and fever when admission. It was only after skin peeling off around fingernails, he was suspected KD. After talking with his mother, we learned more details. Thus, we suggest that if baby fever along with rash without convulsion, chilling, or cyanosis, choosing phenergan injection or chlortrimeton oral would be better.

Hong Wang

2.10 Case 10 KD with CAA After Cease Medicine-2

A previous healthy 4-year-old girl presented with unremarkable past medicine and family history.

She presented at 29 months diagnosed with KD at the local hospital 29 months ago. On Day 12 of illness, she was treated with IVIG. Echocardiography showed coronary artery dilatation, without echocardiography report. After oral aspirin and dipyridamole for 8 months, she followed up in our clinic, and echocardiography showed coronary arteries recovered to normal (Fig. 2.76a, b). Coronary artery CTA was recommended but rejected by her parents. Medications were stopped after returning home. One day before admis-

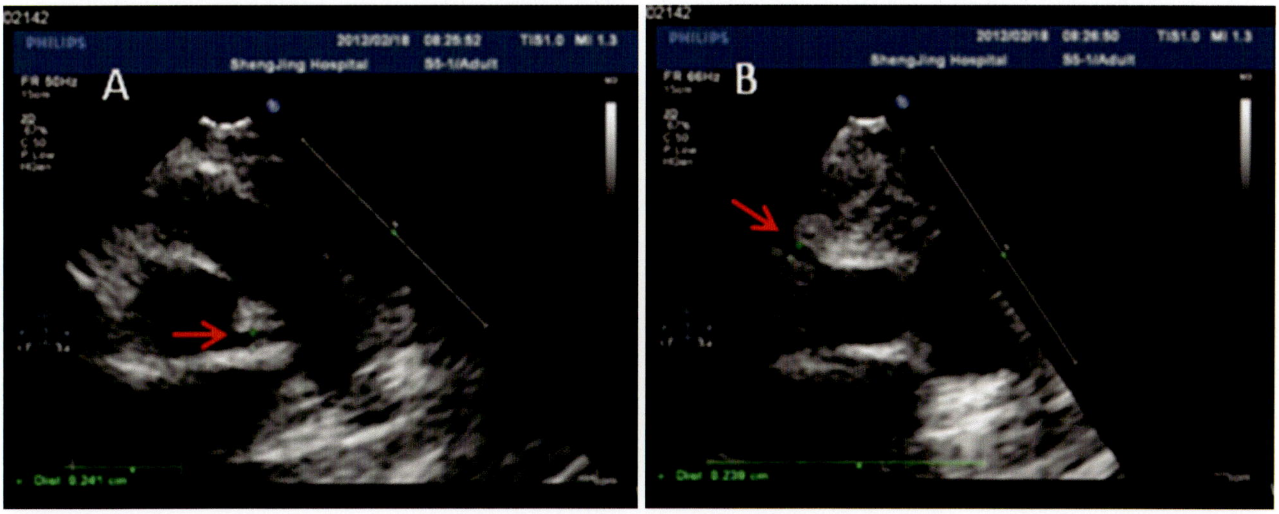

Fig. 2.76 At 8 months of illness, echocardiography showed normal LCA (**a**) and RCA (**b**)

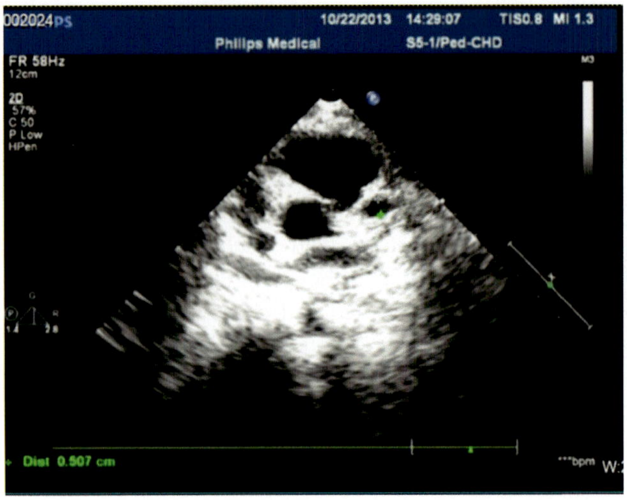

Fig. 2.77 At 29 months of illness, echo showed LAD dilated to 5.0 mm

sion, echocardiography was performed at a local hospital, and it was found that LAD significantly widened. She came to our hospital echocardiography review: confirmed LAD developed CAA. She was admitted in pediatric cardiology ward for coronary artery CTA. Her mental state was stable, with occasional coughing, good diet, and normal urine. Examination showed normal vital signs T 36.1 °C, HR 102 bpm, RR 26 bpm, weight 19 Kg. No significant abnormal signs. Investigation revealed echocardiography showed a LAD dilatation about 5.0 mm (Fig. 2.77). She was treated with (i) reserve coronary artery CTA; (ii) oral aspirin 75 mg/d once per day and dipyridamole 25 mg tid. On Day 3 of admission, coronary artery CT failed due to insufficient sedation. Her parents refused to redo CT. She continued to take oral aspirin and dipyridamole. She was discharged.

At 31 months of illness, she was admitted again for coronary artery CTA. Her examination was normal. CBC revealed WBC 5.5 × 10^9/L, RBC 3.8 × 10^{12}/L, HGB 108 g/L, PLT 265 × 10^9/L. DIC: PT 13.6s, INR 1.2. ECG showed sinus arrhythmia, HR 86–125 beats/min. CTA showed there were no calcified plaques in LAD and RCA. RCA was dominant (Fig. 2.78a). The mid-section of the LAD dilated to 8.5 mm and length 12 mm (Fig. 2.78b). The mid-section of RCA dilated to 4.2 mm and length 5.8 mm (Fig. 2.78c). There were no calcified plaques or stenosis in each segment of LCX (Fig. 2.78d). She had developed a giant CAA and was treated with oral warfarin 1.25 mg/d. On Day 3 of admission, repeated DIC showed INR 1.2. Dose of warfarin was increased to 1.5 mg once daily. On Day 4, INR 2.7. Echocardiography showed LVED 35 mm, LVED 66%, LCA about 2.5 mm, the anterior descending branch obviously widened, about 7.0 mm (Fig. 2.79a). RCA 2.4 mm (Fig. 2.79b). Warfarin was stopped for 1 day. Repeated DIC on Day 5 showed PT 22.5s, INR 2.0. Warfarin was resumed at 1.25 mg once daily.

On Day 6, repeated DIC showed PT 21.5s, INR 1.9. She was discharged.

2.10.1 Follow-Up

At 3 years, she presented with skin freckle for 2 months. Examination was normal (T 36.7 °C, HR 98 bpm, RR 22 bpm, Bp 90/64 mmHg, Weight 21 Kg), except her lower limbs had scattered bleeding spots. CBC at admission revealed WBC 8.0 × 10^9/L, NE 47.3%, HGB 10 g/L, PLT 316 × 10^9/L. DIC showed PT 17.7s, INR 1.6. CK-MB mass, cTnI, NT-pro BNP, and hs-cTnT were normal. ECG showed the sinus rhythm was uneven, 71–94 bpm (Fig. 2.80). Echocardiography showed LVED 34 mm, LVEF 57%, LCA about 2.7 mm. LAD was obviously widened, about 7.2 mm (Fig. 2.81). RCA was normal. She was treated with (i) oral vitamin C; (ii) suspension of oral warfarin; (iii) hematology consultation; she was currently diagnosed properly and control of coagulation disorders. The prolongation of PT was caused by anticoagulant drugs. Due to the characteristics of primary diseases, whether anticoagulant therapy was needed or not requires professional evaluation. If anticoagulant therapy was required, the current state of coagulation was in line with expectations. To prevent thrombosis, her current state of coagulation was safe and did not require treatment, dynamic monitoring of DIC. Continued to take oral warfarin and aspirin. Then was discharged.

At 4 years, echocardiography showed LVED 36 mm, LVEF 67%. LCA about 2.9 mm, LAD 7.0 mm. RCA was normal.

At four and half years, echocardiography showed LVED 36 mm, LVEF 61%. LCA 2.8 mm, LAD 8.0 mm (Fig. 2.81a). RCA 2.6 mm, and 18 mm away from opening dilated to 4.2 mm. No definite plaques and expansions were found in all segments of LCX (Fig. 2.81b).

At 5 years, coronary artery CTA showed there were no calcified plaques in LAD and RCA. RCA distribution was dominant. The proximal section of LAD dilated, the diameter was 10.2 mm, and length was 18.6 mm. The mid-section of LAD was dilated with 5.5 mm in diameter and 5.3 mm in length. The proximal section of RAD was dilated with 5.5 mm in diameter 10.1 mm in length. Mid-section of RCA was dilated with 4.7 mm in diameter and 7.6 mm in length. There were no definite plaques or dilations in each segment of LCX (Fig. 2.82).

Since then, she had never followed up with us.

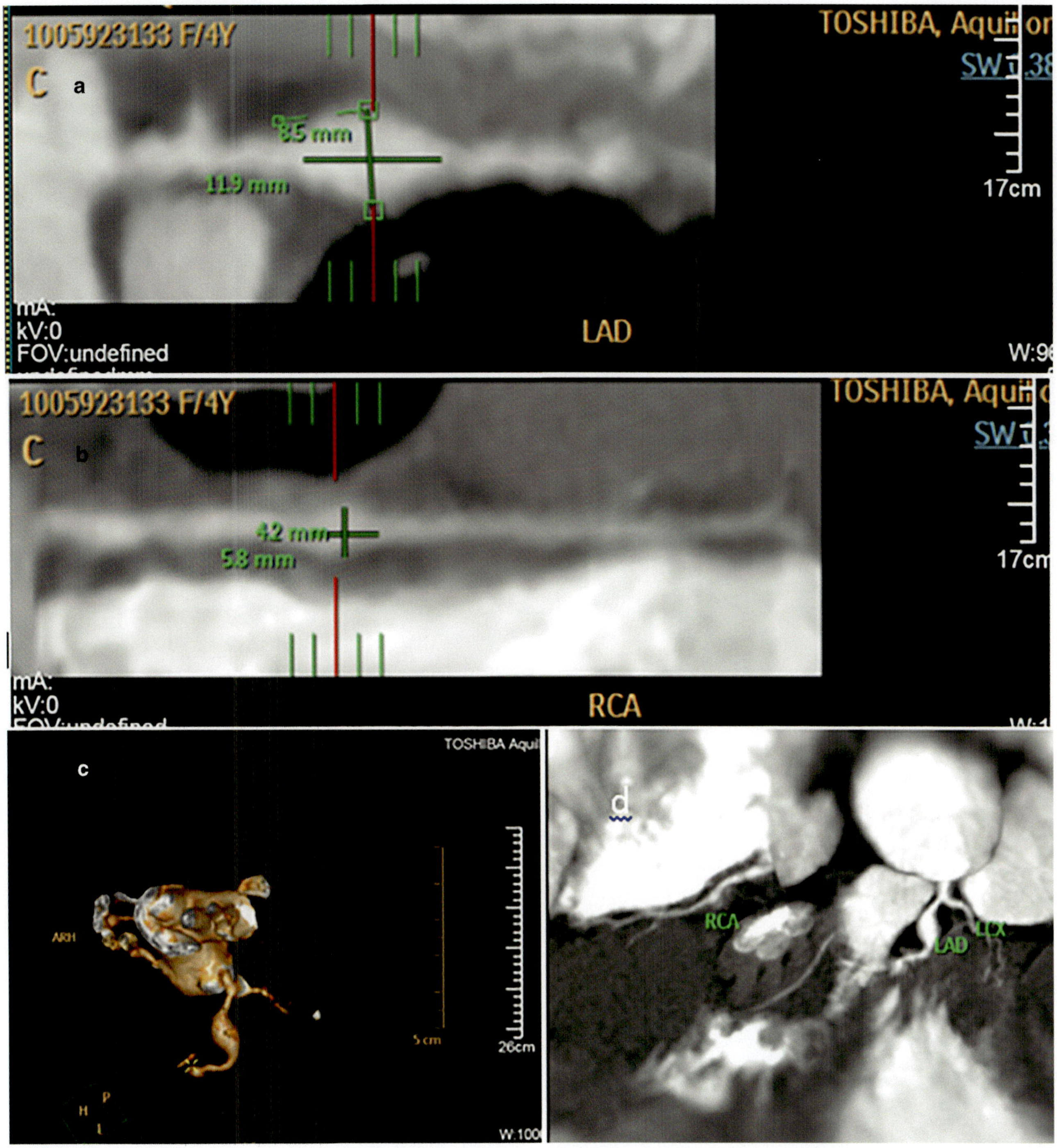

Fig. 2.78 At 33 months of illness, coronary artery CTA showed at middle section of LAD dilatation about 8.5 mm, the length was12 mm (**a**). RCA dilated to 4.2 mm, the length was 5.5 mm (**b**). No calcification plaques were found in LAD, RCA, and LCX (**c**–**d**)

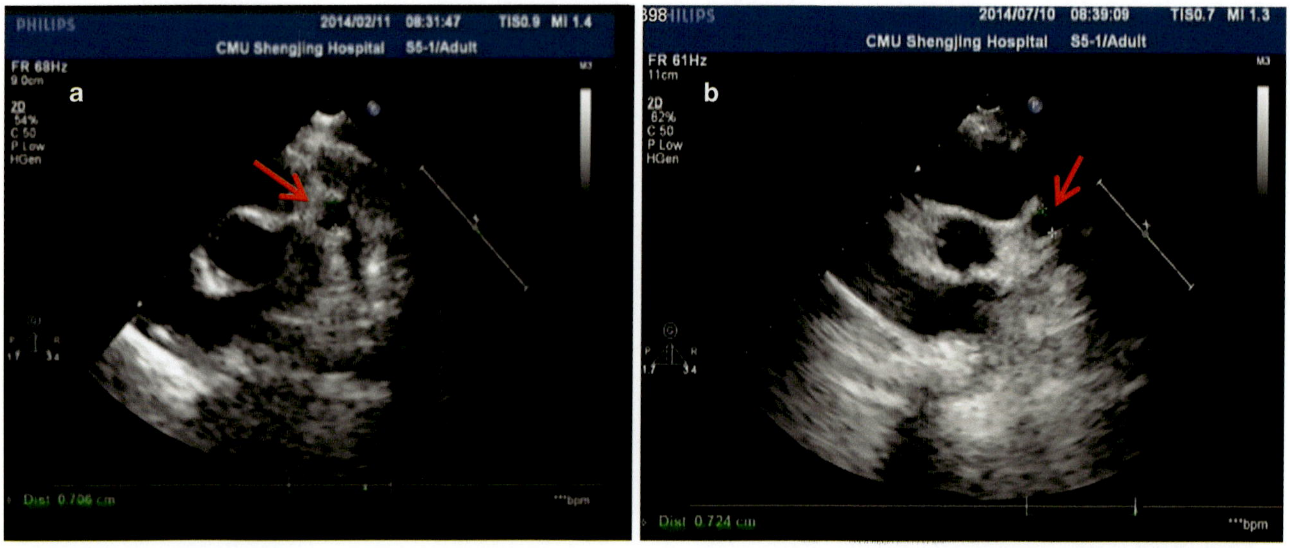

Fig. 2.79 Echocardiography showed LAD was significantly dilated, 7.0 mm at 33 months (**a**) and 7.2 mm at 3 years (**b**)

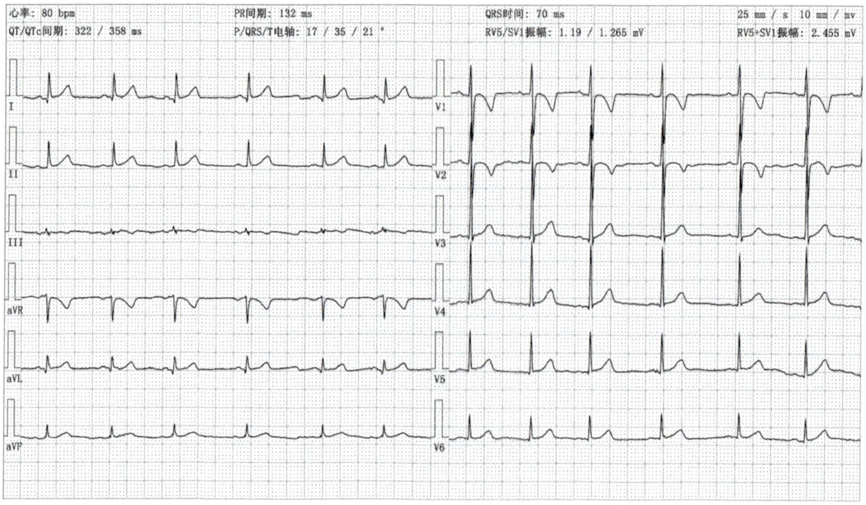

Fig. 2.80 At 3 years of illness, ECG was normal

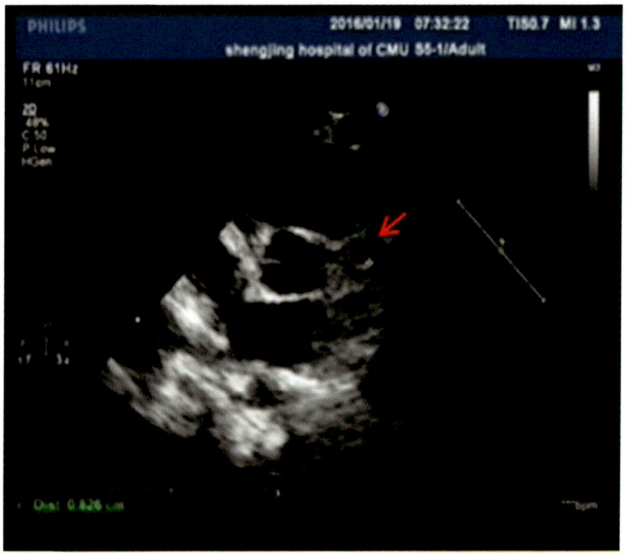

Fig. 2.81 At 4.5 years of illness, echocardiography showed LAD dilated to 8 mm

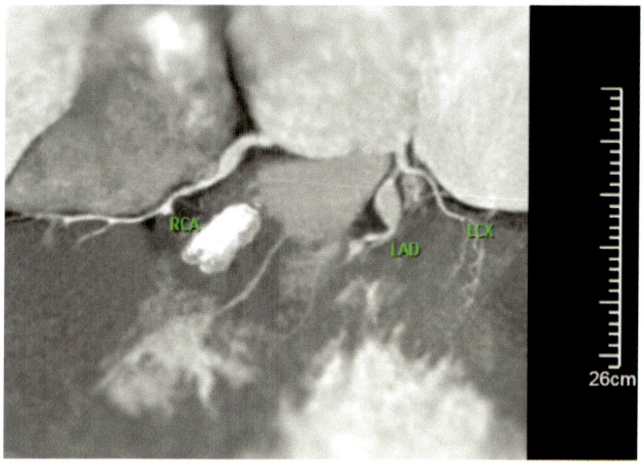

Fig. 2.82 At 5 years of illness, coronary CTA showed LAD dilated to 10.2 mm at proximal section, the length was18.6 mm, 5.5 mm at middle section, the length 5.3 mm. RCA dilated to 4.7 mm at proximal section, the length was 7.6 mm. No calcification plaques were found in LAD, RCA, and LCX

2.10.2 Diagnosis

1. KD
2. Giant Left coronary artery aneurysm

2.10.3 Discussion

She was diagnosed with KD at the local hospital at 4 years old. By now, she was 10 years old. From the dynamic changes of coronary artery, her diagnosis should be unquestionable.

She stopped to take medications after coronary artery recovered which was confirmed by our echocardiography.

2.10.4 Case Specific Clinical Features

1. She had coronary artery lesion at beginning. It may be related to application of IVIG on Day 12 of illness. Medications were stopped after coronary artery recovered.
2. One year after stopping medication, echocardiography found both LCA and RCA dilatation, and it was getting worse.
3. The indications that oral warfarin in KD patient include: (i) giant CAA; (ii) intravascular thrombosis.
4. Once on oral warfarin, DIC should be monitored. The effective index for warfarin is INR 2.0–3.0. But in children with KD they also need oral aspirin. Therefore, for the sake of safety, we usually monitor INR in the range of 1.5–2.5.
5. Warfarin is a strictly controlled class of drugs. Infection, diarrhea, and use broad-spectrum antibiotics all have a greater impact on DIC. If APTT prolong more than 1.5 times, warfarin should be immediately reduced or stopped. Meanwhile, restricting physical activities and preventing contact sharp objects in order to reduce the chance of trauma. If the bleeding tendency cannot be effectively controlled, it requires intramuscular injection of vitamin K_1 2.5–10 mg [48].
6. Chronic vasculitis in KD can last for a long time even without CAA [49]. She had no coronary angiography after ultrasound was confirmed normal, and did not continue to take medication. The interval was nearly 2 years before repeated echocardiography, when LAD widened was found. Although echocardiography did not show LAD lesion before medication discontinuation, from the later imaging data, even if she took the medication again, the condition was deteriorating till 5 years. We inferred that the LAD was not widen or the width was not obvious before stopping medication. Therefore, in children with coronary artery injury, when the ultrasound shows normal coronary arteries, they must take oral aspirin for another 3 months [50]. Even so, several months after stopping medication, we found that some patients developed into small CAA (see case 12). Therefore, it is better to perform coronary angiography before stopping aspirin to prevent the misdiagnosis of distally dilated coronary arteries. At the same time, even if the drug is discontinued according to the routine, long-term follow-up is still necessary.

Hong Wang

2.11 Case 11 KD with CAA, Acute Coronary Artery Thrombus and Thrombocythemia

A previously healthy 2-month-old boy presented with unremarkable antenatal and family history.

He presented on Day 7 of illness with a prolonged fever for 7 days, along with rashes for 5 days, cough for 3 days. He received infusion of ceftizoxime at a local clinic. His fever did not regress, and rashes developed on the trunk on Day 2 of illness. The doctor stopped the infusion immediately. After intramuscular injection of dexamethasone, the rashes improved, but fever was persistent, and he started to have cough. Then he received infusion of erythromycin for 2 days. On Day 5, he had increasing rashes along with mild edema in arms, legs, and scrotum, the doctor stopped giving him intravenous infusion of cefoperazone sodium and sulbactam sodium. Yesterday, the doctor started to give him infusion of meropenem, imipenem, and cilastatin sodium, but his rashes worsened again. Then he was transferred to our clinic and admitted in pediatric respiratory ward as a patient with acute bronchopneumonia. Examination findings include: T 39.1 °C, PR136 bpm, RR30 bpm, weight 7 Kg. His mental stage was stable. He had rashes on the face, trunk, arms, and legs. He had cervical lymphadenectasis about 0.5 × 0.5 cm. Auscultation assessment revealed respiratory rudeness in bilateral pulmonary systems. Examination found normal heart and abdomen. He had edema in the arms and legs, scrotum. Neurological system was normal. On Day 2 of illness CBC revealed WBC 16.5 × 10^9/L, NE 70.3%. On Day 3 of illness, WBC 15.7 × 10^9/L, NE 76.6%. CRP 95.3 mg/L. On Day 5, WBC 11.6 × 10^9/L, NE 82%; CRP 160 mg/L; ESR 40 mm/h. On Day 6, CRP 145 mg/L. Echocardiography revealed a small amount of hydro-pericardium. Chest X-ray revealed bronchopneumonia. After admission, CBC showed WBC 11.5 × 10^9/L, NE 83%, HGB 80 g/L, PLT 231 × 10^9/L. CRP 133 mg/L. PT 16.1s, INR 1.2, APTT 37s, D-dimer 1133 μg/L, FDP 16.5 mg/L. Chest CT presented inflammation at the lower lobes of the lungs. He had (i) acute bronchopneumonia; (ii) sepsis. He was treated with (i) infusion of cefepime hydrochloride and vancomycin after blood sample drawn for culture; (ii) IVIG 2.5 g/d (350 mg/kg/d) for supporting therapy; (iii) infusion of erythromycin.

On Day 9, he still had a fever and the red rashes on the trunk. The dermatologist we consulted with recognized that the patient had erythema multiforme. The dermatologist suggested the patient staying away from possible factors taking low sensitive diet, and having the infection under control. The dermatologist also recommend oral compound glycyrrhizin capsules, half a capsule each time, three times a day; chlorphenamine maleate tablets, 1 mg each time, twice a day. Investigation revealed CKMB 35 U/L; TP 46.4 g/L, ALB 27.20 g/L. CK, ALT, AST, tuberculosis antibody, MP-IgM and MP-IgG antibody were normal. In the night, the rashes were aggravated; they were red spotted rashes, protruded from the surface of the skin and partially merged into pieces, along with eyelid edema. On Day 10, after IVIG, the edema became obvious. To reduce the amount of intravenous infusion, erythromycin and immunoglobulin were left out, and furosemide (2 mg/kg/d, in 2 divided doses) intravenous injection was given. After that, the edema in eyelid was relieved, the edema in the arms and legs was reduced than before. On Day 13, he still had a fever (peak 39 °C). The condition of edema was improved, but there were still rashes. His heart rate was 160–200 bpm. Investigation revealed WBC 38.2 × 10^9/L, NE 67.9%, HGB 85 g/L, PLT 438 × 10^9/L. CRP 133 mg/L. TP 58.2 g/L, ALB 27.4 g/L. Echocardiography showed LVED 17.7 mm, EF 68.4%. RCA dilated to 3.4–5.1 mm (Fig. 2.83) and 12.8 mm in length, LM was about 2.0 mm. ASD 3.1 mm. On Day 14, he was admitted in our pediatric cardiology ward as KD with right CAA. Cervical ultrasonography showed right cervical lymphadenectasis about 2.0 cm × 0.7 cm. He was treated with (i) oral aspirin 30–50 mg/kg/d and dipyridamole 3–5 mg/kg/d, in 3 divided doses; (ii) IVIG 950 mg/kg in 24 h (The total amount of IVIG was 2 g/kg); (iii) oral warfarin 0.1 mg/kg/d. DIC was monitored to keep his INR between 1.5 and 2.5; (iv) infusion of ceftezole for anti-infective therapy; (v) infusion of albumin for 2 days (1 g/kg/d) (vi), oral iron supplements. On Day 15, his fever subsided, but still had cough. He received infusion of erythromycin. On Day 17, he was afebrile over 48 h, aspirin was reduced to one dose 3–5 mg/kg/d.

On Day 19, he had a fever again, fever spiked at 38 °C. There were still some rashes on the trunk; soles were mildly swollen. The cough alleviated. Investigation revealed WBC 11.3 × 10^9/L, NE 55.7%, HGB 71 g/L, PLT 907 × 10^9/L; CRP 46.7 mg/L; TP 58.2 g/L, ALB 27.4 g/L; PT 47.1s, INR 3.0, APTT 49 s. We considered he had (i) thrombocythemia; (ii) IVIG resistance. He was treated with (i) additional single dose of IVIG (1 g/kg); (ii) reduced warfarin at 0.05 mg/kg/d. On Day 21, fever subsided, the cough recovered, and his heart rate was about 110–130 bpm. On Day 22, repeated echocardiography showed RCA dilated to 17 mm × 11 mm

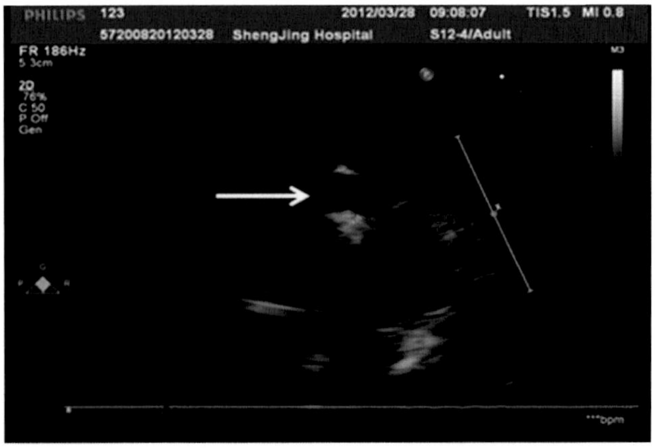

Fig. 2.83 On Day 13 of illness, RCA dilated to 3.4–5.1 mm

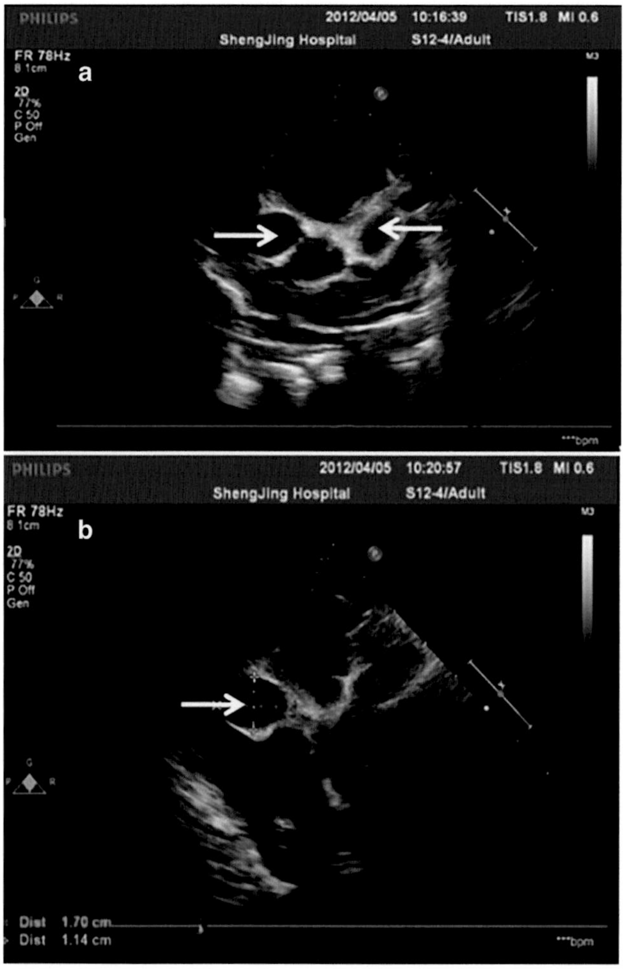

Fig. 2.84 On Day 22 of illness, echocardiography showed both LCA and RCA dilated (**a**), RCA diameter 17 mm (**b**)

(Fig. 2.84a). LM was 2.9 mm, LCX was 1.8 mm, LAD was dilated to 17 mm × 11 mm (Fig. 2.84b). ASD was 3.8 mm. Small amount of hydro-pericardium, an echocardiography-free space of pericardial cavity in the left ventricular posterior wall was about 4 mm; the lateral wall of the left ventricle was 5.5 mm (Fig. 2.85). He had bilateral giant CAA. He was found to have a petechia on the back of his hand after blood sample drawn, and a hemorrhagic spot was also found on the back of the sole. Investigation revealed PT 49.8s, INR 3.1; CRP 9.93 mg/L. We immediately stopped oral warfarin and gave him vitamin K_1 2 mg intramuscular injection.

On Day 24, the fever subsided, the cough recovered, and the rashes reduced. A small hemorrhagic spot could be seen on the arm where the tourniquet pressed. Investigation revealed PT 12.7s, INR 1.0, APTT 28s. Everything went well and he was discharged.

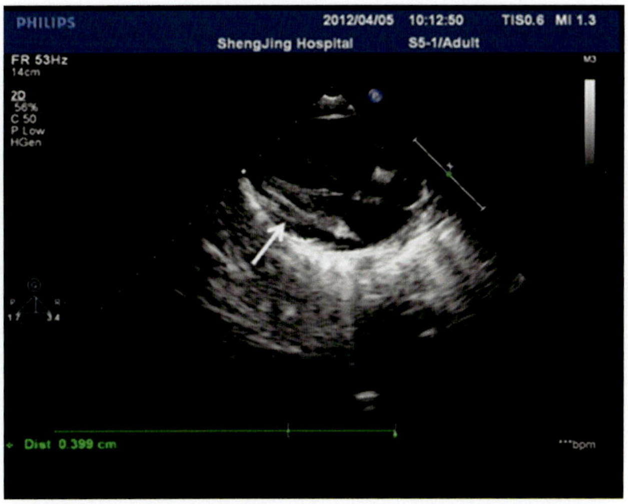

Fig. 2.85 On Day 22 of illness, echocardiography showed 4 mm pericardial effusion behind the posterior wall of the left ventricle

2.11.1 Clinical Course of the Patient

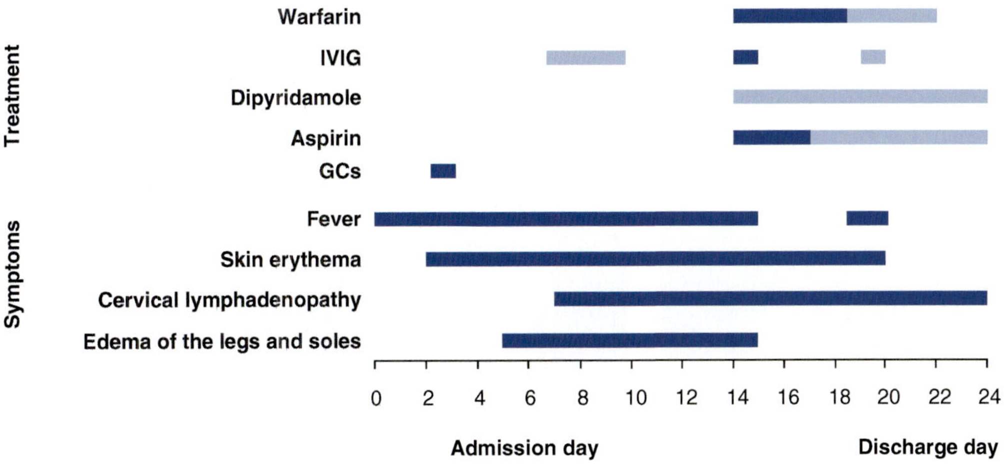

2.11.2 Follow-Up

He followed up with us at out-patient clinic since discharge, and took oral aspirin, warfarin, dipyridamole, and FDP. Echocardiography was performed on schedule.

At 5 months of illness, repeated echocardiography showed LCA dilated to 13 mm at a location 4–5 mm away from opening (Fig. 2.86a), vessel wall was smooth without thrombus. 2–3 mm forward, RCA dilated to 13 mm (Fig. 2.86b), vessel wall was smooth without thrombus. The diameter of each heart chamber was in the normal range. Left ventricular systolic function was normal. The septal of atrium was perfect, without fluid dark area in the pericardial cavity.

At 47 months of illness, repeated echocardiography showed LM was 3.5 mm, the initial segment of RCA was 4.1 mm. 5 mm away, the CAA dilated to 14.4 mm without thrombus (Fig. 2.87). At 50 months of illness, repeated echocardiography showed LM was 3.4 mm; the initial segment of RCA was 4.4 mm. 5 mm away, the CAA dilated to 15 mm; 10 mm away, the CAA dilated to 11.1 mm without thrombus. Left ventricular systolic function was normal. At 63 months of illness, repeated echocardiography showed LM was 3.7 mm, LAD was 3.4 mm; the initial segment of RCA was 4 mm. 5 mm away, the CAA dilated to 14.5 mm without thrombus (Fig. 2.88). At 68 months of illness, repeated echocardiography showed LM was 3.7 mm, LAD was 2.4 mm; the initial segment of RCA was 4–5 mm; 5 mm away, the CAA dilated to 14.3 mm (Fig. 2.89a), 10 mm further away, the CAA dilated to 12.2 mm without thrombus (Fig. 2.89b).

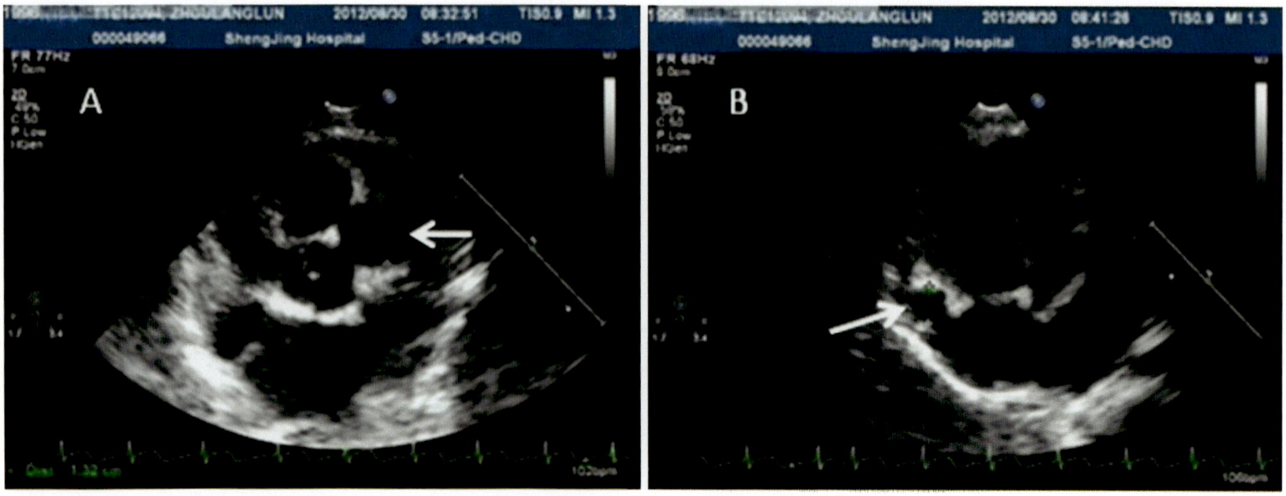

Fig. 2.86 At 5 months of illness, echocardiography showeLCA dilated to 13 mm at middle segment without thrombus (**a**), RCA dilated to 13 mm at right atrioventricular groove (**b**)

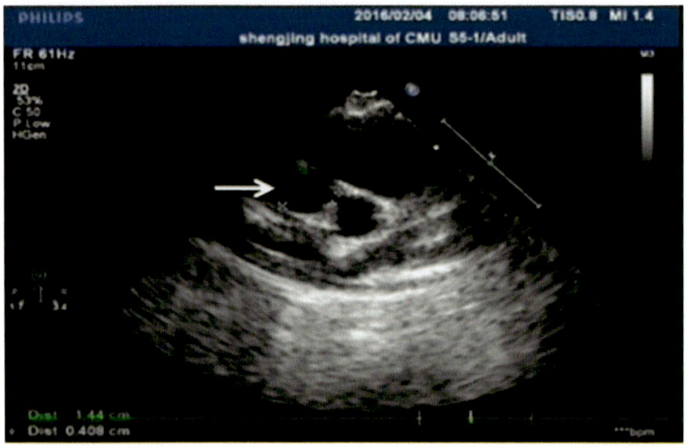

Fig. 2.87 At about 4 years after illness, echocardiography showed the proximal segment of RCA was 4.1 mm, after 5–10 mm the CAA dilated to 14.4 mm without thrombus in it

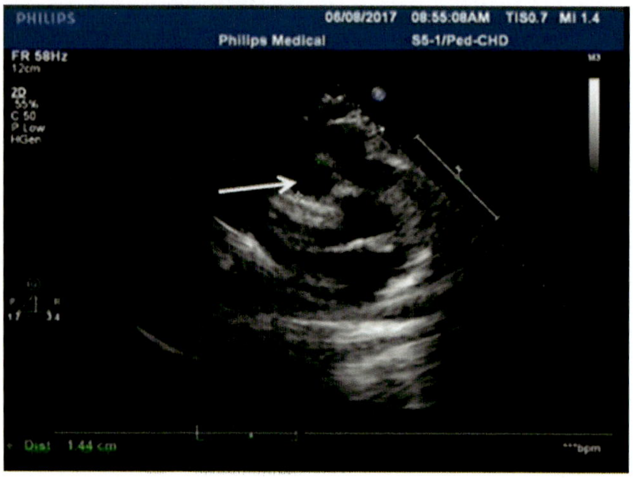

Fig. 2.88 At about 5 years of illness, echocardiography showed RCA dilated to 14.5 mm without thrombus inside

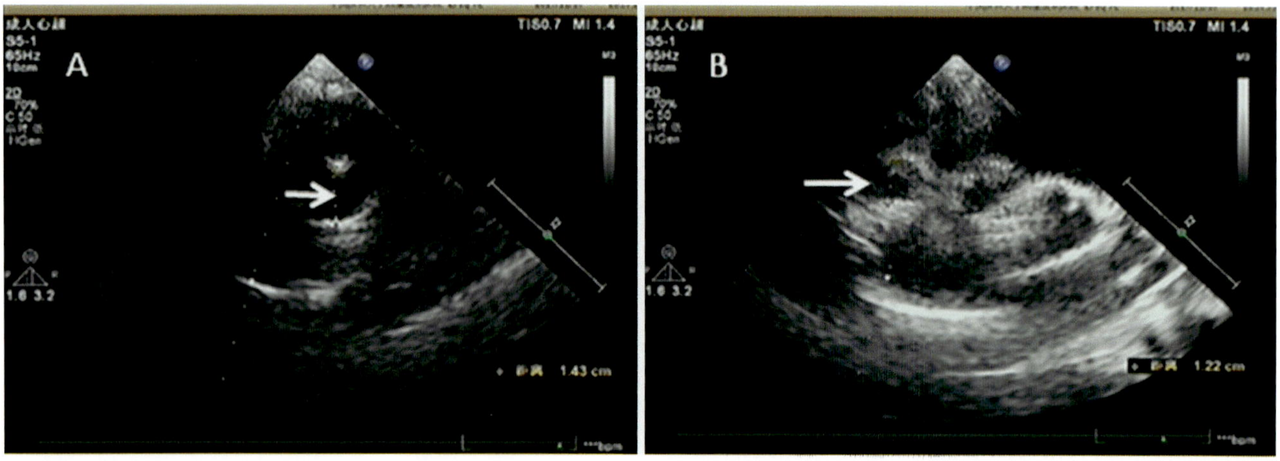

Fig. 2.89 At nearly 6 years of illness, echocardiography showed the proximal segment of RCA was 4–5 mm, after 5 mm the CAA dilated to 14.3 mm (**a**), after 10 mm the CAA dilated to 12.2 mm without thrombus inside (**b**)

2.11.3 Diagnosis

1. KD, IVIG resistance
2. Bilateral giant CAA
3. Hypoproteinemia
4. Thrombocythemia
5. Moderate anemia
6. Acute bronchopneumonia
7. ASD.

2.11.4 Discussion

He had met the criteria of KD for his persistent fever lasting more than 5 days and along with (i) cervical lymphadenopathy; (ii) rashes on the trunk; (iii) slightly swollen soles on Day 19 of illness; (iv) detectable CAA on LCA and RCA; additional: WBC 16.5 × 10^9/L, NE 70.3%; CRP 95.3 mg/L.

KD is an acute self-limited disease, most prognosis is good. CAAs or ectasia develop in 15% to 25% of untreated children with the disease. Treatment with IVIG in the acute phase of the disease reduced the risk to<5% [51]. The rate of recurrence is 1%–2% [29]. In our center, it is common to see that both LCA and RCA dilated. But it is rare to see both LCA and RCA develop giant CAA, especially both over 10 mm in diameters. The classification of CAA was based on Japan standard [51] (see appendix).

Common sites for CAA include the proximal LAD and the proximal RCA, followed by the LM, then LCX, and finally the distal RCA and the junction between the RCA and posterior descending coronary artery. 80% of mild and moderate CAAs subsided within 5 years. The incidence of giant CAAs (diameter >8 mm) is about 5%, and it is almost impossible to subside. The blood flow velocity is low in the CAA and hypostasis may lead to thrombosis, coronary occlusion, even myocardial infarction, and even death [51]. Therefore, long-term anticoagulant therapy is needed in children with CAAs to prevent thrombosis in CAAs. The most common antithrombotic regimen for patients with giant aneurysms is to use low-dose aspirin together with warfarin, maintaining INR of 2–3, and risk management for possible bleeding during the application of warfarin [52].

The conventional time to test INR is usually 5–7 days after taking oral warfarin. But incidence of blood clotting in infants is much less. Once this patient had diarrhea or was treated with large amount of antibiotics, he would soon started to lose vitamin K. If there was a bleeding tendency (skin petechia), vitamin K1 should be injected immediately, which might cause anticoagulation effect falling short. We must prevent the occurrence of intracranial hemorrhage.

When fever persisted after infusion of I, II, III, and IV generation cephalosporin and meropenem or glycopeptide along with elevated CRP, we should concern the possibilities of connective tissue disease and fungal infection.

2.11.5 Case Specific Clinical Features

1. In this case, the boy was young, and was sleeping most of the time. Therefore, it was difficult to identify red conjunctiva. We should make efforts to check the conjunctiva, especially in infants. Also it was difficult to identify edema in legs due to the erythema of the soles in KD. So we considered that it was often difficult to confirm a diagnosis of KD in infants, especially atypical KD. For example, when the patient had diarrhea, the skin around his anus was usually red. We should validate whether there was skin peeling around the anus. Moreover, sometime rashes and conjunctival congestion start shortly after the onset of fever, which makes the KD diagnosis harder. We found that erythema and induration at BCG inoculation site had great significance in diagnosing KD in infants. For the baby younger than 6 months old, when he had a fever for more than 5 days and fever persisted after anti-infection could not be explained by a single cause, he should be on the watch, and coronary artery needed to be assessed and monitored for suspected cases.
2. Patients should be treated with IVIG within the first 10 days of illness and, if possible, within first 7 days of illness [51]. Treated before day 5 of illness, patients have a higher probability to develop IVIG resistance. Treated after day 10 of illness, the incidence of coronary aneurysm increases [53]. In this case, the patient was treated with IVIG on Day 7 of illness, but with an insufficient dose. We did not complement IVIG dose until Day 14 of illness. These all increased the risk of CAA in this case.
3. The risk factors for coronary aneurysm include (i) male; (ii) age <6 months or >3 years; (iii) persistent fever for more than 2 weeks or having a fever again; (iv) cardiac dilatation, arrhythmia; (v) blood work: HBG < 80 g/L; white blood cell count > 16 × 10^9/L-30 × 10^9/L; platelet count > 1000 × 10^9/L; ESR > 100 mm/h; (vi) recurrence case [29]. In this case, he was a 2 months old boy, had persistent fever for more than 2 weeks. Investigation revealed: WBC 38.2 × 10^9/L, HGB 71 g/L. After admission, laboratory presentation marked that ALB 27.20 g/L, but he did not receive infusion of albumin on time. These all induced the injury in his coronary artery.
4. In this case, causes of anemia include: (i) inhibition of infection on bone marrow; (ii) consumption of infection; (iii) reduction of iron intake during infection; (iv) frequent blood drawn. Based on standard treatment, the child should be transfused with red blood cells.

5. It is challenging to treat the giant CAA. But as long as the structure and function of the heart were normal, we could treat the child with anticoagulant and non-specific anti-inflammatory medications until he grow taller, almost as tall as adult. At that time, they can decide whether they need coronary artery bypass grafting.

Le Sun

2.12 Case 12 KD with I°AVB and Urinary Infection

A previous healthy 4-year-old boy presented with unremarkable past medical history or family history.

He presented on Day 4 of illness with fever and lymphadenectasis for 4 days and bilateral conjunctival congestion for 1 day. On Day 1 of illness, he had fever up to 39.5 °C, with cervical lymphadenopathy. He received infusion of second-generation cephalosporin for 3 days in a local hospital; his fever did not regress and developed bilateral conjunctival congestion, strikingly red lips and rashes all over the body on Day 3. Thus, he was admitted in pediatric cardiology ward. In recent 10 days he had occasional cough without sputum. From Day 2, he had stomachache and lost appetite, without vomit and diarrhea. Examination found that he was febrile and his mental state was good; T 39.5 °C, HR 100 bpm, RR 20 bpm, WT 20 kg. There were congestive rashes all over body, no itch. Cervical lympha node was about 2 cm, tenderness tender when touched. He had bilateral conjunctival congestion without purulent secretion; strikingly red lips with strawberry tongue. Others were normal. CBC on Day 2 revealed WBC 16.7 × 10^9/L, NE 67.7%, HGB 124 g/L, PLT 355 × 10^9/L. CRP 57 mg/L. Cervical ultrasound showed cervical lymphadenopathy, and the largest one was 2.1 cm on the left. CBC at admission showed WBC 18.4 × 10^9/L, NE 89.6%, HGB 112 g/L, PLT 442 × 10^9/L. Blood gas analysis revealed PH 7.377, BE −5.1 mmol/L. CRP 75.90 mg/L. NT-pro BNP 659.7 pg/ml. K$^+$, Na$^+$, CK, CKMB, CKMB-M, cTnI, and hs-cTnT were normal. ECG showed sinus tachycardia, HR 150 bpm, I°AVB, low T wave in inferior wall and lateral wall (Fig. 2.90). Cervical ultrasound showed cervical lymphadenopathy, the largest one was 2.2 cm × 1.3 cm on the left. He had met 4 out of 5 criteria for KD. He was treated with infusion of creatine phosphate sodium 1 g/d and levocarnitine 20 mg/kg/d. In addition, he took oral aspirin 30–50 mg/kg/d and dipyridamole 3–5 mg/kg/d.

On Day 5, he continued to have fever and had cough with sputum. Examination found visible jaundice on his face. Investigation revealed TP 57.0 g/L, ALB 32.5 g/L, ALT 300 U/L, AST 69 U/L. AKP 386 U/L, γ-GT 283 U/L, T Bil 75.9 μmol/L, D Bil 58.9 μmol/L, TBA 164.8 μmol/. Glucose and Ca^{++} were normal. MP-IgG 1:40. EBV NA-IgG NE (+/−). Urine test showed protein+g/L, leucocyte esterase +++/μl, urobilinogen + μmol/L, urine bilirubin ++μmol/L, acetone body ++mmol/L, WBC 157.28/HP. Abdominal ultrasound showed liver, gall bladder, and spleen were normal. There were about 1.0 cm free liquid in enterocoelia. He was treated with (i) IVIG 1 g/kg/d for 2 days; (ii) infusion of compound glycyrrhizin and phosphatidylcholine; (iii) oral ursodesoxycholic acid. At night, his jaundice was aggravated, without hepatomegaly. Investigation revealed WBC 10.1 × 10^9/L, NE 86.4%, HGB 103 g/L, RC 0.9%, K$^+$ 3.03 mmol/L, Na$^+$ 127.7 mmol/L, ALT 194 U/L, AST 31 U/L, ALB 32.5 g/L, T Bil 62.2 μmol/L, D Bil 53.1 μmol/L. ECG showed sinus rhythm, HR 113 bpm (Fig. 2.91). He was treated with (i) fluid infusion with Na$^+$ and K$^+$; (ii) infusion of transmetil to promote the bile drainage. On Day 6, after IVIG 1 g/kg, his fever interval extended and abdominal pain was relieved. But he still had cough with sputum. Examination found rashes and jaundice on skin of his trunk still. Investigation revealed that ALB was 27.2 g/L. Chest CT scan was normal. We consulted with a pediatric gastroenterologist who suggested that this boy's

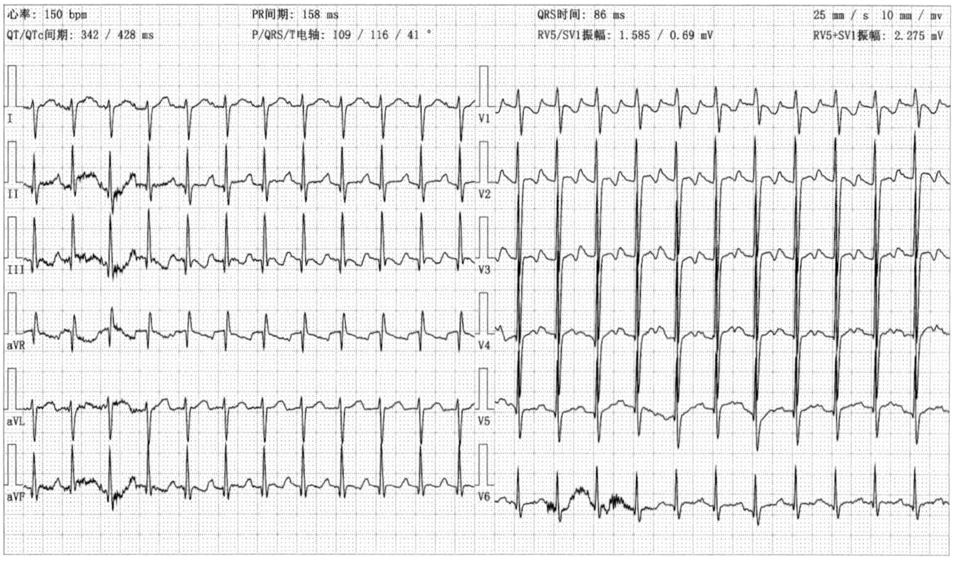

Fig. 2.90 On Day 4 of illness, ECG showed tachycardia, HR 150 bpm, PR interval 158 ms, I°AVB, T wave low-flat on inferior wall and lateral wall

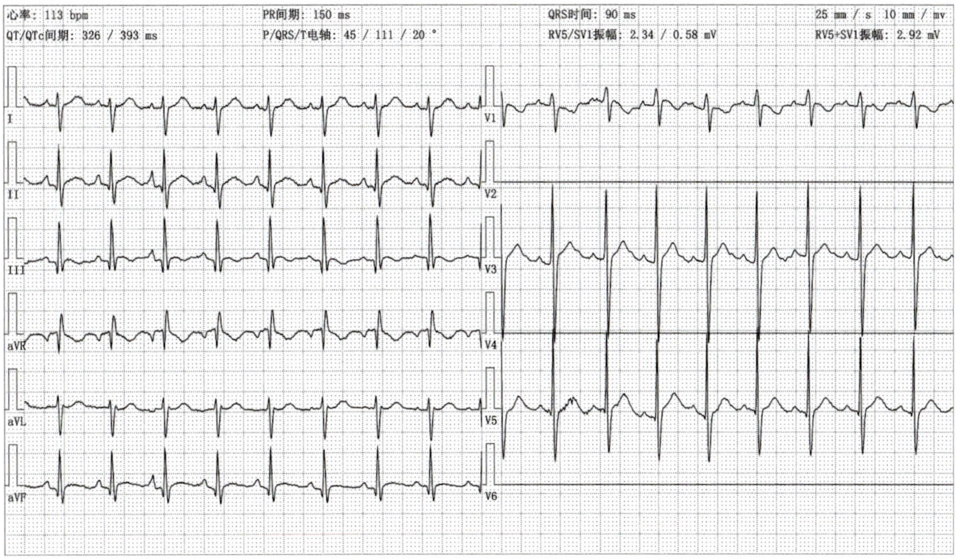

Fig. 2.91 On Day 5 of illness, ECG showed tachycardia, HR 113 bpm, PR interval 160 ms, almost normal

cholestasis was correlated with KD; after treatment, his jaundice had improved; current treatment could be continued. If jaundice aggravates, he could be treated with glucocorticoid infusion under a condition that there was no contraindication. In the presence of significantly increased EBV VCA-IgG and EA-IgG, chronic and active EB virus infection (CAEBV) should be concerned. EBV antibody needed to be retested 1 week later, so did dynamic assessment of liver function. He was treated with albumin 2 g/kg infusion. On Day 7, he was afebrile, abdominal pain was relieved. His appetite was improved. Examination showed mild jaundice on the face. On Day 9, he still had cough. Examination showed bilateral conjunctival congestion disappeared. Investigation revealed WBC 4.95 × 10^9/L, NE 1.0 × 10^9/L, HGB 101 g/L, PLT 558 × 10^9/L. No atypical lymphocyte. Urine WBC 8.59/HP. CRP 25.40 mg/L. NT-pro BNP 1611↑ (<300 pg/ml). ALT 81 U/L, γ-GT 123 U/L. ALB, Bil T, Bil D, TBC, triglyceride, cholesterol, blood gas analysis, and ferritin were normal. Echocardiography showed normal coronary artery. Aspirin dose was reduced to 3–5 mg/kg/d.

On Day 10, peeling skin occurred around fingernails. Examination found no jaundice. Peeling skin occurred around anus, groin, and penis. Investigation revealed WBC 5.72 × 10^9/L, NE 0.8 × 10^9/L, HGB 104 g/L, PLT 615 × 10^9/L. CRP 8.22 mg/L. ALT, AST, ALB, Bile T, and TBC were normal. γ-GT 101 U/L. NT-pro BNP 709.5 pg/ml. EBV EA-IgG (<5.0), EBV NA-IgG (16.0), EBV VCA-IgG (<10.0), EBV-DNA<1.0 × 10^3. These results did not support CAEBV. Hepatobiliary ultrasound result was normal. On Day 11, he was discharged.

2.12.1 Clinical Course of the Patient

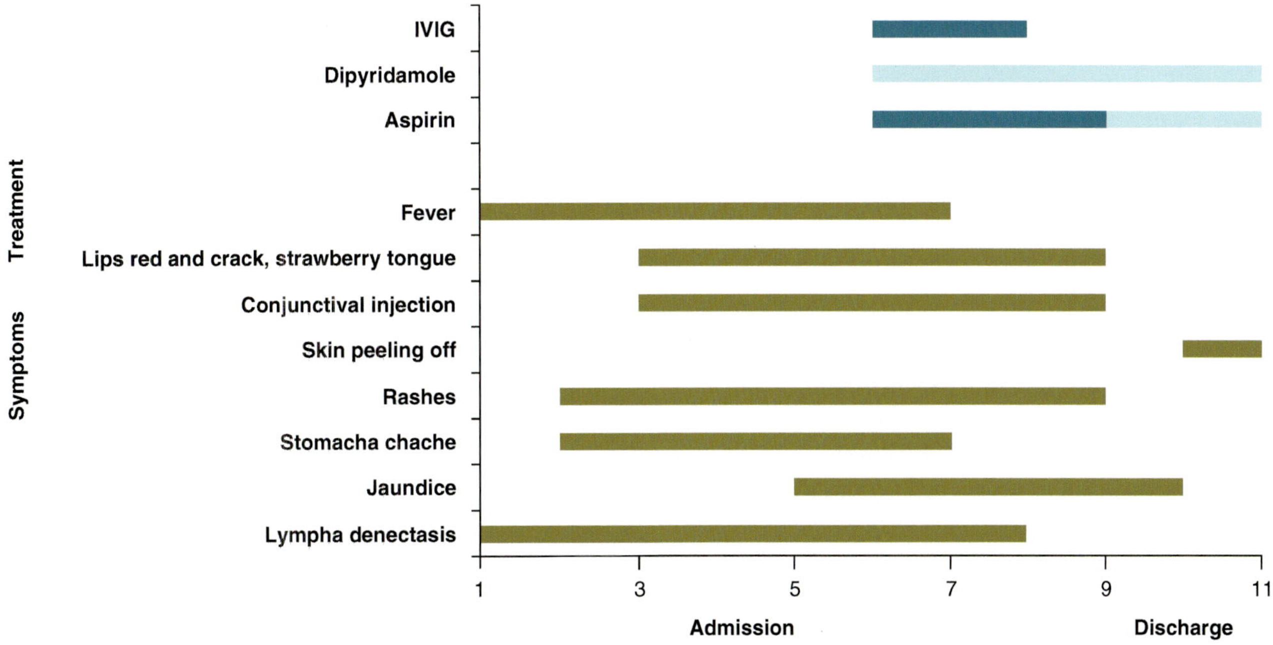

2.12.2 Follow-Up

Since discharge, he took oral Chinese traditional medication to help blood production, along with aspirin, and dipyridamole.

On Day 17, CBC showed WBC and NE were normal, PLT 449 × 10^9/L. NT-pro BNP and γ-GT was normal. EBV IgG revealed post-infection. ESR 34 mm/h. Oral traditional Chinese medicine was stopped. At 2 months, PLT 354 × 10^9/L and ESR 11 mm were almost normal. Echocardiography showed coronary artery was still normal. All medications were stopped.

2.12.3 Diagnosis

1. KD
2. I°AVB
3. Cholestatic hepatitis
4. Aseptic urethritis
5. Seroperitoneum
6. Hyponatremia
7. Hypokalemia
8. Hypoalbuminemia
9. Granulocytopenia.

2.12.4 Discussion

He met all criteria for KD; he had persistent fever over 5 days and was irresponsive to blood sputum antibiotics, along with (i) lymphadenectasis; (ii) bilateral conjunctival congestion; (iii) striking red lips; (iv) rashes all over the body; (v) peeling skin around fingernails on Day 10 of illness.

He also met cholestatic hepatitis criteria [54]: (1) he had KD; (2) jaundice was found on the face and drunk; (3) investigation revealed TP 57.0 g/L, ALB 32.5 g/L, ALT 300 U/L, AST 69 U/L. AKP 386 U/L, γ-GT 283 U/L, T Bil 75.9 μmol/L, D Bil 58.9 μmol/L, TBA 164.8 μmol/L. Urine test showed protein +g/L. Leucocyte esterase +3/μl. Urobilinogen +μmol/L, urine bilirubin ++μmol/L; (4) after IVIG and aspirin treatment, skin jaundice disappeared, and both liver function and urine routine were recovered to normal.

Differential diagnosis for CAEBV and hepatitis A or B should be considered.

2.12.5 Case Specific Clinical Features

1. KD results in cardiac damage including myocarditis (case 1), abnormal cardiac conduction system [55] (case 14), changes in valves, pericardial effusion (see case 4), and so on. This boy had I°AVB (PR interval should be less than 120 ms in a 4-year-old child with HR 150 bpm) and transient T wave inversion on Day 5. On Day 6, both ABV (PR interval should be less than 140 ms in a 4-year-old child with HR 113 bpm.) and T wave was improved. On Day 7, his ECG was normal. These data indicated myocardium damage, but insufficient for myocarditis. I°AVB means PR interval is over normal high value, usually over 180 ms in children and over 200 ms in adult. Additionally, though some PR interval was not over normal high value, the PR interval was prolonged by 10 ms when HR remained the same or higher. Most I°AVB happened in the condition of infection, some happened in congenital heart disease, digitalism, hypokalemia, or increased vagal tone [57]. This boy was found to have I°AVB on Day 4 and K^+ was normal. He developed hypokalemia and hyponatremia, his ECG recovered later. ASO was normal. We could not explain his symptoms using other conditions but KD only.
2. Jaundice often occurs in KD when complicated with cholesterol hepatitis, but jaundice on the skin is often misdiagnosed as hepatitis A, as reported in literature [57]. Cholesterol hepatitis is caused by small vessel vasculitis. This boy had acute cholangitis complication. Although glucocorticoid can relieve cholestasis, it is considered as one of the independent risk factors causing coronary artery lesion. Therefore, we could not use it to treat the patient. After IVIG and oral aspirin, his vessel vasculitis was under control and his cholangitis settled subsequently. Thus, he did not need to undergo surgery operation, but need to stay away from fatty food. It is necessary to limit fat intake for patients like him. With liver dysfunction, as soon as his temperature was under control in 36–48 h or even shorter, aspirin dose should be reduced soon to prevent the dysfunction aggravated.
3. Okano lay out the criteria for chronic active EB virus infection (CAEBV) in 2005 [58]. This boy had severe hepatic dysfunction at onset of illness. EBV IgG was dubious. Gastroenterologist was concerned about possible CAEBV, which was under special condition of an individual without clear immune dysfunction. EBV infection may result in chronic and recurrent symptoms of infectious mononucleosis syndrome, and corresponding EBV-Ab changes were called CAEBV [59]. Retested EBV revealed he had no recent infection and no elevated atypical lymphocyte. Therefore it was not sufficient to make the diagnosis of CAEBV. However, it was necessary to be careful. After all, the prognosis was not so well.

Hong Wang

2.13 Case 13 KD with Frequent Premature Ventricular Contraction

A previously healthy 3-year-old boy had no significant past medical and family history.

He presented on Day 4 of illness with a diarrhea and intermittent fever for 4 days along with bilateral conjunctival hyperemia, dry and cracked lips history. **Examination** revealed he had fever (38.9 °C), smooth breath (HR 116 bpm, RR 24 bpm), warm hands and feet (BP 85/50 mmHg). A few congest papules on his forehead. Cervical lymphadenectasis was found on the left side. He had non-purulent bilateral conjunctival hyperemia, dry and cracked lips with strawberry tongue. He had hepatomegaly (liver edge from right costal margin was 2 cm andIIcirrhosis). In addition, auscultation assessment revealed that his heart rhythm was irregular, 2 premature pbm without murmur. Others were normal. Blood test at admission revealed WBC 9.36×10^9/L, NE 61.87%, HB 123 g/L, PLT 164×10^9/L, CRP 14.7 mg/L, ESR 13 mm/h, normal cTnI and hs-cTnT, elevated NT pro-BNP (499 ng/ml), ECG sinus rhythm, HR 93 bpm, frequent PVC (Fig. 2.92a, b). Liver function and routine stool tests were normal. Rotavirus antibodies were negative. MP-IgM was positive. Due to continuous fever for 2 days, with no other obvious diagnosis, he was treatment with (i) infusion of ceftezole and erythromycin; (ii) infusion of nutritional creatine phosphate sodium 1 g/d and levocarnitine 20 mg/kg/d; (iii) oral montmorillonite and bifidobacterium tetravaccine tablets.

On Day 7, he still had fever but diarrhea was relieved. Cervical ultrasound: the largest cervical lymph node was 3 cm × 1 cm on the left. Echocardiography showed RCA and LCA were normal. Abdominal ultrasound was normal. He had met full criteria for KD, and he was treated with (i) oral aspirin 30–50 mg/kg/d and dipyridamole 3–5 mg/kg/d, in three divided doses; 2) IVIG 1 g/kg/d for 2 days (but his parents refused to receive this treatment until on Day 8). On Day 9, his fever and conjunctivitis were settled. On Day 11, aspirin was decreased to 3–5 mg/kg/d after afebrile over 48 h. Retested blood work revealed normal CBC, CRP, and NT pro-BNP (Table 2.10). On Day 12, peeling skin occurred around fingernails. Holter showed sinus rhythm, the total HR was 134,404 with the highest HR at 141 bpm, the lowest HR was 58 bpm, the average HR was 94 bpm, and the total PVC was 10,777 times, ventricular trigeminy was 66 times, first degree atrioventricular block (AVB) (Fig. 2.93) (Fig. 2.94a, b). On Day 14, he was discharged.

2.13.1 Clinical Course of the Patient

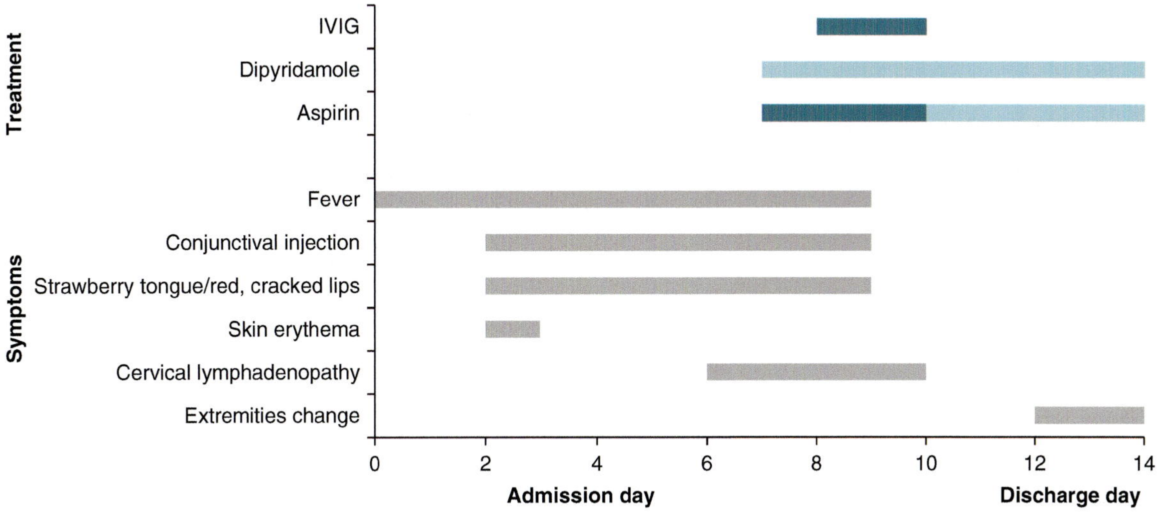

2.13.2 Follow-Up

Since discharged, she took (i) oral aspirin and dipyridamole 3–5 mg/kg/d about 2 months; (ii) FDP and levocarnitine for management of myocardial nutrition about 2 months.

At 2 months of illness, repeated echocardiography showed normal results. Until 5 years after the onset, his coronary artery was still normal, but he has not had Holter recorded, ECG was normal on 4 and 5 years of illness (Fig. 2.95a, b) (Fig. 2.96). Auscultation assessment for 1 min did not find premature contraction.

2.13.3 Diagnosis

1. KD
2. Arrhythmia: frequent PVC

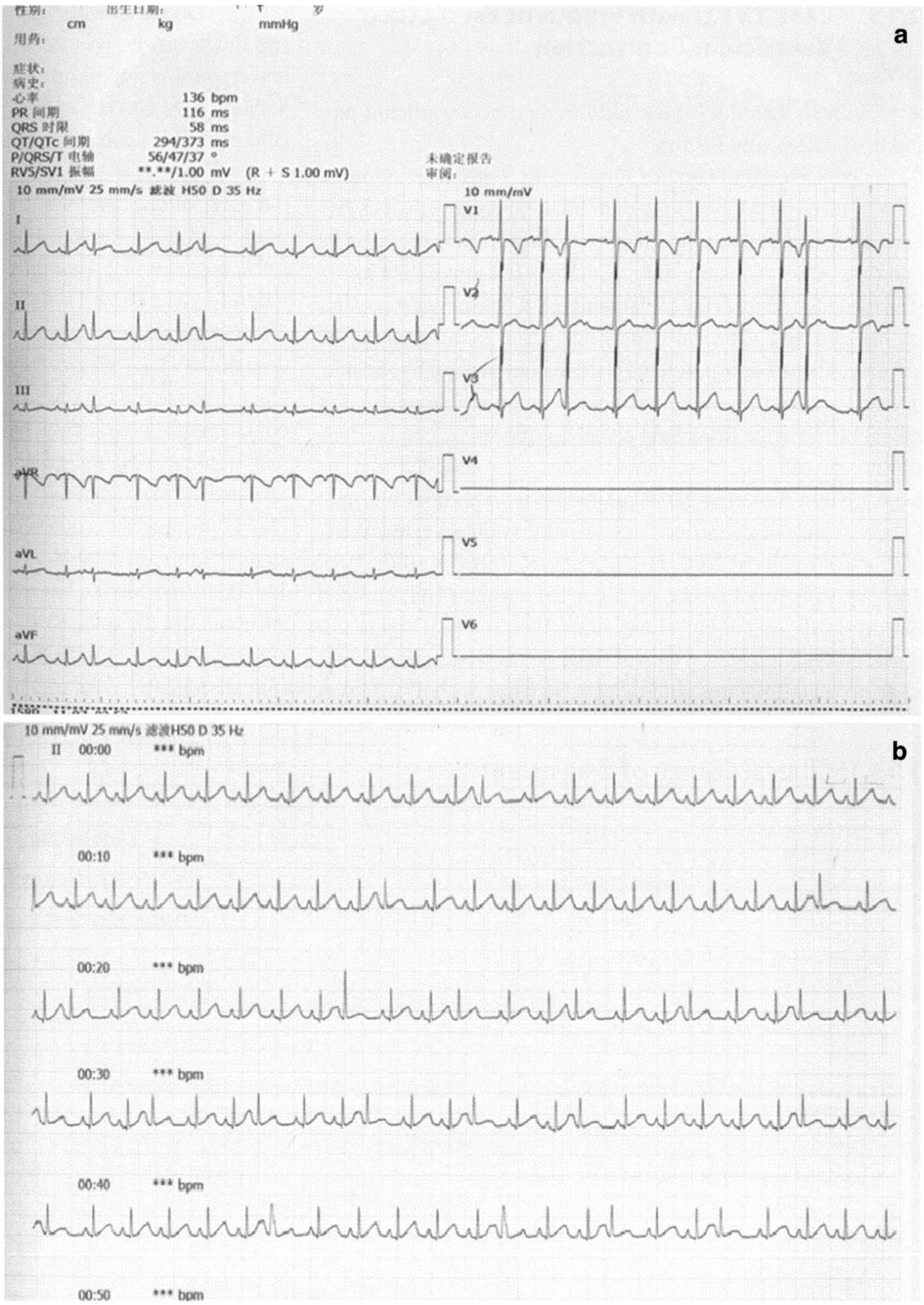

Fig. 2.92 On Day 4 of illness, 12 lead ECG (**a**) and long II (**b**) showed sinus rhythm, HR 93 bpm, frequent PVC

心律失常数据统计表

Hour	HR n/min	MinHR n/min	MaxHR n/min	VE n	VE Pair n	VE Run n	VE Big n	VE Trig n	SVE n	SVE Pair n	SVE Run n	SVE Big n	SVE Trig n	L n
08:30 09:30	137	113	173	0	0	0	0	0	422	0	0	2	36	0
09:30 10:30	127	112	146	0	0	0	0	0	1091	0	0	0	85	0
10:30 11:30	130	116	146	0	0	0	0	0	738	0	0	1	55	0
11:30 12:30	146	127	169	0	0	0	0	0	567	0	0	1	51	0
12:30 13:30	146	133	160	0	0	0	0	0	91	0	0	2	2	0
13:30 14:30	130	122	139	0	0	0	0	0	1051	0	0	5	106	0
14:30 15:30	130	118	142	0	0	0	0	0	840	0	0	1	67	0
15:30 16:30	146	134	157	0	0	0	0	0	287	0	0	0	19	0
16:30 17:30	141	125	162	0	0	0	0	0	351	0	0	14	19	0
17:30 18:30	133	118	151	0	0	0	0	0	662	0	0	29	19	0
18:30 19:30	136	125	150	0	0	0	0	0	173	0	0	2	6	0
19:30 20:30	130	111	155	0	0	0	0	0	391	0	0	2	21	0
20:30 21:30	116	103	131	0	0	0	0	0	445	0	0	0	28	0
21:30 22:30	120	109	134	0	0	0	0	0	462	0	0	0	19	0
22:30 23:30	121	110	134	0	0	0	0	0	527	0	0	0	24	0
23:30 00:30	126	112	142	0	0	0	0	0	577	0	0	0	47	0
00:30 01:30	130	114	151	0	0	0	0	0	984	0	0	0	15	0
01:30 02:30	123	112	136	0	0	0	0	0	919	0	0	3	27	0
02:30 03:30	120	108	134	0	0	0	0	0	659	0	0	1	54	0
03:30 04:30	122	107	142	0	0	0	0	0	966	0	0	0	60	0
04:30 05:30	137	117	164	0	0	0	0	0	705	0	0	0	31	0
05:30 06:30	139	121	162	0	0	0	0	0	1101	0	0	1	75	0
06:30 07:30	134	122	150	0	0	0	0	0	1144	0	0	2	101	0
07:30 08:07	144	127	176	0	0	0	0	0	557	0	0	1	27	0
All	131	109	176	0	0	0	0	0	15710	0	0	67	994	0

Fig. 2.93 On Day 12 of illness, the counting table of Holter

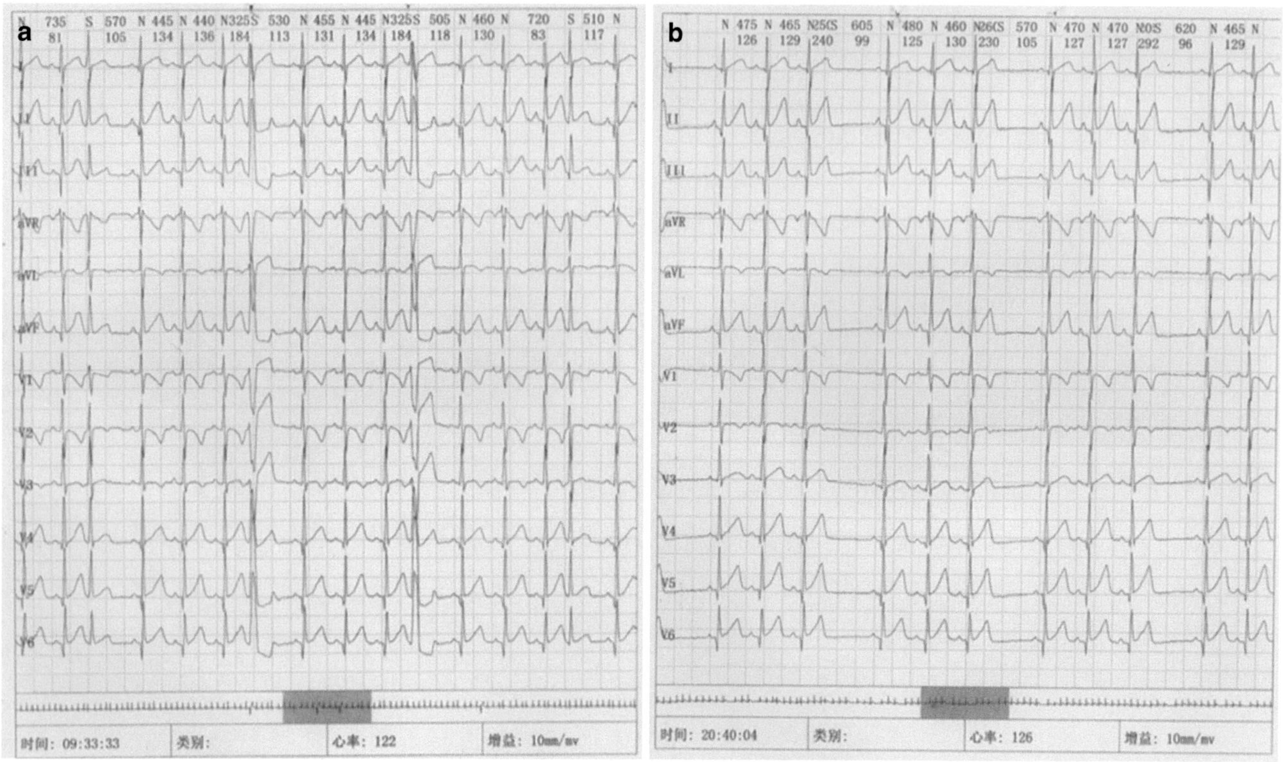

Fig. 2.94 On Day 12 of illness, Holter sinus rhythm, HR 80 bpm, PVC trigeminy (**a**), I°AVB (PR interval 210 ms) (**b**)

Table 2.10 The dynamic changes of lab parameters

Day	2	4	5	6	8	11	12	19	58
WBC ($\times 10^9$/L)	16.7	18.4			4.95		5.72		
NE (%)	67.7	89.6			21.1		18		
RBC ($\times 10^{12}$/L)		3.85			3.5		3.7		
HGB (g/L)	124	112			101		104		
PLT ($\times 10^9$/L)	355	442			558		615	449	354
CRP (mg/L)	57	75.9			25.4	12.1	8.22		
ALT (U/L)			300	194	81		40		
ALB (g/L)			32.5	27.2	37.7		37		
T Bile (mmpl/L)			75.9	62.2	18.3		10.5		
D Bile (mmpl/L)			58.9	53.1	11.8		8.2		
TBA (mg/L)			164.8		12.5		5.5		
γ-GT (U/L)			283		123		101	50	
NT-pro BNP (pg/ml)	659.7				1611	1034	709		

3. I°AVB
4. Acute diarrhea
5. MP infection

2.13.4 Discussion

KD is a type of febrile systemic vasculitis. Coronary artery aneurysms (CAA) or dilatation are the most common associated complications in KD, and may lead to myocardial infarction, sudden death, or ischemic heart disease. In addition, other relatively infrequent heart complications, especially cardiac arrhythmia have been noted which consist of premature contraction, atrioventricular heart block, ventricular tachycardia, ventricular fibrillation, those complications maybe life threatening sometimes. A study including 508 cases of KD showed 5.5% patients developed arrhythmias, and ST changes incidence rate was 5.6% [60]. The possible mechanism in KD leading to arrhythmia was that myocardial ischemia, myocardial interstitial edema, and micro-thrombus formation. Some patients even had normal ECG in the acute phase of KD, but developed arrhythmia several years later [61]. In our center there was a 2-year-old boy with IRBBB, QRS 98 ms at initial and developed CRBBB 10 years later, QRS 136 ms (see case 14). The prev-

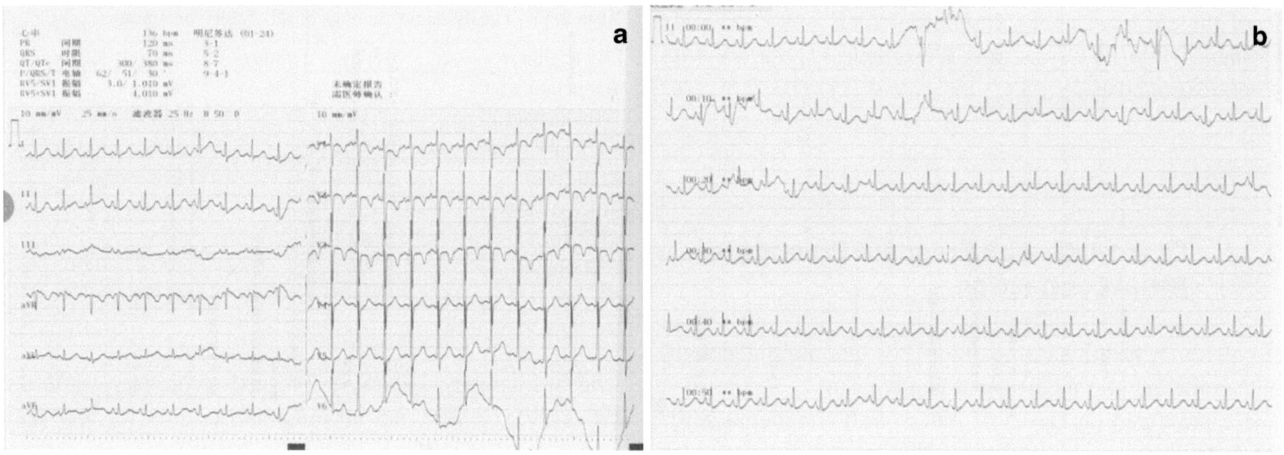

Fig. 2.95 At 4 years of illness, 12 leads ECG (**a**) and long II lead (**b**) were normal

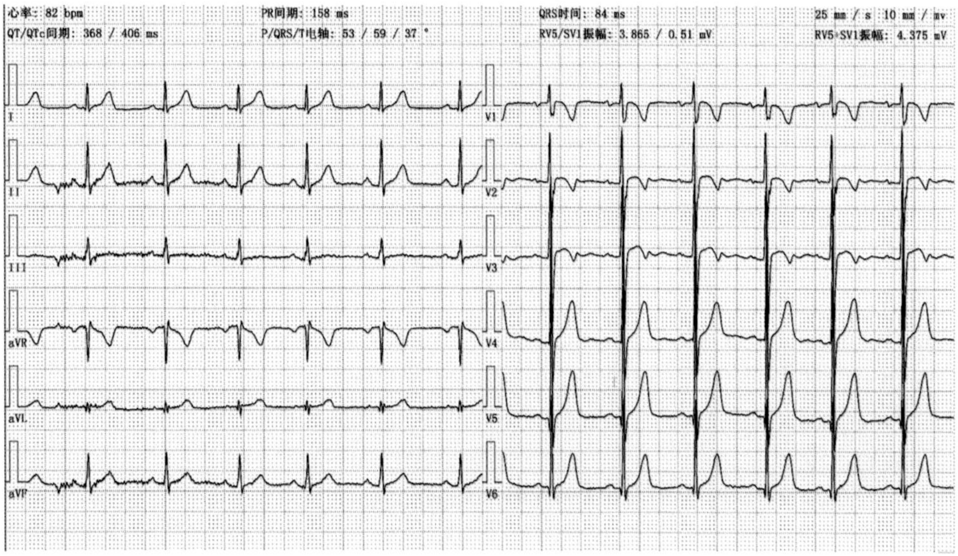

Fig. 2.96 At 5 years of illness, ECG was normal

alence of arrhythmia in adults who had been diagnosed with KD in childhood was higher than healthy people [61]; so regular follow-up must be performed on patients with a history of KD.

He was diagnosed with KD on the basis of the presence of fever over 5 days and the other clinical features (i) rashes; (ii) bilateral conjunctival hyperemia; (iii) dry and cracked lips with strawberry tongue; (iv) cervical lymphadenopathy >1.5 cm; (v) peeling skin around fingernails.

Arrhythmia may occasionally present in long-term follow-up KD patients with compromised left ventricular function and CAA, coronary artery stenosis, and thrombosis. Premature ventricular contraction (PVC) usually occurs in children with structural heart disease but can occur in up to 15% of infants, and 35% of children and adolescents without heart disease [62].

2.13.5 Case Specific Clinical Features

1. In this case, no coronary artery injury showed in echocardiography, PVC could be caused by myocardial ischemia due to myocardial damage and peripheral coronary artery stenosis [55], and these pathological changes cannot be found in routine investigation. Along with disappearance of vasculitis, myocardial ischemia was improved and PVC disappeared. In this case, Holter recorded PR interval was 210 ms, therefore I°AVB was diagnosed. KD could affect the atrioventricular conduction system, leading to sinus node dysfunction and atrioventricular block. This dysfunction and block were thought to be caused by ischemia of the sinus node and atrioventricular node, or caused by perivascular edema, cell infiltration, compression of conduction cells, and decreased microcirculation

of the coronary artery. In clinic, I°AVB was commonly seen, while PVC was rare. Nevertheless, both are with good prognosis.

Yan-qiu Chu

2.14 Case 14 KD with Frequent Premature Atrial Contraction

A previously healthy 11-month-old boy was presented without significant past medical and family history.

He presented on Day 5 of illness with continuous fever for 5 days along with bilateral conjunctival hyperemia, dry and cracked lips for 3 days, and a transient rash. **Examination** revealed T38 °C, smooth breath. HR 120 bpm, RR 35 bpm, BP 85/50 mmHg. He had bilateral conjunctival congestion and red lips. Erythema was found around BCG scar, palms, and soles. Hands were swollen. Anus was red without peeling skin. Cervical lymphadenectasis was found on both sides. Auscultation assessment revealed irregular heartbeats about 6 bpm, without murmur. Others were normal. Admission blood test revealed WBC, CRP, and NT-pro BNP elevation shown in Table 2.11. MP-IgG 1:640. Cervical ultrasound detected lymphadenectasis 2.9 cm × 0.9 cm on the left side, 2.0 cm × 0.8 cm on the right side. ECG showed sinus tachycardia, HR 136 bpm. Frequent premature atrial contraction (PAC). Atrial trigeminy, intraventricular aberrant conduction were identified (Figs. 2.97 and 2.98).

Table 2.11 The dynamic changes of laboratory parameters

Day of illness	5day	8day	11day	21day
Temperature (°C)	39.6	36.5	36	36.2
WBC ($\times 10^9$/L)	19.4		12.1	8.9
NE (%)	53.4		23.6	32
HGB (g/L)	106		115	126
PLT ($\times 10^9$/L)	325		532	337
CRP (mg/L)	60.2		8.56	3.6
ESR (mm/h)	61		79	20
NT pro-BNP (pg/ml)	428.9		161.8	

Echocardiography showed normal coronary arteries (Fig. 2.99). He had met all diagnosis criteria for KD, and treated with (i) IVIG 1 g/kg/d for 2 days; (ii) oral aspirin 30–50 mg/kg/d; dipyridamole 3–5 mg/kg/d, both in 3 divided doses; (iii) infusion of the second-generation of cephalosporin and erythromycin after blood sample taken to culture.

On Day 8, fever, conjunctivitis, and swollen hands were subsided. Holter showed sinus rhythm. The total HR was 186,697, the highest HR was 176 bpm, the lowest HR was 109 bpm, the average HR was 131 bpm (Fig. 2.100). The total PAC was 15,710 times. Atrial bigeminy was 67 times (Fig. 2.101a), atrial trigeminy was 994 times (Fig. 2.101b). Some PAC were accompanied with aberrant conduction, some were not transmitted. On Day 11, skin peeled off around finger nails on the right hand. Aspirin was reduced to one dose 3–5 mg/kg/d from last day. Re-evaluation of blood revealed ESR 79 mm/h, CRP 8.56 mg/L. NT pro-BNP 161.8 pg/ml. He was discharged.

2.14.1 Clinical Course of the Patient

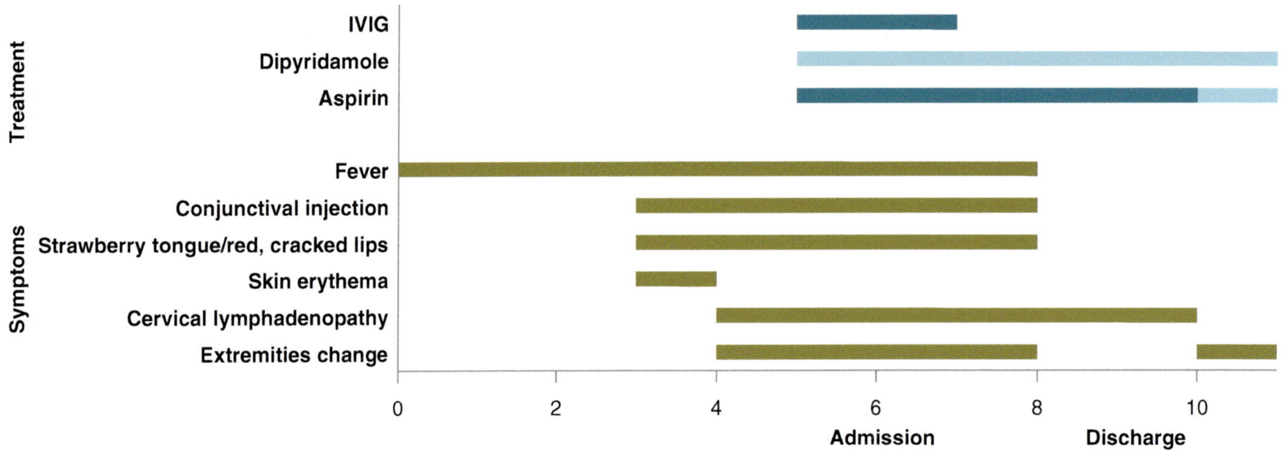

2.14.2 Follow-Up

Since discharged, he was on oral aspirin and dipyridamole 3–5 mg/kg/d. At 3 weeks of illness, routine blood test and CRP were normal. ESR was 20 mm/h. At 2 months of illness, LCA and RCA were still normal, and all medication were stopped. Without Holter recorded, both ECG (Fig. 2.102) (Fig. 2.103) and echocardiography were normal at 4 years of illness.

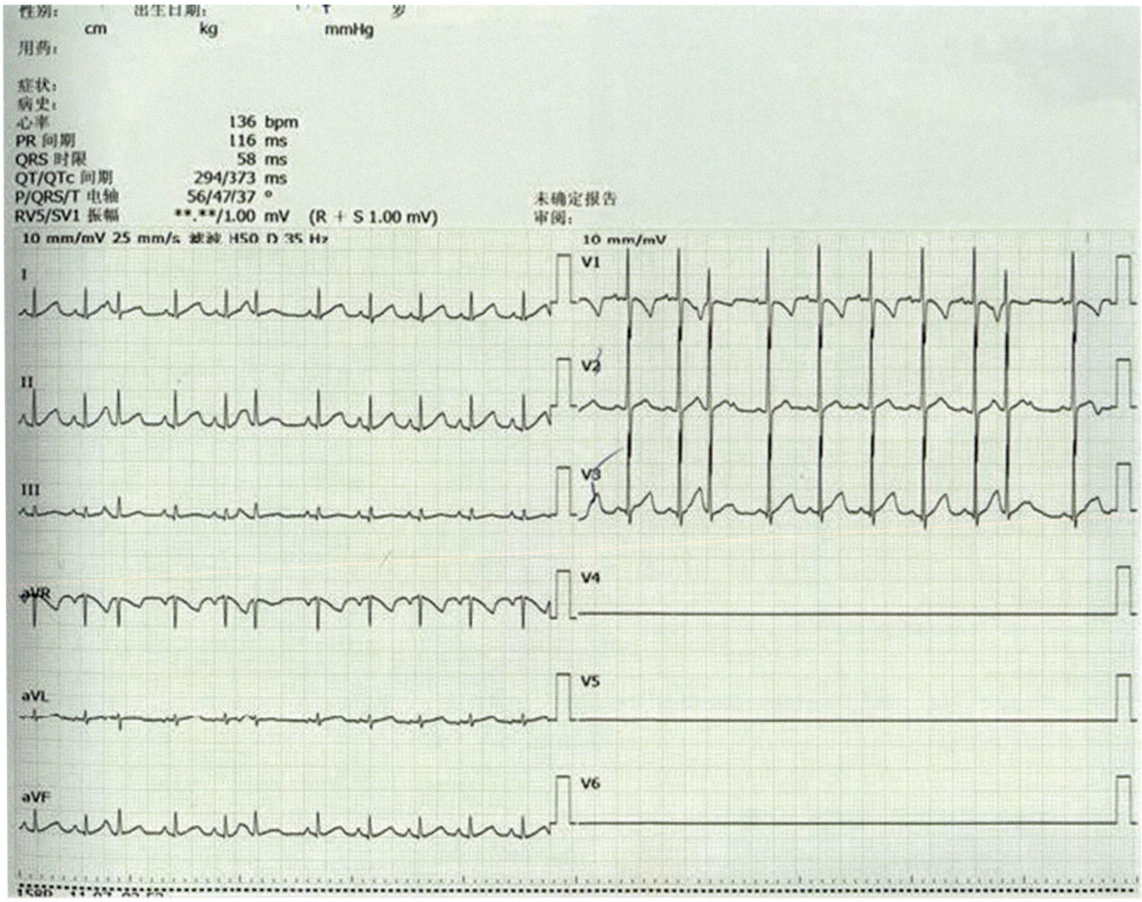

Fig. 2.97 On Day 5 of illness, ECG showed frequent PAC

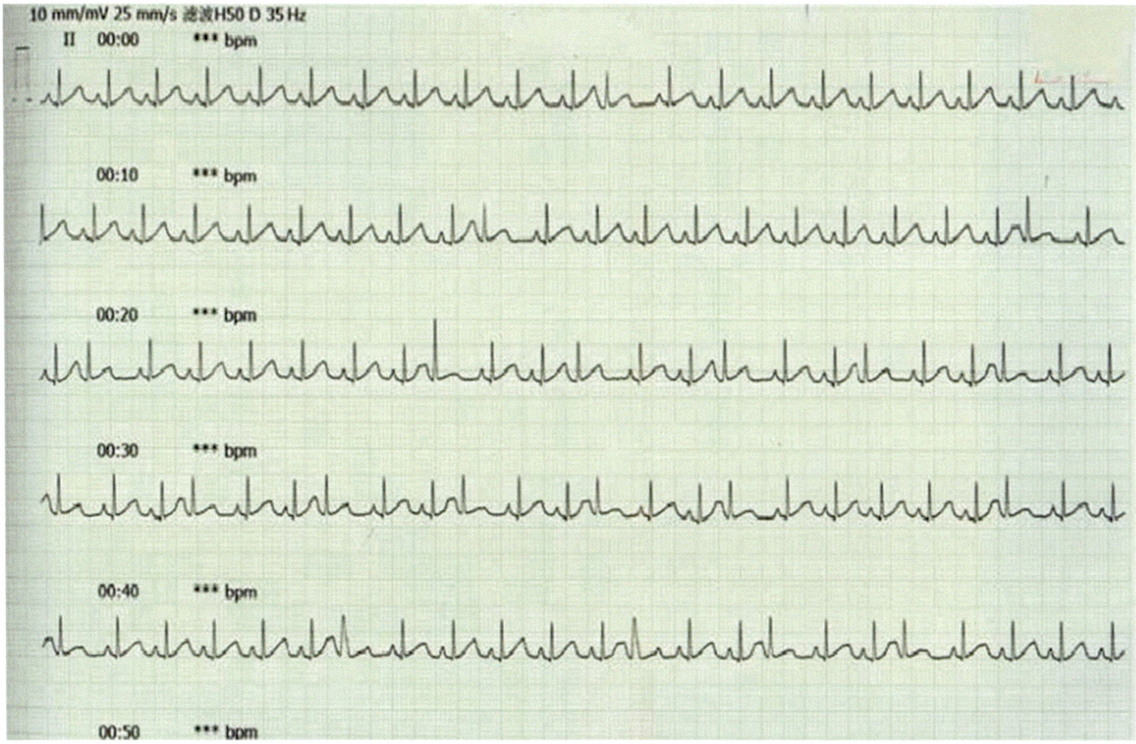

Fig. 2.98 On Day 5 of illness, ECG II showed frequent PAC, atrial trigeminy, intraventricular aberrant conduction

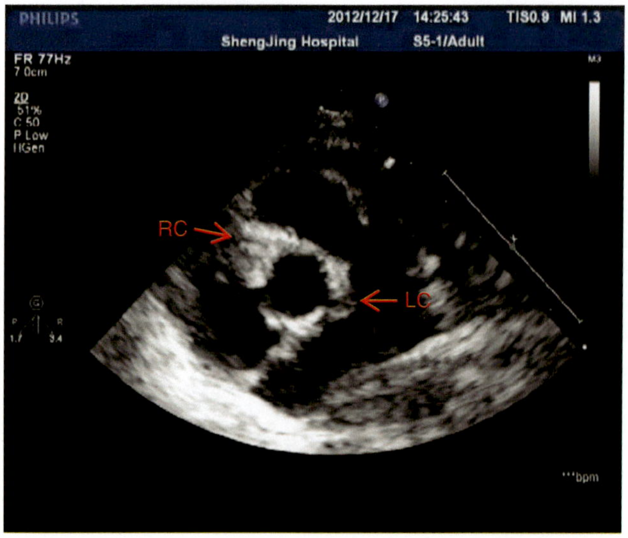

Fig. 2.99 On Day 5 of illness, echocardiography showed both LCA and RCA were normal

Fig. 2.100 On Day 9 of illness, counting table of Holter

Hour	HR n/min	MinHR n/min	MaxHR n/min	VE n	VE Pai n	VE Run n	VE Big n	VE Trig n	SVE n	SVE Pa n	SVE Ru n	SVE Bi n	SVE Trig n	L n
08:30 09:30	137	113	173	0	0	0	0	0	422	0	0	2	36	0
09:30 10:30	127	112	146	0	0	0	0	0	1091	0	0	0	85	0
10:30 11:30	130	116	146	0	0	0	0	0	738	0	0	1	55	0
11:30 12:30	146	127	169	0	0	0	0	0	567	0	0	1	51	0
12:30 13:30	146	133	160	0	0	0	0	0	91	0	0	2	2	0
13:30 14:30	130	122	139	0	0	0	0	0	1051	0	0	5	106	0
14:30 15:30	130	118	142	0	0	0	0	0	840	0	0	1	67	0
15:30 16:30	146	134	157	0	0	0	0	0	287	0	0	0	19	0
16:30 17:30	141	125	162	0	0	0	0	0	351	0	0	14	19	0
17:30 18:30	133	118	151	0	0	0	0	0	662	0	0	29	19	0
18:30 19:30	136	125	150	0	0	0	0	0	173	0	0	2	6	0
19:30 20:30	130	111	155	0	0	0	0	0	391	0	0	2	21	0
20:30 21:30	116	103	131	0	0	0	0	0	445	0	0	0	28	0
21:30 22:30	120	109	134	0	0	0	0	0	462	0	0	0	19	0
22:30 23:30	121	110	134	0	0	0	0	0	527	0	0	0	24	0
23:30 00:30	126	112	142	0	0	0	0	0	577	0	0	0	47	0
00:30 01:30	130	114	151	0	0	0	0	0	984	0	0	0	15	0
01:30 02:30	123	112	136	0	0	0	0	0	919	0	0	3	27	0
02:30 03:30	120	108	134	0	0	0	0	0	659	0	0	1	54	0
03:30 04:30	122	107	142	0	0	0	0	0	966	0	0	0	60	0
04:30 05:30	137	117	164	0	0	0	0	0	705	0	0	0	31	0
05:30 06:30	139	121	162	0	0	0	0	0	1101	0	0	1	75	0
06:30 07:30	134	122	150	0	0	0	0	0	1144	0	0	2	101	0
07:30 08:07	144	127	176	0	0	0	0	0	557	0	0	1	27	0
All	131	109	176	0	0	0	0	0	15710	0	0	67	994	0

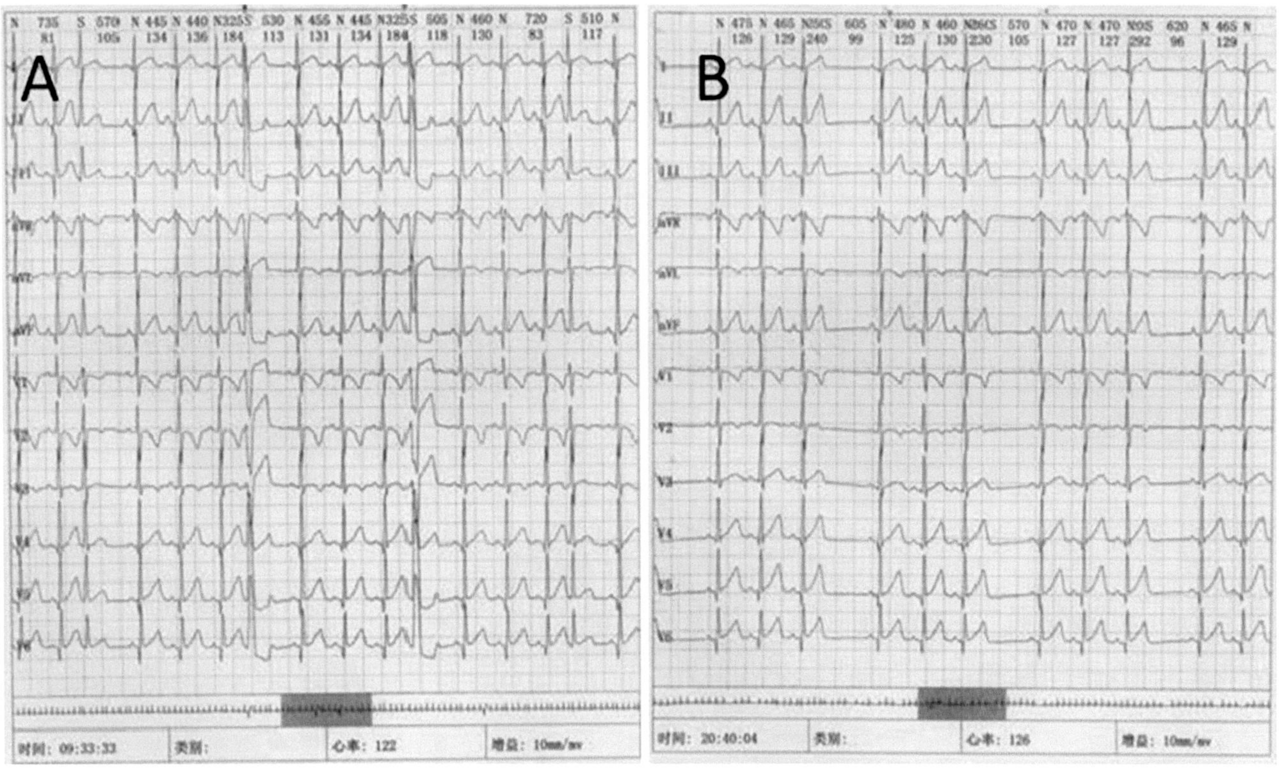

Fig. 2.101 On Day 9 of illness, some PAC accompanied with aberrant conduction (**a**), frequent PAC, some were not transmitted (**b**)

2.14.3 Diagnosis

1. KD
2. Frequent PAC
3. MP infection.

2.14.4 Discussion

He was diagnosed with KD on the basis of the presence of fever over 5 days and the presence of other clinical features; (i) he had transient rashes and around BCG scar erythema; (ii) bilateral conjunctival congestion, without purulent secretions; (iii) red and cracked lips; (iv) red palms and soles, edema hands and later peeling skin around fingernails; (v) cervical lymphadenopathy over 1.5 cm. As well as elevated WBC, CRP, and NT-pro BNP.

This 11-month-old boy developed a reaction at the BCG inoculation site. BCG reaction has been reported as a common finding in young patients with KD where BCG vaccination is mandatory. Edema, redness, ulcer changes, or crust formation at the BCG inoculation site were listed as a symptom or finding both on the fifth revised edition of the diagnostic guidelines of KD in Japan and in the American Heart Association Scientific Statement [63], but is not included in the diagnostic criteria. It was postulated that the erythematous changes at the BCG site are part of a generalized activation of the immune system and that molecules cross-reacting between the infectious agent involved and mycobacterial BCG antigens contribute to the inflammatory process. Reaction at the BCG inoculation site could be a useful diagnostic sign for KD, and it occurs more frequently in younger patients, especially in those less than 27 months of age. It would be a more useful sign than cervical lymphadenopathy for diagnosis of KD in this age group [64].

2.14.5 Case Specific Clinical Features

1. In this case, ECG was not performed before he was diagnosed with KD and did not have Holter recorded after discharged. Thus, we cannot determine whether PAC was related to KD. But ECG was normal at 4 years of illness.
2. KD can lead to arrhythmia, and the mechanism is not very clear yet. Most scholars believe that arrhythmia is related to myocardial inflammation, cell edema, and myocardial ischemia. Unlike other arrhythmias, PAC is more likely to be related to myocardial ischemia [55]. Furthermore, as an inflammatory disease, KD can lead to a series of inflammatory factors releasing that may possibly cause immune injury of the cardiac conduction system, contributing to cardiac arrhythmia [65].

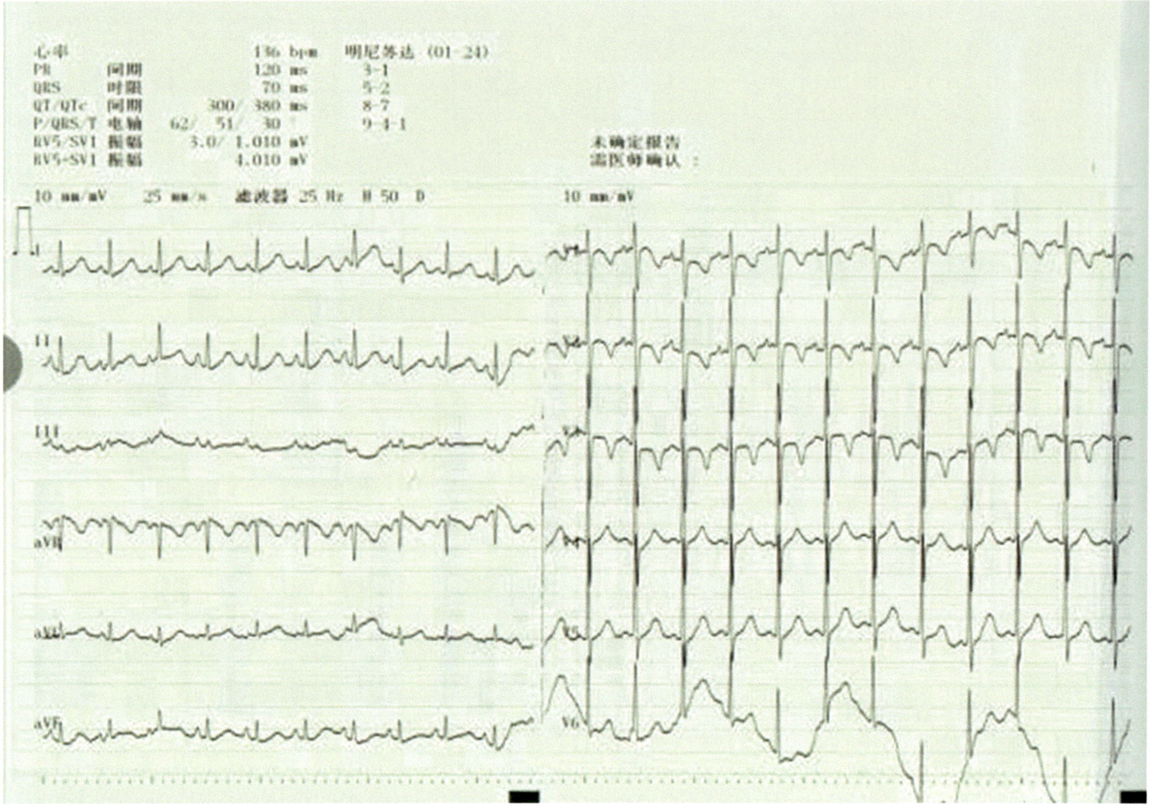

Fig. 2.102 At 4 years of illness, ECG was normal

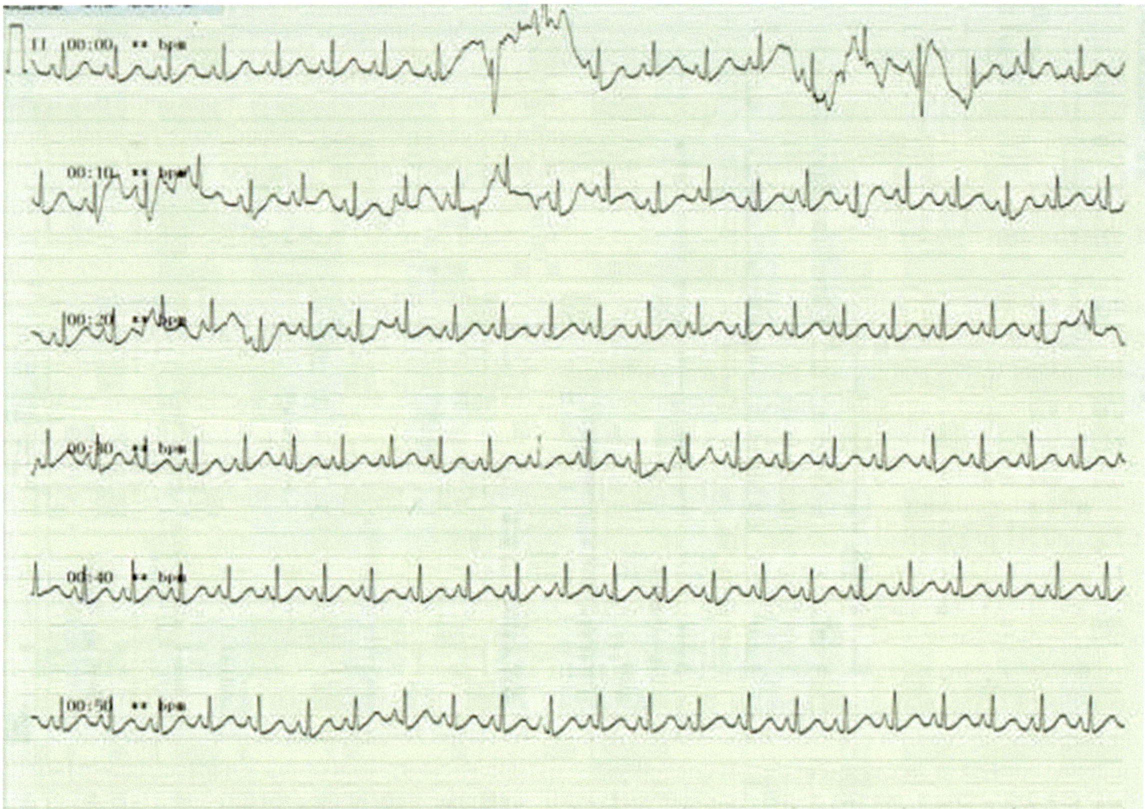

Fig. 2.103 At 4 years of illness, ECGIIwas normal

Yan-qiu Chu

2.15 Case 15 KD with CRBBB

A previous healthy 2-year-old boy had no significant past medical and family history.

He presented on Day 9 of illness. His fever started 6 h after DPT vaccination and last for 9 days along with rashes for 3 days and red conjunctiva, red lips for 1 day. Since the onset, his mental state was nice. He lost appetite, without vomit or diarrhea. Examination revealed cervical lymphadenectasis about 2 cm on the left, rashes on the back, red conjunctiva with red and dry lips. His liver was enlarged 2 cm below right costal margin. Others were normal. After 9 days of fever and 5 criteria reached for KD, he was given IVIG 2 g/kg, oral aspirin 30–50 mg/kg/d, and dipyridamole 3–5 mg/kg/d. Auxiliary examinations revealed normal complete blood count. ECG showed incomplete right bundle branch block (IRBBB) (Fig. 2.104). Echocardiography showed no coronary damage (Fig. 2.105a). Lung CT scan indicated acute bronchial pneumonia. He was treated with infusion of erythromycin.

On Day 11, fever was settled while rashes and red conjunctiva also subsided. Investigation revealed ALB 28.4 g/L; MP IgG 1:40. Twenty grams of albumin was infused to the patient. On Day 12, he got fever again, with cough. Retested WBC was normal. Infusion of erythromycin and oral antiviral drugs were continued. On Day 15, he was afebrile over 48 h, additional congestive rash appeared on his upper limbs. Drug related rash was considered after consulting with dermatologist. Thus, we switched the intravenous erythromycin to oral azithromycin, and reduced aspirin to one dose of 3–5 mg/kg/d. On Day 16, repeated echocardiography showed LCA was mild dilated to LCA 3.1 mm (Fig. 2.105b). On Day 22, retested blood work showed PLT 652 × 10^9/L. CK 254 IU/L, CK-MB 33 IU/L. He started to take oral coenzymum Q10 and fructose sodium diphosphate.

On Day 24, all symptoms subsided. Repeated chest CT showed inflammation was absorbed, coronary artery CTA showed normal result, LCA 2.8 mm, RCA 1.7 mm (no image saved). He was discharged.

2.15.1 Clinical Course of the Patient

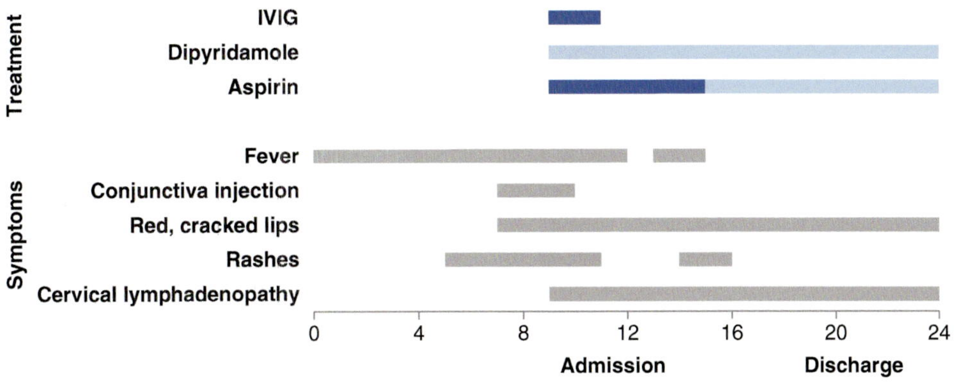

2.15.2 Follow-Up

Since discharge, he was prescribed with daily oral aspirin and dipyridamole. Echocardiography was performed at 1, 2, and 3 months. The coronary artery remained normal, without ECG being recorded. He stopped taking any medication at 3 months of illness.

Ten years later, the boy felt hard to breath and chest pain on the left during running. Therefore, he went to local hospital. Abnormality was found in ECG. Then he came back to our clinic. ECG showed CRBBB (Fig. 2.106). Echocardiography was normal (Fig. 2.107a–c). Coronary artery CTA showed normal (Fig. 2.108). At 11 years of illness, echocardiography showed normal result (Fig. 2.109a, b). At 13 years of illness, ECG showed CRBBB) (Fig. 2.110).

2.15.3 Diagnosis

1. KD
2. LCA dilation
3. CRBBB
4. Hypoalbuminemia
5. Thrombocytosis
6. HyperCKemias
7. Acute bronchopneumonia

2.15.4 Discussion

The boy had met the criteria of KD 12 years ago. He had persistent fever for 9 days, along with (i) rashes on face and trunk; (ii) cervical lymphadenopathy; (iii) lips red and

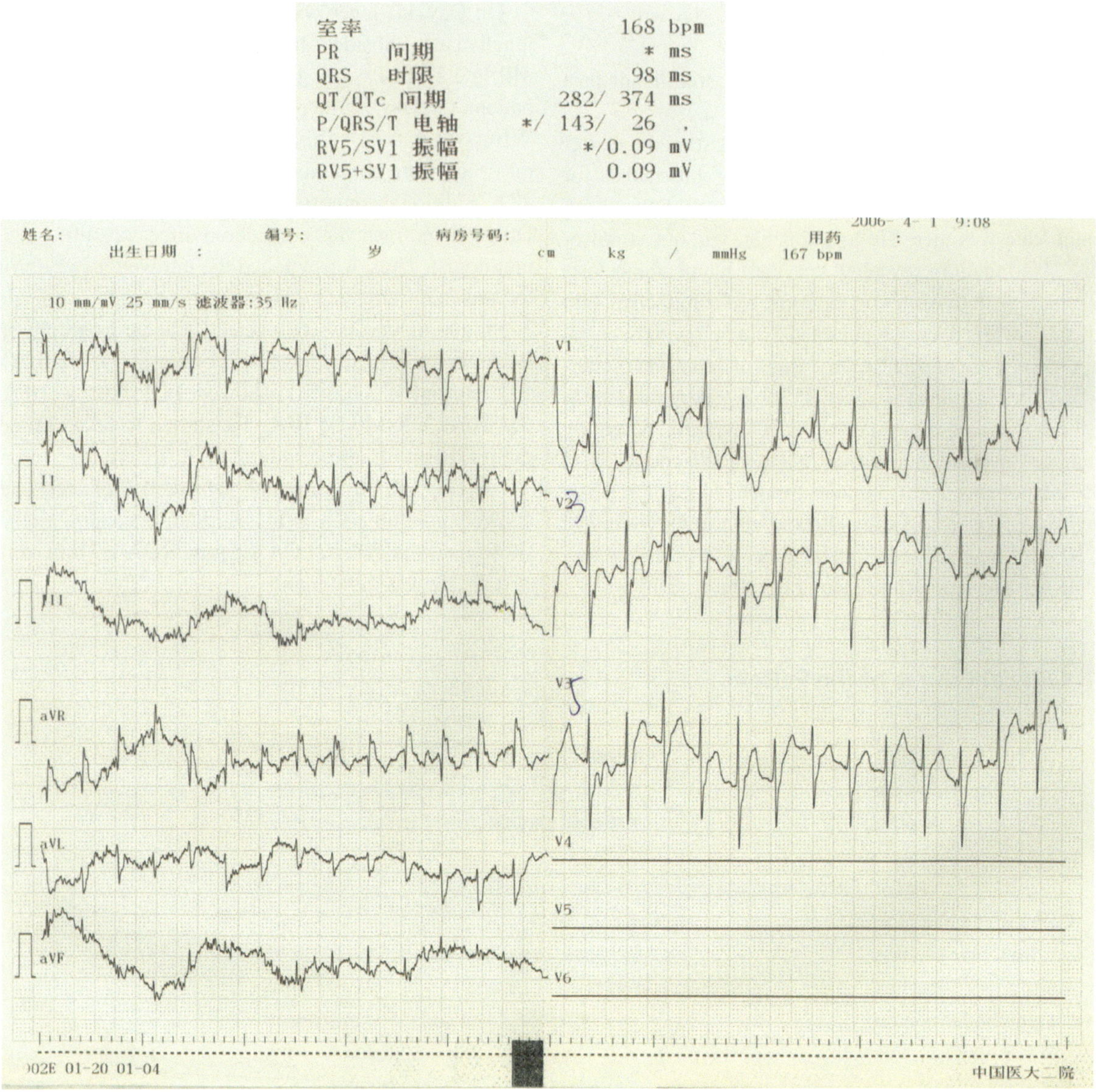

Fig. 2.104 On Day 9 of illness, ECG showed IRBBB, QRS 98 ms

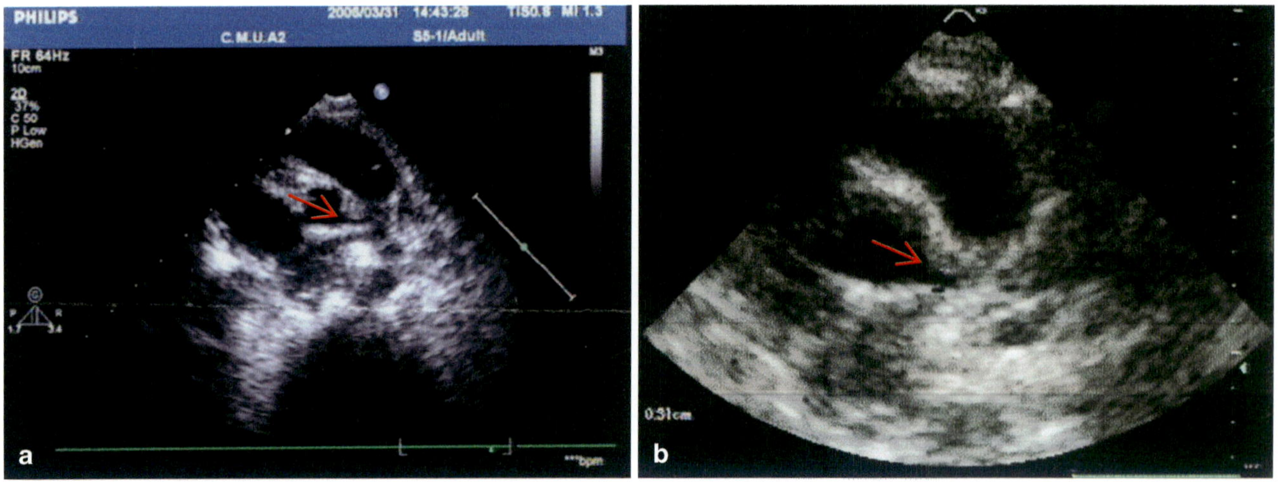

Fig. 2.105 On Day 9, echocardiography showed normal LCA (a), while it slightly dilated to 3.1 mm on Day 16 (b)

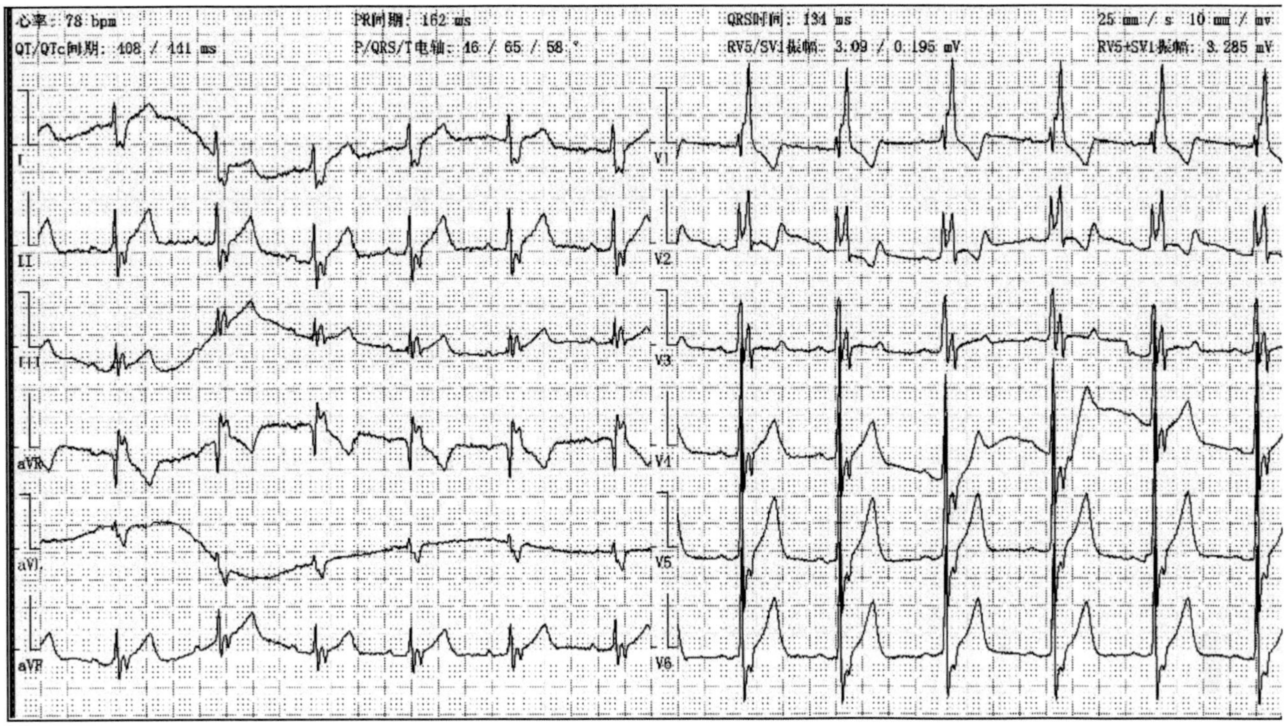

Fig. 2.106 At 10 years of illness, ECG showed CRBBB, QRS 134 ms

cracked; (iv) bilateral conjunctival congestion; (v) Echocardiography showed his LCA was mildly dilated.

The differential diagnosis from measles should be assessed. Firstly, he had vaccination of measles 1 year ago; secondly, his rashes appeared on Day 6 of fever; last, his blood test result was no measles-antibody detected at the third day after admission.

2.15.5 Case Specific Clinical Features

1. The atrioventricular bundle is divided into two branches from the front of the interventricular septum. The right bundle branches go along the right ventricular septum and the right ventricular wall. CRBBB is commonly seen in rheumatic heart disease, pulmonary heart disease, ventricular septum defect, coronary heart disease, and sometimes also in healthy people. The IRBBB was common in the ASD. However, his echocardiography failed to detect the atrial septum defect. Thus, we did not record it again since he was discharged.
2. Previous literature reported sudden cardiac arrest in an adolescent Chinese boy 11 years after KD [66], but without CRBBB. It may be related to inflammation aggravates heterogeneity of ventricular repolarization [67], or may be related to the changes of QT interval dispersion [68]. The ECG of this boy at the onset showed R_{V1} wave with a shape like M, but the QRS duration was only 96 ms. The S_{V5} wave was less than 40 ms without electrical axis bias. Thus, it belonged to normal ECG after echocardiography showed no ASD. Therefore when his coronary artery recovered, we usually did not ask for re-recording ECG after his discharge (this case happened in 2006). But 10 years later, when he felt hard breath during running, his ECG showed typical CRBBB, with the QRS duration194 ms. Then he came back to our clinic to follow up with examination. His coronary artery and systolic function were normal. His coronary artery CTA was normal as well. It coordinated with the literature that the small vasculitis can last for a long time [67], even with no known sequelae. Since then, repeated ECG together with echocardiography were performed regularly at our clinic as follow up procedures. We do not know when his ECG aggravation happened. Since his repeated ECG 1 year later remained unchanged, we deduced that his CRBBB may exist forever. We assumed that the scar maybe formed around the right bundle branch.

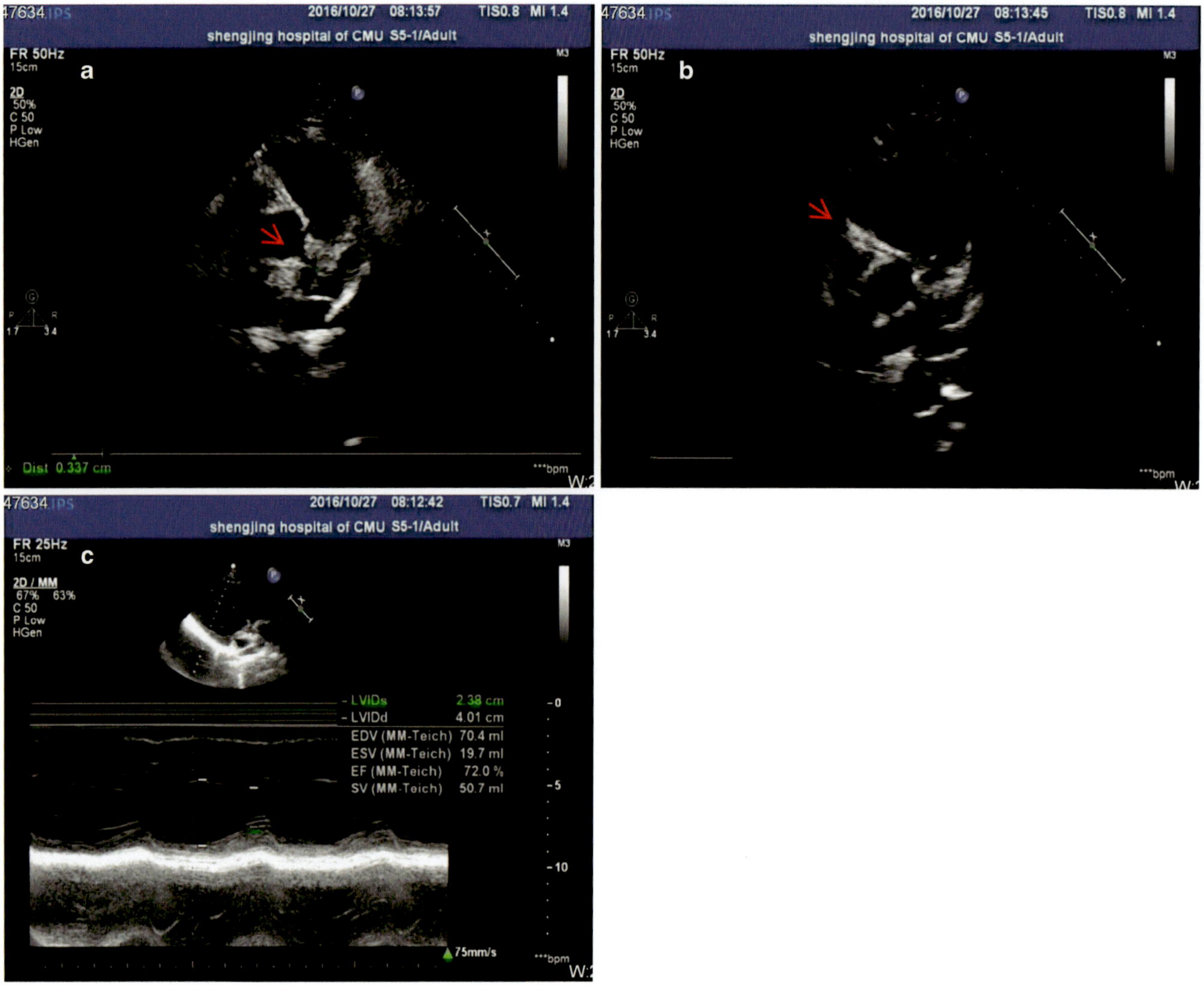

Fig. 2.107 At 10 years of illness, echo showed normal LCA (**a**), RCA (**b**), and LVEF (**c**)

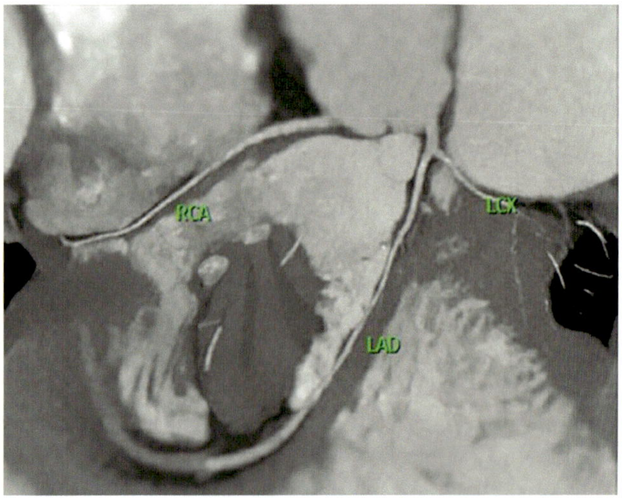

Fig. 2.108 At 10 years of illness, coronary artery CTA showed normal LCA and RCA

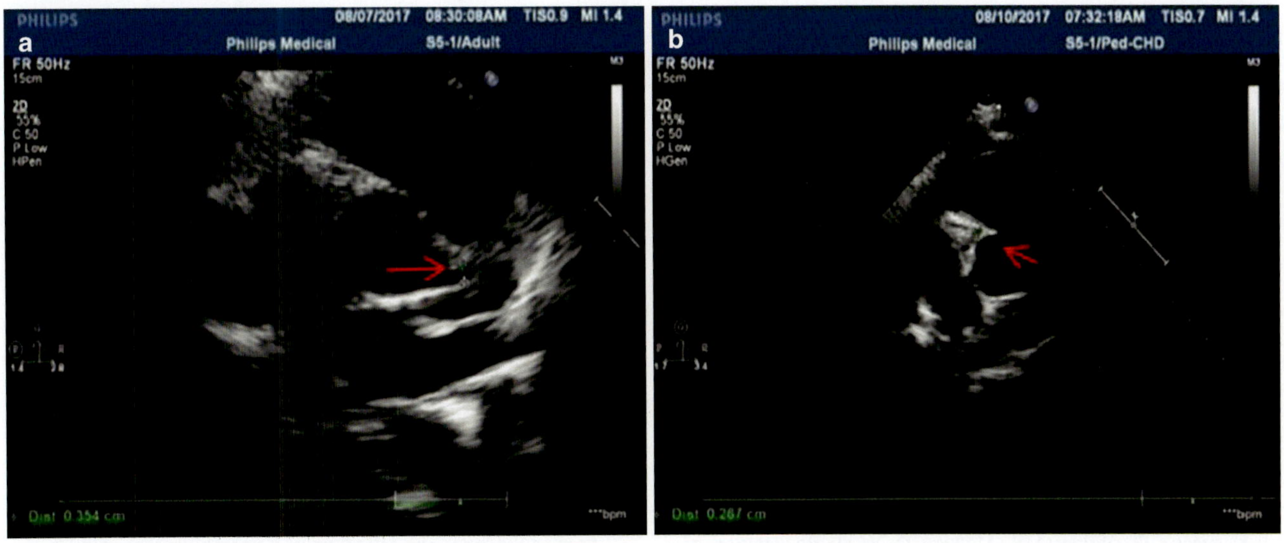

Fig. 2.109 At 11 years of illness, Echo showed normal LCA (**a**), RCA (**b**)

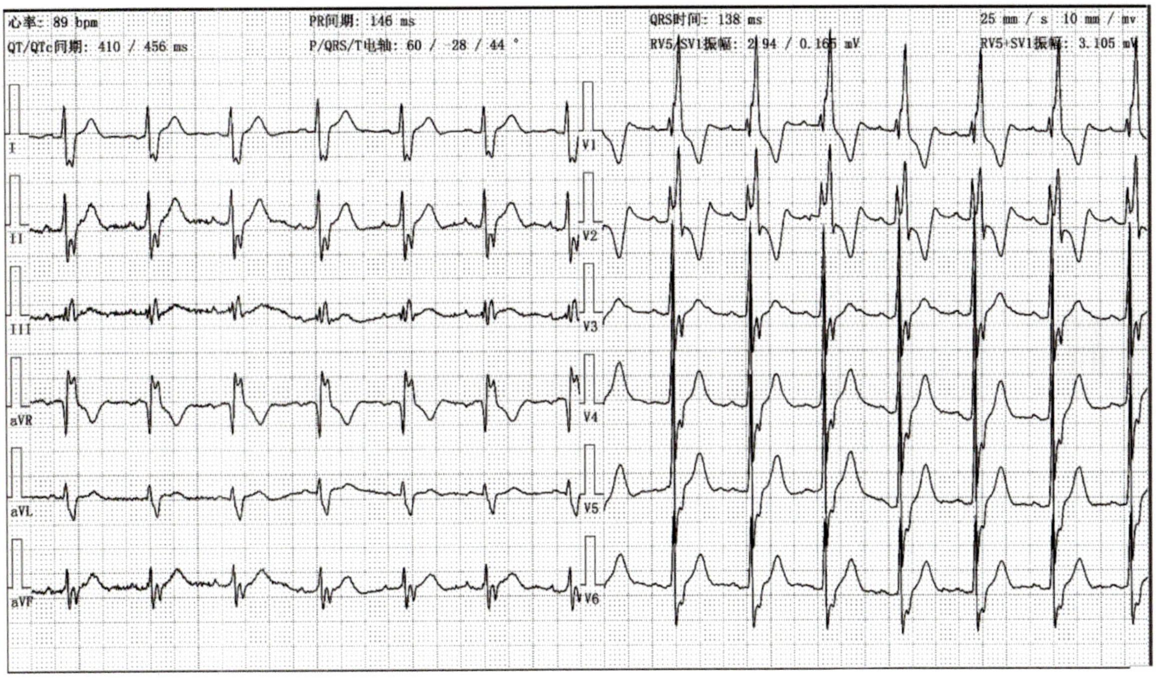

Fig. 2.110 At 11 years of illness, ECG showed CRBBB, QRS 138 ms

Yun-ming Xu

References

1. Research Committee of the Japanese Society of Pediatric Cardiology; Cardiac Surgery Committee for Development of Guidelines for Medical Treatment of Acute Kawasaki Disease Guidelines for medical treatment of acute Kawasaki disease: report of the Research Committee of the Japanese Society of Pediatric Cardiology and Cardiac Surgery (2012 revised version). Pediatr Int. 2014;56(2):135–58.
2. Sandeep S, Peter P, Leslie T. Myocarditis. Lancet. 2012;379(9817):738–47.
3. Yutani C, Go S, Kamiya T, et al. Cardiac biopsy of Kawasaki disease. Arch Pathol Lab Med. 1981;105:470–3.
4. Aggarwal P, Suri D, Narula N, et al. Symptomatic myocarditis in Kawasaki disease. Indian J Pediatr. 2012;79(6):813–4.
5. Yonesaka S, Takahashi T, Eto S, et al. Biopsy-proven myocardial sequels in Kawasaki disease with giant coronary aneurysms. Cardiol Young. 2010;20(6):602–9.
6. Zhang YL, Wang H, Yu XX, et al. Comparison analysis of muscle enzymes in children with myocarditis and Duchene/Becker muscular dystrophy. J Cent South Univ (Med Sci). 2016;41(9):984–91.

7. Numano F, Shimizu C, Tremoulet AH, et al. Pulmonary artery dilation and right ventricular function in acute Kawasaki disease. Pediatr Cardiol. 2016;37(3):482–90.
8. Richards JB, Wilcox SR. Diagnosis and management of shock in the emergency department. Emerg Med Pract. 2014;16(3):1–22.
9. Gámez-González LB, Murata C, Muñoz-Ramírez M, et al. Clinical manifestations associated with Kawasaki disease shock syndrome in Mexican children. Eur J Pediatr. 2013;172(3):337–42.
10. İşgüder R, Doksöz Ö, Bağ Ö, et al. Kawasaki disease shock syndrome: a severe form of Kawasaki disease. Turk J Pediatr. 2013;55(3):319–21.
11. April MM, Burns JC, Newburger JW, et al. Kawasaki disease cervical lymphadenopathy. Arch Otolaryngol Head Neck Surg. 1989;115(3):512–4.
12. Zhang MM, Shi L, Li XH, et al. Clinical analysis of Kawasaki disease shock syndrome. Chin Med J (Engl). 2017;130(23):2891–2.
13. Kurokawa Y, Masuda H, Kobayashi T, et al. Effective therapy with infliximab for clinically mild encephalitis/encephalopathy with a reversible splenial lesion in an infant with Kawasaki disease. J Med Invest. 2017;40(3):190–5.
14. Kanegaye JT, Wilder MS, Molkara D, et al. Recognition of a Kawasaki disease shock syndrome. Pediatrics. 2009;123:e783–9.
15. Gatterre P, Oualha M, Dupic L, et al. Kawasaki disease: an unexpected etiology of shock and multiple organ dysfunction syndrome. Intensive Care Med. 2012;38:872–8.
16. Gao SY, Li XA, Li RY, et al. The relationship between viral infection and Kawasaki disease. Shandong Pharm. 2014;54(10):66–7.
17. Li YH, Wu BQ, Huang RG, et al. Kawasaki disease complicated with Mycoplasma pneumoniae in children with laboratory tests and clinical features. Chin Gen Pract. 2012;15(88):2649–51.
18. Kusakawa S, Heiner DC. Elevated levels of immunoglobulin E in the acute febrile mucocutaneous lymph node syndrome. Pediatr Res. 1976;10(2):108–11.
19. Wang H, Liu S, Xing YL, et al. The limitation of MB isoenzyme of creatine kinase mass in assess myocardial injury with muscular disease. Zhongguo Wei Zhong Bing Ji Jiu Yi Xue. 2011;23(12):723–6.
20. Tsai YJ, Lin CH, Fu LS, et al. The association between Kawasaki disease and allergic diseases, from infancy to school age. Allergy Asthma Proc. 2013;34(5):467–72.
21. Woon PY, Chang WC, Liang CC, et al. Increased risk of atopic dermatitis in preschool children with Kawasaki disease: a population-based study in Taiwan. Evid Based Complement Alternat Med. 2013;605123
22. Terai M, Shulman ST. Prevalence of coronary artery abnormalities in Kawasaki disease is highly dependent on gamma globulin dose but independent of salicylate dose. J Pediatr. 1997;131(6):888–93.
23. Zhou YC, Guo WX. Ultrasonic medicine. 4th ed. Beijing: Scientific and Technological Literature Press; 2003. p. 649–52.
24. Kato H, Koike S, Yokoyama T. Kawasaki disease: effect of treatment on coronary artery involvement. Pediatrics. 1979;63(2):175–9.
25. Kobayashi T, Saji T, Otani T, et al. Efficacy of immunoglobulin plus prednisolone for prevention of coronary artery abnormalities in severe Kawasaki disease (RAISE study): a randomized, open-label, blinded-endpoints trial. Lancet. 2012;379(9826): 1613–20.
26. Athappan G, Gale S, Ponniah T. Corticosteroid therapy for primary treatment of Kawasaki disease-weight of evidence: a meta-analysis and systematic review of the literature. Cardiovasc J Afr. 2009;20(4):233–6.
27. Newburger JW, Takahashi M, Gerber MA, et al. Diagnosis, treatment, and long-term management of Kawasaki disease: a statement for health professionals from the Committee on Rheumatic Fever, Endocarditis, and Kawasaki Disease, Council on Cardiovascular Disease in the Young. Am Heart Assoc Pediatr. 2004;114(6):1708–33.
28. Singh S, Newburger JW, Kuijpers T, et al. Management of Kawasaki disease in resource-limited settings. Pediatr Infect Dis J. 2015;34(1):94–6.
29. Xue XD. Pediatrics [M]. Beijing: People's Medical Publishing House; 2005. p. 201.
30. Kobayashi T, Inoue Y, Takeuchi K, et al. Prediction of intravenous immune globulin unresponsiveness in patients with Kawasaki disease. Circulation. 2006;113(22):2606–12.
31. Xing YL, Wang H, Yu XY, et al. Assessment of coronary artery lesions in children with Kawasaki disease: evaluation of MSCT in comparision with 2-D echocardiography. Pediatr Radiol. 2009;39(11):1209–15.
32. Sugahara Y, Ishii M, Muta H, et al. Warfarin therapy for giant aneurysm prevents myocardial infarction in Kawasaki disease. Pediatr Cardiol. 2008;29(2):398–401.
33. Xing YL, Wang H, Yu XY, et al. Assessment of coronary artery lesions in children with Kawasaki disease: evaluation of MSCT in comparison with 2-D echocardiography. Pediatr Radiol. 2009;39(11):1209–15.
34. Dadlani GH, Gingell RL, Orie JD, et al. Coronary artery calcifications in the long-term follow-up of Kawasaki disease. Am Heart J. 2005;150(5):1016.
35. Orenstein JM, Shulman ST, Fox LM, et al. Three linked vasculopathic processes characterize Kawasaki disease: a light and transmission electron microscopic study. PLoS One. 2012;7(6):e38998. https://doi.org/10.1371/journal.pone.0038998.
36. Kamiya T, Suzuki A, Ono Y, et al. Angiographic follow-up study of coronary artery lesion in the cases with a history of Kawasaki disease–with a focus on the follow-up more than ten years after the onset of the disease. In: Kato H, editor. Kawasaki Disease. Proceedings of the fifth International Kawasaki Disease Symposium, Fukuoka, Japan, May 22–25, 1995. New York, NY: Elsevier Science; 1995. p. 569–73
37. Yokoi H. Long-term clinical follow-up after rotational atherectomy to coronary arterial stenosis in Kawasaki disease. Nihon Rinsho. 2008;66(2):373–9.
38. Soriano M, Martínez E, Negreira S, et al. Risk of coronary artery involvement in Kawasaki disease. Arch Argent Pediatr. 2016;114(2):107–13.
39. Zhao CN, Du ZD, Gao LL. Corticosteroid therapy might be associated with the development of coronary aneurysm in children with Kawasaki disease. Chin Med J. 2016;129(8):922–8.
40. Kim JJ, Hong YM, Yun SW, et al. Assessment of risk for Korean children with Kawasaki disease. Pediatr Cardiol. 2012;33(4):513–20.
41. Kobayashi T, Inoue Y. Takeuchi, et al. Prediction of intravenous immunoglobulin unresponsiveness in patients with Kawasaki disease. Circulation. 2006;113(22):2606–12.
42. Yonesaka S, Nakada T, Sunagawa Y, et al. Endomyocardial biopsy in children with Kawasaki disease. Acta Paediatr. 1989;31(6):706–11.
43. Newburger JW, Takahashi M, Burns JC. Kawasaki disease. J Am Coll Cardiol. 2016;67(14):1738–49.
44. Shen XM, Wang WP. Pediatrics (version 7) [M]. Beijing: People's Medicine Publishing House; 2008.
45. Yang SY, Chen SB. Pediatric cardiology (version 4) [M]. Beijing: People's Medicine Publishing House; 2012.
46. Baumer JH, Love SJ, Gupta A, et al. Salicylate for the treatment of Kawasaki disease in children. Cochrane Database Syst Rev. 2006;4:CD004175.
47. Holve TJ, Patel A, Chau Q, et al. Long-term cardiovascular outcomes in survivors of Kawasaki disease. Pediatrics. 2014;133(2):e305–11.
48. Qilu Pharmaceutical, Warfarin User's Manual, 2012.
49. Shah V, Christov G, Mukasa T, et al. Cardiovascular status after Kawasaki disease in the UK. Heart. 2015;101(20):1646–55.
50. Yang S, Shubao C. Pediatric Cardiology. 4th ed. Beijing: People's Medical Publishing House; 2012.

51. McCrindle BW, Rowley AH, Newburger JW, et al. Diagnosis, treatment, and long-term management of Kawasaki disease: a scientific statement for health professionals from the American Heart Association. Circulation. 2017;135(17):941.
52. Suganara Y, Ishii M, Koizum IH, et al. Warfarin therapy improves clinical outcome of Kawasaki disease patients with giant coronary aneurysm. J Am Coll Cardiol. 2003;41(6):485.
53. Hu YM, Jiang ZF, Futang Z. Practice of Pediatrics [M]. Beijing: People's Medical Publishing House; 2015. p. 786.
54. Wei GY, Like Y. Integrative Medicine cholestatic hepatitis clinical observation of 26 cases [J]. Medicinal. 2002;17(5):39.
55. Sumitomo N, Karasawa K, Taniguchi K, et al. Association of sinus node dysfunction, atrioventricular node conduction abnormality and ventricular arrhythmia in patients with Kawasaki disease and coronary involvement. Circ J. 2008;72(2):274–80.
56. Liang YC, Wu MC. Practical Pediatric Electrocardiogram. [M]. Beijing: People's Medical Publishing House; 1981.
57. Majumdar I, Wagner S. Kawasaki disease masquerading as hepatitis: a diagnostic challenge for pediatricians. Clin Pediatr (Phila). 2016;55(1):73–5.
58. Okano M, Kawa K, Kimura H, et al. Proposed guidelines for diagnosing chronic active Epstein-Barr virus infection. Am J Hematol. 2005;80(1):64–9.
59. Ito Y, Suzuki M, Kawada J, et al. Diagnostic values for the viral load in peripheral blood mononuclear cells of patients with chronic active Epstein-Barr virus disease. J Infect Chemother. 2016;22(4):268–71.
60. Garrido-García LM, Peña-Juárez RA, Yamazaki-Nakashimada MA. Cardiac manifestations in the acute phase of Kawasaki disease in a third level children's hospital in Mexico City. Arch Cardiol Mex. 2018 Apr 9. pii: S1405-9940(18)30035-1.
61. Komaki H, Nakashima T, Minatoguchi S. Radiofrequency catheter ablation for ventricular tachycardia in ischemic cardiomyopathy due to Kawasaki disease. Cardiol Young. 2018;28(6):890–3.
62. West L, Beerman L, Arora G. Ventricular ectopy in children without known heart disease. J Pediatr. 2015;166(2):338-42.e1.
63. Ayusawa M, Sonobe T, Uemura S, et al. Revision of diagnostic guidelines for Kawasaki disease (The 5th Revised Edition). Pediatr Int. 2005;47(2):232–4.
64. Garrido-García LM, Castillo-Moguel A, Vázquez-Rivera M, et al. Reaction of the BCG Scar in the acute phase of Kawasaki disease in Mexican Children. Pediatr Infect Dis J. 2017;36(10):e237–41.
65. Wang M, Li S, Zhou X, et al. Increased inflammation promotes ventricular arrhythmia through aggravating left stellate ganglion remodeling in a canine ischemia model. Int J Cardiol. 2017;248:286–93.
66. Halliday B, Murgatroyd F, Whitaker D, et al. Sudden cardiac arrest in adolescence: the case of ventricular fibrillation 11 years after presenting with Kawasaki's disease. Heart. 2012;98(23):1756.
67. Fujino M, Hata T, Kuriki M, Horio K, et al. Inflammation aggravates heterogeneity of ventricular repolarization in children with Kawasaki disease. Pediatr Cardiol. 2014;35(7):1268–72.
68. Ghelani SJ, Singh S, Manojkumar R. QT interval dispersion in North Indian children with Kawasaki disease without overt coronary artery abnormalities. Rheumatol Int. 2011;31(3):301–5.

KD with Nervous System Involvement

3

Ce Wang, Hong Wang, Yanqiu Chu, and Bai Gao

Abstract

KD is an acute, self-limited febrile illness. Although significant long-term sequelae are confined to the coronary arteries, multiple other organs and tissues are inflamed during the acute illness and causing clinical symptoms. Likewise, irritability and a culture-negative pleocytosis of the cerebrospinal fluid in infants with prolonged fevers suggest that aseptic meningitis may develop in patients with KD. But it is usually overlooked. Common complications of nervous system in KD children include: aseptic meningitis as the most common one, seizures, temporary hemiplegia, facial paralysis, ataxia, hearing impairment, visual abnormalities, and behavioral abnormalities can also be associated (Alves et al., Rev Assoc Med Bras 57(3):299–300, 2011; Poon et al., Hong Kong Med J 6(2):224–226, 2000; Knott et al., Am J Otolaryngol 22(5):343–348, 2001). Neurological involvement in children with KD may be due to ischemic effects of small vessel inflammation which cause neuritis, ischemia, and increased intracranial pressure. The symptoms of abducens nerve palsy in some children with KD recovered after 2–6 weeks of treatment (Amano and Hazama, Acta Pathol Jpn 30(3):365–373, 1980). Histopathological examination of KD nervous system showed edema, necrosis, glial cell hyperplasia, lymphocyte invasion, etc. (Guven et al., Pediatr Int 52(2):334, 2010; Rodríguez-Lozano et al., Allergol Immunopathol (Madr) 42(1):82–83, 2014). In our department, aseptic meningitis is the most common one. We saw abduction nerve paralysis in one KD patient, and abnormal EEG lasted over 4 months in another patient. In most of the children, neurological impairments were recovered within one month.

C. Wang · H. Wang (✉) · Y. Chu
Department of Pediatric Cardiology, Shengjing Hospital of China Medical University, Shenyang, P.R. China

B. Gao
Department of Neurology function, Shengjing Hospital of China Medical University, Shenyang, P.R. China

3.1 Case 16: KD with Aseptic Meningitis (CSF Cell Count Elevated)

A previously healthy 4-year-old girl enjoying regular sport fun had no significant past medical and family history.

She presented on Day 7 of illness with remittent fever, along with conjunctiva congestion for 5 days, without chills or convulsions. She had occasional cough, diarrhea for 2 days, and was prescribed with azithromycin for 2 days, erythromycin for 3 days, and methylprednisolone 1mg/kg for 1 day. *Examination* revealed fever 37.5°C, pulse rate 105 bpm, RR 20 bpm, BP 103/63mmHg, weight 17.5 kg, cervical lymphadenectasis about 1.5 cm on the right, bilateral conjunctival congestion without pus secretions, red lips, strawberry tongue. Peeling skin around right thumb fingernail. Others were normal. *Admission* blood test revealed WBC 22.14 × 10^9/L, NE 83.6%, CRP 174mg/L, ALT 92U/L. MP-IgM was mildly positive. cTnI, CKMB mass, hs-cTnT, and NT-pro BNP were normal. Chest X-ray film showed slightly enlarged heart shadow. Cervical ultrasound showed lymphadenectasis about 2.0cm×0.8cm on the left. She had met 5 criteria for the KD, and she was treated with (1) IVIG 1g/kg/d for 2 days; (2) oral aspirin 200mg tid, dipyridamole 25mg tid; (3) infusion of azithromycin 175mg/day, for 3 days.

On Day 8, her body temperature was 36.8°C. ALB 28.1g/L, ALT 57U/L. ASO 85.5 IU/ml. She had developed hypoproteinemia and received infusion of 20-gram albumin. On Day 9, her highest body temperature was 37.6°C at night. Echo showed that RCA was dilated about 4.0 mm (Fig. 3.1a) and spreading to 17 mm (Fig. 3.1b), and LCA was 2.7 mm. She got headache and was treated with mannitol and furosemide. On Day 11, her temperature was 37.3°C. Retested blood work revealed ALB, ALT, and AST were normal. NT-pro BNP 2147pg/ml. ASO 104IU/ml. CRP 37.50mg/L, ESR 88mm/h. She was suspected of having streptococcal infection and received infusion of cefazolin sodium

On Day 12, she was afebrile, but still had headache. Meningeal irritation sign was negative. EEG showed bilateral

H. Wang (ed.), *Paediatric Kawasaki Disease*, https://doi.org/10.1007/978-981-15-0038-1_3

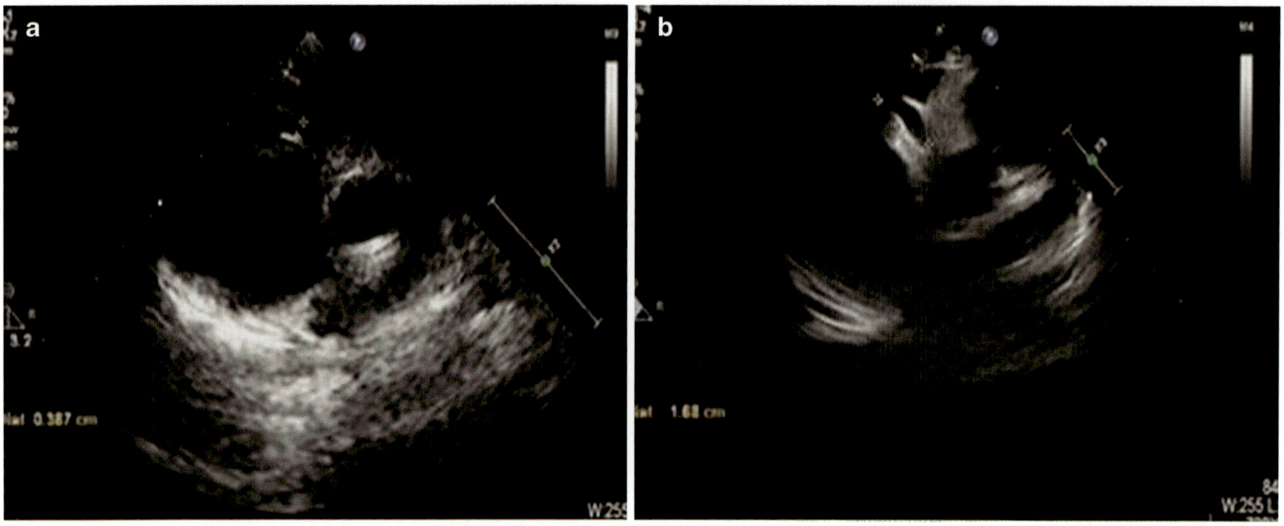

Fig. 3.1 On Day 9 of illness, RCA 4.0 mm (**a**), and spread length about 17 mm (**b**)

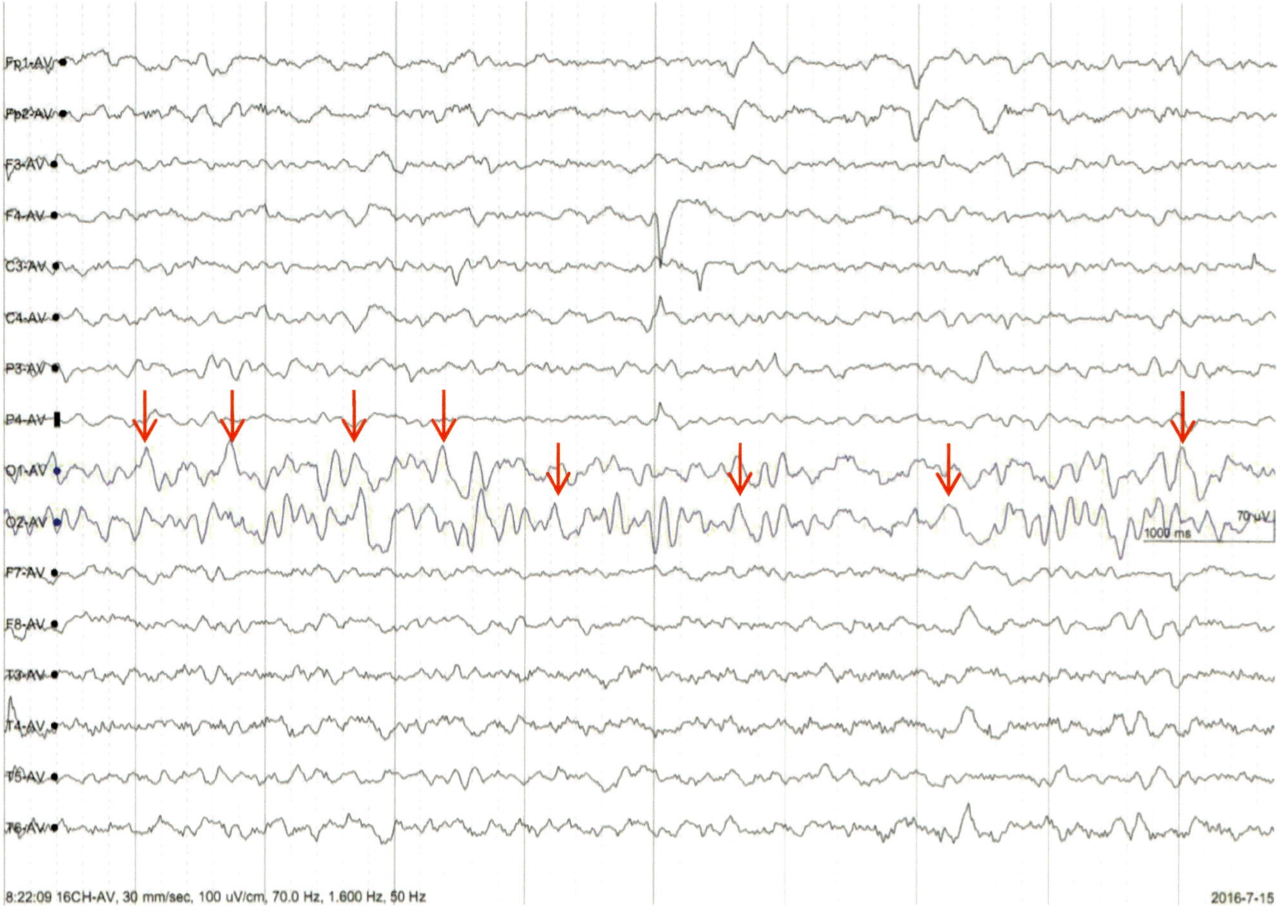

Fig. 3.2 On Day12, EEG showed bilateral occipital region was the main amplitude of amplitude 6–7 Hz theta waves

occipital region was the main amplitude of amplitude 6–7Hz theta waves (Fig. 3.2). Lumbar puncture showed CSF pressure 30 drops/min. CSF was clear. Pandy's test was negative. The total number of cells 41 × 10^6/L, WBC 41 × 10^6/L, NE 2.4%, M 97.6%, RBC 0 × 10^6/L. CSF chlorine 123.8mmol/L, glucose 3.00 mmol/L, protein 0.14g/L. She developed aseptic

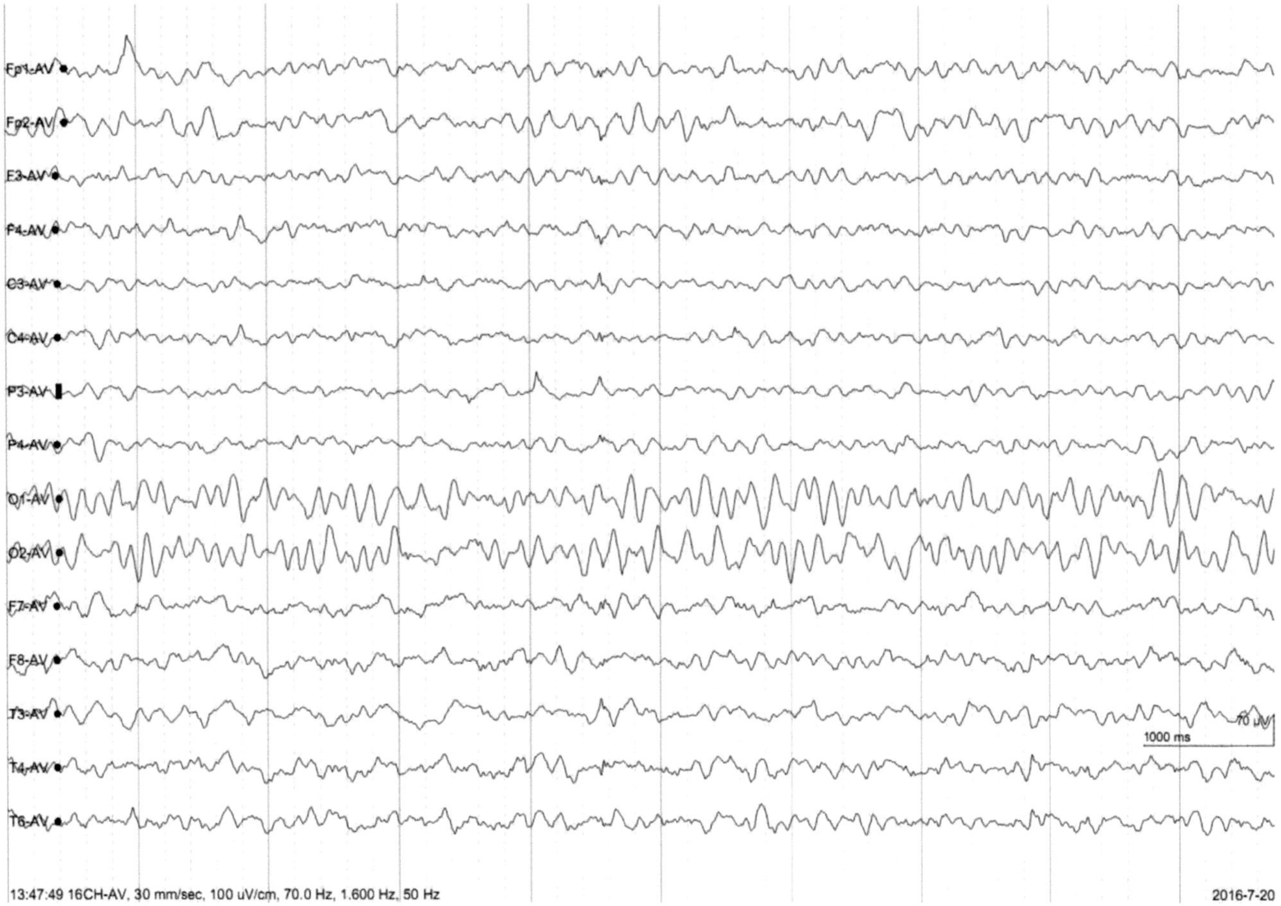

Fig. 3.3 On Day 15 of illness, EEG showed bilateral occipital area was improved to 8 Hz, medium amplitude was normal

meningitis and was given infusion of deproteinized calf blood extract and cefuroxime sodium. Aspirin was reduced to one dose 75 mg per day. On Day 13, she felt well. Repeated blood work showed WBC 10.89×10^9/L, NE 44%, HBG 113g/L, PLT 450×10^9/L. Liver function and NT-pro BNP were normal. CRP 8.23mg/L, ESR 62mm/h. On Day 14 of illness, repeated echo showed RCA widen two sections, 3.1 mm at opening and 4.3 mm at middle part, while LM 2.7 mm and LAD 2.3 mm without dilation. On the following day, EEG showed bilateral occipital area was improved to 8 Hz, medium amplitude was normal (Fig. 3.3). On Day 20, the patient's temperature was normal, without any discomfort. Blood test showed WBC 7.56 × 10^9/L, NE 51.9%, HGB 107g/L, PLT 286×10^9/L. The patient was discharged. On Day 28, repeated echo in clinic showed LAD was 4 mm and RCA had aneurysm dilatation about 9.3mm. She was admitted again: WBC 7.82 × 10^9/L, NE 67.5%, HGB 120g/L, PLT 267 × 10^9/L. CRP 1.29mg/L. Troponin I, CKMB-Mas, NT-pro BNP, hs-cTnT, and DIC were normal. On Day 29, repeated echo showed LVED 33mm, LVEF 69%. RCA was normal at opening, 4 mm away from opening, it dilated about 5.3 mm, and aneurysm dilated about 9 mm to 9.5 mm at distal (Fig. 3.4). She took warfarin orally, with the initial dose at 0.05 mg/kg/day, and the INR was 1.1. After 3 days, warfarin dosage was adjusted to 0.1 mg/kg/day. On Day 30, INR was 1.2. Coronary artery CTA failed due to recurrent urticarial on her face and trunk. She was discharged.

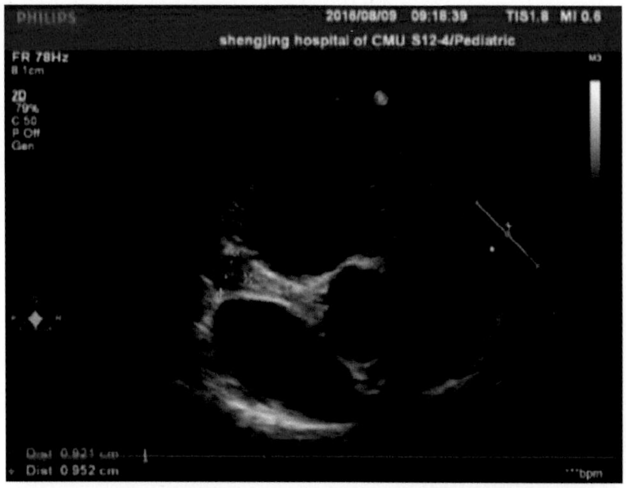

Fig. 3.4 Four weeks after the onset, RCA dilated to 9–9.5 mm at distal

3.1.1 Clinical Course of the Patient

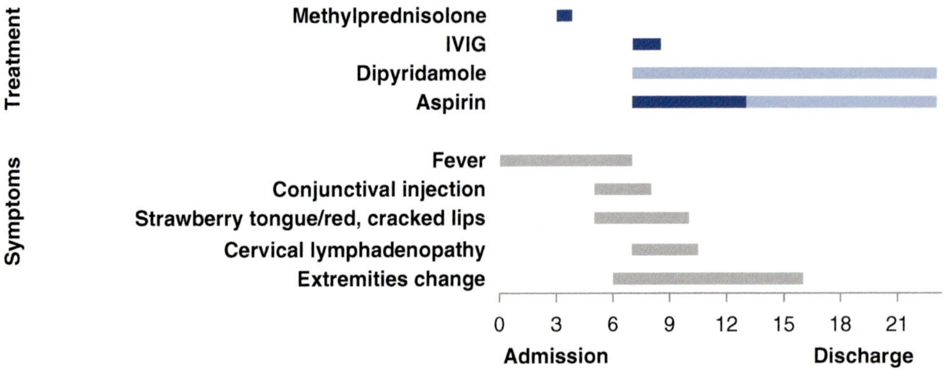

Table 3.1 Coronary artery changes and drug dosage adjustment

Time of illness	1.5 M	2.5 M	3 M	4 M	5 M	9 M	1Y	14 M	20 M
INR	1.1	1.1	1.2	1.1	1.2	1.2	1.4	2	1.7
Warfarin(mg/kg)	0.13	0.11	0.12	0.125	0.14	0.14	0.15	0.15	0.15
Aspirin(mg/kg)	3	3	3	3	3	3	3	3	3.5
LM(mm)	2.5	2.5	2.6	2.6	2.6	2.1	2.4	2.6	2.6
LAD(mm)	2.8	2.7	2.3	2.3	2				
RCA-1(mm)	5.6	5.5	5	5	5.3	4.4	4.1	4	3.9–5.1
RCA-2(mm)			10	Fig. 6A–B	Fig. 7-A	Fig. 7-B	Fig. 8-A	Fig. 8-B	Fig. 8-C

RCA-1: the opening of RCA, RCA-2: the distal of RCA

3.1.2 Follow-up

She was followed up for over 2 years, and DIC was monitored in clinic monthly (Table 3.1). Coronary artery CTA was attempted but failed again for her skin allergy. Four months later: the EEG showed sinus bradycardia (Fig. 3.5). The echo showed LVED 38 mm, LVEF 59%. RCA opening widened about 2.6mm, after extending 5 mm, the diameter of the inner diameter was about 5mm, and the width of the distal end was about 10 mm (Fig. 3.6a, b). No exact thrombus was found in it. LCA was about 2.6 mm, and LAD was about 2.3 mm. INR was 1.1. Warfarin was adjusted to 1.6 mg for 1 day and 2.5 mg for 2 days alternately, a period of 3 days. From 4 months to 20 months, echo was repeated (Fig. 3.7–3.8), warfarin was adjusted according to INR (Table 3.1).

3.1.3 Diagnosis

1. KD (Giant Right CAA)
2. Aseptic meningitis
3. Liver dysfunction
4. Hypoalbuminemia
5. MP infection
6. Streptococcus infection didn't exclude.

3.1.4 Discussion

Her diagnosis of KD was based on she had persistent fever for 7 days, antibiotic treatment was ineffective and along with (1) bilateral conjunctiva hyperemia, no purulent secretion; (2) non-suppurative swelling of the neck lymph nodes; (3) lips red, bayberry tongue; (4) echo showed giant CAA on the right. Differential diagnosis should be assessed from sepsis, suppurative meningitis, and viral meningitis.

3.1.5 Case Specific Clinic Features

1. The most common nervous system manifestations of KD is aseptic meningitis [1]. It is found that this kind of nervous system is often involved in the stage of temperature fading. Most of them first appear somnolence or headache, and abnormal slow wave can be recorded in the EEG. Generally, children with these conditions have meningeal irritation sign, positive PAP's sign, or positive metacarpal mental reflex. This child had transient headache without positive sign in physical examination. CSF puncture result showed only increased number of cells but mainly mononuclear cells. Because CSF pressure was normal, we did not give the patient mannitol and furosemide; we replaced antibiotics with second-generation

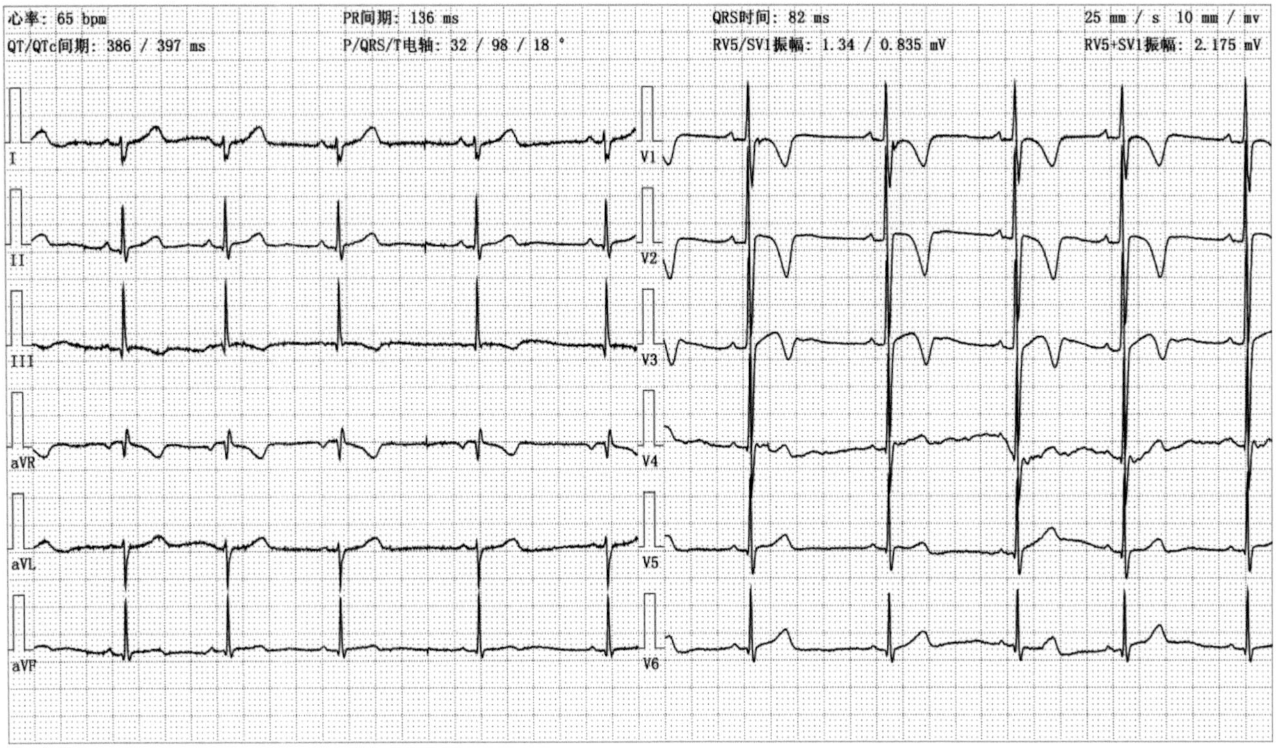

Fig. 3.5 Four months after the onset, ECG showed sinus bradycardia (HR 65bpm)

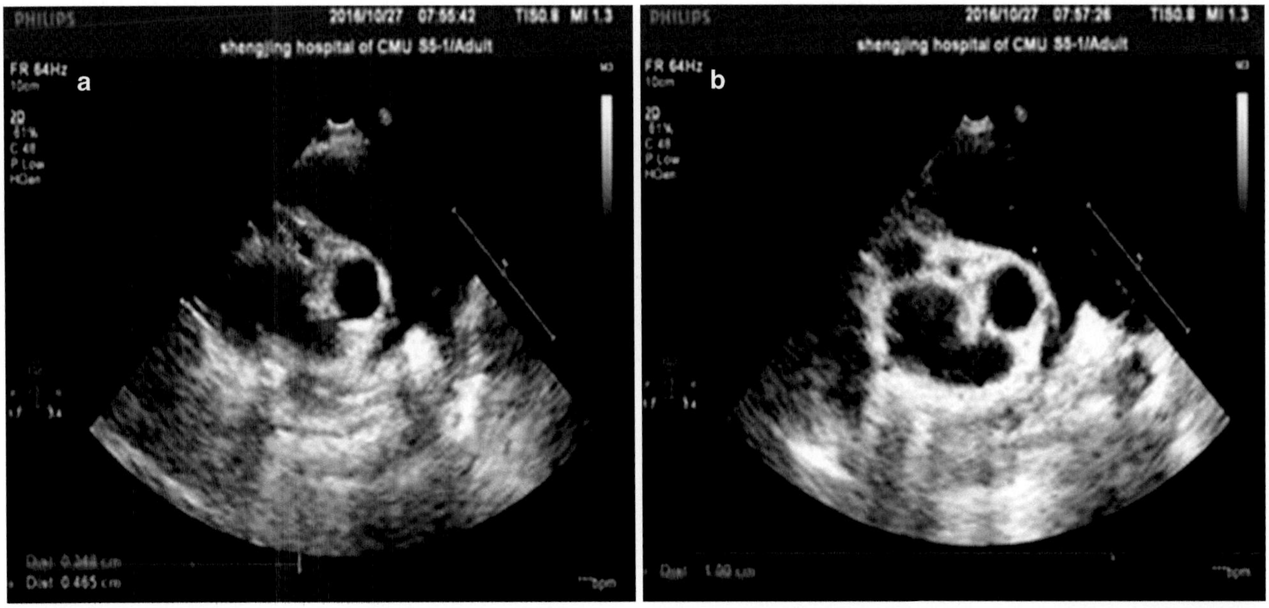

Fig. 3.6 Four months after the onset, RCA opening dilated to 3.5–4.7 mm (**a**), about 10 mm at distal (**b**)

cephalosporin, which is able to penetrate the blood–brain barrier for anti-inflammatory.

2. Transient slow waves in EEG without clinic symptom is meaningless. Sometimes, normal people can have slow waves when they are sleepy. But if, in addition to the primary disease, the slow wave persists over 3 days, combined with facts including headaches, increased CSF cell number, mononuclear cells in majority, complication with nervous system should be considered.
3. Aseptic meningitis, as the name suggests, is characterized by negative results in CSF culture test. But once cell number in CSF is increased, treatment should include antibiotics,

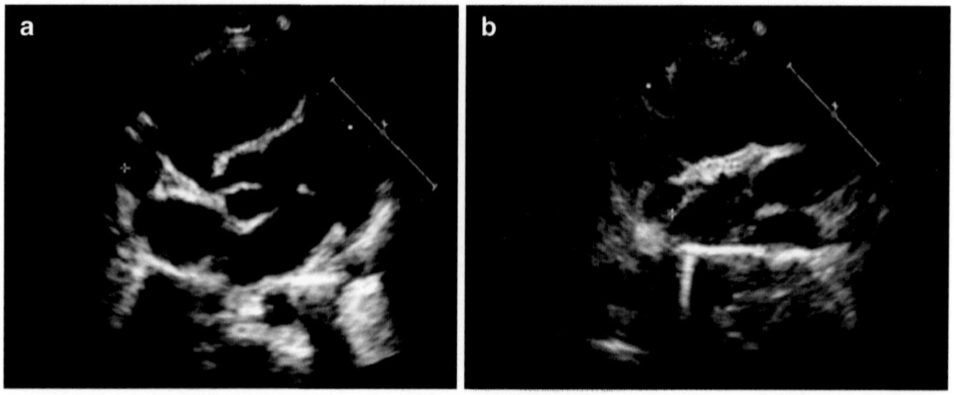

Fig. 3.7 Five months after the onset, RCA dilated about 10 mm at distal (**a**). Nine months after the onset, RCA dilated to 9–10mm at distal (**b**)

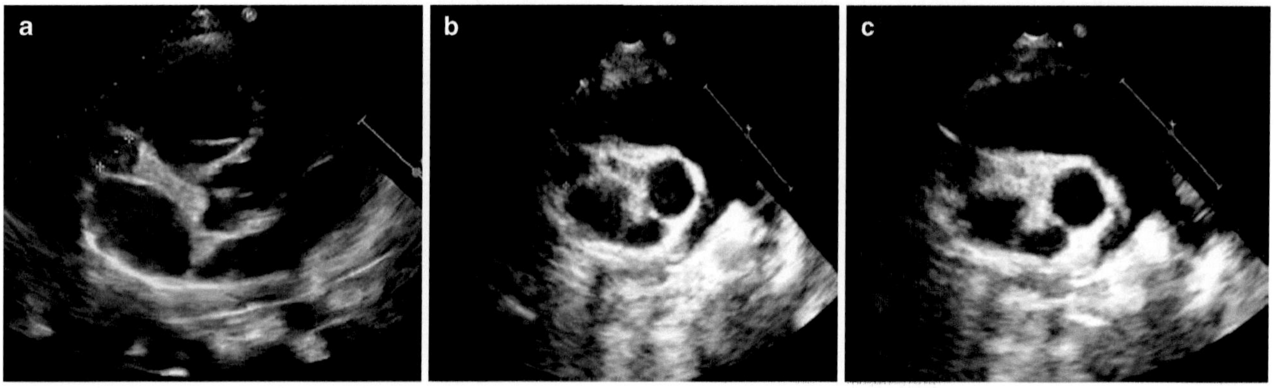

Fig. 3.8 Echocardiography showed distal RCA dilated to 10–11 mm at 1 year (**a**), 11–12 mm at 14 months (**b**) and 20 months (**c**) of illness

and antibiotics that can pass blood–brain barrier should be selected. As to whether the CSF needs to be reexamined, it should be assessed by clinical fever, headache, or somnolence symptoms improvement. In this case, the number of cerebrospinal fluid cells was slightly increased and was not under re-examination. Antibiotics should be used for 1–2 weeks in children. Sometimes CSF test need to be repeated before making decision on the time to stop antibiotics.

4. ASO in the uninfected population is less than 25IU/L. ASO in this patient had a trend of increasing after IVIG. Thus, we could not exclude the input antibody. It continued to rise three days after the treatment, although less than 200IU/L, we considered that she had primary infection. Antibiotics or penicillin should be given for at least a week, then check it again. If over the normal high value, especially when combined with increasing CRP and ESR, intramuscular injection of long-acting penicillin must be given, and follow-up. When admitted to the hospital, the child had fever for only 7 days with peeling skin already, which usually occurred 9–11 days in KD, and the part of the desquamation was not around fingernails. Therefore, a streptococcus infection should be considered and kept in the check list.

Ce Wang

3.2 Case 17: KD with Aseptic Meningitis and Acute Cholestatic Hepatitis

A 14-month-old girl was previously healthy without significant past medical and family history.

She presented on Day 4 of illness with remittent fever, along with conjunctival congestion for three days. On Day 2 of illness, she developed a large number of congestive rashes on the back without itch. In a local hospital, she received infusion of erythromycin for one day, and monophosphate adenosine and azithromycin for another day. Since the onset, she was sleepy with lack of appetite, without cough or vomiting. Examination revealed fever (39.1°C), PR 120bpm, RR 22 bpm, a lot of rashes on the back, the larger bilateral cervical lymphadenopathy about 1.5cm, conjunctival congestion without purulent secretions, red and cracked lips. Auscultation assessment on lungs and heart were normal, without hepatosplenomegaly. Nervous system was normal. Admission blood test revealed WBC 20.2×10^9/L, NE 73.3%. CRP 107mg/L. NT-pro BNP 3225pg/ml. cTnI, CKMB mass, and hs-cTnT were normal. Cervical ultrasound showed multiple enlarged lymph nodes on the left, the larger one was about 2.0cm×0.8cm. She had met 5 criteria for the

KD and treated with aspirin 150mg, three times daily, dipyridamole 25mg, twice a day.

On Day 5, her body temperature was 39.5°C, bilateral Babinski signs were suspected positive. Retested blood work revealed WBC 24.0×10^9/L, NE 92.3%, HGB 113g/L, PLT 253×10^9/L. ESR 61mm/h. Liver function ALB 34.7g/L, ALT 103U/L, AST 57U/L, TBA 252.0μmol/L. MP-IgG antibody 1:160. Treatment included (1) IVIG 1g/kg for two days. (2) azithromycin 100mg/day IV for three days; (3) polyene phosphatidylcholine 5ml/day IV; (4) adenosine succinate 250mg/day IV. On Day 6, her rash and conjunctivitis were subsided, but fever was still up to 39.5°C along with lethargy. Bilateral Babinski signs were suspected positive. EEG was normal. Lumbar puncture result revealed: CSF pressure 100 drops/min, CSF colorless and transparent. Pandy's test was negative, total number of cells 28×10^6/L, WBC 28×10^6/L, NE 70%, RBC 0×10^6/L. CSF biochemistry: chlorine 117.9mmol/L, glucose 3.45mmol/L, protein 0.74g/L. Treatment included (1) ceftriaxone sodium 80mg/kg once a day, intravenous infusion; (2) because the patient's stool was black, oral aspirin was suspended; (3) mannitol 2.5ml/kg Q12h; (4) calf serum deproteinized 0.4g/time IV once a day. On Day 7, the temperature was regressed to 38.5°C. The stool was black with negative occult blood. On Day 8, her fever stayed at 38.5°C, and the stool color recovered to yellow. Retested blood revealed WBC 23.2×10^9/L, NE 77.2%, HGB 88g/L, PLT 246×10^9/L; NT-pro BNP 1077pg/ml; hs-cTnT 0.078ng/ml; CRP 103mg/L. Liver function ALB 25.1g/L, ALT 26U/L, TBA 13.5μmol/L. Regular occult blood was weakly positive (non-occult blood diet). ECG was normal; brain MRI identified right axillary arachnoid cyst, bilateral mastoiditis. ECHO: both LCA and RCA were normal (Fig. 3.9) Liver ultrasound was normal (Fig.3.10). Pediatric neurologist suggested IV naloxone 0.4mg/time, once a day, for 5 days. Thus, treatment was adapted to (1) IVIG another 2g/kg in 24 hours; (2) infusion of albumin 1g/kg, for two days; (3) naloxone 0.4mg/time, q8h IV for 4 days; (4) oral ferralia plus vitamin C for anemia. On Day 9, she still had fever, and received methylprednisolone 1mg/kg/day IV for 5 days. On Day 11, her fever settled over 48 hours, her mental state was nice. Aspirin was reduced to 50 mg/time, once a day. On Day 12, peeling skin occurred around fingernails. Retested blood revealed WBC 14.8×10^9/L, NE 54.7%, HGB 84g/L, PLT 433×10^9/L. NT-pro BNP 355.4pg/ml. hs-cTnT 0.033ng/ml; CRP 28.2mg/L. Liver function ALB 32.5g/L. Conventional occult blood was negative. On Day 13, fever again went up to 38.5°C, red rash appeared again, but mental state was good. Dermatologist suggested drug rashes. Treatment was adapted to (1) switching from ceftriaxone sodium to erythromycin; (2) mannitol and furosemide changed to once a day; (3) naloxone stopped. On Day 14, fever and rash subsided. Methylprednisolone was reduced to 0.5 mg/kg/day. On Day 17, the temperature was about 37.5–37.9 °C for two days. The mental state was good. CSF pressure 80 drops/min (children crying slightly), colorless and transparent. Pandy's test was negative, total number of cells 5×10^6/L, WBC 5×10^6/L, NE 10.0%, M 90.0 %, RBC 0×10^6/L. CSF biochemical showed no obvious abnormalities, CSF etiology was negative. Blood routine WBC 6.8×10^9/L, NE 22.5%, HGB 90g/L, PLT 293×10^9/L (Table 3.2). NT-pro BNP 77.12pg/ml. hs-cTnT was normal. ESR 41mm/h. Echo showed normal result (Fig. 3.11). Treatment included: (1) Stopping prednisolone, mannitol, and furosemide; (2) The patient had been using prednisolone and antibiotics for one week, could not be excluded from fungal infection, so oral fluconazole 5mg/kg/day for three days. On Day 20, desquamation around fingernails. The patient was discharged.

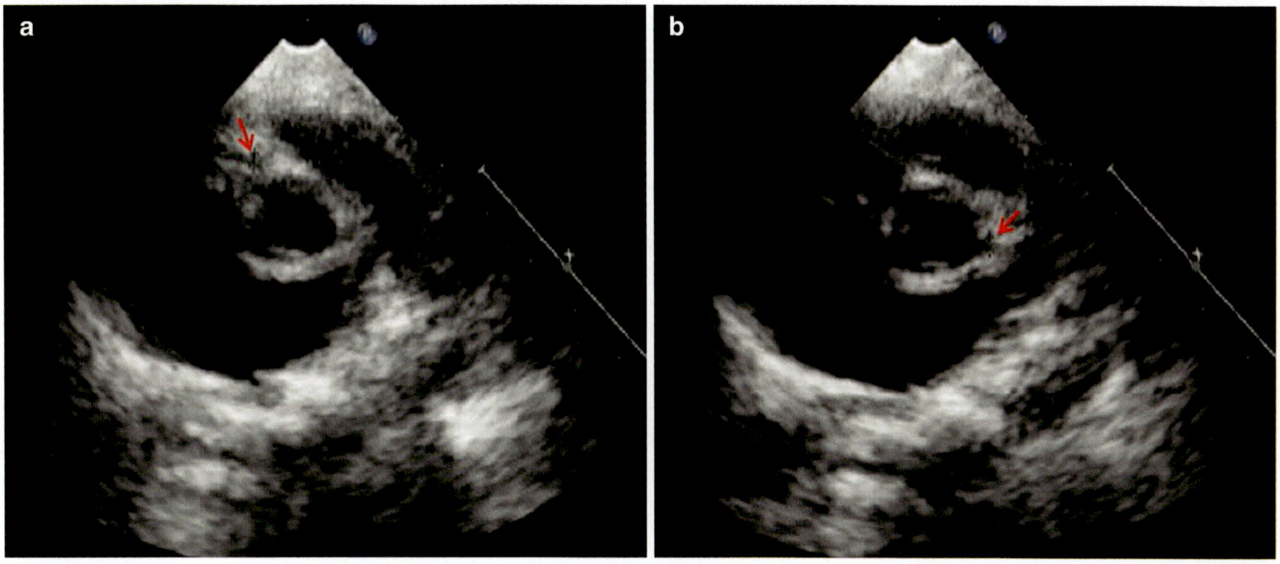

Fig. 3.9 On Day 8 of illness, echo showed RCA (**a**) and LCA (**b**) were normal

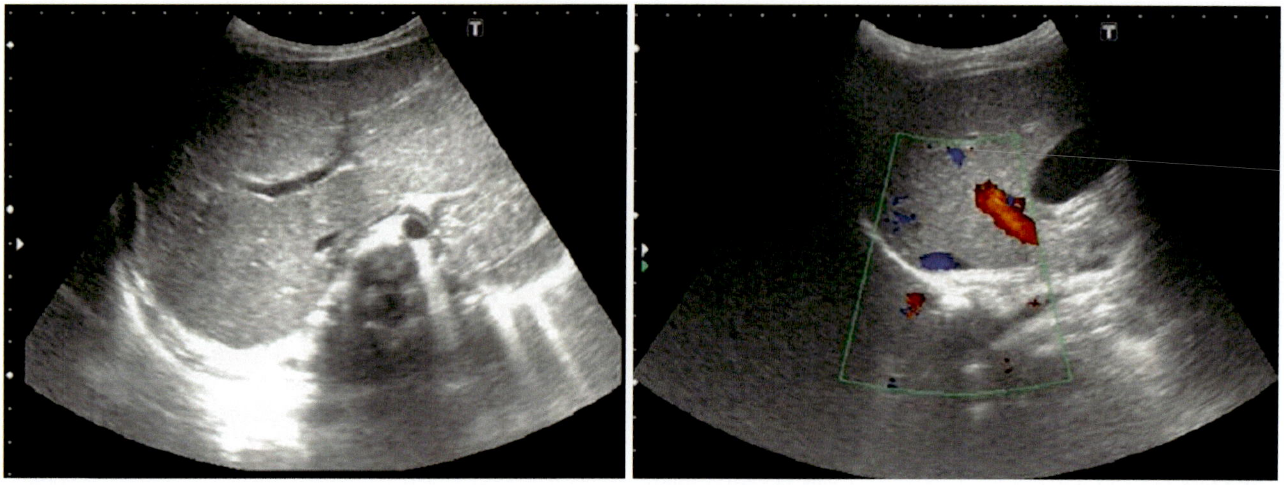

Fig. 3.10 On Day 8 of illness, liver ultrasound was normal

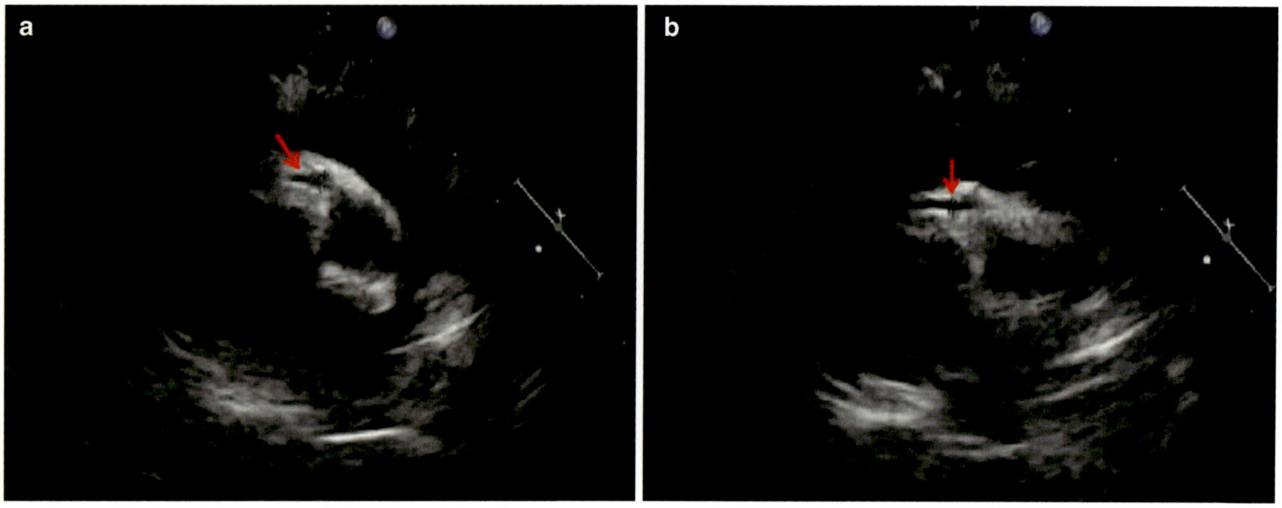

Fig. 3.11 On Day 17 of illness, RCA (**a**) and LCA (**b**) were normal

3.2.1 Clinical Course of the Patient

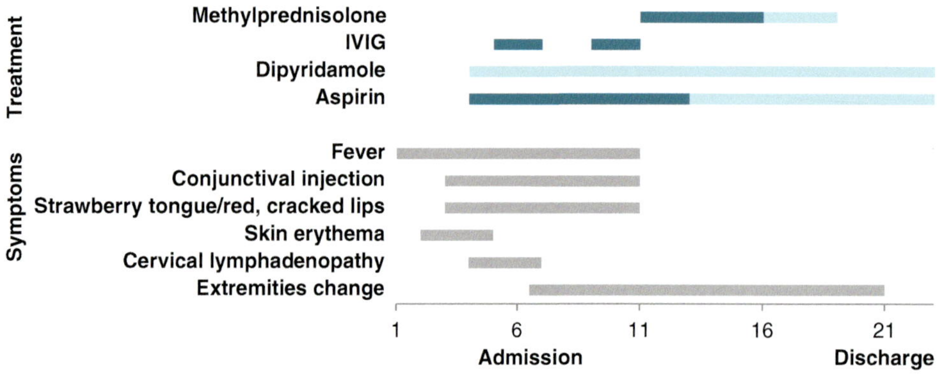

Table 3.2 The dynamic changes of Lab parameters

Time of illness	Day 5	Day 6	Day 8	Day 12	Day 17
Blood WBC×10⁹ /L	24	-	23.2	14.8	6.8
PLT×10⁹ /L	253	-	246	433	293
CRP mg/L	107	-	103	28.2	10
ALB g/L	34.7	-	25.1	32.5	35
TBA μmol/L	252	-	13.5	10	5.2
CSF WBC×10⁶/L	–	28	–	–	5
NE%	–	70	–	–	10
M%	–	30	–	-	90
chlorine mmol/L	–	117.9	–	–	120
sugar mmol/L	–	3.45	–	–	3.5
protein mmol/L	–	0.74	–	–	0.32

3.2.2 Follow-up

Echo was performed at 1, 2, and 5 months and all had normal result, brain protein hydrolysate tablets and multivitamin B were stopped at one month of illness, and aspirin and dipyridamole were stopped at two months with normal ESR.

3.2.3 Diagnosis

1. KD, IVIG resistance
2. Aseptic meningitis
3. Hypoproteinemia
4. Moderate anemia
5. Right axillary arachnoid cyst
6. Bilateral mastoiditis

3.2.4 Discussion

The KD diagnose was sufficient. She had persistent fever over 5 days, which was irresponsive to antibiotics, along with (1) rashes in the course of the disease; (2) bilateral bulbar conjunctival congestion without exudate, (3) erythema on hands; (4) cervical lymphadenopathy. Others included leukocytosis and significantly elevated CRP.

Differential diagnosis of suppurative meningitis should be considered. Supporting points were based on: the patient got fever, rash, and lethargy. Physical examination suggested suspected positive Babinski signs. WBC and CRP were significantly high after IV antibiotics treatment. The first CSF test showed increase in cell numbers mainly in NE. However, the fact that CSF was clear, sugar and chlorine levels were normal, and the bacterial culture test showed negative results in blood and CSF, did not support a possible meningitis.

3.2.5 Case Specific Clinic Features

1. The child was always sleepy when she was admitted in our hospital. Bilateral Babinski signs were suspected positive. The lumbar puncture was still needed although EEG was normal. CSF indicated slight increases in the number of cells and protein amount. Aseptic meningitis diagnosis was made.
2. The neurological involvement in children with KD is varied. The most common cases are aseptic meningitis, epileptic seizures, temporary hemiplegia, facial paralysis, ataxia, hearing impairment, abnormal visual acuity, and abnormal behavior are also reported [1]. Based on the physical signs, auxiliary examination, and symptomatic treatment, we used the third-generation cephalosporin anti-infective treatment which could pass through the blood–brain barrier, and observed dynamic changes in CSF.
3. After treated with 2g/kg IVIG twice, patient's fever was only regressed to 38.5 °C, along with rashes and conjunctivitis which meet the criteria of IVIG resistance. For the treatment, IVIG can be combined with glucocorticoid, which is beneficial to reduce vascular inflammation and reduce brain edema [2].
4. After the patient received infusion of 4g/kg of IVIG, CRP elevated again. Antibiotics and glucocorticoids were used in the treatment for one week. At the same time, diarrhea occurred, and fungal infection could not be excluded. Considering a large dose of IVIG had been used, it was not suitable to test 1-3-β-D glucan, so oral fluconazole for 3 days was given to the patient for experimental treatment, and it had a nice effect.
5. When the patient was admitted in hospital, the inflammatory reaction was severe. Hepatic function was damaged and albumin was significantly reduced, which was the risk factor of CAA [3]. Although echo showed coronary artery was normal during the hospitalization, long-term dynamic follow-up was still needed.

Ce Wang

3.3 Case 18: KD with Aseptic Meningitis-Abnormal EEG for Four Months

A three-year-old boy was previously healthy without significant past medical and family history.

He presented on Day 7 of illness with remittent fever. On Day 2 of illness, he came to our clinic for fever along with cough and abdominal pain. Abdominal ultrasound indicates lymphadenectasis, with significantly elevated CRP. Thus, he was admitted in our PICU as sepsis. Since the onset of illness, he was in poor mental state, had lethargy, lost appetite, was sleepy, and urinated less urine. Examination revealed the following results: body temperature 36.9°C, pulse PR 138bpm, RR 25bpm, bilateral cervical lymphadenectasis, obvious pain when touched on the right side. Others were normal. *Admission* blood test revealed WBC 32.3×10⁹/L, NE 90.2%, HGB 117g/L, PLT 315×10⁹/L. CRP 175mg/L. PCT 1.98ng/ml. ALT 63U/L. MP-IgM(+), HSV-IgM(+). Abdominal ultrasound revealed abdominal lymphadenectasis. Lumbar puncture test showed that CSF pressure was 80 drops/min, negative in Pandy's test, the total number of cells 1900×10⁶/L, WBC 17×10⁶/L, NE 40%, L 60%, RBC 1883×10⁶/L (puncture bleeding). CSF biochemistry panel showed: glucose 5.53mmol/L, chlorine 118.6mmol/L, protein 0.16g/L. There was no exact abnormality found in head CT scan. Pulmonary CT showed mild inflammation in the middle lobe of the right lung and the upper lobe of the left lung. He was diagnosed with: (1) sepsis; (2) aseptic encephalitis; (3) HSV infection; (4) acute bronchopneumonia; (5) MP infection; and he was treated with (1) IVIG 7.5g on the first day; (2) infusion of erythromycin; (3) medication and supplements for preserving liver function and nourishing brain cells. On Day 8, he still had fever and retested blood work revealed WBC 17.5×10⁹/L, NE 94.4%, HGB 109g/L, PLT 405×10⁹/L, CRP 168mg/L. ALT 417U/L, AST 295U/L, ALB 33.7g/L, TBA 213.5μmol/L. On Day 9, fever persisted. Retested blood revealed WBC 19.5×10⁹/L, NE 90.7%, HGB 102g/L, PLT 317×10⁹/L. CRP 65.3mg/L. On Day 10, he presented bilateral conjunctival erythema and cracking lips, strawberry tongue and a lot of rashes on face and back. Laboratory parameters were shown as: WBC 17.7×10⁹/L, NE 85.6%, HGB 107g/L, PLT 337×10⁹/L. CRP 53.5mg/L. ALT 233U/L, AST 66U/L, ALB 27.3g/. He had met 4/5 criteria for the KD and was treated with (1) IVIG 15g/day, for 2 days; (2) aspirin 150mg, three times a day, dipyridamole 25mg, three times a day; (3) albumin 10g/day for 2 days; (4) methylprednisolone 1mg/kg/day for 5 days. On Day 11, he still had fever, but rashes were regressed. Retested CBC showed WBC 19×10⁹/L, NE 85.3%, HGB 95g/L, PLT 304×10⁹/L. CRP 66mg/L. ALT 135U/L, AST 19U/L, ALB 30.8g/L. NT pro-BNP 55.7ng/ml. ESR 47mm/h. On Day 13, he had no fever over 48 hours. Blood work was retested and revealed WBC 19.3×10⁹/L, NE 78.5%, HGB 93g/L, PLT 351×10⁹/L; CRP 34.5mg/L. Repeated echo showed normal results. Aspirin was reduced to 50mg/day. On Day 14, he was still afebrile, the rashes subsided, the lips remained dry and red; WBC 26.5×10⁹/L, NE 71.9%, HGB 101g/L, PLT 371×10⁹/L, CRP 10.6mg/L, ALT 50U/L, AST 19U/L, ALB 29.0g/L. Intravenous infusion of albumin 10g was given to the patient. On Day 17, he had fever again, along with bilateral conjunctival congestion, with blood test results shown as follows: WBC 20.6×10⁹/L, NE 62.1%, HGB 93g/L, PLT 425×10⁹/L. CRP 35.5mg/L. Liver function test showed ALT 19U/L, ALB 31.8g/l. ESR 48mm/h. ASO 225IU/ml. He was diagnosed with (1) IVIG resistance; (2) streptococcus infection; and he was transferred to the pediatric cardiology department. On Day 18, he was treated with: (1) antibiotics infusion for one week to anti-streptococcus infection; (2) continuous low-dose aspirin and dipyridamole; (3) methylprednisolone 15mg for 4 days; (4) repeated infusion of erythromycin; (5) infusion of mannitol (20%). On Day 19, he had fever to 37.6 °C with cough. Both hands had periungual desquamation. Retested blood revealed WBC 13.2×10⁹/L, NE 62.7%, HGB 90g/L, PLT 586×10⁹/L, CRP 14.80mg/L. ALB 32.7g/L. Repeated EEG identified the bilateral occipital leads the alpha wave of medium amplitude 8.0Hz, and the two leads were scattered in the low medium amplitude theta wave. Conclusion: the background rhythm was slightly slower (Fig. 3.12a). And he was treated with (1) interferon intramuscular injection once a day; (2) oral azithromycin 150mg for 3 days; (3) Diflucan 70mg/day for 3 days to prevent fungal infection.

On Day 24, his fever was up to 38 °C. Repeated echo showed normal result. On the follow 2 days, the highest temperature was 37.6°C. Fever settled down on Day 27, but he developed nasal congestion and runny nose. Retested blood revealed WBC 4.6×10⁹/L, NE 39%, L 52.3%, HGB 83g/L, PLT 581×10⁹/L. CRP 12.80mg/L. ASO 167 IU/ml (Table 3.3). Re-recorded EEG revealed abnormal signals (Fig. 3.12b). Bilateral occipital lead dominated with moderate amplitude of θ activity, each lead was scattered in low amplitude β wave. He was discharged.

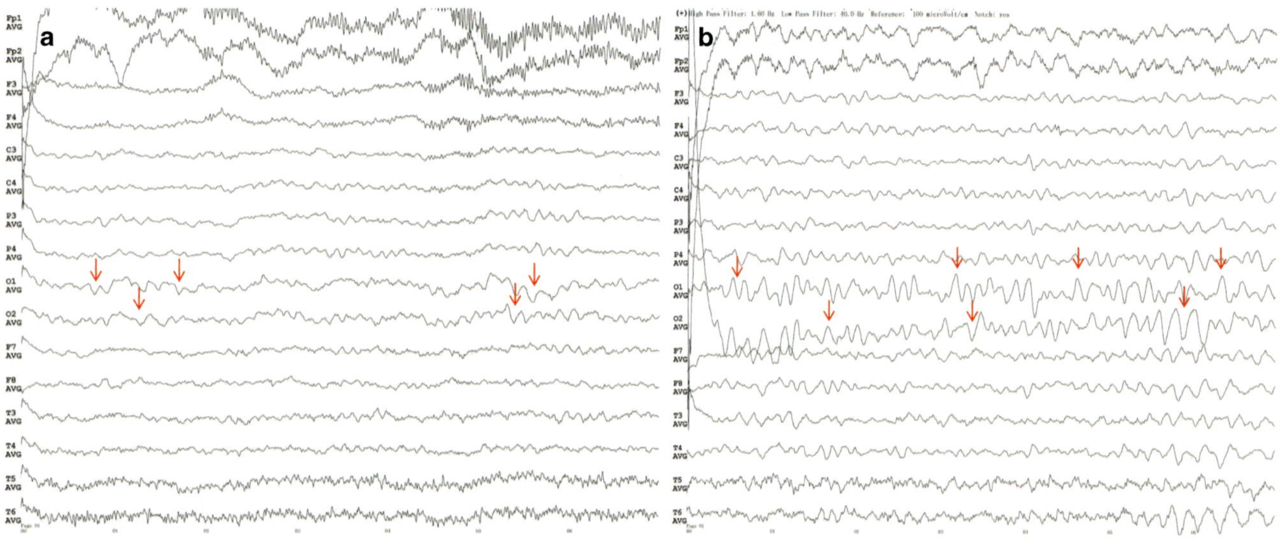

Fig. 3.12 On Day 19 of illness, the bilateral occipital leads showed the alpha wave of medium amplitude 8.0 Hz, and the two leads were scattered in the low medium amplitude theta wave (a). On Day 27 of illness, EEG: moderate amplitude of θ activity (b)

3.3.1 Clinical Course of the Patient

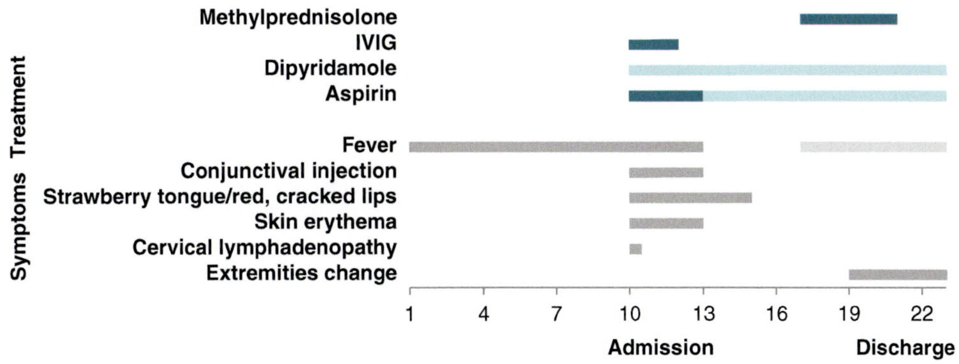

3.3.2 Follow-up

On Day 28, he got fever of 38.4°C again, and periungual desquamation of both hands. After 2 days of oral antivirus medicine, the fever subsided. At 2 months of illness, the coronary artery remained normal, ESR was normal, aspirin and dipyridamole were stopped. Re-recording EEG showed the moderate amplitude 6–7Hz of the bilateral occipital lead was mainly theta wave, and the left and right are roughly symmetrical, there is no obvious amplitude difference, each lead scattered in the low amplitude theta wave, and the dispersion was in the low amplitude beta wave (Fig. 3.13a). Continue oral brain protein hydrolysate tablets and compound vitamin B. At 3 and 4 months of illness, EEG kept abnormal (Fig. 3.13b–3.14a).

At 5 months, EEG recovered to normal (Fig. 3.14b) and the brain protein hydrolysate tablets and compound vitamin B were stopped. He followed up for 1.5 years, and the coronary artery kept normal (Table 3.3).

3.3.3 Diagnosis

1. KD, IVIG resistance
2. Aseptic encephalitis
3. Herpes simplex virus infection
4. Acute bronchopneumonia;
5. MP infection;
6. Liver dysfunction;
7. Streptococcus infection;
8. Moderate anemia.

3.3.4 Discussion

The diagnosis of KD was sufficient. He had persistent fever over 5 days, oral and infusion of antibiotics were ineffective. He also had the following symptoms: (1) rashes on face and back during the fever, (2) bilateral conjunctival congestion without exudate, (3) erythema on hands; (4) cervical lymphadenopathy.

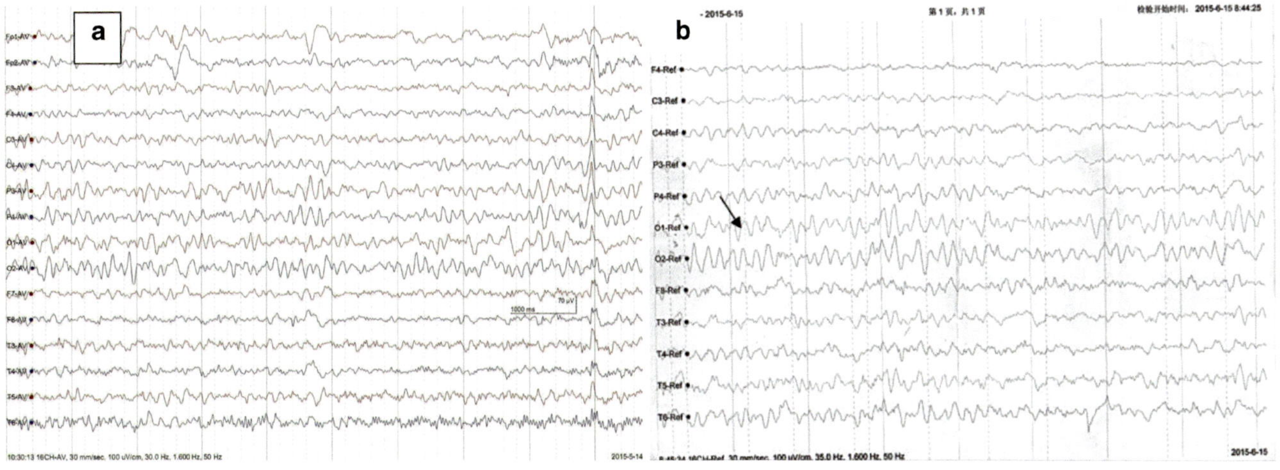

Fig. 3.13 EEG at 2 months of illness, background rhythm was slightly slower (**a**). At the three months of illness, the EEG was still abnormal (**b**)

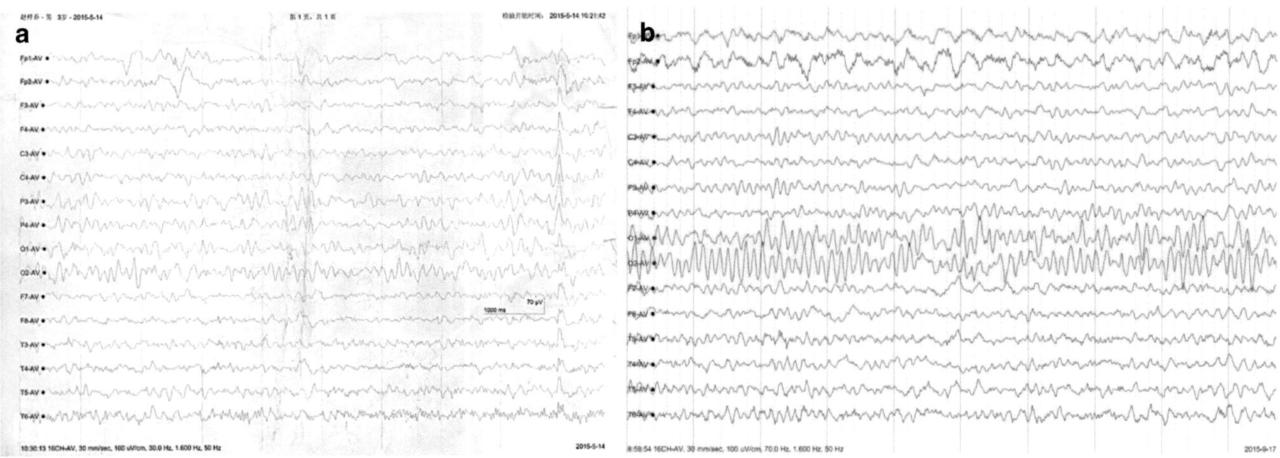

Fig. 3.14 At 4 months of illness, EEG was still abnormal (**a**). At 5 months, the EEG was normal (**b**)

Table 3.3 The dynamic changes of lab parameters

Time of illness	7 days	8 days	9 days	10 days	11 days	13 days	14 days	17 days	19 days	27 days
WBC ($\times 10^9$/L)	32.3	17.5	19.5	17.7	19	19.3	26.5	20.6	13.2	4.6
PLT ($\times 10^9$/L)	315	105	317	337	304	351	371	425	586	581
CRP (mg/L)	175	168	65	53.5	66	34.5	10.6	35.5	14.8	12.8
ALB (g/L)	35	33.7	–	27.3	30.5	–	29	31.8	32.7	–
ALT (U/L)	40	417	–	233	135	–	50	19	20	–
TBA (μmol/L)	–	213.5	–	–	15	–	–	–	–	–

Leukocytosis was positive, and mainly in NE. There was significantly elevated CRP. Differential diagnosis of sepsis should be considered. For children with fever, a diagnosis of KD at early stage combined with IVIG treatment timely can dramatically reduce the incidence of coronary artery lesion. The child was admitted in the hospital as a patient with infection, and he was given IVIG at 400mg/kg/day. It was reported that admission of gamma globulin can inhibit the inflammatory reaction and improve the prognosis [4]. After diagnosis of KD was made, IVIG was administered in a single dose at 2g/kg.

Differential diagnosis of streptococcus infection is often needed to be made from KD. Before the patient receiving IVIG, his ASO had a rising trend. After the infusion of IVIG, it continued to rise over 200IU/L, and then decreased. We could not confirm where source of infection came from, it was impossible for us to distinguish between natural and artificial infections. Thus he was treated with first-generation antibiotics for one week for anti-streptococcus infection purpose. After that, ASO was reduced to less than 200IU/L. Therefore, additional long-acting penicillin was not required to be used.

3.3.5 Case Specific Clinic Features

1. The nervous system involvement in KD can be characterized by irritability, lethargy, aseptic meningitis, abductor nerve paralysis, and so on. The incidence is 1–30% in children with KD [5, 6]. The child was sleepy when he was admitted to our hospital, and the neurological examination revealed positive for bilateral Babinski signs. The Corning's puncture examination suggested a majority of lymph with slightly elevated CSF cells. If eliminating the fact of bleeding during the procedure, the cells were in normal range and the pathogen was negative. No exact abnormality was found in the brain CT scan. EEG showed slightly slower background rhythm. The patient was diagnosed with KD combined with aseptic meningitis for this patient was established.
2. Neurological involvement in children with KD may be due to ischemic effects of small vessel inflammation that cause neuritis, ischemia, and increased intracranial pressure [7]. The symptoms of abducens nerve palsy in some children with KD could be recovered after 2 to 6 weeks of treatment [8–10]. The first abnormal EEG of the child was on Day 16–17 of illness. During the outpatient follow-up, EEG remained abnormal until 5 months later. Nevertheless, most of the children recovered within one month.
3. The child had aseptic meningitis. On Day 4, we treated him with a small dose of glucocorticoid to control the inflammation and alleviate cerebral edema. He received infusion of methylprednisolone at 1mg/kg/day for 5 days.

His fever regressed and stable for 4–5 days, then his fever came back again. Two days later, his cough was aggravated, along with conjunctival congestion and red lips. The diagnosis of IVIG resistance was established. For he had IVIG total 4g/kg. Thus, GC was added in the treatment plan. At that time, the lung CT suggested that inflammation scattered in both lungs. Additional infusion of 1mg/kg/day methylprednisolone was given to him for 4 days. After afebrile for 2 days, he had low fever along with nasal congestion and runny nose, symptoms of respiratory infection. Considering a complication with upper respiratory infection, we prescribed medication for him to take at home for 2 days. taking-home medicine for 2 days. His fever settled.

Ce Wang

3.4 Case 19: KD with Aseptic Meningitis-Peripheral Facial Nerve Palsy

A 5-month-old boy presented with unremarkable past medical history and family history.

He presented on Day 12 of illness (in 1998), with a history of continuous fever for 12 days, along with bilateral conjunctival congestion, red lips for 2 days and peeling skin around fingernails for one day. His body temperature was between 38 °C and 39 °C. After receiving infusion of penicillin and second-generation cephalosporin for 2 days, he developed congest rashes on the back on Day 5 of illness. Local pediatrician suspected they were drug related rashes and switched antibiotics to fosfomycin sodium for one day. Those rashes increased and he developed strikingly red lips and bilateral conjunctival congestion on Day 10. Antibiotics was switched again to cefobid and dexamethasone 5 mg. Fever only settled for 30 hours. On Day 11, fever recurred and he developed peeling skin around fingernails. On Day 12, he was admitted in our pediatric cardiology ward. He had diarrhea 3–4 times per day since antibiotics infusion, without vomiting or coughing. Examination revealed T36.5°C, smooth breath (PR 120bpm, RR 30bpm), weight 7kg. General condition was well. He had red lips and erythema around BCG scar. Hepatomegaly was 2 cm below right costal margin. Others were normal. CBC on Day 7 revealed WBC16.7×10^9/L, NE 47%. Cold agglutinin test and MP-IgM were negative. RSV-IgA was positive. Echo showed coronary artery was normal. He was given infusion of second-generation cephalosporin.

On Day 13, fever recurred to 39°C.Laboratory findings revealed WBC 25.9×10^9/L, RBC 4.38×10^{12}/L, HGB 10.5gm%, PLT 959×10^9/L. Urine and stool routine tests were normal. Stool culture was negative and intestinal flora analysis was normal. ESR 81mm. CRP 45.7mg/L. ALT 41U/L. ALB, CK, CKMB, and ASO were normal. Echo showed LCA was dilated about 4.3mm (Fig. 3.15a), RCA 2.7mm (Fig. 3.15b), LVED 24 mm. Chest DR was normal. For he had met all criteria of KD, he was treated with oral aspirin 50mg/kg/day and dipyridamole 3–5 mg/kg/day, both in 2 to 3 divided doses. On Day 14, fever stayed between 38°C and 38.5°C, with mild coughing. ECG showed ST section elevation 2mm on lead II, III, aVF (Fig.3.16). He was given infusion of FDP and erythromycin. On Day 15, fever was still 38.5°C and left eye could not close and his mouth drooped toward to right when crying. Examination found that erythema around BCG disappeared. He had developed left infranuclear facial palsy. He was given infusion of vitamin B. Meanwhile head MRI was ordered. On Day 17, his body temperature was about 38°C. EEG showed normal results (Fig. 3.17). The lumbar puncture failed due to bleeding. On Day 19, he still had a fever about 38.2°C. Conjunctival congestion regressed, but left red lips remained. Peeling skin occurred around toenails. Investigation revealed WBC 15.6×10^9/L, NE 55%, RBC 4.14×10^{12}/L, HGB 92g/L, PLT 739×10^9/L. Blood cul-

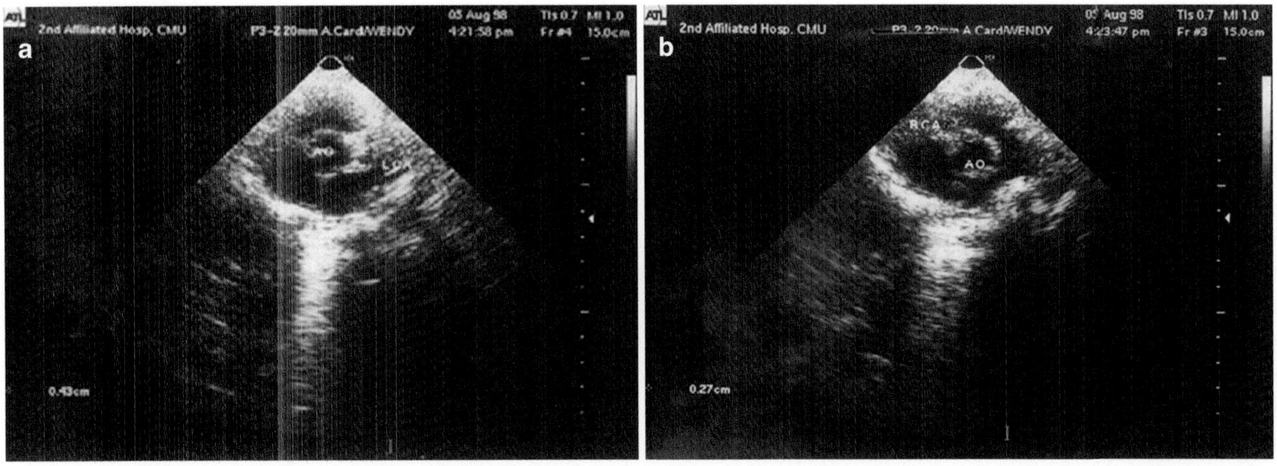

Fig. 3.15 On Day 12 of illness, echo showed LCA dilated about 4.3mm (**a**). RCA was 2.7mm (**b**)

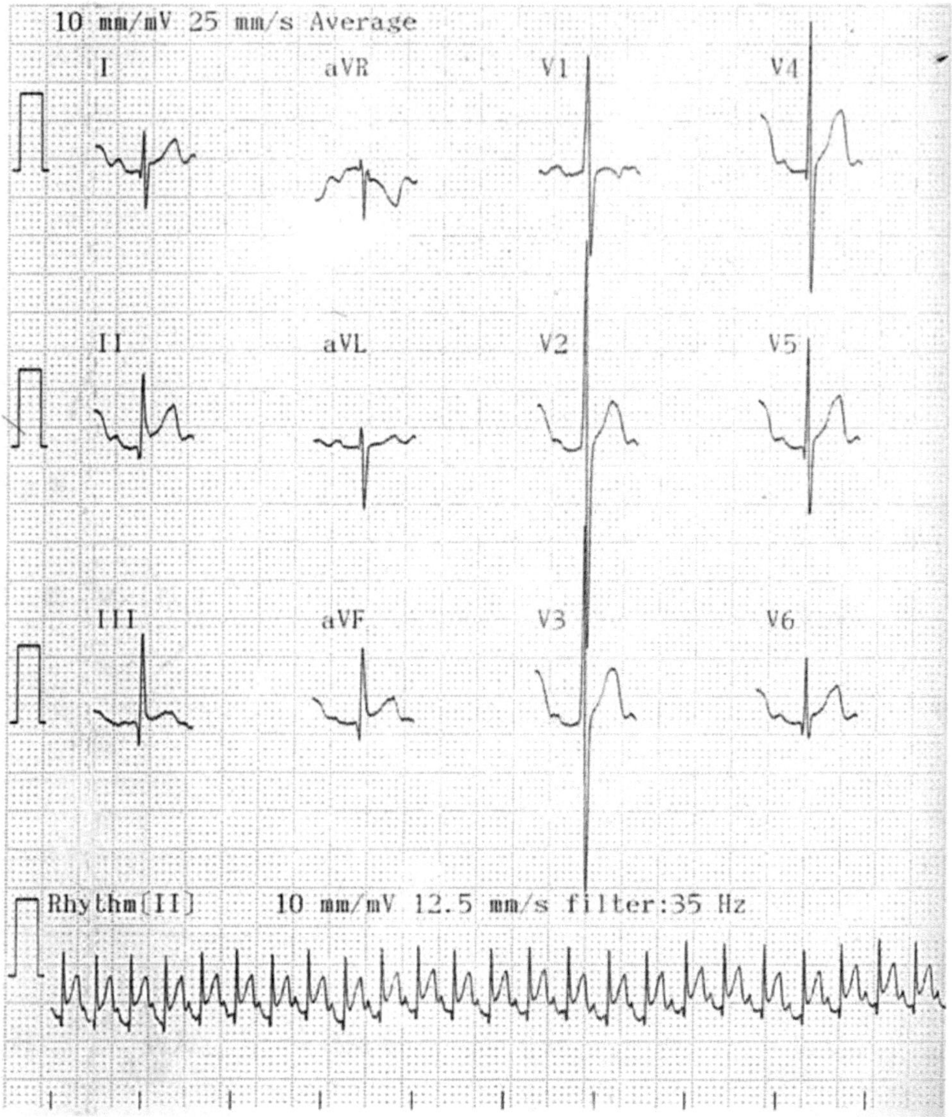

Fig. 3.16 On Day 14 of illness, ECG showed ST section elevated 0.2mv on leads II, III, and aVF

ture was negative. His TCD showed there was insufficient blood supply in bilateral cerebral artery and left anterior artery (Fig. 3.18). Lumbar puncture was re-performed. CSF was slightly yellow and mixed. The CSF dropping velocity was at 100 drops/min. The protein test was positive with WBC 32×10^6/L, NE 70%; protein 1.96g/L, Glu 4.4mmol/L, Cl^-119mmol/L, which indicated aseptic meningitis. His head MRI showed there was a 7mm cystic lesion in left paracele, and the subarachnoid space of frontal lobe was slightly widened (images lost during the transition of system upgrading). He was treated with fast infusion of 20% mannitol 25ml every 12 hours. That night, he developed polypnea, RR was up to 60 bpm, along with cyanosis and edema on his face, oliguria, low-dull heart sounds, HR 140 bpm. Hepatomegaly mark was 5cm below right costal margin and 5cm below the xiphoid, spleen was 2cm below left costal margin. He had edema in lower limbs extremity. ECG showed elevated ST section 0.2mv on lead II, III, and aVF (Image was not scanned due to weak signals). Chest DR showed enlarged heart, and the cardio-thoracic ratio was 0.62, indicating pulmonary edema. He had developed acute heart failure, and aseptic meningitis. Thus, he was transferred to PICU and treated with cediland fast saturation in half dose, furosemidum infusion and reduced mannitol at dose of 2.5ml/kg, every 12 hours. He was sedated using 5% chloral hydrate. Nasal tubing was used for oxygen inhaling. FDP infusion was given to him, and zinacef infusion was changed from twice per day to every 8 hours. On Day 21, his general state was improved. Peeling skin settled. He had fever at 38.5°C occurring two times a day, along with red lips, vomiting (once coffee like content). Blood sample analysis revealed WBC 21.7×10^9/L, RBC 4.6×10^{12}/L, HGB 91g/L, PLT 528×10^9/L, CRP 235mg/L. He had developed delayed vitamin K deficiency. Intramuscular

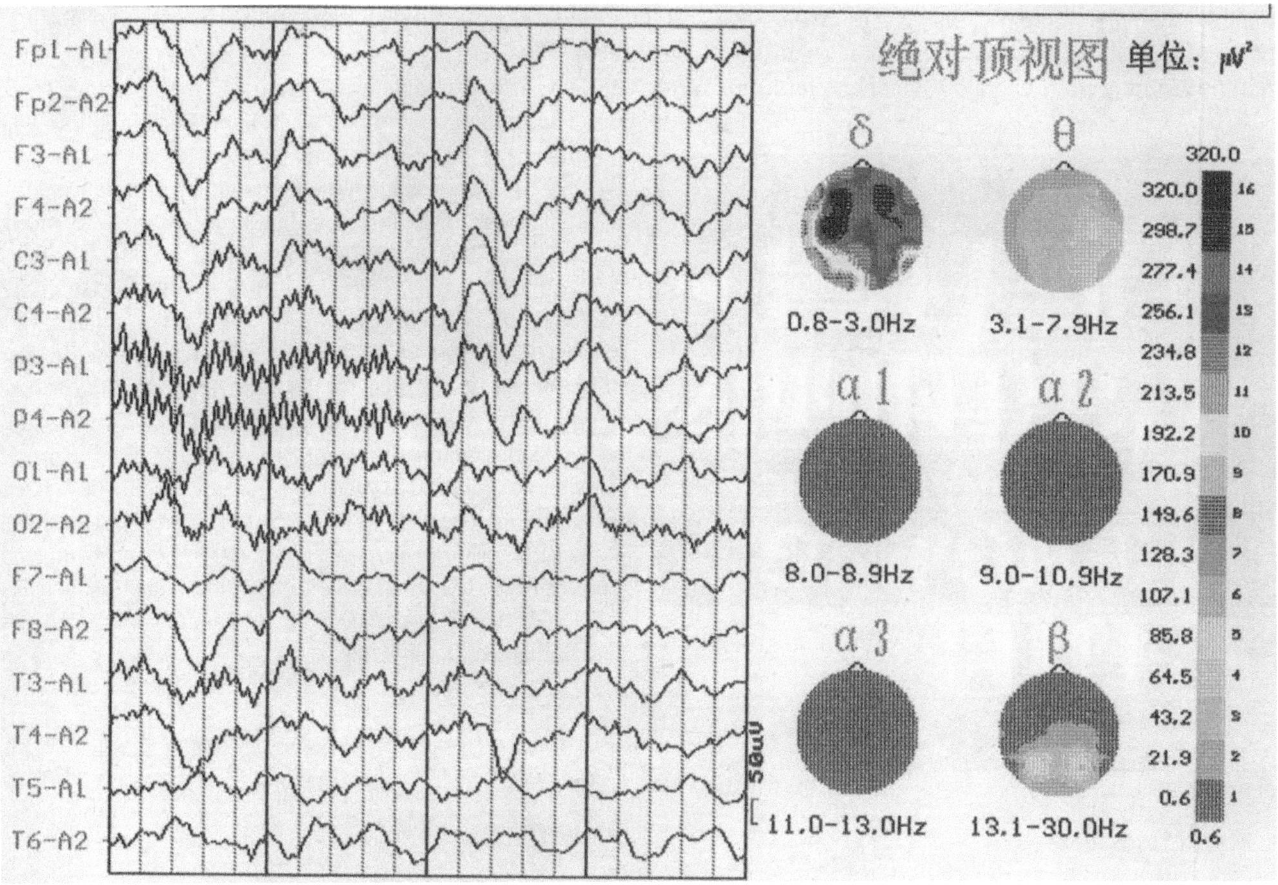

Fig. 3.17 On Day 16 of illness, EEG was normal

Exam 3

2 MHz Temporal (velocities in cm/s)

Depth	Vm	Vs	Vd	PI	RI	Right	Depth	Vm	Vs	Vd	PI	RI
34	38	65	24	1.10	0.63	MCA	36	44	80	17	1.42	0.79
32	38	65	22	1.16	0.66	MCA	32	41	70	18	1.28	0.74
30	37	60	22	1.09	0.64	MCA	30	34	62	12	1.57	0.80
30	40	65	23	1.10	0.64	ACA	44	-40	-50	-32	0.39	0.36
46	-22	-41	-11	1.03	0.73	ACA	42	-41	-53	-32	0.45	0.39
44	-23	-47	-10	1.24	0.79	ACA	40	-41	-55	-34	0.43	0.38
44	-24	-45	-14	0.98	0.68	ACA	38	-46	-58	-38	0.37	0.34
42	-24	-43	-13	1.00	0.70	ACA	36	-46	-59	-38	0.40	0.35
40	-24	-43	-13	1.00	0.70	ACA	34	-37	-49	-29	0.45	0.40
38	-21	-38	-8	1.13	0.79							
36	-23	-42	-14	0.94	0.66							
34	-22	-38	-12	0.97	0.69							

Fig. 3.18 On Day 17 of illness, TCD showed blood supply was insufficient in bilateral cerebral artery and left anterior artery

injection of 7mg vitamin K_1 was given for three days. He never vomited again. On Day 27, he had fever at 39.5°C. His red lips improved. Laboratory findings revealed WBC 17.7×10^9/L, NE 50.2%, RBC 4.94×10^{12}/L, HGB 108g/L, PLT 208×10^9/L. ESR12mm.TB 51.8g/L, ALB 28.6g/L. Blood sample was taken again for culturing. There was Klebsiella growing one week later. Intestinal flora was normal.

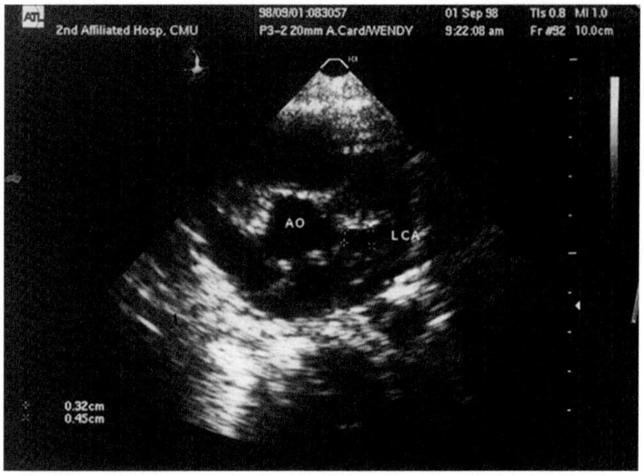

Fig. 3.19 On Day 12 of illness, echo showed RCA was 3.2–4.5 mm

On Day 37, his fever settled. His mouth still deflected to right side when crying, but his eyes closed very well. Investigation revealed WBC 15.6×10^9/L, NE 47.2%, RBC 4.32×10^{12}/L, HGB 96g/L, PLT 829×10^9/L. CRP 13.7mg/L. Echo showed 5mm ASD. LCA was dilated 3.2–4.2mm (Fig. 3.19), RCA 2.6mm. Chest DR showed the ratio of heart/chest was normal. On the following 2 days, the dosage of aspirin was reduced to 3mg/kg/day. On Day 42, he was afebrile and his mouth was symmetry when he cried. Zinacef infusion was reduced to every 12hours per day. Six days later, investigation revealed WBC 15.3×10^9/L, NE 41.1%, RBC 4.53×10^{12}/L, HGB103g/L, PLT 832×10^9/L. Zinacef infusion was stopped. ECG showed ST section elevation 2mm on leads II, III, aVF (Fig. 3.20). On Day 52, he was afebrile for 2 weeks and discharged (Table 3.4).

Fig. 3.20 On Day 47 of illness, ECG showed ST section elevated 0.2 mv on leads II, III, and aVF

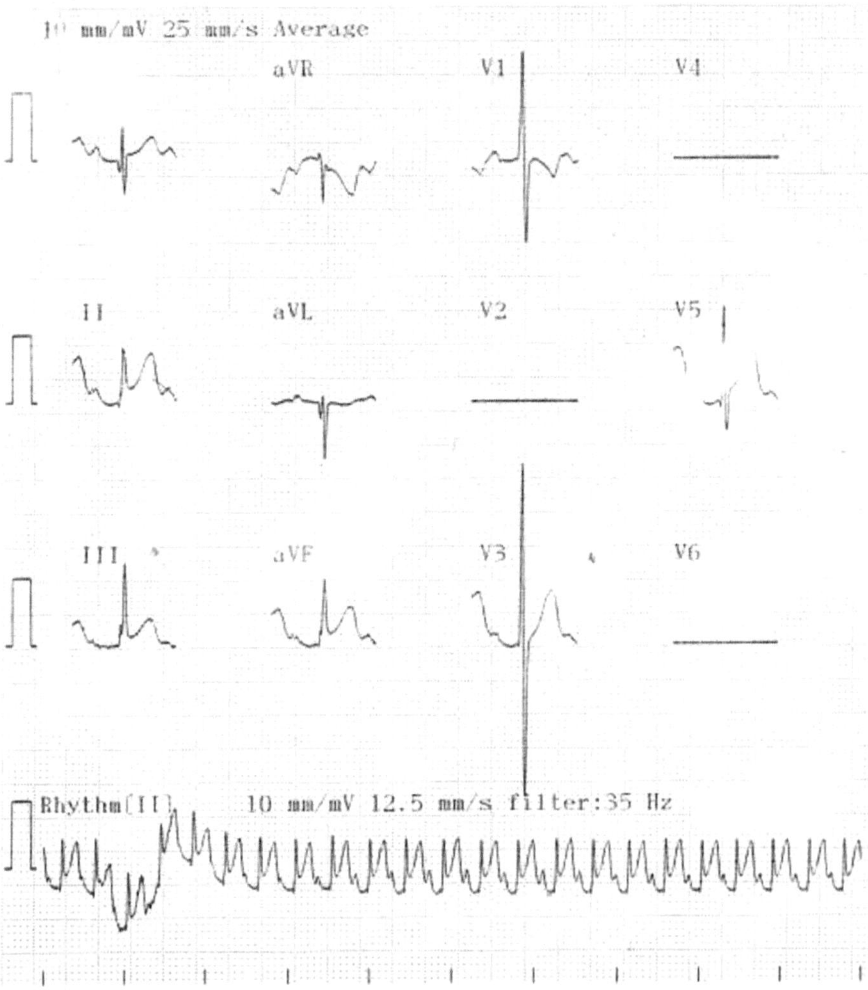

3.4.1 Clinical Course of the Patient

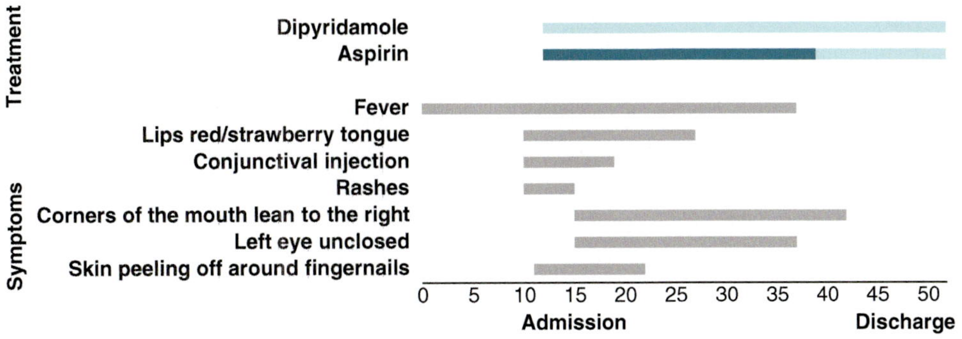

Table 3.4 The dynamic changes of laboratory parameters

Type of Illness	7 days	13 days	19 days	21 days	27 days	37 days	48 days
WBC ($\times 10^9$/ml)	16.7	25.9	15.6	21.7	17.7	15.6	15.3
NE (%)		75	55	75	50.2	47.2	41.1
HGB (g/L)		105	92	91	108	96	103
PLT ($\times 10^9$/ml)	470	959	739	528	208	828	832
CRP (mg/L)		45.7		235		13.7	
ESR (mm/h)		81					

3.4.2 Follow-up

After discharge, he was never followed up again (Table 3.4).

3.4.3 Diagnosis

1. KD
2. Left CAA
3. Peripheral facial nerve palsy
4. Aseptic meningitis
5. Acute heart failure
6. Anemia
7. Thrombocytopenia
8. Liver dysfunction
9. Delayed vitamin K deficiency
10. Hypoalbuminemia

3.4.4 Discussion

He had met the diagnosis criteria of atypical KD. He had continuous fever for 12 days, and the fever was not under control by broad-spectrum antibiotics, along with (1) bilateral conjunctiva; (2) peeling skin around fingernails; (3) red lips; (4) congestion around BCG scar; (5) coronary artery dilatation; in addition, his WBC increased and mainly in NE, with anemia and thrombocytopenia, elevated ESR and CRP.

3.4.5 Case Specific Clinical Features

1. The mechanism of KD is unclear. It has been commonly recognized that the trigger for KD could be a bacterial superantigen. KD may result in multiple organ lesions. To author's best understanding in 1998 when KD was first defined, there is no literature reporting KD with facial nerve paralysis [11]. Though this patient was diagnosed with aseptic meningitis, and he was given second-generation antibiotics infusion based on septic meningitis for total 36 days. Secondly, until acute heart failure occurred we could not confirmed for sure that all his symptoms were caused by KD. After treatment, his clinic-laboratory reports showed good results except LCA lesions when he was discharged.
2. According to literature reports and our center's data, KD with aseptic meningitis usually showed a mild protein elevation in CSF. This child's protein content was significantly higher, which might be related to bleeding in CSF during lumbar puncture procedure 2 days ago or/and due to KD itself.
3. Second blood culture showed positive results in one battle, which happened after all symptoms improved, except high-level fever only for one day. We did not exclude possibilities that it might come from either sample contamination or inter-hospital cross-infection. Therefore, we did not change antibiotics, and the changes later confirmed our conjecture.
4. He was admitted in our ward on Day 12 of illness, and overdue on IVIG treatment time (<10days). Therefore, we did not treat him with IVIG; and this treatment plan was accepted in 1998. Now the guideline has been modified, that if he still had fever, or still showed elevated inflammatory bio-markers, such as ESR or CRP, he should be treated with IVIG even past optimal treatment

period [12]. If IVIG was not effective, TNF inhibiter [13] or plasma exchange [14] could be adopted; thus, organ lesions maybe diminished or slightly.

5. With dilated coronary artery and abnormal ECG, injured myocardium was sensitive to digoxin. Therefore, reduction in digoxin dose was proper. At meanwhile, the mechanism of mannitol in reducing intracranial pressure was through transient hyperosmotic diuresis (over 20 years ago, mannitol dose was 5ml/kg). It can result in transient hypervolemia, increasing heart burden, and inducing heart failure. The current guideline has been changed to reduce the mannitol dose to 2.5ml/kg, with furosemidum infusion 30 minutes later. Thus, heart failure would not happen again in our center, and headache symptom also could be reduced.
6. It has been reported, as early as 1984, that the facial never was involved in KD [15]. About 3.5 years ago, a KD child with abductor never involved (see case 24) presented in our center. Fortunately, both kids recovered soon without permanent sequela.

Hong Wang

3.5 Case 20: KD with Aseptic Meningitis-Abducens Nerve Injury

A healthy 26-month-old boy presented with unremarkable past medicine history or family history.

He presented on Day 6 of illness with fever for 6 days, and erythema and edema in his hands and feet for 3 days, rashes and bilateral bulbar conjunctival congestion for 4 days. He went to the local hospital and was treated with second-generation cephalosporin and vitamin C for 3 days. Then he was transferred to our pediatric cardiology ward as a KD patient. Examination revealed the following: T38.4°C, HR 130 bpm, irritable, rashes on his face, bilateral conjunctival congestion without exudate, erythema and cracking lips with strawberry tongue, bilateral cervical lymphadenopathy with the largest one about 1.5cm in diameter, enlarged liver under rib margin 4cm, qualitative II degree, erythema palms, edema in hands and feet, positive bilateral Babinski signs. *Admission* blood test showed WBC 13.8x10^9/L, NE 82%, HGB 87g/L, PLT 73x10^9/L. CRP 198mg/L. ALB 22.1g/L. cTnI 0.133μg/L, NT-pro BNP>35000pg/ml, hs-cTnT 0.016 ng/ml. Cervical ultrasound showed that lymphadenectasis was about 1.7cmx0.7cm on the left. He had met full criteria for KD, and was treated with (1) IVIG 1.0g/kg/day for 2 day; (2) aspirin 200mg and dipyridamole 25mg, three times daily oral; (3) myocardial nutrition therapy; (4) mannitol 32ml intravenous fast infusion, qd; (5) cefuroxime sodium intravenous drip, q12h; (6) 10g albumin IV; (7) all solution limit speed at 40ml/h.

On Day 6, he was sleepy and irritated. His total urination was 200ml through the whole night. Examination found swollen face and feet and positive bilateral Babinski sign. On Day 7, his mental state was not improved. Retested blood sample showed WBC 11.8x10^9/L, NE 78.5%, HGB 84g/l, PLT 215x10^9/L. CRP 196mg/L, NT-pro BNP>35000pg/ml, weak positive TB antibody, positive MP-IgM. Lumbar puncture test showed CSF pressure was high (80drops/min). Pandy's test was negative. The total number of cells was 246x10^6/L, WBC 246x10^6/L, NE 78.4%, L 25.2%. Glucose 3.7mmol/L, chlorine 119mmol/L, protein 0.9g/L. Pulmonary CT showed bilateral pleural effusion (Fig. 3.21), inferior lobe of right lung with inflammation. ECG showed low-flat T wave in the inferior wall of myocardium (Fig. 3.22). He was treated with: (1) IVIG 1g/kg for two days; (2) mannitol (20%) and furosemide q12h to reduce craniofacial pressure; (3) deproteinized calf serum infusion to nourish brain cells; (4) intravenous albumin; (5) replacing antibiotics with ceftriaxone sodium; (6) azithromycin infusion for three days; (7) improving anemia. On Day 8, his fever regressed to once per day, with normal urine volume and improved edema, but he still had drowsiness. Blood test showed positive PINF. Head MRI, EEG, and TCD were normal. The thoracic cavity ultrasound showed effusion only 1.2cm on the left and 0.8cm on the right, and puncture was not required to perform. Repeated ECG showed T wave was still lower (Fig. 3.22). On Day 11, his mental state was significantly improved, though he still had medium fever and edema in feet. Furthermore, he developed internal strabismus in both eyes and could not look outward; his limbs motion was very well. Examination found positive neck rigidity. Retested blood showed WBC 13x10^9/L, HGB 84g/L, PLT 173x10^9/L. CRP 105mg/L. cTnI 0.117μg/L, NT-pro BNP 23381pg/ml, hs-cTnT 0.027ng/ml. ALB 29.0g/L. D-D 3373μg/L, FDP 21.1μg/L. Re-recorded ECG was normal (Fig. 3.23).

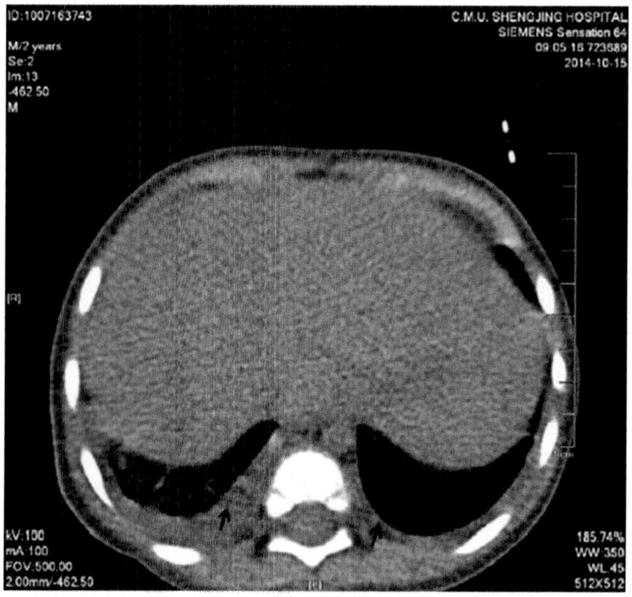

Fig. 3.21 On Day 7 of illness, pulmonary CT showed bilateral pleural effusion

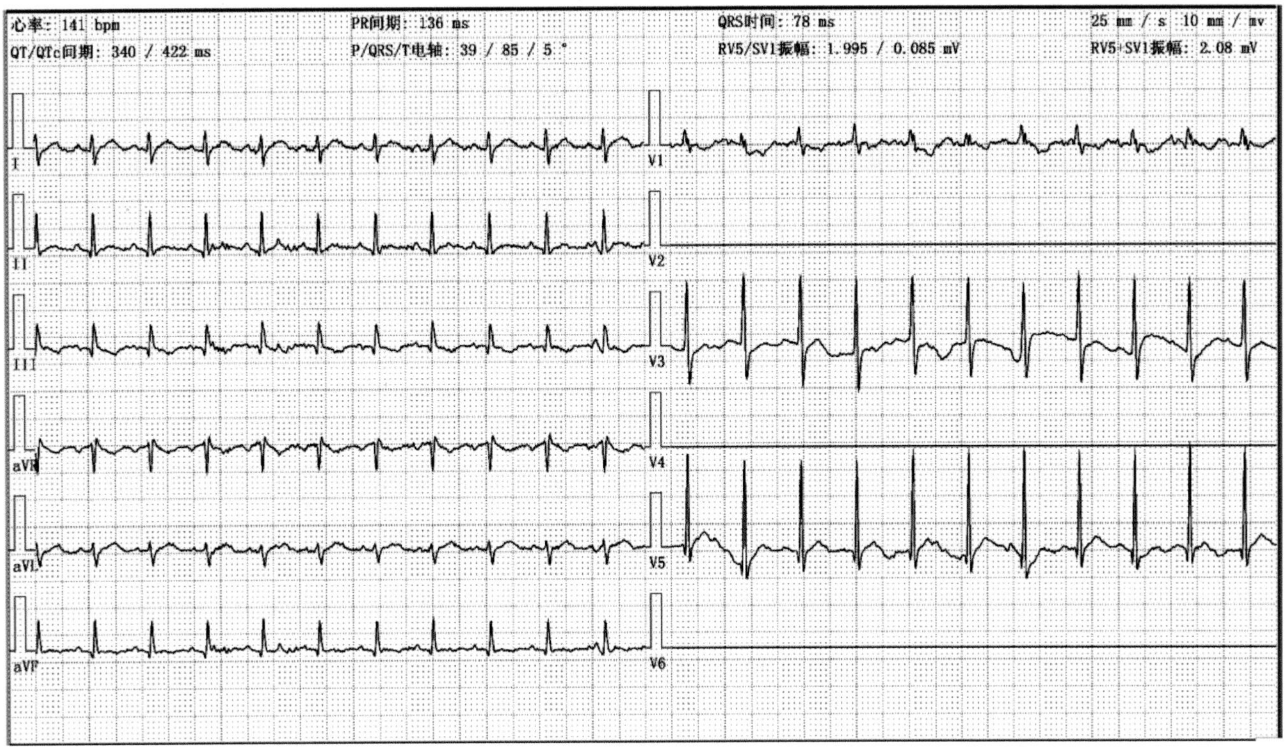

Fig. 3.22 On Day 7 of illness, ECG showed low level of T wave in the inferior wall of myocardium

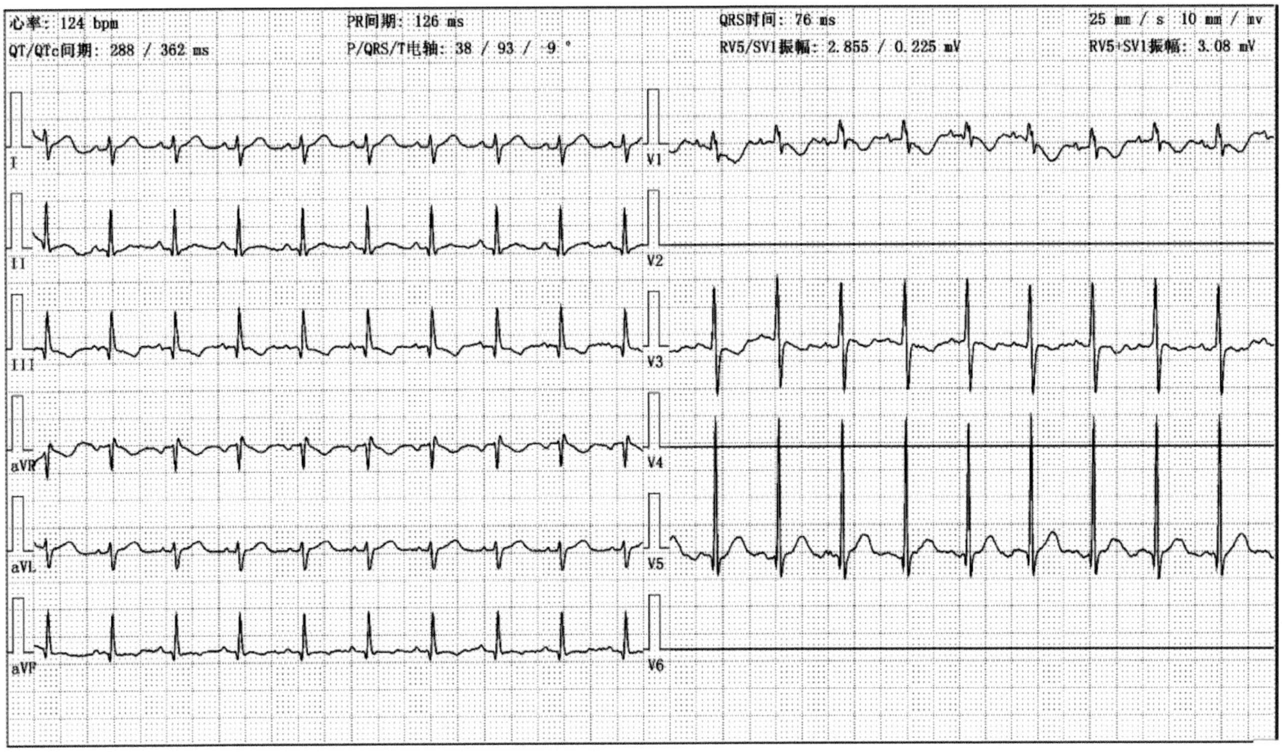

Fig. 3.23 On Day 8 of illness, ECG showed T wave still lower in the inferior wall of myocardium

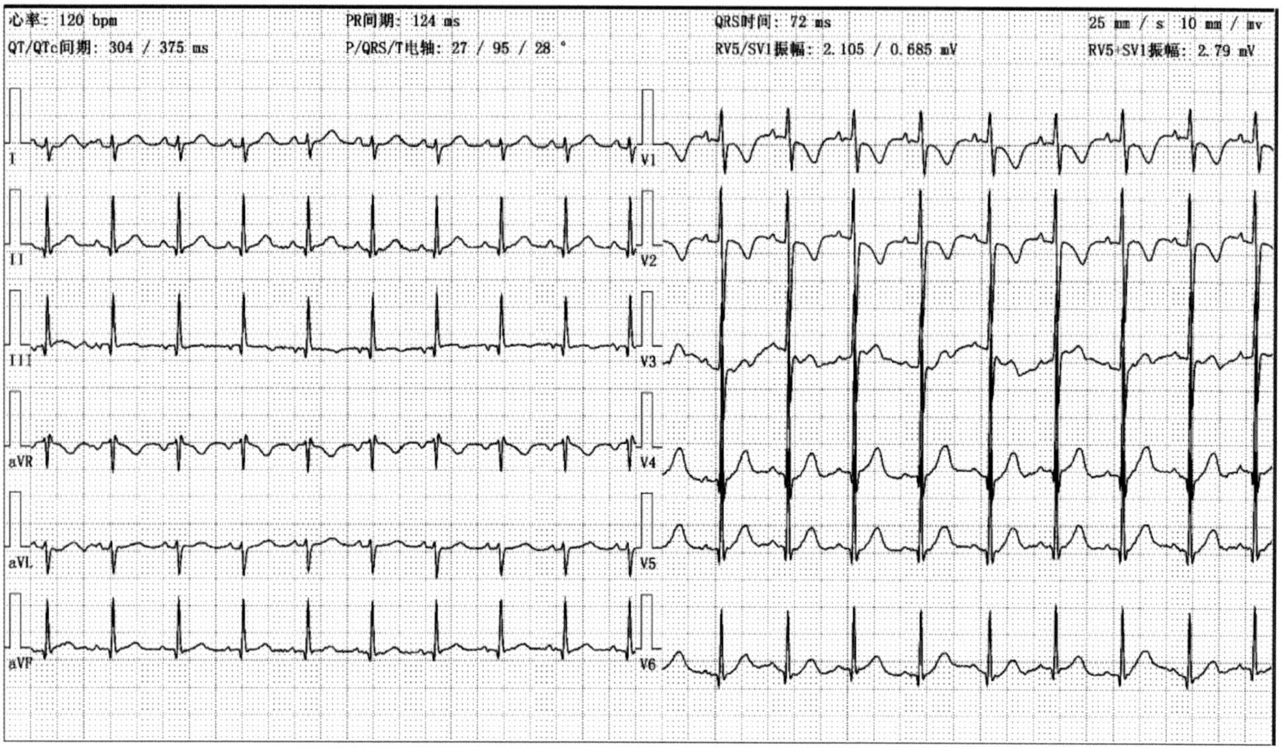

Fig. 3.24 On Day 11 of illness, ECG showed normal

Echo showed LCA 3.4mm, RCA 3.5mm (Fig. 3.24). He was treated with (1) neurology consultation and was recommended to have dynamic EEG performed; (2) IVIG another 2g/kg in 24 hours. On Day 12, the fever interval was prolonged, the fever peak was down to 37.7°C. Examination found edema hand and foot alleviated but still somnolence, neck stiffness, and eyes convergence. Abdominal ultrasound revealed 2.4cm of peritoneal effusion. Retested blood showed WBC 12×10^9/L, NE 55.7%, HGB 88g/L, PLT 488×10^9/L. Non-fasting glucose 6.9mmol/L, potassium 2.9mmol/L, sodium 134mmol/L. Pediatric neurology consultation opinion: diagnosis with meningoencephalitis, and he was given: (1) intravenous combined with oral potassium supplement; (2) lumbar puncture, retesting for blood bacteria and tuberculosis; (3) ABEP and the brain MRI; (4) consulting ophthalmologist and tuberculosis specialist; (5) effective antibiotics and supportive treatment. CSF pressure was normal (30 drops/points). Pandy's test was positive, the total number of cells was 20×10^6/L, WBC 10×10^6/L. CSF biochemistry: protein 0.86g/L. MP-IgM in CSF negative. On Day 13, retested CRP 17mg/L. NT-pro BNP 1991 pg/ml, hs-cTnT 0.014 ng/ml. DIC: D-Dimer 928μg/L, FDP 6.1mg/L. Liver function: ALB 30.7g/l. Troponin I was normal. On Day 15, CSF culture was negative and repeated BAEP was normal. Fever regressed to 37.3°C but he still had binocular convergence and was sleepy. On Day 17, repeated ECG was normal. Rechecked echo showed LCA about 3–3.4mm, LAD 3.3mm, RCA 3–3.5mm (Fig. 3.25). Dynamic EEG showed bilateral hemispherical δ wave (Fig. 3.26). Head MR was normal, MRA showed the right vertebral artery was slenderer than the left one (Fig. 3.27). Consulting pediatric neurology specialist, and he suggested to improve the brain blood supply for treatment. On Day 18, he was afebrile. We switched medication from ceftriaxone to cefuroxime sodium. On the following day, repeated lumbar puncture showed CSF WBC 7×10^6/L. Pandy's test was negative. CSF protein was 0.77g/L. Laboratory parameter revealed WBC 3.1×10^9/L, NE 8.8%. CRP, NT-pro BNP, hs-cTnT, and liver function were normal. On Day 22, his right eye recovered and mental state improved. Retested blood

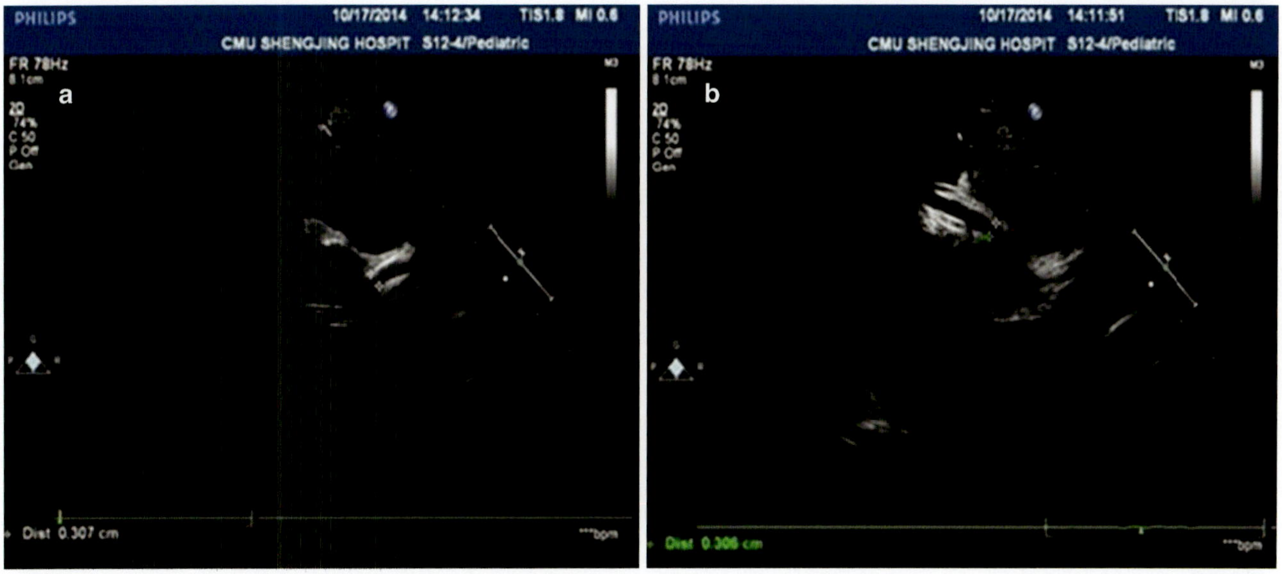

Fig. 3.25 On Day 11 of illness, echo showed: LCA 3.4mm (**a**), RCA 3.5mm (**b**)

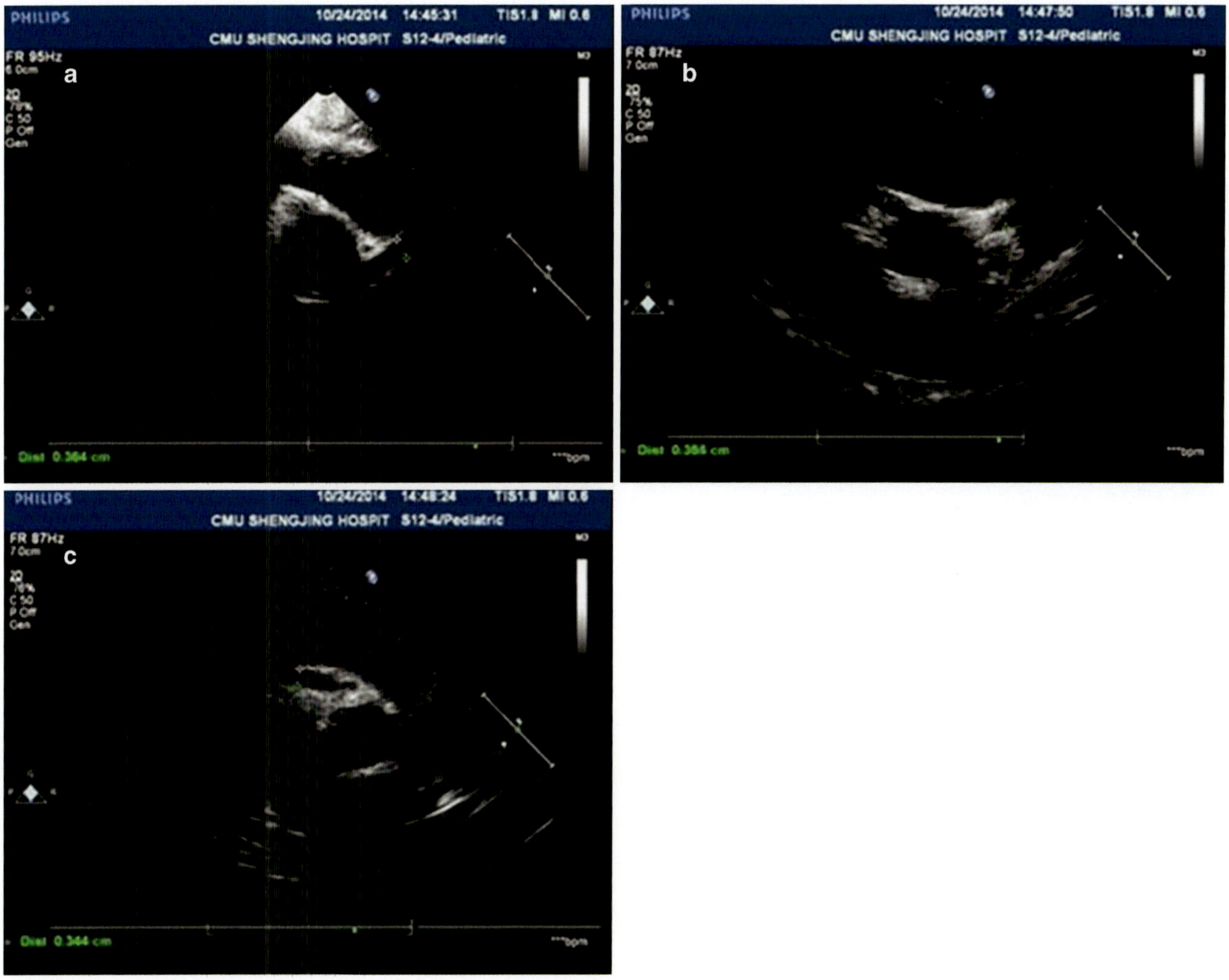

Fig. 3.26 On Day 17 of illness, echo showed: LCA 3.6mm (**a**), LAD 3.6mm (**b**), RCA 3.4mm (**c**)

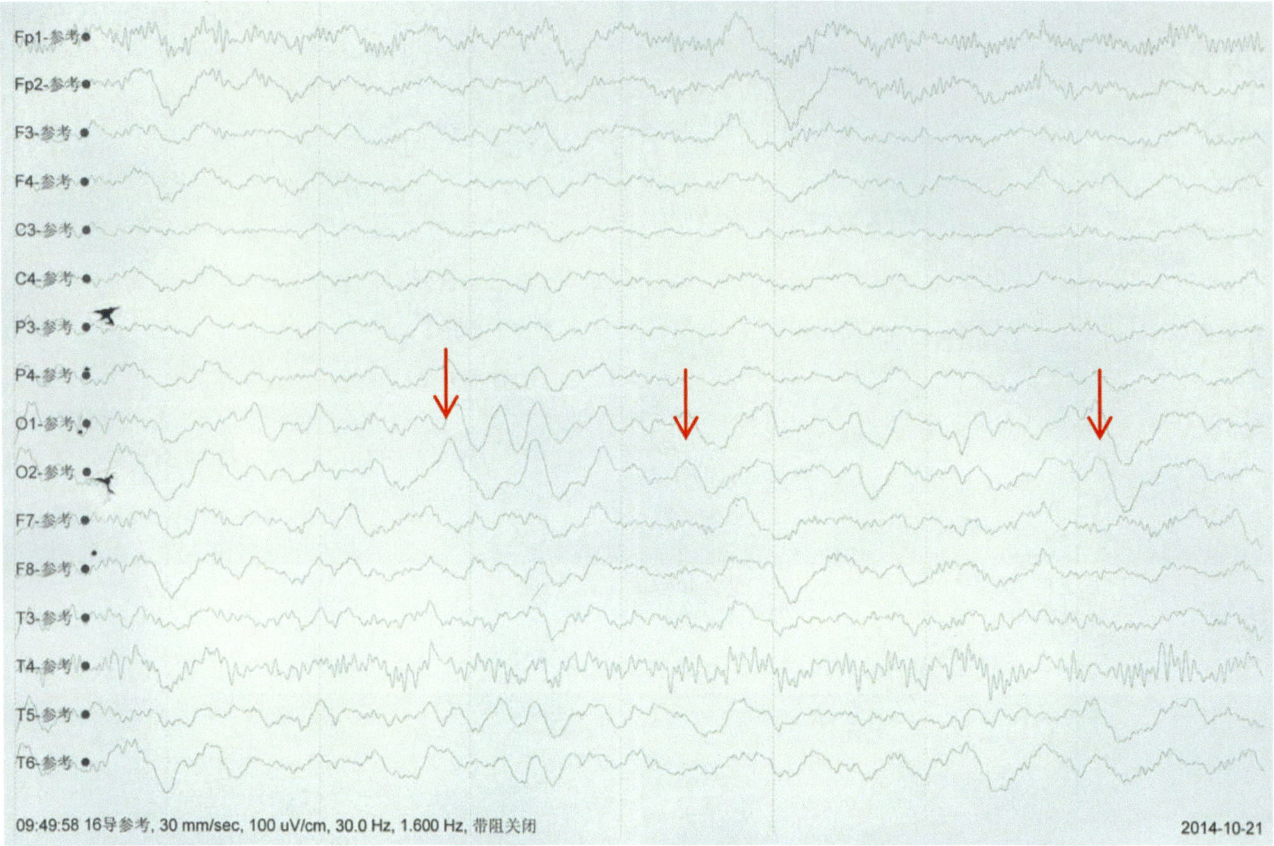

Fig. 3.27 On Day 17 of illness, dynamic EEG: bilateral hemispherical δ wave.

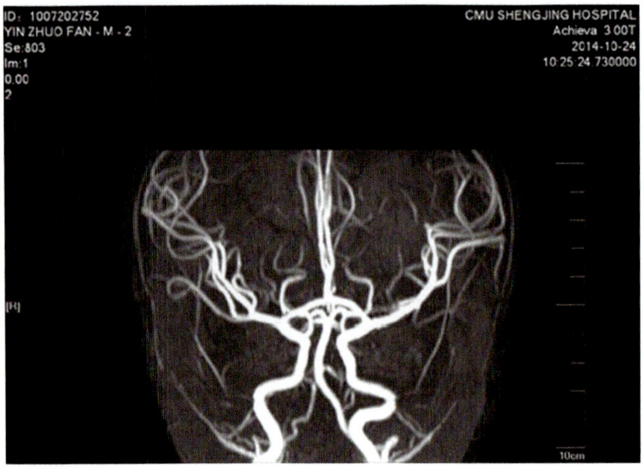

Fig. 3.28 On Day 17 of illness, MRA showed right vertebral artery was slenderer than left

showed WBC 3.2×10^9/L, NE 30%, HGB 95g/L, PLT 473×10^9/L. Pediatric neurologist consultation suggested the patient had KD and aseptic meningoencephalitis. He was treated with lysine inositol vitamin B_{12} orally and mannitol used once a day for 3 days. On the following two days, rechecked echo showed LCA 3.3–3.8mm, LAD normal, RCA 2.9–3.3mm (Fig. 3.28). Repeated lung CT showed decreased bilateral lung permeability (Fig. 3.29a). The left lung slanting crack increased slightly and no effusion was found (Fig. 3.30b).

On Day 25, everything went well except for left eye convergence. Retested blood revealed WBC 3.6×10^9/L, NE 35%, HGB 100g/L, PLT 332×10^9/L. ESR 41mm/h. The patient was discharged.

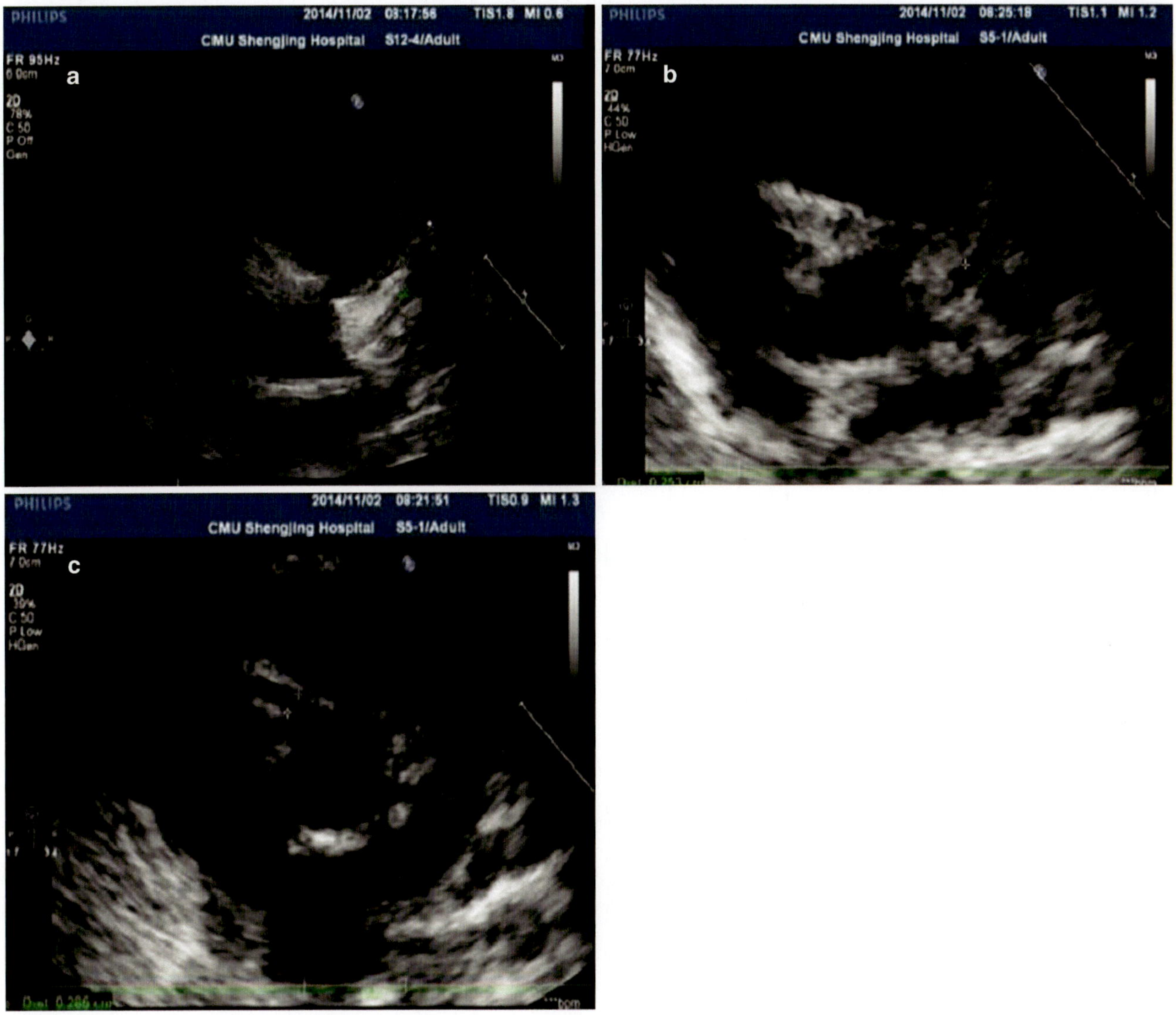

Fig. 3.29 On Day 26 of illness, echo showed: LCA 3.7mm (**a**), LAD 2.5mm (**b**), RCA 3.3mm (**c**)

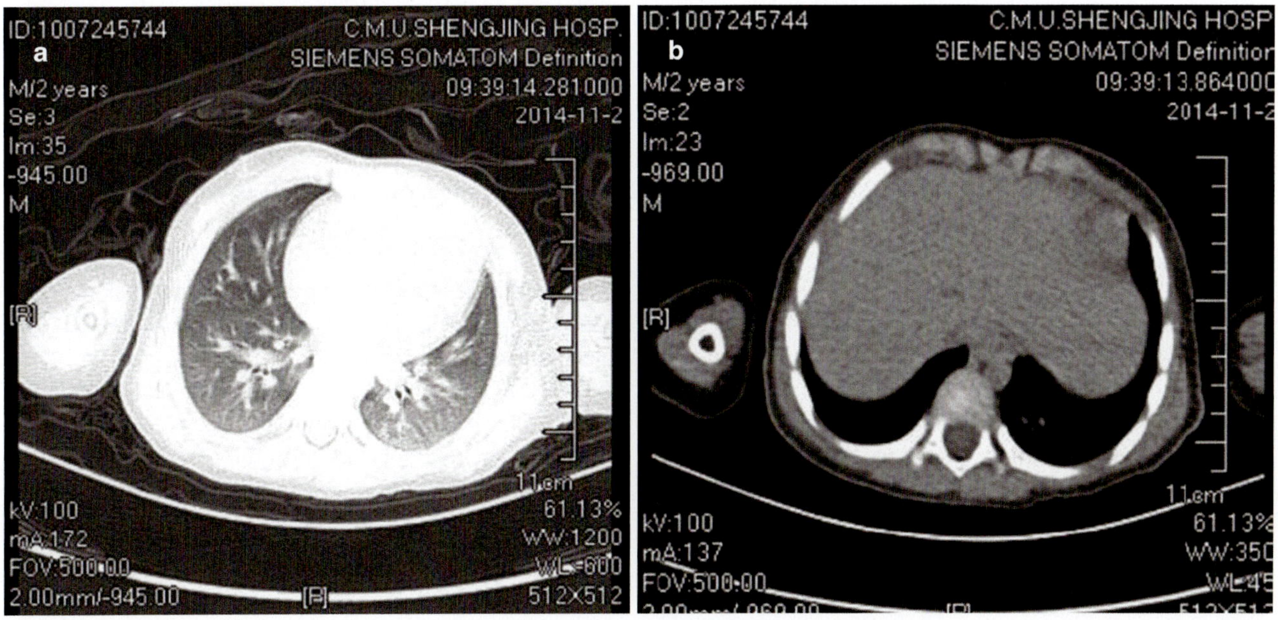

Fig. 3.30 On Day 26 of illness, bilateral lung permeability decreased (**a**), no effusion was found (**b**).

3.5.1 Clinical Course of the Patient

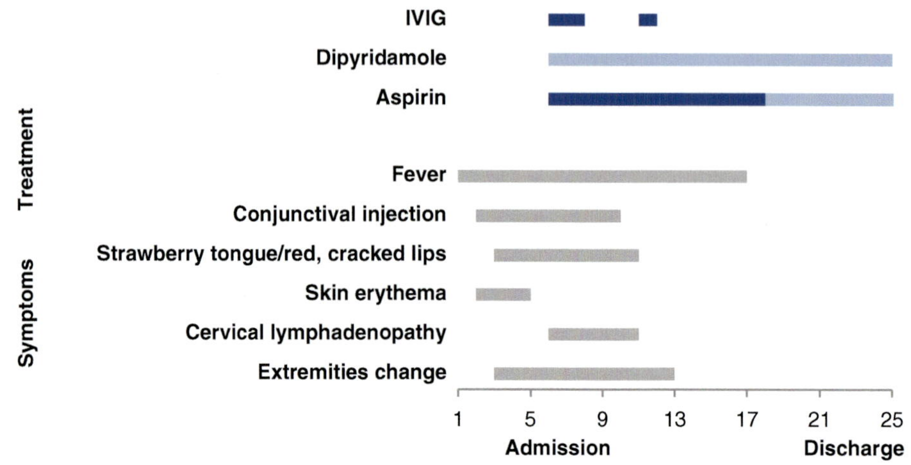

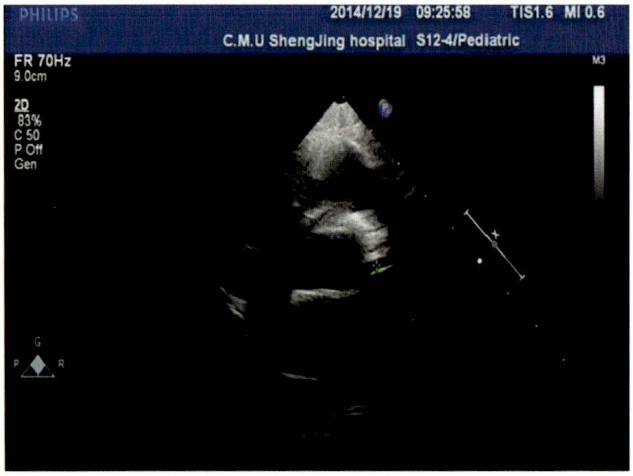

Fig. 3.31 Two months later: echo showed LCA normal

3.5.2 Follow-Up

Since discharge, he was given intramuscular injection of monosialotetrahexosylganglioside Sodium qod for 2 months until his left eye recovered. Echo was performed at 1, 2, 5, and 24 months, and LCA recovered at 2 months (Fig. 3.31) and remained normal to 2 years. RCA recovered at 5 months of illness. He stopped taking aspirin orally. EEG was not recorded again after he was discharged.

3.5.3 Diagnosis

1. KD
2. Bilateral coronary artery dilatation
3. Myocardial injury
4. Aseptic meningoencephalitis
5. Abduction nerve paralysis
6. Hypoproteinemia
7. Bilateral pleural effusion
8. Peritoneal effusion
9. Acute bronchitis
10. MP infection
11. Moderate anemia
12. Thrombocytopenia
13. Myelocytic deficiency
14. Parainfluenza virus infection
15. Hypokalemia

3.5.4 Discussion

The diagnostic basis of KD was enough: He had prolonged fever over 5 days and the fever could not be under control when treated with antibiotics. He also had (1) rashes during the course of the disease; (2) bilateral bulbar conjunctival congestion without exudate, (3) erythema of the hands; (4) cervical lymphadenopathy, and CRP 198mg/L.

Differential diagnosis of scarlet fever, sepsis, and purulent meningitis should be considered. After the first 2g/kg gamma globulin was given to the child, his fever was not obviously regressed, and had feet edema and significantly elevated CRP, which belonged to IVIG resistance, then additional 2g/kg IVIG was given. After the initial IVIG treatment, he still had persistent fever and CRP remained high. According to the literature report, this is a high-risk index for IVIG resistance. Thus, patient can be treated with IVIG combined with corticosteroids [2].

This patient had severe KD with complications in multiple organs, liver dysfunction, and decrease in albumin, the latter may be associated with the pleural and abdominal effusion. When hypoalbuminemia (albumin below 30g/L) occurred, the patient needs intravenous infusion of albumin to relieve the edema in the inner wall of the coronary artery [16].

3.5.5 Case Specific Clinic Features

1. The neurological involvement of children with KD is varied: the most common cases are aseptic meningitis, epileptic seizures, temporary hemiplegia, facial paralysis, ataxia, hearing impairment, abnormal visual acuity, and abnormal behaviors were also reported [1, 17–21]. This boy's eyes were normal at admission, and then gradually developed into binocular convergence after admission. After treatment, the right eye was recovered first, and about one month later the left one also recovered. These changes supported KD with oculomotor nerve involvement.
2. Suppression in bone marrow after infection, and medications such as antibiotics, aspirin and dipyridamole, may contribute to the leukocytic reduction and neutrophils deficiency. Traditional Chinese medication was given orally to increase leukocyte.
3. Echo was rechecked at three weeks of illness, and LAD was wider than before. For it was within one month of disease onset, and it belonged to the progressive period of inflammation, so it was necessary to recheck echocardiography weekly.
4. The child had bilateral coronary dilation. He needed to take oral aspirin until coronary arteries became normal, continue to take it for another three months, in addition to repeated echo for dynamic follow-up. Taking aspirin to normalize coronary arteries and another 3 months are required. Thus, it was necessary to perform echo check regularly. It is recommended that computed tomographic angiography should be performed within one month of onset during the acute phase (one month) in patients with CAA or coronary artery dilatation [17]. According to guidelines, IVIG, aspirin, and regular ECHO can significantly reduce the incidence of CAA [18].

Ce Wang

References

1. Alves NR, Magalhães CM, Almeida Rde F, et al. Prospective study of Kawasaki disease complications: review of 115 cases. Rev Assoc Med Bras. 2011;57(3):299–300.
2. Nakagama Y, Inuzuka R, Hayashi T, et al. Fever pattern and C-reactive protein predict response to rescue therapy in Kawasaki disease. Pediatr Int. 2016;58(3):180–4.
3. Newburger JW, Takahashi M, Gerber MA, et al. Diagnosis, treatment, and long-term management of Kawasaki disease: a statement for health professionals from the Committee on Rheumatic Fever, Endocarditis and Kawasaki Disease, Council on Cardiovascular Disease in the Young, American Heart Association. Circulation. 2004;110(17):2747–71.
4. Soares MO, Welton NJ, Harrison DA, et al. An evaluation of the feasibility, cost and value of information of a multicenter randomized controlled trial of intravenous immunoglobulin for sepsis (severe sepsis and septic shock): incorporating a systematic review, meta-analysis and value of information analysis. Health Technol Assess. 2012;16(7):l–186.
5. Stowe RC. Facial nerve palsy, Kawasaki disease, and coronary artery aneurysm. Eur J Paediatr Neurol. 2015;19(5):607–9.
6. Emiroglu M, Alkan G, Kartal A, et al. Abducens nerve palsy in a girl with incomplete Kawasaki disease. Rheumatol Int. 2016;36(8):1181–3.
7. Amano S, Hazama F. Neural involvement in Kawasaki disease. Acta Pathol Jpn. 1980;30(3):365–3.
8. Guven B, Tavli V, Mese T, et al. Isolated abducens palsy in adolescent girl with Kawasaki disease. Pediatr Int. 2010;52(2):334.
9. Rodríguez-Lozano A, Juárez-Echenique JC, Rivas-Larrauri F, et al. VI nerve palsy after intravenous immunoglobulin in Kawasaki disease. Allergol Immunopathol (Madr). 2014;42(1):82–3.
10. Wurzburger BJ, Jeffrey RA. Lateral rectus palsy in Kawasaki disease. Pediatr Infect Dis J. 1999;18(11):1029–31.
11. Wang H, Yu XY, Piao YA. A case report about Kawasaki Disease with multi organs lesions. Pediatric Emerg Med. 2000;7(3):165.
12. Kuo HC, Yang KD, Chang WC, et al. Kawasaki disease: an update on diagnosis and treatment. Pediatr Neonatol. 2012;53(1):4–11.
13. Xue LJ, Wu R, Du GL, et al. Effect and safety of TNF inhibitors in immunoglobulin-resistant Kawasaki disease: a meta-analysis. Clin Rev Allergy Immunol. 2017;52(3):389–400.
14. Matsui M, Okuma Y, Yamanaka J, et al. Kawasaki disease refractory to standard treatments that responds to a combination of pulsed methylprednisolone and plasma exchange: Cytokine profiling and literature review. Cytokine. 2015;74(2):339–42.
15. Sabatino G, Midulla M, Morgese G, et al. Kawasaki's syndrome: description of 4 cases. Pediatr Med Chir. 1984;6(4):521–7.
16. Miura M, Kobayashi T, Kaneko T, et al. Association of severity of coronary artery aneurysms in patients with Kawasaki disease and risk of later coronary events. JAMA Pediatr. 2018;172(5):e180030.
17. Grande Gutierrez N, Shirinsky O, Gagarina N, et al. Assessment of coronary artery aneurysms caused by Kawasaki disease using Transluminal attenuation gradient analysis of computerized tomography angiograms. Am J Cardiol. 2017;120(4):556–2.
18. Michihata N, Matsui H, Fushimi K, et al. Guideline concordant treatment of Kawasaki disease with immunoglobulin and aspirin and the incidence of coronary artery aneurysm. Clin Pediatr. 2015;54(11):1076–80.
19. Poon LK, Lun KS, Ng YM. Facial nerve palsy and Kawasaki disease. Hong Kong Med J. 2000;6(2):224–6.
20. Knott PD, Orloff LA, Harris JP, et al. Kawasaki disease multicenter hearing loss study group. Sensorineural hearing loss and Kawasaki disease: a prospective study. Am J Otolaryngol. 2001;22(5):343–8.
21. Amano S, Hazama F. Neutral involvement in Kawasaki disease. Acta Pathol Jpn. 1980;30(3):365–73.

KD with Digestive System Involvement

4

Xuexin Yu, Xuemei Li, Hong Wang, Yue Zhang, and Yunlong Huo

Abstract

Gastrointestinal symptoms or signs are not part of the diagnostic criteria for KD. However, many patients with KD have abdominal complaints as part of their presentation. Actually, a retrospective research revealed about 6% KD patients consulted gastroenterologist initially (Ohnishi et al., J Med Ultrason (2001) 45(2):381–384, 2018). Their median duration of illness at gastroenterology consultation was 5 days, whereas median duration of illness at infectious disease consultation was 6 days. It is interesting that patients in this series with gastrointestinal presentation were male, older, and had lower inflammatory markers and peripheral blood eosinophilia.

Gastrointestinal symptoms, notably are diarrhea, abdominal pain, and frequently occurred vomiting. Furthermore, elevated serum aminotransferases, gallbladder hydrops, and rarely other forms of gastrointestinal involvement such as ischemic colitis, intussusception, hepatic necrosis, splenic infarct, intestinal pseudo-obstruction, colitis, and colon edema are also reported (Newburger et al., Circulation 110(17):2747–2771, 2004). The severity of these symptoms is highly variable among patients. Acute abdominal pain and distension, vomiting, hepatomegaly, and jaundice were the most common symptoms at onset. In most cases, gastrointestinal symptoms gradually resolve after the treatment of KD itself. Surgical abdominal complications of KD have rarely been reported in the literature. These complications include gallbladder hydrops with cholestasis, small intestinal occlusion, paralytic ileus ischemic colitis and massive liver necrosis, hemorrhagic duodenitis, and appendicular vasculitis (Bagrul et al., Cardiol Young 28(8):1070–1073, 2018). Zulian et al. reported that 10 of 219 patients (4.6%) presented with severe abdominal complaints required surgical intervention or endoscopy (Zulian et al., J Pediatr 142(6):731–735, 2003). The postoperative diagnoses were gallbladder hydrops, paralytic ileus, appendicitis, and hemorrhagic duodenitis. Garnett described two cases with acute surgical abdomen in whose acute appendicitis was histologically confirmed (Garnett et al., Pediatr Surg Int 30(5):549–552, 2014). If abdominal symptoms are predominant and features typical of KD are not evident, initiation of appropriate medical treatment may be delayed, with potential consequences for the development of cardiac sequelae (Zulian et al., J Pediatr 142(6):731–735, 2003). Abdominal ultrasonography can help evaluate the gastrointestinal complications of KD. Unexplained gastrointestinal symptoms in the presence of fever and rash and at least 1 or 2 of the major clinical signs of KD (especially non-exudative conjunctivitis, mucocutaneous changes) should prompt consideration of KD in the differential diagnosis.

In this chapter, we listed 6 KD cases accompanied with gastrointestinal involvement including liver, gallbladder, intestinal tract, and pancreas. None of them required surgical intervention, and the prognosis was well.

X. Yu · X. Li · H. Wang (✉) · Y. Zhang
Department of Pediatric Cardiology, Shengjing Hospital of China Medical University, Shenyang, China

Y. Huo
Department of Pathology, Shengjing Hospital of China Medical University, Shenyang, China

4.1 Case 21 KD with Gastrointestinal and Liver Dysfunction

A previously healthy 2-year-old male presented to hospital with unremarkable past medical and family history.

He presented to our hospital on Day 9 of illness with a history of fever for 9 days, abnormal liver function and ventosity, congested rashes on the back for 2 days, and feet edema for 4 days. In local hospital, he was treated with IVIG 15 g (average 400 mg/kg/day), erythromycin, cephalosporin, and liver-protecting drug. *Examination* revealed the following results: afebril, smooth breath (HR 110 bpm, RR 24 bpm), warm hands and feet (BP 90/60 mmHg), enlarged

H. Wang (ed.), *Paediatric Kawasaki Disease*, https://doi.org/10.1007/978-981-15-0038-1_4

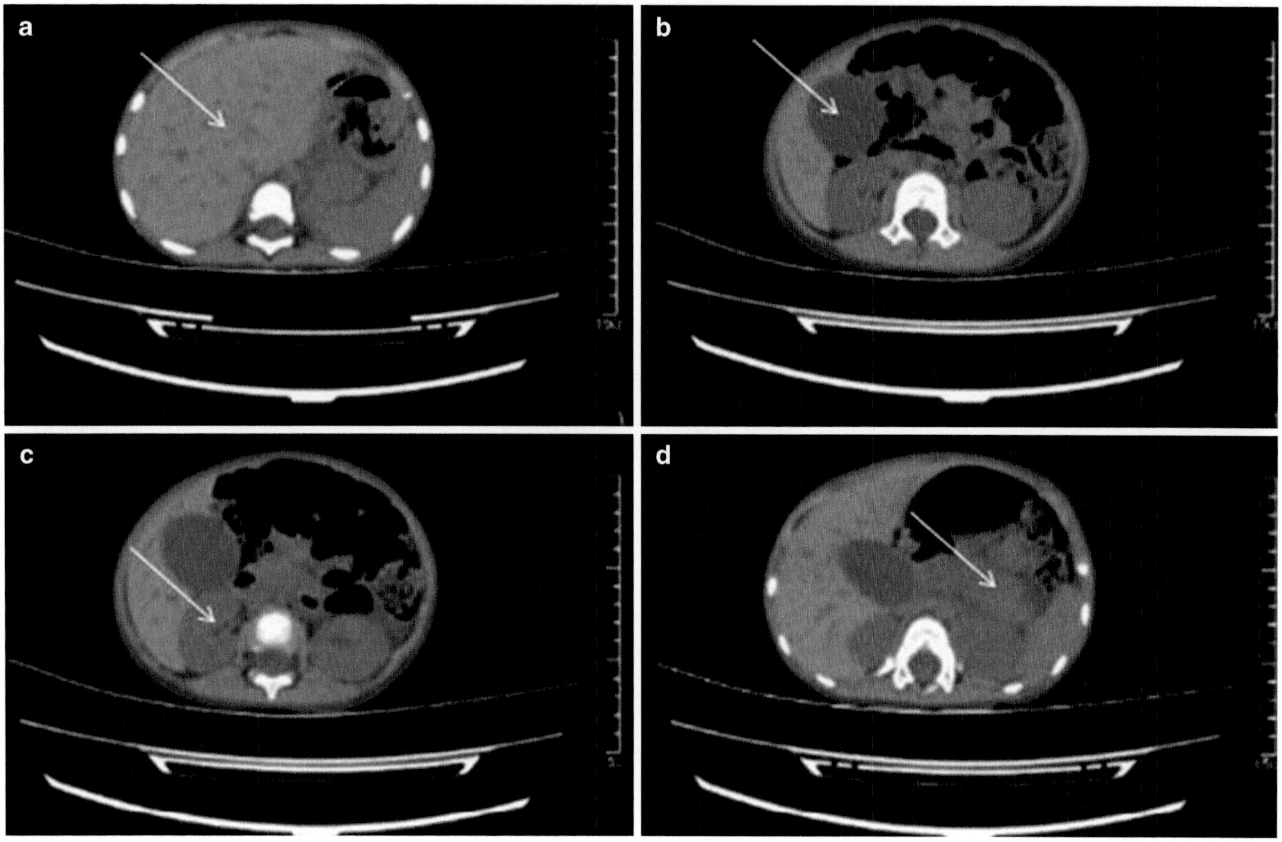

Fig. 4.1 On Day 9 of illness, abdominal CT scan showed hepatomegaly (**a**), gallbladder enlargement (**b**), mild pyelectasis (**c**), the pancreatic parenchyma is full and mild edema maybe (**d**)

liver 3.0 cm below right costal margin (moderate hard), and enlarged spleen 1.0 cm below left costal margin (moderate hard). He had ventosity in the abdomen (soft at touch) along with hypoactive bowel sounds. He had edema in lower limbs and feet. Others were normal. *Admission blood* test revealed a normal complete blood count, slightly elevated CRP (14.5 mg/L); liver function TP 51.28 g/L, ALB 23.42 g/L, ALT 57 U/L, AST 200 U/L, blood amylase 28 U/L, lipase 56.3 U/L, blood glucose 4.9 mmol/L, serum potassium 2.88 mmol/L. Urinalysis, kidney function, and myocardial enzyme were normal. Abdominal CT scan showed (1) hepatomegalia (Fig. 4.1a), gallbladder enlargement (Fig. 4.1b); (2) mild pyelectasis (Fig. 4.1c); (3) the pancreatic parenchyma being full and showing mild edema (Fig. 4.1d); (4) ascites (Fig. 4.2). She was treated with (1) fasting, hypovolemia correction, fluid infusion; (2) zinacef infusion; (3) albumin infusion.

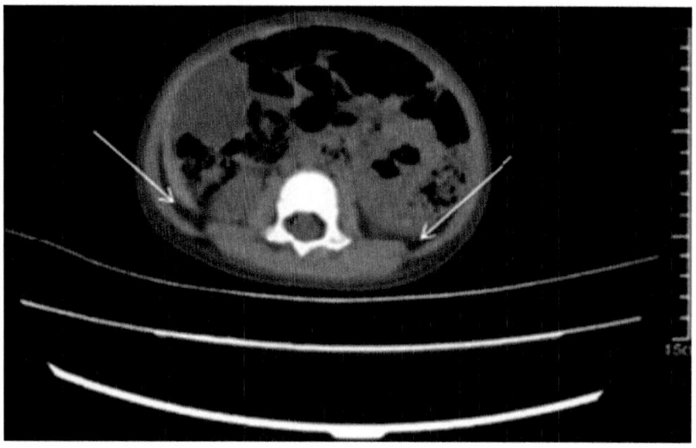

Fig. 4.2 On Day 9 of illness, abdominal CT scan showed ascites

On Day 10, he was feverish again spiking to 39 °C. Investigation revealed: ESR 41 mm/h. ALB 25 g/L, ALT 41 U/L, AST 21 U/L. Serum potassium 4.12 mmol/L; MP-IgM and CP-IgM negative, MP-IgG positive (1:160). Chest DR was normal. Abdominal ultrasound revealed hepatomegaly, enlarged 2.0 cm below right costal margin, and the echo was homogeneous (Fig. 4.3a). The gallbladder was about 10.5 cm × 3.3 cm and the wall was thickened about 0.2 cm (Fig. 4.3b). Hypogastric effusion was about 1.6 cm (Fig. 4.3c). He received infusion of azithromycin 10 mg/kg/day for 3 days. On Day 11, gastroscopy showed erythematous gastritis (Fig. 4.4a) and duodenum inflammation (Fig. 4.4b). Biopsy histopathology presented glands in regular shape, interstitial infiltration of lymphocytes and plasma cells, minor vessel expansion, and fibrous hyperplasia. It did not find significant dilation of lymphatic vessels (Fig. 4.5).

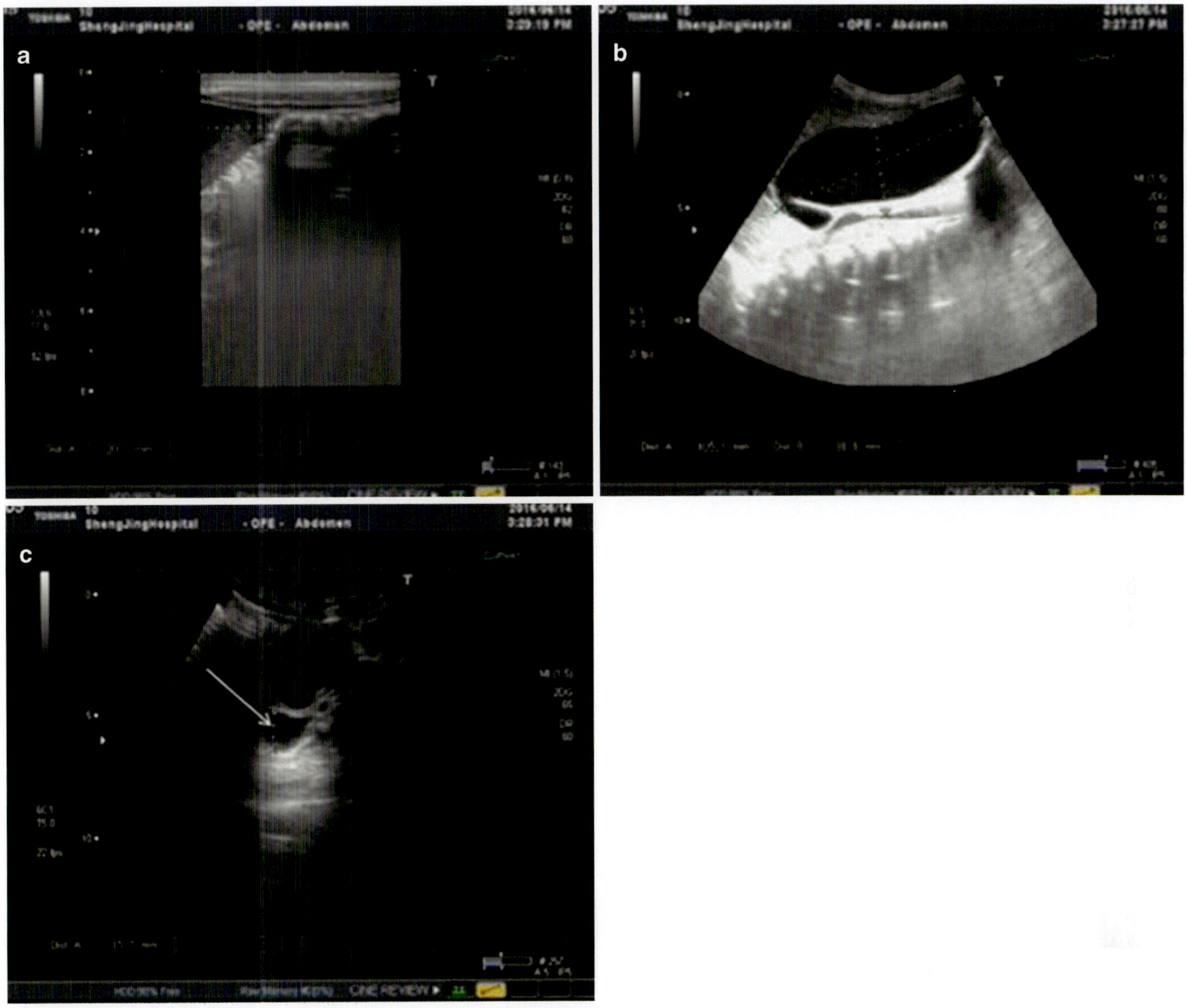

Fig. 4.3 On Day 10 of illness, abdominal ultrasound revealed hepatomegaly, which enlarged 2.0 cm below right costal margin and the echo was homogeneous (**a**), gallbladder was about 10.5 cm × 3.3 cm and the wall was thickness about 2 mm (**b**), hypogastric effusion was about 1.6 cm (**c**)

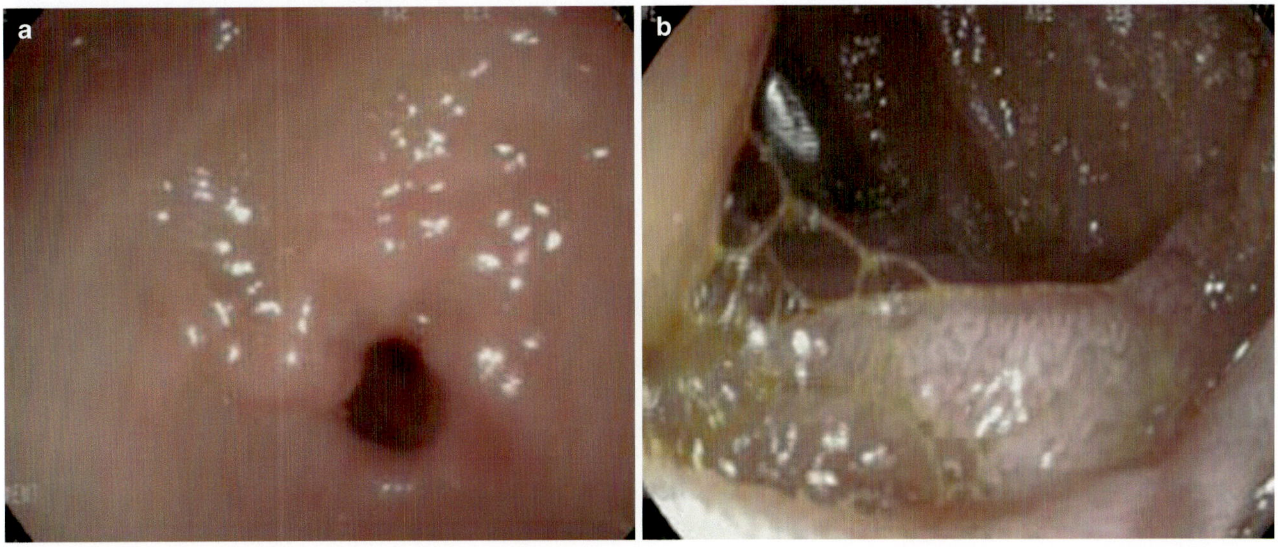

Fig. 4.4 On Day 11 of illness, gastroscopy showed erythematous gastritis (**a**), duodenum inflammation (**b**)

His mother confirmed he had bilateral conjunctival congestion, red lips, and edema in hands and feet before he was admitted. Cervical ultrasound showed lymphadenectasis on the left side, and the biggest one was 1.4 cm × 0.6 cm. He had met all the criteria for KD. He was treated with (1) IVIG 2 g/kg/day; (2) oral aspirin 30–50 mg/kg/day and dipyridamole 3–5 mg/kg/day in three divided doses; (3) infusion of creatine phosphate sodium 1 g/day. On Day 14, after IVIG, his fever was settled over 48 h and ventosity in abdomen was relieved. The dosage of aspirin was reduced to 3–5 mg/kg/day. Echo showed the LCA dilated about 3.3 mm (Fig. 4.6a), and RCA dilated about 3.2 mm (Fig. 4.6b).

On Day 16, he was in good condition. Retested blood work showed: WBC 6.34 × 10^9/L, NE% 91.6%, Hb100g/L, PLT 226 × 10^9/L, CRP 4.55 mg/L; normal ALB, ALT, and AST in liver function panel. He was discharged.

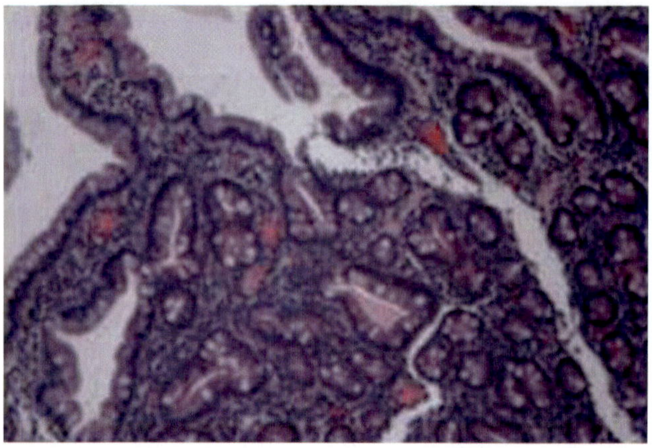

Fig. 4.5 Biopsy of gastric mucosa showed regular glandular shape, lymphocytes and plasma cell infiltrated interstitial, the minute vessel expands, fibrous hyperplasia, but no significant dilation of lymphatic vessels

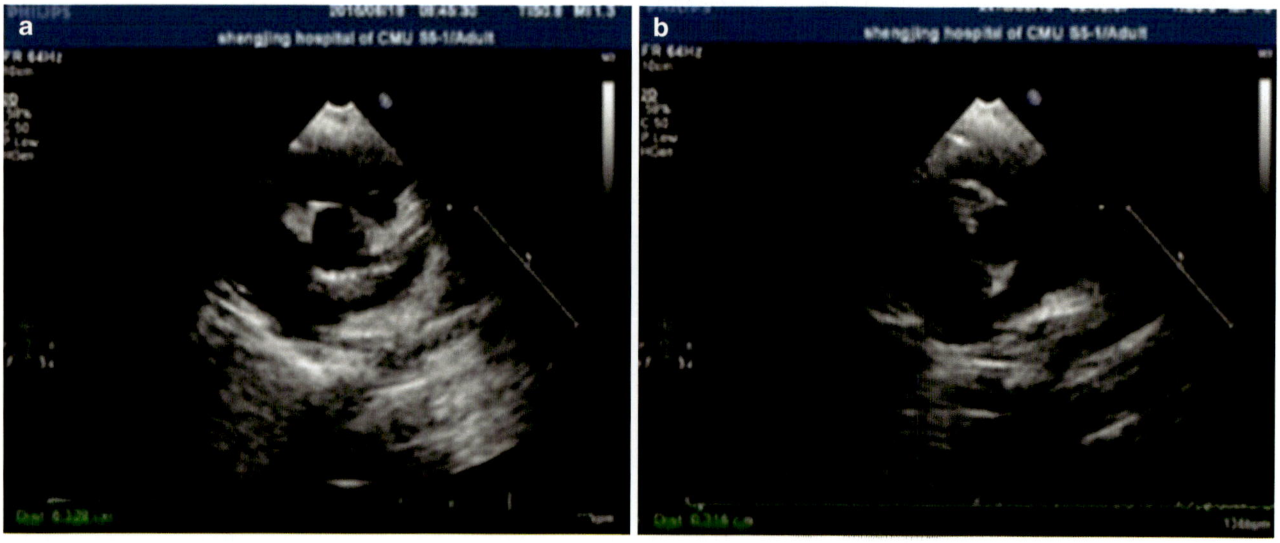

Fig. 4.6 On Day 14 of illness, echo showed the LCA dilated about 3.3 mm (**a**), RCA dilated about 3.2 mm (**b**)

4.1.1 Clinical Course of the Patient

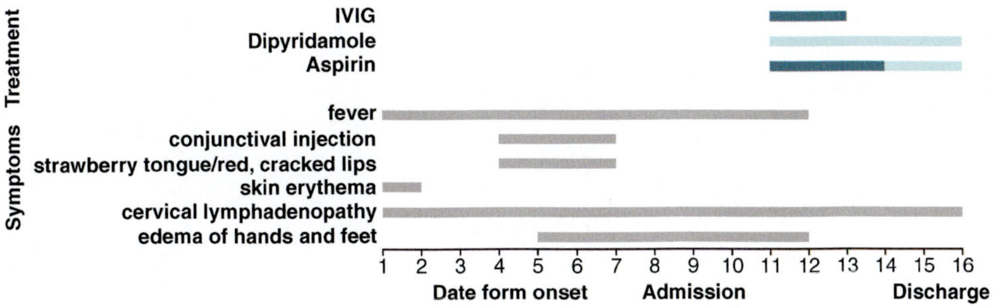

4.1.2 Follow Up

Since discharged, he continued to take: (1) aspirin and dipyridamole; (2) FDP and levocarnitine. Echo was performed 3 weeks later. LCA was regressed to 3.1 mm (Fig. 4.7). RCA was normal. 4 weeks later, LCA was 3.0 mm. Both LCA (Fig. 4.8a) and RCA (Fig. 4.8b) recovered at 5 weeks of illness.

On Day 60, he had normal PLT, ESR, and echo. Then he stopped medication except aspirin until at 4 months of illness.

4.1.3 Diagnosis

1. KD.
2. Bilateral coronary artery dilatation.
3. Hypoalbuminemia.
4. Liver dysfunction.
5. Hypokalemia.
6. Mild anemia.
7. MP infection.

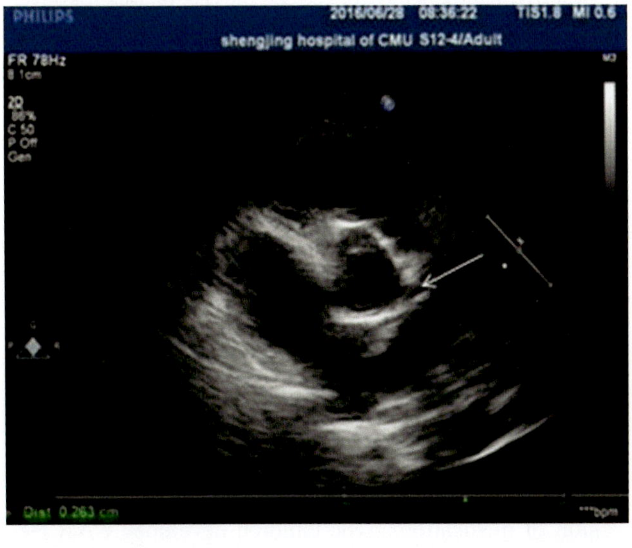

Fig. 4.7 2D echo performed at 3 weeks of illness, LCA was regressed to 3.1 mm (arrow), RCA was normal

4.1.4 Discussion

He had met the criteria of KD for he had continuous fever lasting more than 5 days, along with (1) conjunctival congestion without exudation; (2) generalized rashes; (3) red lips; (4) edema in hands and feet; (5) bilateral coronary artery dilatation shown in echo.

4.1.5 Case Specific Clinic Features

1. KD is an inflammatory disease mostly happening in childhood. Patients can present with complications with multi-systems involved, often vasculitis in small-medium sized arteries. The most common pathologic findings are systemic vasculitis and a high incidence of inflammatory lesions affecting various organs, such as liver, kidney, lungs, and nervous system. The most serious and life-threatening complication in KD is the development of angitis and aneurysmal dilation in the coronary arteries accompanied by thrombosis. In some cases, patients die from coronary artery disease. However, the inflammatory lesions occur not only in coronary arteries but also in abdominal arteries. Liver dysfunction may be mild with slightly elevated transaminase, or severe with cholestasis hepatitis, cholecystitis, and so on [1–3]. The mechanism of liver dysfunction in KD has not been fully established. Hypotheses include generalized inflammation, vasculitis in small and medium sized vessels, congestive heart failure secondary to myocarditis, non-steroidal anti-inflammatory antipyretics, toxin-mediated effects, or a combination of above events [4].
2. Although the association between hypoalbuminemia and coronary artery abnormalities has been reported previously, the mechanism of hypoalbuminemia in KD is not completely understood. Inflammatory processes have

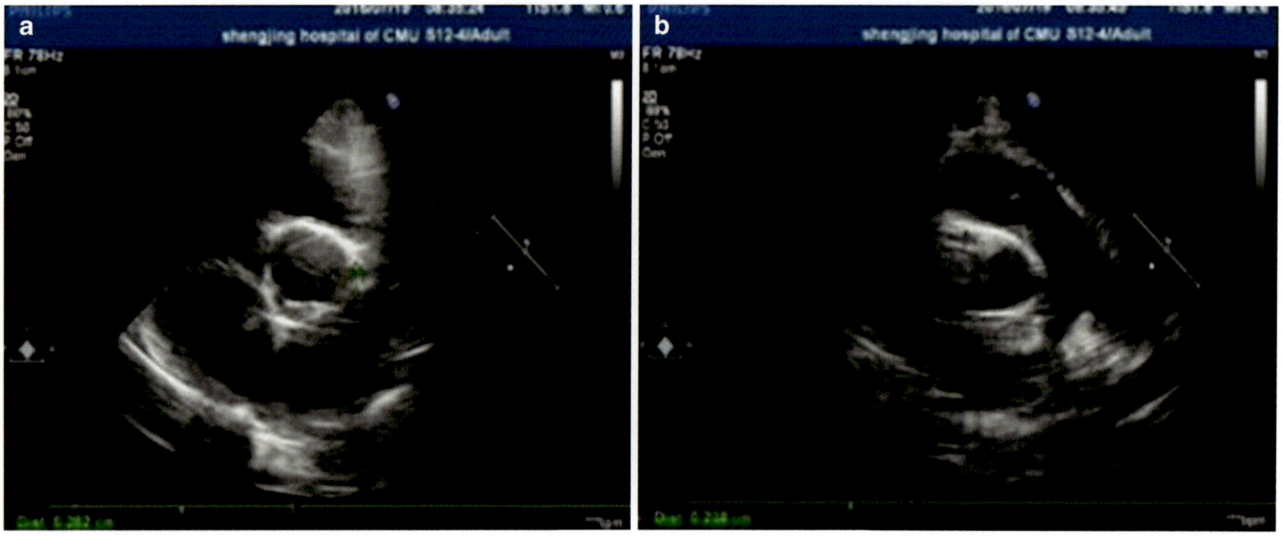

Fig. 4.8 At 5 weeks of illness, both LCA (**a**) and RCA (**b**) were normal

been associated with hypoalbuminemia and appear to be mediated, at least in part, by inflammatory cytokines directing protein synthesis toward increased production of acute phase proteins (i.e., CRP), followed by subsequent decreases in production of other proteins such as albumin. Additionally, during acute inflammation, there may be increased albumin escaping from inflamed vessels, often referred as capillary leak. Finally, an inflammation reaction at acute phase can change matrix structure of intestine, leading to increases in interstitial space of intestine [5–7].

3. The mechanism of anemia caused by KD is not very clear. Some believe that non-bacterial inflammatory reactions inhibit hematopoietic function of bone marrow. After all, inflammation-associated anemia represents a significant andhighly prevalent problem in clinic [8]. Chronic disease anemia is often observed in various inflammatory states, such as infections, inflammatory disorders, and certain cancers [9]. Of course, anemia caused by KD can be subsided in the self-recovery process.
4. In this case, the boy was nonresponsive to broad-spectrum antibiotics. Laboratory investigations showed elevated transaminases and reduced albumin. On Day 6–7 of illness, IVIG 400 mg/kg was administered, and it rapidly ameliorate the overall condition and regressed fever. However, he was feverish again, along with edema on feet 3 days later. After further enquiry with his parents, we confirmed that he had all major symptoms of KD, especially bilateral coronary artery dilation. These confirmed the diagnosis. Second fever was thought to be related to the insufficient dosage of gamma globulin. So he was treated with IVIG 2 g/kg/day and oral aspirin and persantine. He recovered soon and was discharged.
5. Gastrointestinal symptom is a common feature of KD. Children with KD have decreased appetite that is associated with fever and with gastrointestinal reaction to oral aspirin. This symptom occurs almost in every infant with nausea and vomiting. The diagnosis for this patient was not finalized. We decided to performgastroscopy. Because of this, we know that inflammation in vascular system in KD patients could be associated with a variety of complications in digestive system, such as gastritis, duodenitis, gallbladder wall edema, pancreatic edema, peritoneal effusion, abdominal wall edema, etc. These symptoms subsided after IVIG treatment and did not require treatment for gastric mucosa protection. The cause of hypokalemia in children was also associated with poor appetite.
6. Some researchers have described the risk factors for developing coronary artery injuries as the followings: being male, age <12 months, hypoalbuminemia, persistent fever for more than 2 weeks, WBC >30.0 × 10^9/L, ESR >100 mm/h, CRP >100 mg/L and non-responsive to IVIG. In this case, this patient was a boy and had hypoalbuminemia. On Day 6–7 of illness, IVIG 400 mg/kg was administered which ameliorated overall condition rapidly and controlled fever transiently. But CRP didn't drop to normal level and he was feverish again 3 days later. So he was treated with IVIG 2 g/kg/day and recovered. On Day 14, echo showed bilateral coronary artery dilatation. He continued to take oral aspirin and dipyridamole. Echo showed coronary artery dilatation returned gradually to normal. It is generally required to give patients oral aspirin and dipyridamole for another 3 months. Even with extension of medication, some children developed CAA (see the section of CAA) in the first year of illness. It indicates that in the cases of KD with persistent fever within

2 weeks, the timely and adequate treatment of IVIG is effective and could reduce the risk of coronary artery injury. To be safe, patients still need long-term follow-up.

Xue-mei Li

4.2 Case 22 KD with Acute Peritonitis

A previously healthy 5-year-old boy had no remarkable antenatal, family, and post medical history.

He presented on Day 3 of illness with diarrhea for 3 days along with stomachache and fever for 2 days. On the first day of illness, he had mucous stool 4–5 times and improved after he took some yeast. On Day 2 of illness, he developed fever (39.1 °C) and had paroxysmal stomachache on the right lower abdomen, without nausea or vomiting. He took first generation antibiotics and Ibuprofen at home. Fever, stomachache, and diarrhea were not regressed. He was brought to our clinic. After blood examination and abdominal CT scanning, he was admitted to pediatric surgery and was diagnosed with acute appendicitis. He lost appetite and slept poorly. His urine was normal. *Examination* showed that his spirit was nice, breath smoothly, and had afebrile (36.2 °C), P 90 bpm, R 24 bpm, Bp 73/57 mmHg, W 19.8 kg. Auscultation revealed normal heart and lung. Abdomen was flat, without varicose veins, ventosity, gastrointestinal type, or peristaltic wave. Right lower abdomen tenderness was obvious, without muscle tension or rebound tenderness, untouched package or hepatosplenomegaly. Shifting dullness was negative and the bowel sounds were 4 times/min. *Admission blood* test revealed WBC 20.06 × 10^9/L, NE 88.8%, RBC 4.3 × 10^{12}/L, HGB 115 g/L, PLT 425 × 10^9/L. CRP 103 mg/L. cTnI <0.01ug/L. pH 7.372, HCO_3^- 9.9 mmol/L, SBC 20.6↓mmol/L, ABE −4.2 mmol/L, SBE −4.5 mmol/L, K^+ 3.4 mmol/L, Na^+ 135 mmol/L, Anion gap (K+) 12.3 mmol/L; blood amylase hemodiastase (AMY) 14(20–129)U/L, lipase (LPS) 14.1(0–60) U/L. Feces were normal. Rotavirus titer was negative. Abdominal 3-D color ultrasound revealed no obvious effusion and mass image. Abdominal CT scan showed the gastrointestinal tract at the middle and upper abdomen was slightly dilated and aerated (Fig. 4.9a). Sigmoid colon cavity was empty and the wall was thickened. Lymphadenectasis was found in posterior of peritoneum, mesenterium (Fig. 4.9b), and around bilateral iliac artery. His chest DR was normal (Fig. 4.10). He was given II antibiotics infusion, fasting water and fluid infusion, preparation for preoperative.

On Day 4 of illness, he continued on fasting (food and liquid), and received anti-inflammation and fluid supplement. He was afebrile, without vomiting or nausea. Laparoscopic appendectomy and peritoneal lavage and drainage were performed under general anesthesia in the afternoon.

Surgical procedure in brief: took the arc incision at umbilical edge which is about 1.0 cm in length, cut open the skin and subcutaneous parts, blunted separation to the peritoneum step by step, clipped peritoneum and cut it open, placed a Trocar which was 10 cm in diameter to set up a pneumoperitoneum where the pressure was 9 mmHg and made sure laparoscope through it, put the 5 mm trocar on left middle and lower abdomen. There was thin purulent secretion at right lower abdominal cavity and pelvic. The appendix was hyperemia and edema at posterior of caecum and with purulent on the surface. It was about 8 cm long (Fig. 4.11c), 1.0 cm tips diameter. Electric cut mesentery and one-time ligatured 1 cm from root, cutting the appendix between two ligatures (distal end was 0.3 cm). After cauterization of the damaged end of the appendix, the vermix was put into a pathological bag, and it was taken out by Trocar from umbilicus. Examination was performed for no Meckel's diverticulum and other abnormalities on the about 100 cm of terminal ileum. Laparoscopic view revealed that the 100 cm long wall at the junction of sigmoid colon and

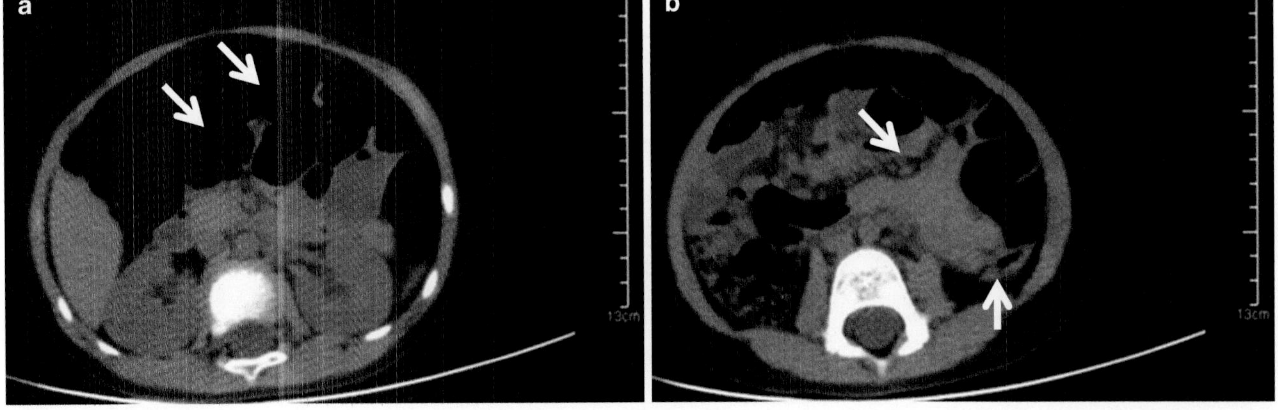

Fig. 4.9 On Day 3 of illness, abdominal CT showed slight expansion and flatulence of the middle upper intestine (**a**). Sigmoid colon cavity was empty and the wall was incrassated. Lymphadenectasis was found on posterior of peritoneum, mesenterium (**b**), and around bilateral iliac artery

rectum was congestive, edema and pus moss adhesion of the surface, but had no perforation. 500 ml normal saline was used to douche the abdominal and pelvic cavity, and relieved pneumoperitoneum after confirming no bleeding. A drainage tube (front plane, 5 side holes) was left in pelvic cavity for drainage and immobilized to left lower abdomen. Suture the incision layer by layer with absorbable line and conglutinated with medical glue on the skin. Numbers of gauze and equipment were matched. Examination found green watery stool in the rectum, but no mass and bloody stool. The surgery was completed. Antibiotics was changed to third generation.

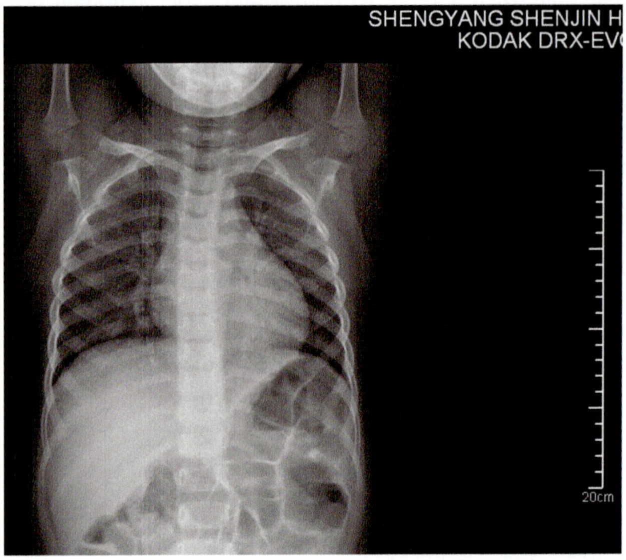

Fig. 4.10 On Day 3 of illness, chest DR was normal

On Day 5 of illness, he had fever again (38.5 °C) and unresponding to physical cooling. Lysis in aspirin 0.2 g was intravenous injected to antipyretic treatment. Pathological report of appendectomy: Inflammatory cells infiltrated the serosa layer of appendix (Fig. 4.11d).

On Day 6 of illness, in addition to ongoing fever (38.5 °C), he had loose stools but normal urine. Physical examination showed he had normal mind, spirit and heart, and lung auscultation. His abdomen was soft but not tenderness and no pressing pain. The dressing on the incision was clean and no exudation.

On Day 7 of illness, he had no vomiting but still had loose light yellow fluid stool, and persistent fever to 39 °C at night. Congestive rashes developed on his back, neck, and limbs,

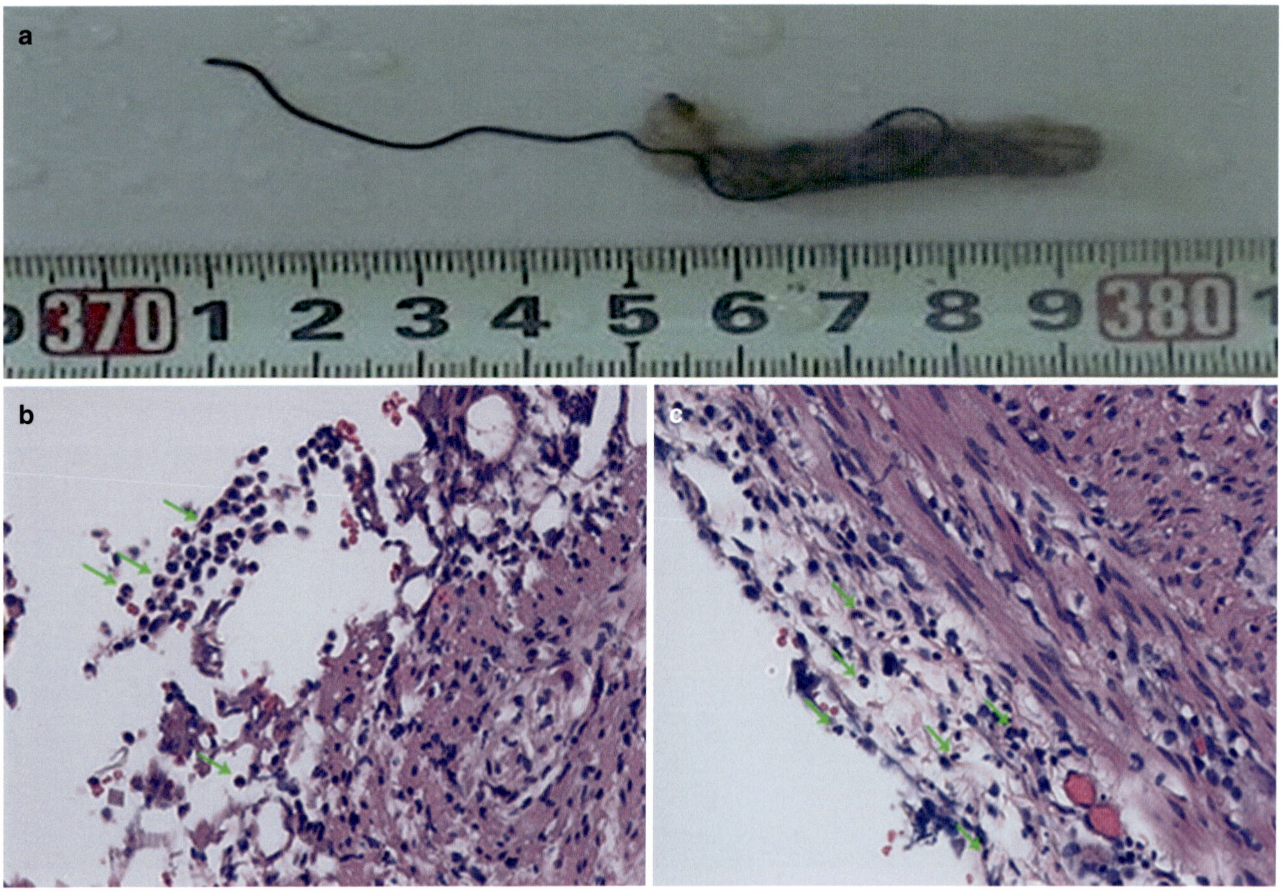

Fig. 4.11 On day 4 of illness, the appendix was hyperemia and edema, with purulent exudation on the surface, its length was about 8 cm (**a**). Pathological examination of HE staining showed inflammatory cells infiltrated serous layer. Serous layer of appendix (**b** and **c**-green arrow)

he had red palm without itching. His drainage liquid was about 2 ml. Physical examination was normal. CBC revealed WBC 16.17 × 10^9/L, NE 88.2%, HGB106g/L, PLT 508 × 10^9/L; CRP 65.40 mg/L. Dermatologist diagnosis included (1) Allergic dermatitis; (2) Drug eruption? He suggested (1) avoiding allergens; (2) taking the clarityne half pill per day; intravenous glycyrrhizin and Vitamin C once a day; (3) hydrocortisone cream for external use twice per day; (4) he was at the state of acute sensitization and the injury of skin was continuing, monitoring the EO\IgE and CRP; (5) changed antibiotics to Mepem; (6) hip bath twice a day and fasting today.

On Day 8 of illness, he still had watery stools. Rashes were mildly regressed but fever was persistent, and he developed bilateral conjunctival congestion, without purulent discharge. The drainage leads 2 ml of light yellow liquid. Physical examination found normal abdomen. The dressing at incision site was clean and no exudation. Abdominal ultrasound showed cholestasis in the cholecyst (Fig. 4.12), no hydrops in enterocoelia. There was no swelling around drainage tube. Drainage tube was removed, and dressing was changed.

On Day 9 of illness, patient still had fever 38.5 °C at night. After consultation with pediatric cardiologist, KD was diagnosed. Thus, he was transferred to pediatric cardiovascular ward for further treatment. The cervical ultrasound revealed lymphadenopathy, with larger ones about 1.2 × 0.7 cm on the left and about 1.2 × 0.4 cm on the right. He was given (1) IVIG 2 g/kg over 12 hours; (2) IV Mannitol (2.5 ml/kg) and torsemide (0.5 mg/kg) one time when half of IVIG finished; (3) oral aspirin 30 mg/kg/day in 3 divided doses and dipyridamole 3–5 mg/kg/day in 2 divided doses; (4) metronidazole and gentamicin suppository clysis. His fever settled on the Day 10 of illness. On Day 12 of illness, he was afebrile over 48 h. Examination found rashes still all over body. Lips and mouth were red and dry, with strawberry tongue (+). Liver was enlarged 3–4 cm from right rib, moderate hard. He moved joints of limbs freely and had no peeling skin around fingernails. Lab investigation revealed WBC 6.27 × 10^9/L, NE 65.5%, RBC 3.5 × 10^{12}/L, HGB 93 g/L, PLT 662 × 10^9/L. CRP 8.37 mg/L. ESR 44 mm/h. ALB 28.2 g/L. NT-pro BNP 590.1 pg/ml. Echo showed normal LVED (Fig. 4.13a), LVEF (Fig. 4.13b), LCA (Fig. 4.13c), and RCA (Fig. 4.13d). He received infusion of albumin 20 g for 2 days, and aspirin reduced to one dose 75 mg.

On Day 13, he was afebrile. Physical examination did not find significant progress except regressed bilateral conjunctiva congestion. Liver ultrasound showed the liver was enlarged at the distance of 1.3 cm from rib lower margin (Fig. 4.14a). Gallbladder was recovered (Fig. 4.14b).

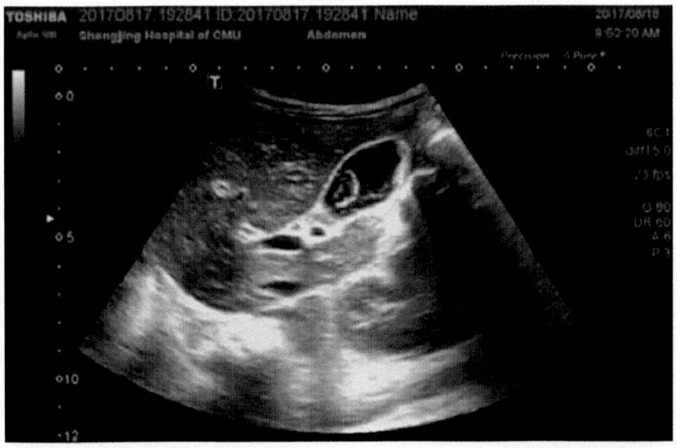

Fig. 4.12 On Day 8 of illness, cholestasis in the cholecyst

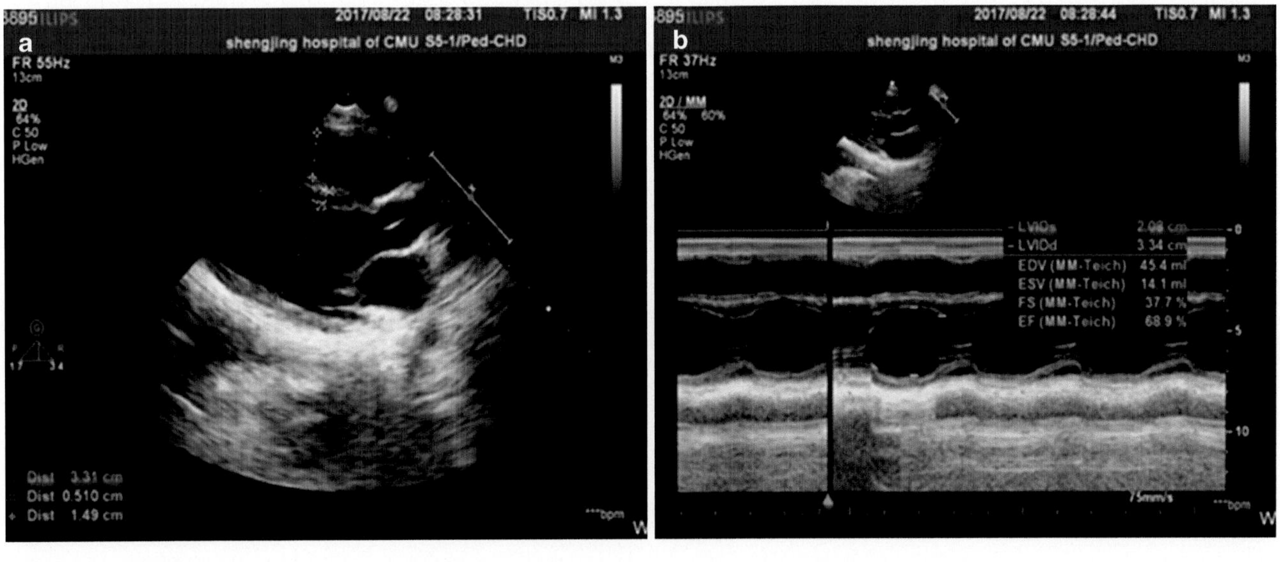

Fig. 4.13 On Day 12 of illness, echo showed normal LVED (**a**), LVEF (**b**), LCA (**c**), and RCA (**d**)

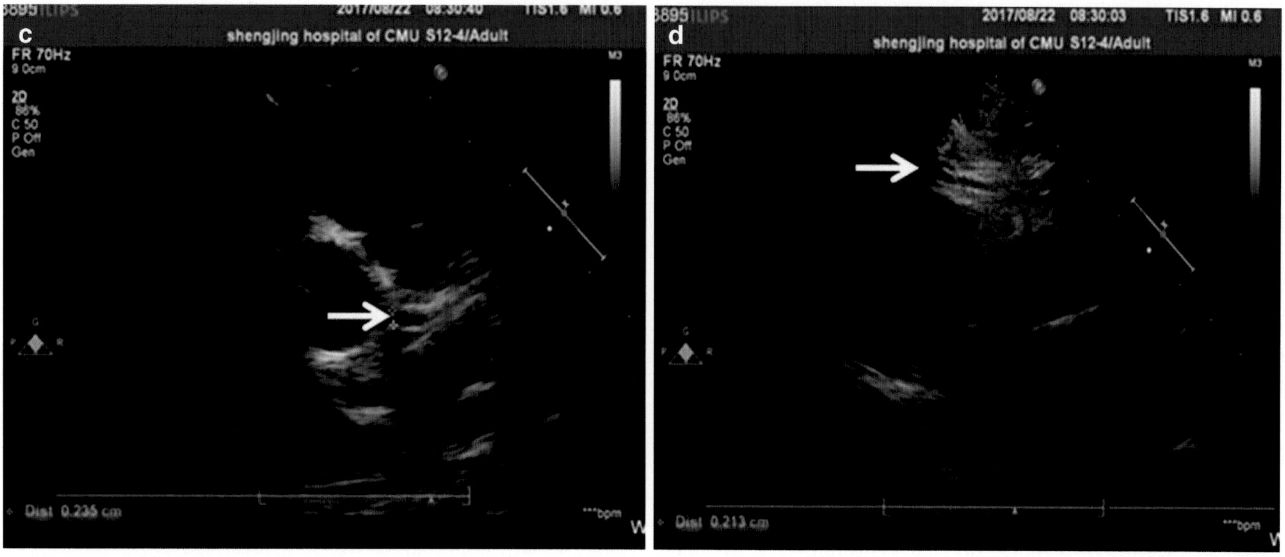

Fig. 4.13 (continued)

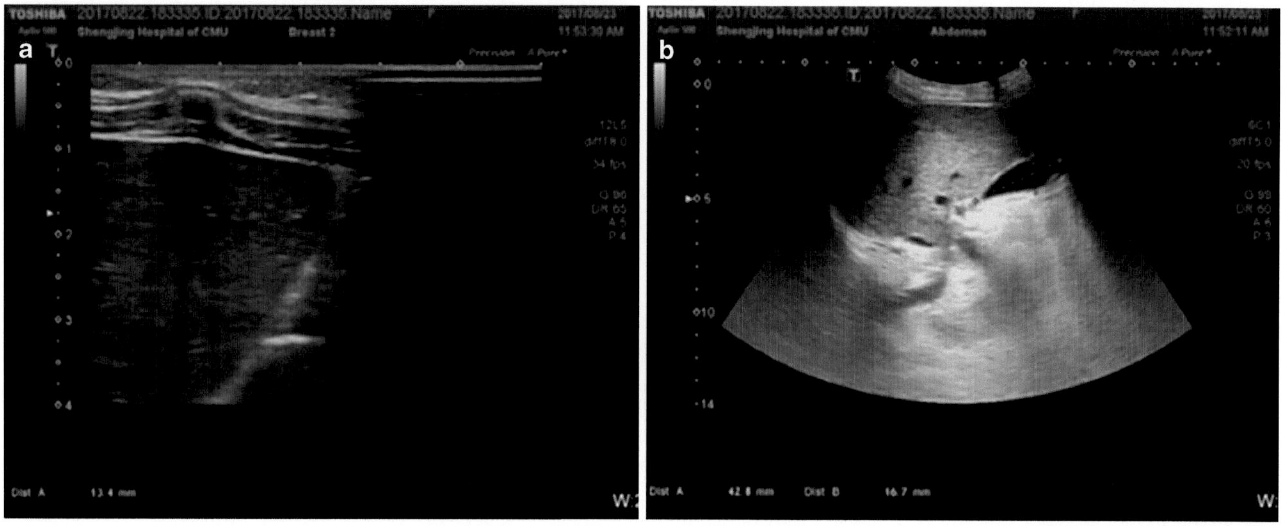

Fig. 4.14 On Day 12 of illness, liver ultrasound showed liver was swelling of 1.3 cm from the margin of right costal (**a**). Gallbladder was normal (**b**)

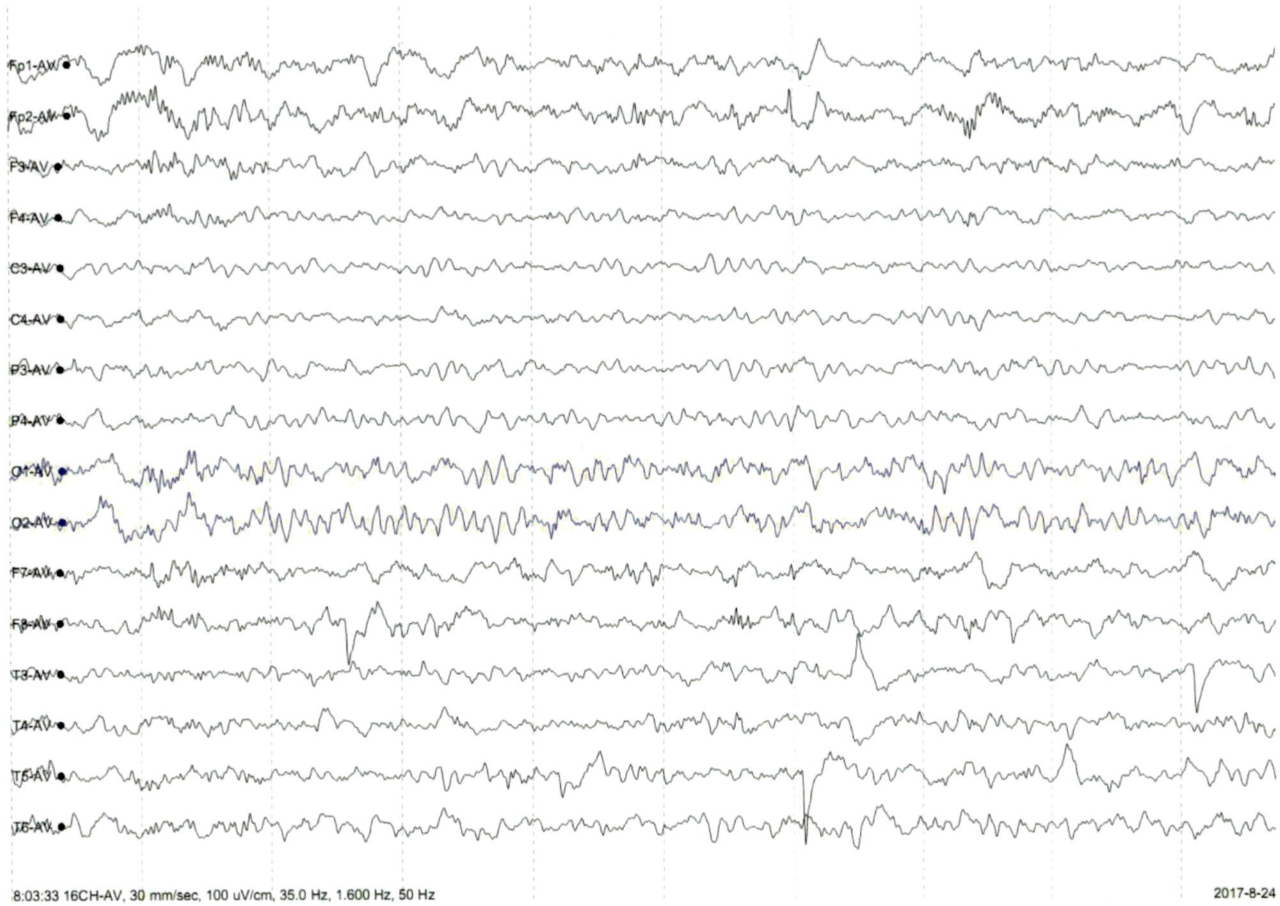

Fig. 4.15 On Day 13 of illness, EEG was normal

On Day 15, he was afebrile over 48 hours. Examination showed rashes were regressed and lips redness disappeared. Liver was regressed to 2–3 cm under margin of right rib, and he had peeling skin around fingernails. Albumin was recovered to 38 g/L. EEG was normal (Fig. 4.15). He was discharged.

4.2.1 Clinic Course of the Patient

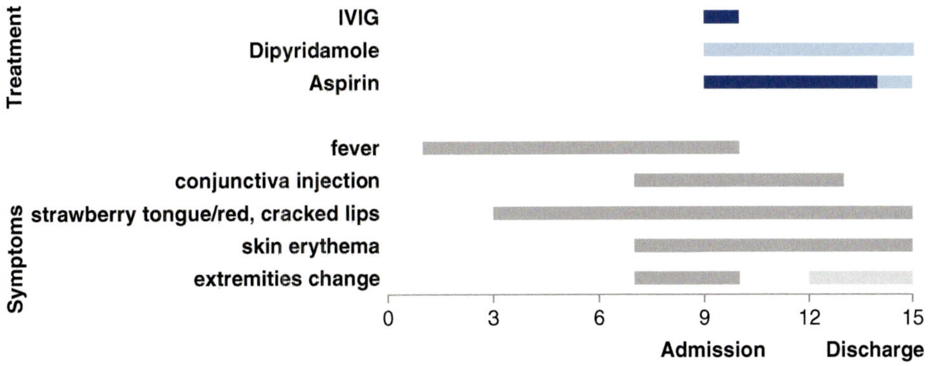

4.2.2 Follow Up

Since discharged, he took oral aspirin 75 mg once daily and dipyridamole 75 mg divided in 3 doses, also Niferex 150 mg once per day. At 1 month of illness, NT-pro BNP settled. At 2 months of illness, the ESR and PLT were almost normal. ECG was normal (Fig. 4.16). Echo performed at 3 weeks, 1, 2, 6, and 12 months showed normal coronary artery. Liver ultrasound showed liver regressed at 2 months. All medications were stopped at 2 months of illness (Table 4.1).

4.2.3 Diagnosis

1. KD.
2. Peritonitis.
3. Hypoproteinemia.
4. Mild anemia.

4.2.4 Discussion

The patient met at least 4 out of 5 criteria for KD, he had a continuous fever for 9 days, and the antibiotic treatment was ineffective, with the following clinical manifestations: (1) rashes all over the body; (2) bilateral conjunctival congestion, without purulent secretion; (3) red and dry lips, with strawberry tongue; (4) palm congestion during fever, and peeling skin around fingernails on Day 13 of illness; as to the lymphadenopathy it was still 1.2 cm on Day 13 of illness (it is usually the most swelling at the beginning of the fever) [10].

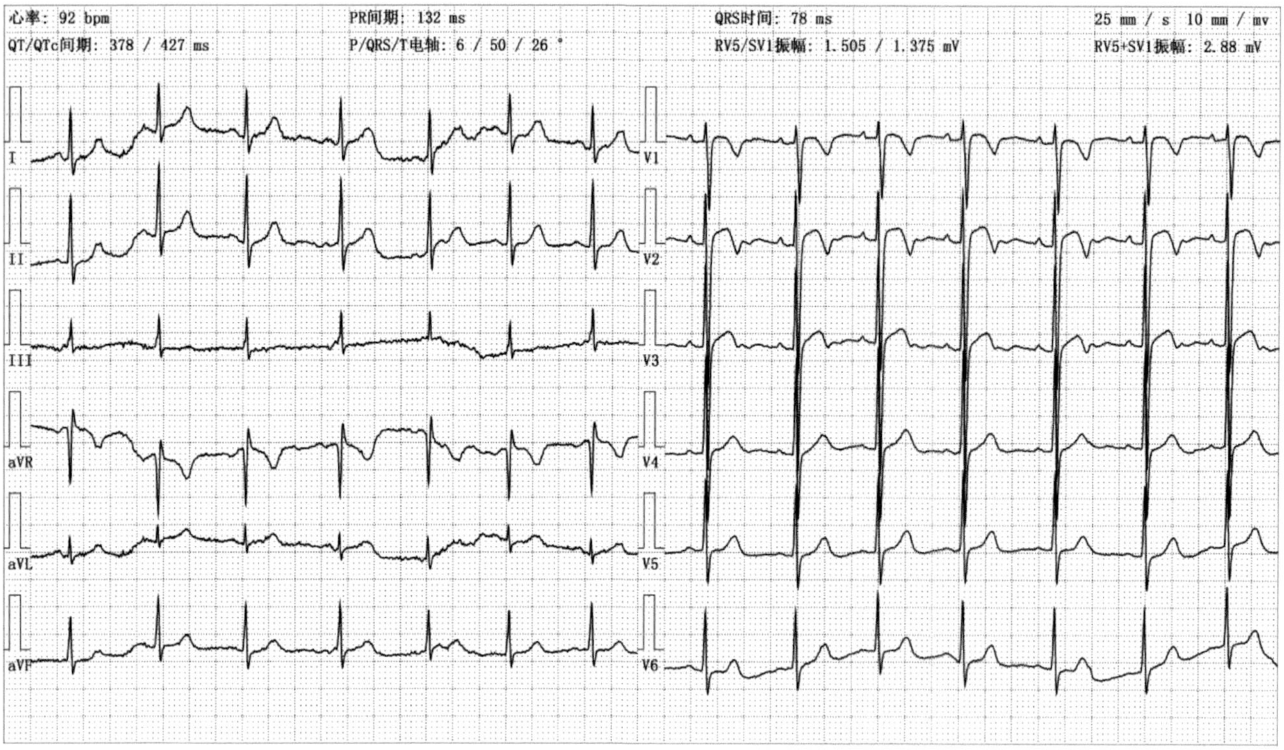

Fig. 4.16 At 2 months of illness, ECG was normal

Table 4.1 The dynamic changes of lab parameters

Lab parameters	4 days	5 days	8 days	10 days	13 days	21 days	30 days	60 days	71 days
WBC ($\times 10^9$/L)	20.06		16.17	13.88	6.27	5.15	4.32	5.3	
NE (%)	88.8		88.2	77.6	56.5	39	45.1	51.9	
RBC ($\times 10^{12}$/L)	4.3		3.9	3.89	3.5	3.5	3.8	3.8	
HGB (g/L)	115		106	103	93	97	10.6	10.7	
PLT ($\times 10^9$/L)	425		508	550	662	629	484	354	
CRP (mg/L)	103	96	65.4	75.2	8.37	1.08			
ESR (mm/h)				61	48		34	20	4
ALB (mg/L)	42.5			28.2	38.4				
NT-pro BNP (pg/ml)				483.6	590		49		

The patient had normal liver function and liver size at admission. With persistent fever, albumin leaked and he developed hypoproteinemia. Then liver was enlarged. While liver ultrasonic echo was normal, which was different from hepatitis B. After treatment with IVIG and IV albumin, oral aspirin, and broad-spectrum antibiotics infusion, his appetite was improved, leakage was reduced, albumin was recovered, and the liver retracted to normal size, too [4].

4.2.5 Case Specific Clinical Features

1. The patient met the diagnostic criteria of cholestasis cholecystitis: he had stomachache, and abdominal CT revealed the flatulence of middle upper abdomen. Liver ultrasound showed cholestasis in gallbladder on Day 9 of illness (the enlargement of gallbladder with the thickened wall of gall was only found transiently at beginning). On the Day 8, it may be recovered (see the case 19). The gallbladder recovered after IVIG and broad-spectrum antibiotics infusion.
2. The patient met the diagnostic criteria of peritonitis: He was admitted to hospital with 3 days' intermittent pain at right lower abdomen. Physical examination found obvious tenderness. Laparoscopic examination found that there was purulent secretion on general specimen appendix and the colon 100 cm long intestinal wall at the junction of sigmoid colon and rectum was congestive, edema and pus moss adhesion of the surface. Pathological examination on HE staining showed the inflammation cells infiltrated serous layer. The whole abdominal CT scan revealed swollen mesenteric lymph nodes. It was possibly that the KD children were easier to have intestinal invagination (see case 20).
3. The differential diagnosis of acute suppurative appendicitis should be considered. The inflammation of acute suppurative appendicitis started from the inner membrane of appendix, gradually spreaded to serosa layer. In some cases the serosa was normal [11]. This boy only had inflammation cells infiltration on serosa layer, which indicated it was not the suppurative appendicitis but the complication of KD on peritoneum.
4. 8–9 days after diagnosed with KD, he did not developed coronary artery dilation.

Yue Zhang

4.3 Case 23 KD with Acute Cholecystitis

A previous healthy 3-year-old boy had an unremarkable antenatal, family history. His past medical history showed that he had significant allergy to milk.

He presented on Day 4 of illness with a history of persistent fever for 4 days and rashes for 1 day. He had received infusion of second-generation cephalosporin for 3 days. Fever did not regress. He was admitted to our pediatric gastrointestinal ward for liver dysfunction and KD to be excluded. Since the onset of illness, he was sleepy and had poor appetite. *Examination* revealed fever (38.7 °C), mild bilateral conjunctivitis, rashes all over body with pruritus. Cervical lymphadenectasis about 2 cm on the left, red fissuring lips with strawberry tongue. Others were normal. *Admission blood* tests revealed WBC 19.5 × 10^9/L, NE 89.3%, HGB 120 g/L, PLT 262 × 10^9/L. TP 60.7 g/L, ALB 39.4 g/L, ALT 628 U/L, AST 195 U/L, Bil T 44.5 μmol/L, BilD 32.9 μmol/L. CRP 76.9 mg/L, ASO, rheumatoid factors, and IgE were normal. EBV-IgM(−). He was given infusion of polyene phosphatidyl choline 5 ml/day and compound glycyrrhizin 20 ml/day, adenosine monophosphate 5 mg/kg/d, as well as glucose:NS 1:1 solution.

On Day 5, his fever interphase was 5–6 hours with diluted stool. Tests revealed serum ammonia 64.7 μmol/L. NT-pro BNP 724.6 pg/ml (<300 pg/ml). CKMB mass, cInI, and hs-InT were normal. NSE 26.900 ng/ml, ALT 418 U/L, AST 91 U/L, ALB 28.2 g/L, Bil T 24.6 μmol/L, Bil D 17.5 μmol/L, TB 98 μmol/L, γ-GT 274 U/L. D-Dimer 1334 μg/L. CRP 78.5 mg/L, ESR 53 mm/h. Chest DR was normal. As a result of consulting to pediatric cardiologist, the boy met the 5 criteria for KD and then was transferred to pediatric cardiology ward and treated with IVIG 1 g/kg/day for 2 days. He was given aspirin 30–50 mg/kg/day and dipyridamole 3–5 mg/kg/day, in two or three divided doses. Creatine phosphate sodium 1.0 g/day was then prescribed.

On Day 6, tetraflux bifidobacterium was applicated to relieve ventosity and constipation. Abdominal examination found positive Murphy's sign, suspicious positive tenderness at right lower portion, no rebound tenderness and muscular tension palpable, hypoactive bowl sounds. Abdominal ultrasound detected dilated plump gallbladder 12.3 cm × 4.6 cm (Fig. 4.17), and the wall thickness was 2 mm (Fig. 4.18). Cervical ultrasound revealed bilateral lymphadenectasis, the largest was 2.1 cm × 1.0 cm on the left and 1.7 cm × 0.5 cm on the right, in regular shape with clear border. ECG was normal. We consulted pediatric general surgeon, he suggested fasting and switching to third-generation cephalosporin infusion q12h. On Day 7, he was afebrile. Investigation revealed TP 73.5 g/L, ALB 28.2 g/L, ALT 164 U/L, AST 24 U/L, γ-GT 157 U/L. TB and TBA were normal. Repeated abdominal ultrasound showed the enlarged gallbladder size of 13.1 cm × 4.2 cm (Fig. 4.18) and the wall thickness was less than 2 mm. He was given albumin 20 g infusion for 2 days and omeprazole 1 mg/kg/day infusion. On Day 9, he had been afebrile more than 48 h, all the symptoms disappeared except Murphy sign and abdominal tenderness on right lower portion. Retested blood work revealed WBC 10.04 × 10^9/L, NE 58.3%, HGB 108 g/L, PLT 373 × 10^9/L. Serum ammonia 43.3μmol/L. CRP 25.3 mg/L. NT-pro BNP

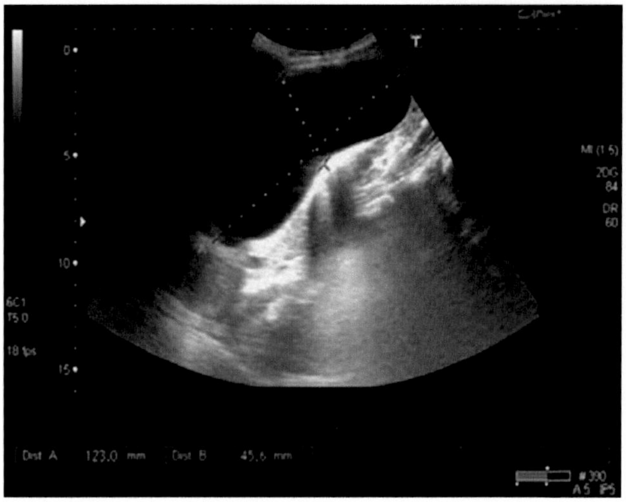

Fig. 4.17 On Day 6 of illness, gallbladder was markedly enlarged about 12.3 cm × 4.6 cm, the wall thickness was 2 mm

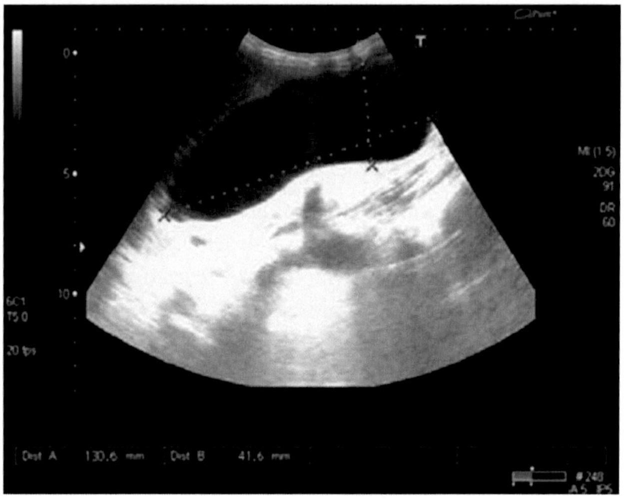

Fig. 4.18 On Day 7 of illness, gallbladder was markedly enlarged about 13.1 cm × 4.2 cm, the wall thickness was less than 2 mm

432 pg/ml. NSE 33.270 ng/ml. ALT 79 U/L. AST, T Bil, and D Bil were normal. TBA 15.3 μmol/L, γ-GT 106 U/L. Repeat abdominal ultrasound revealed gallbladder was 10.8 cm × 4.2 cm (Fig. 4.19) and the wall was less than 2 mm. Aspirin was reduced to 3–5 mg/kg/day. Ursodeoxycholic acid was adapted to 10 mg/kg in three divided dose.

On Day 11, his ventosity was relieved. Thus liquid diet was permitted. Blood culture was negative of bacteria. Repeated abdominal ultrasound revealed gallbladder had regressed to 11.6 cm × 3.8 cm (Fig. 4.20), the wall was less than 2 mm and there was retroperitoneal lymphadenectasis.

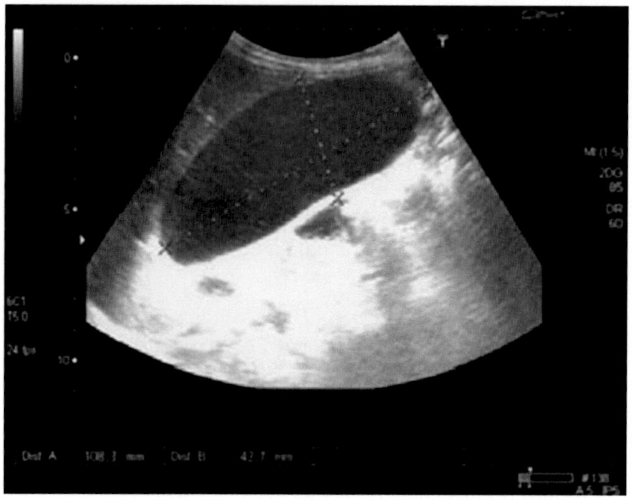

Fig. 4.19 On Day 9 of illness, gallbladder was regressed to 10.8 cm × 4.2 cm and the wall thickness was less than 2 mm

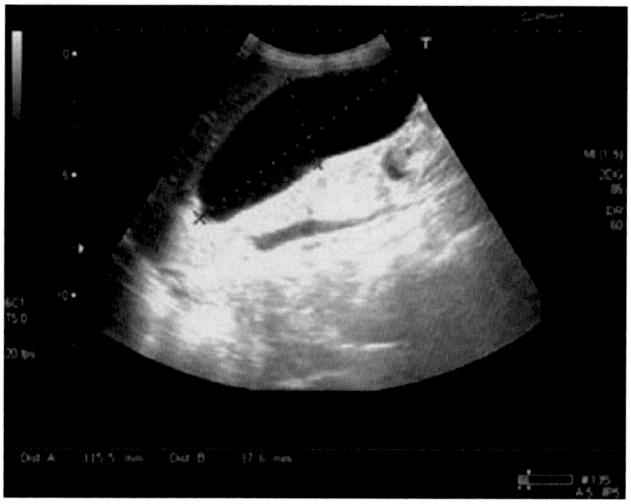

Fig. 4.20 On Day 11 of illness, gallbladder was regressed to 11.6 cm × 3.8 cm, the wall thickness was less than 2 mm and lymphadenopathy retroperitoneal

On Day 12, abdominal pain was settled. Liquid food was tolerated, although Murphy sign was still positive. Investigation revealed WBC 9.88 × 10^9/L, NE 47.4%, HGB 10^9 g/L, PLT 520 × 10^9/L. CRP 7.39 mg/L. NT-pro BNP 407.5 pg/ml. On Day 13, he took half-liquid diet without abdominal pain. Murphy sign was negative. Desquamation appeared around the fingernails. Ultrasound showed normal bilateral adrenal glands. On Day 14, investigations revealed normal ALB, ALT, and AST. TBA 22.9/L, γ-GT 69 U/L. ESR 28 mm/h. Echo showed coronary artery was normal. He was discharged.

4.3.1 Clinical Course of this Patient

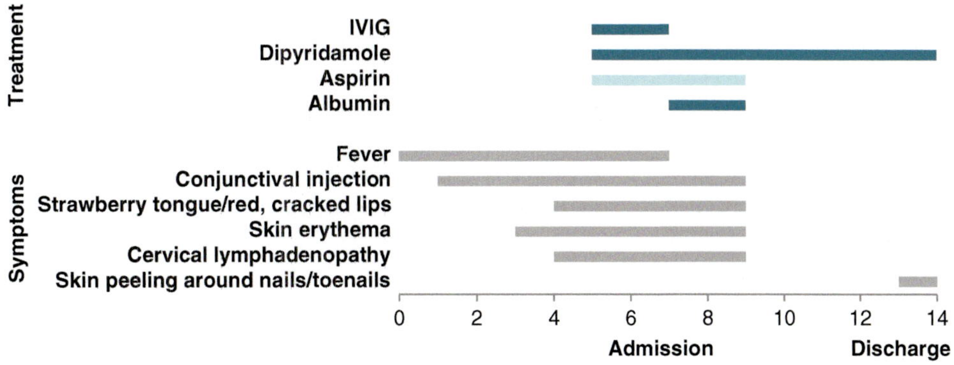

4.3.2 Follow Up

TBA and ESR were subsided in 1 week and 1 month later, respectively. All the medications were stopped for normal coronary artery at 2 months.

4.3.3 Diagnosis

1. KD.
2. Acute cholecystitis.
3. Liver dysfunction.
4. Hypoalbuminemia.

4.3.4 Discussion

The diagnosis of KD was based on the following: he had persisted fever for more than 5 days; antibiotics were ineffective, along with (1) congestive rashes all over the body; (2) bilateral conjunctivitis without purulent excretion; (3) cervical lymphadenopathy over 1.5 cm; (4) dry and cracked lips with strawberry tongue; (5) swelling palms and subsequent desquamation around fingernails.

4.3.5 Case Specific Clinic Features

1. In this special case, the KD patient had a complication of acute cholecystitis. The initial symptoms include fever, rashes, and liver dysfunction. He was admitted to pediatric gastrointestinal ward for easing acute cholecystitis. However, dry fissuring lips, cervical lymphadenopathy detected by ultrasound, and bilateral conjunctivitis emerged in succession. They completely met the criteria of KD. The patient was transferred to our pediatric cardiovascular ward.
2. Acute cholecystitis was defined as inflammation of gallbladder caused by bacteria invasion to gallbladder wall or gallbladder duct obstruction. According to pathogenesis of cholecystitis, it can be categorized into two types, calculus and non-calculus. Most acute cholecystitis is caused by calculus, whereas non-calculus cholecystitis is only responsible for 4–8% of acute cholecystitis. For its complicated inducements, it is hard to make calculus cholecystitis diagnosis.
3. This boy's case was categorized in non-calculus cholecystitis aseptic, which is referred as acute cholecystitis in which gallstone was not found by imageological or surgery pathological examinations. Inducements of non-calculus cholecystitis were generally classified into (1) gallbladder hemodynamic disorder, which was subsequent to sympathetic excitement after severe trauma or major surgery, gallbladder artery contraction leading to ischemia, or ischemia and necrosis of gallbladder caused by vasoactive agent; (2) cholestasis: post-operative fasting, usage of analgesic, gallbladder evacuation disturbance caused by abdominal infection, elevated intensity of bile salt which provoked acute inflammation of gallbladder; (3) overload of bile pigment caused by severe trauma, absorption of retroperitoneal hematoma, and quantity transfusion; (4) XII factor activated by transfusion. Blood vessel of gallbladder was injured by activation of XII factor-dependent pathway. The blood vessel spasm leads to ischemia, necrosis even penetration of gallbladder; (5) bacterial infection, mucous membrane damage would facilitate bacterial infection. In patients with abdominal purulent infection, bacteria can be displaced to gallbladder causing purulent infection. The cause of cholecystitis in KD patients was mostly from hemodynamic disorder.
4. The symptoms of acute cholecystitis including sudden extremely severe pain or colic on the right upper portion of abdominal, which radiating to right shoulder and right subscapular angle, with nausea, vomiting, fever reaching

39 °C, and shiver in severe cases. Jaundice may present if liver dysfunction or common bile duct is involved. The signs include muscle tension, tenderness, rebound tenderness on right and middle portion of upper abdomen, positive Murphy sign, mild jaundice, peripheral circulation failure, and infectious shock in severe cases. In this case the patient met the typical criteria of acute cholecystitis, which reminded us a differential diagnosis of acute cholecystitis.

5. The liver function varies with the state of cholecystitis. Antibiotics and medications for liver function protection were effective. The initial liver function change showed elevated transaminases while increased TBA which indicated severe cholecystitis and extrahepatic cholangitis. The chronic intermittent cholecystitis, severe gastrointestinal symptoms, and malnutrition would result in decreased ALB, usually as a result of albumin leak of vasculitis in KD, which represent marked liver dysfunction. The liver function would regain swiftly. AST and ALT were quick except for ALB. Infusion of albumin was necessary sometimes. Abnormality of above four parameters at the same time indicated that the patient in a critical condition. Clinician should be alert of the severity.
6. The etiology of LFT abnormality in KD patients is also not clear yet. Hypotheses were proposed including generalized inflammation, vasculitis, congest heart failure secondary to myocarditis, non-steroidal anti-inflammatory antipyretics, toxin-mediated effects, or a combination of these events [3]. It is found that in patients with KD, AAC on abdominal USG, especially with gallbladder distension, was a meaningful finding that was associated with the development of CAA in patients with KD by using both simple and multiple logistic regression analysis [4].
7. The most effective diagnostic method is to take various imageological examinations including abdominal ultrasound, CT, MRCP, and ERCP. Typical ultrasound images present: (1) increased volume of gallbladder, prolonged short axis was more diagnostic than long axis; (2) oval or pear-shaped gallbladder; (3) the wall was usually thin<0.3 cm; (4) bile transparency was high (80%); (5) Murphy sign positive; (6) calculus or constriction of duct neck. Gallbladder wall thickening, rough or "double ring" sign, poor transparency or blurred profile are not diagnostic. Diagnosis based on abdominal CT relies on calculus in bile duct or gallbladder, dilation of gallbladder and widespread wall thickening (significantly increased in enhanced scan). Examination using MRCP and ERCP is critical in cases complicated with calculus associated bile obstruction. In cases with simple cholecystitis, they are unnecessary.
8. Once cholecystitis identified, fasting, anti-infection, liver-protecting, and cholagogic measures were added on the treatment list besides the standard treatment for KD. Routine treatment excludes both MRCP and ERCP that require surgical operation. Symptoms and liver dysfunction could be settled by conservative medicine. Antibiotics should be selected according to CRP and blood bacteria culture results. In this case infusion of albumin was given after IVIG to prevent high colloid osmotic pressure, though hypoalbuminemia was found on Day five of the illness.
9. For the patient presented persistent fever, we tested NSE to exclude possible neuroblastoma. NSE was progressively elevated afterwards, thus, we examined adrenal gland using ultrasound. After KD was diagnosed, neuroblastoma was excluded. Mediastinum CT was also disregarded. The reason for elevated NSE remained unidentified.

Xue-xin Yu

4.4 Case 24 KD with Acute Cholecystitis and Pancreatitis

A previous healthy 4-year-old boy presented without significant past medical history and family history.

He presented on Day 4 of illness with high fever (40 °C) and cervical lymphadenectasis and pain. On Day 2, after receiving infusion of secondary-generation cephalosporin, azithromycin, vidarabine monophosphate, vitamin C, and dexamethasone, his fever interval was prolonged, but he developed persistent severe abdominal pain, without vomit or diarrhea. On Day 3, he was transferred to our clinic, where laboratory tests showed elevated CBC, ALT, and CRP. Abdominal CT results, bilateral parotid gland, and abdominal ultrasound results were all abnormal. On Day 4, rashes developed on his trunk, thus he was admitted to our pediatric gastrointestinal ward as a patient with cholestatic hepatitis, sepsis, and acute pancreatitis. Since the onset of illness, he had paroxysmal abdominal pain, lost appetite. *Examination* revealed he was irritable with fever (38 °C), had rashes scattering on the trunk, cervical lymphadenectasis (2 cm), dry and red lips, and congestive pharynx. His abdomen was soft, without tenderness, rebound tenderness or muscular tension palpable. The bowel sound was 4–5 times per minute. Others were normal. *Admission blood* tests revealed WBC 13.9 × 10^9/L, NE 80.5%, HGB 116 g/L, PLT 291 × 10^9/L. CRP 87.1 mg/L. TP 60.5 g/L, ALB 37.6 g/L, ALT 519 U/L, AST 938 U/L, T Bil 26.6 μmol/L, D Bil 20.3 μmol/L. Serum lipase 210.6 U/L, serum amylase 95 U/L. D-dimer 930 μg/L. Abdominal CT revealed hepatosplenomegaly, multiple lymphadenectasis of mesentery, and retroperitoneum with pelvic effusion. Ultrasound of parotid gland showed echo enhancement of left parotid gland (Fig. 4.21) with left cervical lymphadenectasis (Fig. 4.22). Abdominal ultrasound revealed gallbladder wall edema (Fig. 4.23). Compound glycyrrhizin 5 ml/day and polyene phosphatidyl choline 20 ml/day were given to protect liver, lansoprazole 1 mg/kg/day was given to inhibit excretion of gastric acid and pancreatin indirectly, ademetionine (to promote bile drainage) and secondary-generation-cephalosporin infusion were given.

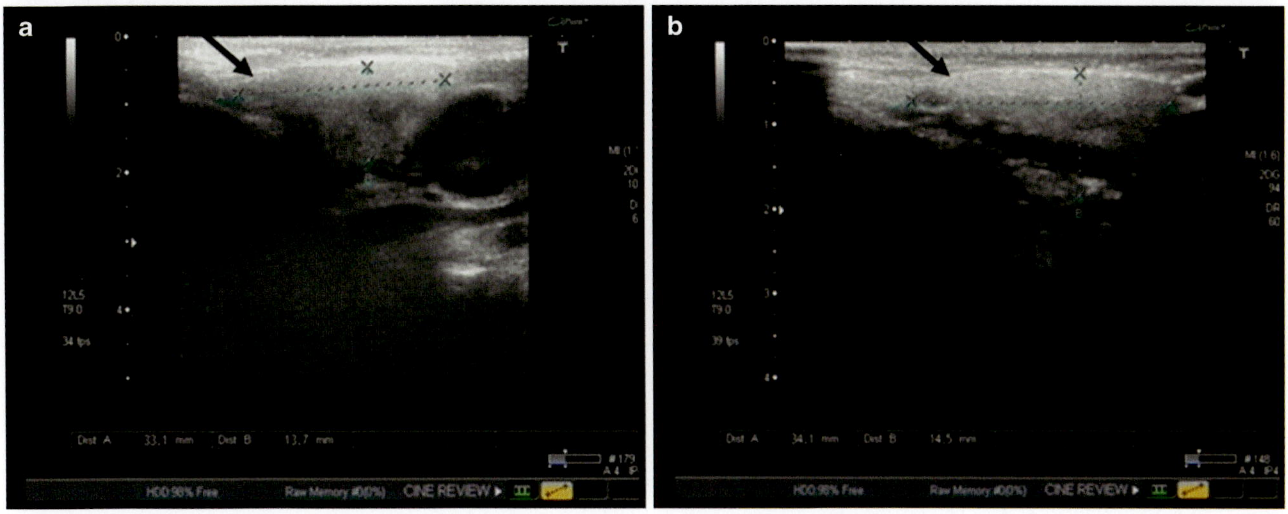

Fig. 4.21 On Day 3 of illness, the left parotid gland was 3.3 cm × 3.2 cm × 1.4 cm (**a**) and the right parotid gland was 3.4 cm × 2.1 cm × 1.5 cm (**b**) in size with alleviated internal echo signal, no mass detected, and the blood supply was normal

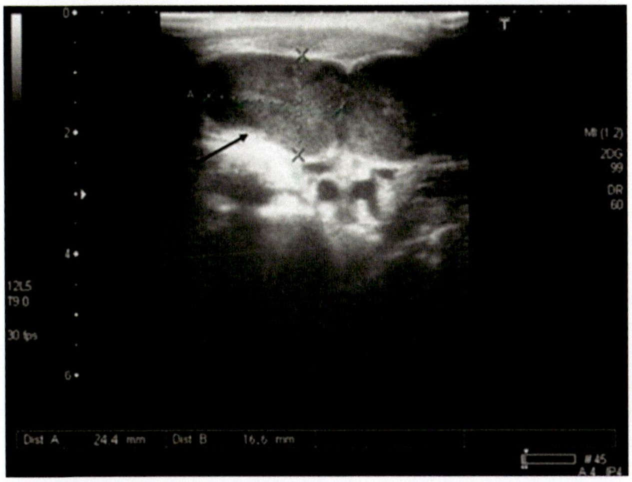

Fig. 4.22 On Day 3 of illness, cervical ultrasound showed cervical lymphadenectasis, the largest one was 1.7 cm × 0.6 cm on the right

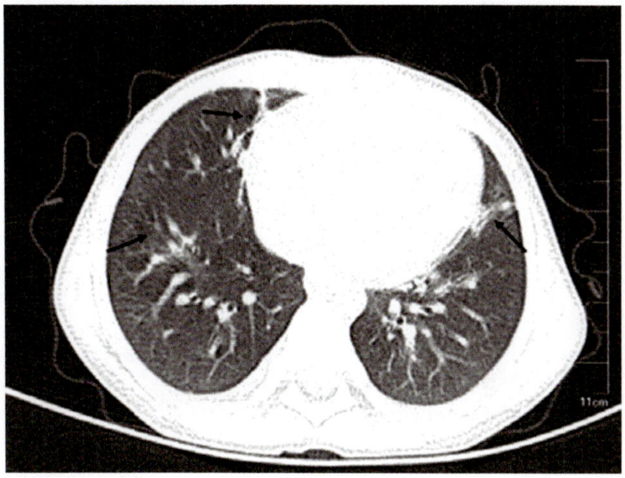

Fig. 4.24 On Day 5 of illness, chest CT scan showed bilateral multi lobular pneumonia

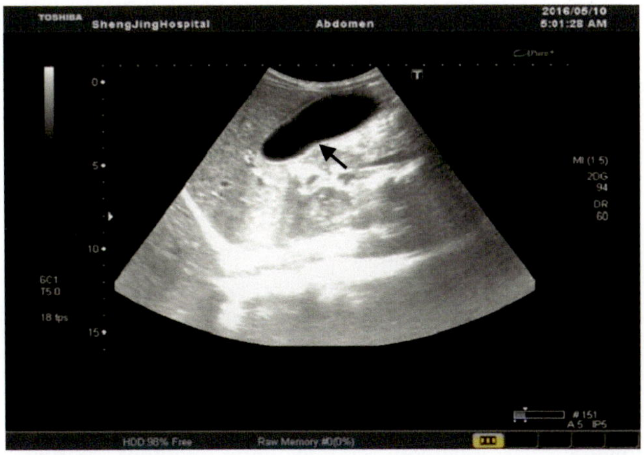

Fig. 4.23 On Day 3 of illness, abdominal ultrasound showed gallbladder wall edema 2 mm

On the Day 5 of illness, he developed bilateral conjunctivitis and strawberry tongue, his abdominal discomfort was relieved after diluted defecation. Investigations revealed WBC 12 × 10^9/L, NE 86.5%, HGB 112 g/L, PLT 238 × 10^9/L. CRP 121 mg/L. TP 54.5 g/L, ALB 32.3 g/L, ALT 219 U/L, AST 88 U/L, T Bil 54.0 μmol/L, D Bil 44.7 μmol/L, TBA 229.4 μmol/L, γ-GT 386 U/L. Serum lipase 113.1 U/L. NT-pro BNP 4402 pg/ml. MP-IgG1:80. Chest CT detected bilateral multi-lobe and segment pneumonia (Fig. 4.24). After consultation with pediatric cardiologist, he was diagnosed with KD and transferred to pediatric cardiology ward. He was treated with (1) IVIG 1 g/kg/day for 2 days; (2) oral aspirin 30–50 mg/kg/day and dipyridamole 3–5 mg/kg/d, both in two or three divided doses; (3) azithromycin 10 mg/kg/day for 3 days. On the Day 6, his abdominal pain was intermittent, and fever interval was prolonged. Tests revealed positive PINF-IgA. ECG was normal.

His fever was subsided on the Day 7, but he was still dispirited, meningeal irritation sign was negative. Babinski signs were negative. Retested results revealed serum lipase 72.3 U/L. TP 70.2 g/L, ALB 27.9 g/L, ALT 111 U/L, AST 41 U/L, γ-GT 219 U/L, TBA 28.3 μmol/L. EEG revealed bilateral occipital portion was mainly medium amplitude θ wave, mixed with a little δ wave. Abdominal ultrasound was normal (Fig. 4.25). He was treated with (1) albumin 1 g/kg/day for 2 days; (2) deproteinized calf blood extract 0.4 g/day to nourish brain cells; (3) 20% mannitol 2.5 ml/kg, qd, and furosemide 1 mg/kg infused 30 min after mannitol. On the Day 9, he had been afebrile more than 48 hours. Mental state was significantly improved. Rashes and conjunctivitis regressed. Echo revealed small shunt at atrial level and coronary artery was normal. Rechecked EEG was normal. We reduced aspirin dose to 3–5 mg/kg/day.

On the Day 10, blood bacteria culture was negative. On the Day 11, all the symptoms disappeared. Laboratory tests revealed WBC 9.62 × 10e^9/L, NE 46.7%, HGB 95 g/L, PLT 541 × 10^9/L. CRP 11.70 mg/L. ALT 37 U/L, AST 27 U/L. Serum lipase 122.9 U/L. NT- pro BNP 689.5 pg/ml. MP-IgG 1:160. He was discharged.

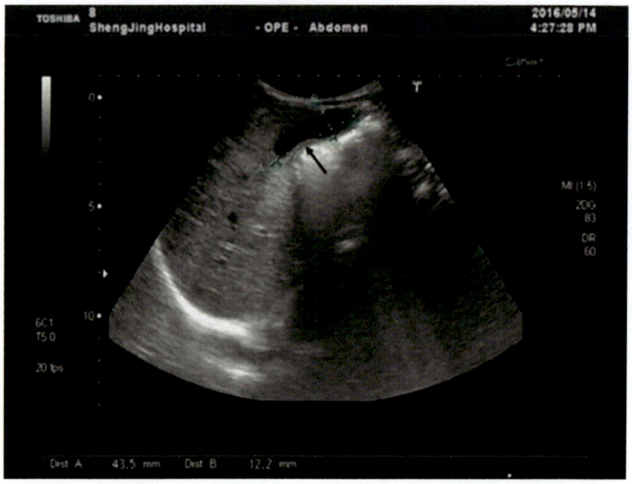

Fig. 4.25 On Day 7 of illness, abdominal echo showed gallbladder was recovered

4.4.1 Clinical Course of this Patient

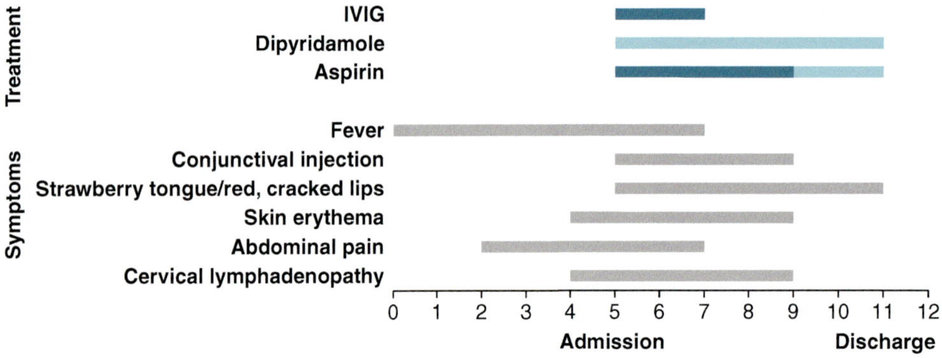

4.4.2 Follow Up

Serum lipase and NT-pro BNP recovered 1 week later, no dilation of coronary artery detected after 1 month and 2 months, thus, discontinued all medicine. Six months and 1 year later, his coronary artery was kept normal.

4.4.3 Diagnosis

1. KD.
2. Cholestatic hepatitis.
3. Acute cholecystitis.
4. Acute pancreatitis.
5. Hypoalbuminemia.
6. Neurological system involvement need to excluded.
7. Acute bronchopneumonia.
8. MP infection.
9. PINF virus infection.
10. ASD.

4.4.4 Discussion

The diagnosis of KD was identified: he had persistent fever over 5 days, antibiotics were ineffective; along with (1) sporadic red rashes on the trunk; (2) cervical lymphadenectasis over 1.5 cm on left; (3) red and cracked lips and strawberry tongue; (4) bilateral conjunctivitis without purulent excretion.

4.4.5 Case Specific Clinic Features

1. This is a rare case of KD with cholestasis, cholestatic hepatitis, and pancreatitis. According to the guideline, cholestasis is referred to T Bil < mg/DL (85.5 μmol/L) and D Bil >1.0 mg/DL(17.1 μmol/L), or T Bil >5 mg/DL and D Bil/ T Bil>20%. This patient met the first criterion.
2. Patients with cholestatic jaundice and fevers are mostly seen in virus infection, and secondarily seen in KD [12]. Although gastrointestinal symptoms were beyond diagnosis criteria of KD, they can be symptoms belonging to KD. Abdominal pain in patients with febrile and cholestatic jaundice may be the initial symptoms of KD. Ultrasound of gallbladder might be normal, or with hydrocholecystis/gallbladder wall thickening. Increased activity of ALT and γ-GT along with elevated serum TB, normal liver function except hypoalbuminemia are atypical symptoms of KD. And which may delay the diagnosis and subsequent treatment.
3. Electron microscope reveals giant mitochondria in liver autopsy samples from KD patients with cholestasis. This may be caused by oxidative damage to DNA, cell membrane, and protein. In the acute stage of KD, the level of serum TBI is markedly elevated, followed by gradual reducing to normal after IVIG treatment. It was speculated that elevated TBI could promote synthesis of cholesterol via bile acid, and is also associated with activation of bile duct cytokines in biliary system [13].
4. To be diagnosed with acute pancreatitis, patients must meet at least 2 criteria of the following: (1) classic symptoms or signs (abdominal pain, vomiting, or ileus); (2) serum amylase elevated three times higher than normal or lipase in the upper limits; (3) evidences of pancreatic edema or inflammation, hemorrhage, or necrosis shown in abdominal ultrasound and computed tomography [14]. In this case the boy presented abdominal pain, normal serum amylase but markedly elevated lipase. Ultrasound detected gallbladder wall edema. Therefore, he met the diagnosis criteria.
5. Pancreatitis and common bile duct stenosis (with or without obstructive jaundice) tend to occur in older and severe KD patients. Pancreatitis and bile duct lesion in KD may be self-limited, and the cholecystectomy and pancreatic duct drainage procedures need to be determined with caution [15].
6. Children pancreatitis was mainly caused by systemic disease, trauma, medication, bile duct disease, and infection, though the etiology of 30% patients was unclear. In this case the patient had no history of trauma or special medication. Abdominal ultrasound revealed he had no bile duct disease. So we considered the pancreatitis was the compliment of the blood vessel inflammation of KD.
7. Gastrointestinal symptoms especially liver dysfunction, cholecystitis, and pancreatitis are commonly seen in KD patients. Liver and gallbladder might be involved in KD patients with pancreatitis. The potential mechanisms include (1) CD8-T cell and macrophage infiltration in pancreas [16]; (2) vasculitis of middle artery and vein of pancreas; (3) polymorphonuclearcyte selectively infiltrated epithelial cell of bile duct [17]. In cases initially not meeting criteria of KD or IKD, we should look into other systems such as symptoms of cardiovascular system, gastrointestinal system, articular, urinary system or neurological system. Severe abdominal signs of KD might be commonly seen in 5-year-old patients, which should be considered as cholecystitis and pancreatitis. Immediate tests in serum and urine amylase, and serum lipase, and abdominal ultrasound were recommended. KD should be included in differential diagnosis in patients of acute cholecystitis and pancreatitis.
8. It is worth noting for elevated serum amylase, which is common, but not enough to diagnose pancreatitis. Clinical symptoms or image evidence were necessary. Elevated serum lipase was a more specific indication than serum amylase, it is referential for pancreatitis. When febrile potential KD children developed abdominal signs, intensive examinations were needed. Cholecystitis and pancreatitis should be considered as soon as possible; serum and urine amylase, serum lipase and abdominal ultrasound were helpful in early stage. Early diagnosis and treatment would improve the prognosis.
9. Mechanism of pancreatitis in KD patients was still ambiguous. Pathological basis may be general vasculitis. Small and medium vessel vasculitis in pancreas may cause vasoactive substance released, which disrupt capillary integrity and thus increase the permeability of blood vessel. Edema of pancreas tissue and relative narrow of blood vessel cause pancreas ischemia, the inflammation is provoked. It is suggested that T cell activated by some product of microorganism, and abnormal activation of T cell and monocyte releases large amount of cytokines and mediators of inflammation, which provoke cascade amplification effect. The release of cytokines leads to inflammation injury of general epithelial cells and full-thickness of blood vessel, the collagen on the blood vessel wall is exposed, where platelet is adhered and activated. The active platelet releases multiple vasoconstrictors, in additional to the effect of inflammatory transmitters, the blood perfusion of pancreas is reduced, which leads to microcirculation disturbance, and then hypoxic-ischemic injury and ischemic reperfusion injury.

10. According to reported cases by far, KD patients combined with pancreatitis were all seen in patients older than 3 years old. In another word, pancreatitis tends to happen to older children. Biopsy findings confirm that pancreas damages may happen in infants [18]. This may be because the clinical symptoms of infants were too atypical to be identified as pancreatitis, or the severe cases combined with pancreatitis quickly lead to death. Vomiting, abdominal pain, and jaundice may be the initial manifestations of KD accompanied with pancreatitis, which could be misdiagnosed. When acute abdomen pain happened together with febrile and multi-system involved, clinician should consider possible diagnosis of KD. In this case, the initial abdominal ultrasound was not targeting on pancreas; the following ultrasound showed pancreas was normal after treatment.
11. Parotitis was reported scarcely as a trigger of KD, which is caused by *staphylococcus aureus* and sensitive to antibiotics [19, 20]. Typical features of parotitis are a warm, red, tense, painful, and tender swollen parotid gland and, in the more severe cases, patients have fever. The regional lymph nodes may also become swollen and tender. The typical ultrasound image shows that the glands are swollen, indistinct, and the internal echo is weakened, colored blood flow is abundant in glands. As to our case, absence of elevated amylase and normal echo of glands excluded the diagnosis of parotitis. However, the parotitis patients who are insensitive to antibiotics with persistent fever should be carefully considered as a possible IKD.

Xue-xin Yu

4.5 Case 25 KD with Acute Intussusception

A previously healthy 14-month girl presented on Day 12 of illness; she had high fever (39.9 °C) with shivering for 12 days, without convulsion. Her fever was not regressed after taking oral cephalosporin for 3-day and second-generation cephalosporin for subsequent 6-day. On Day 10 of illness, she had additional bilateral conjunctivitis without purulent excretion. She was given infusion of second-generation cephalosporin and vitamin C, but her symptoms were not improved. She was admitted to our pediatric cardiology ward as KD. She had mild cough and nausea since her illness. *Examination* revealed acute febrile face (38.3 °C), cervical lymphadenectasis, clear boundary and high mobility, conjunctivitis without purulent excretion, red and cracked lips, and strawberry tongue, along with red and swollen extremities. Others were normal. *Admission blood* tests revealed WBC 18.9 × 10^9/L, NE 73.5%, HGB 98 g/L, PLT 977 × 10^9/L. cTnI, hs-TnT, CKMB mass, NT-pro BNP, MYO and ECG were normal. Cervical ultrasound revealed bilateral lymphadenectasis, 1.8 cm × 0.8 cm on left, 1.5 cm × 0.7 cm on right. She was given oral aspirin 30–50 mg/kg/d, dipyridamole 3–5 mg/kg/day, both in two or three divided doses; IVIG 2 g/kg within 24 hours, and started to take oral erythromycin. She received infusion of 20% mannitol (2.5 ml/kg) followed by furosemide (1 mg/kg) 30 minutes later after half course of IVIG.

On Day 13, she had fever only once. Tests revealed CRP 52 mg/L. ESR 55 mm/h. ALB 28 g/L. MP-IgG 1:160. She was given infusion of erythromycin 20–30 mg/kg/day and albumin 1 g/kg/day for 2 days. On Day 14, she had afebrile for 48 h, was irritated with lack of appetite. Examination found that strawberry tongue was regressed, with desquamation of fingers around nails. Investigations revealed positive CP-IgM. Echo showed bicuspid valve mono-wave (Fig. 4.26); coronary artery and LV function were normal. Pneumonia was detected by chest DR (Fig. 4.27). We reduced the dosage of aspirin to 3–5 mg/kg/day. Considerating her intolerance to erythromycin infusion, we changed it to oral. First-generation cephalosporin infusion was given.

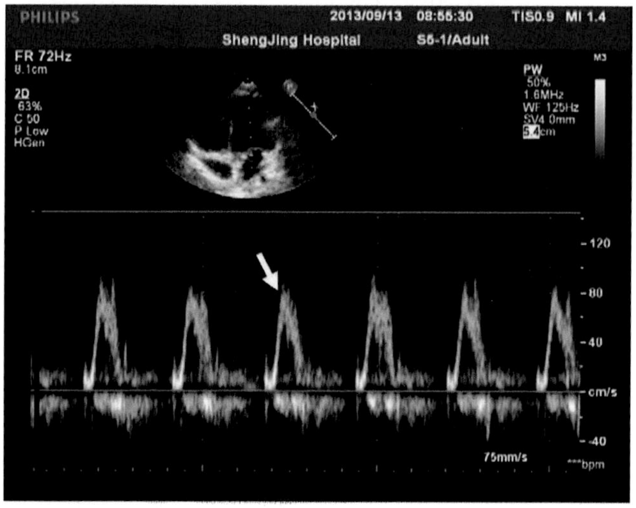

Fig. 4.26 On Day 14 of illness, echo showed bicuspid valve mono-wave

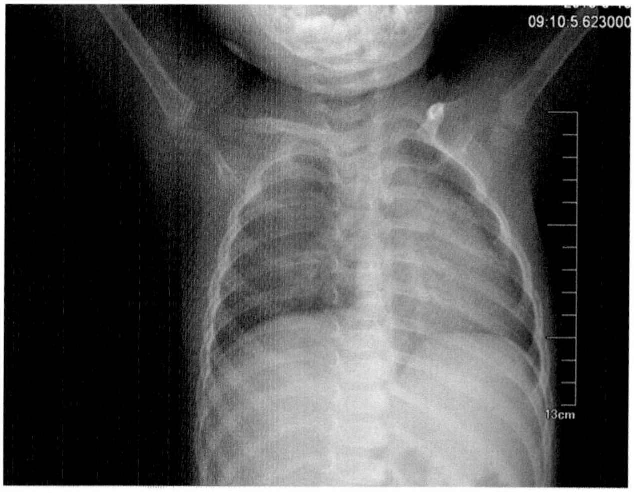

Fig. 4.27 On Day 14 of illness, chest DR presented pneumonia

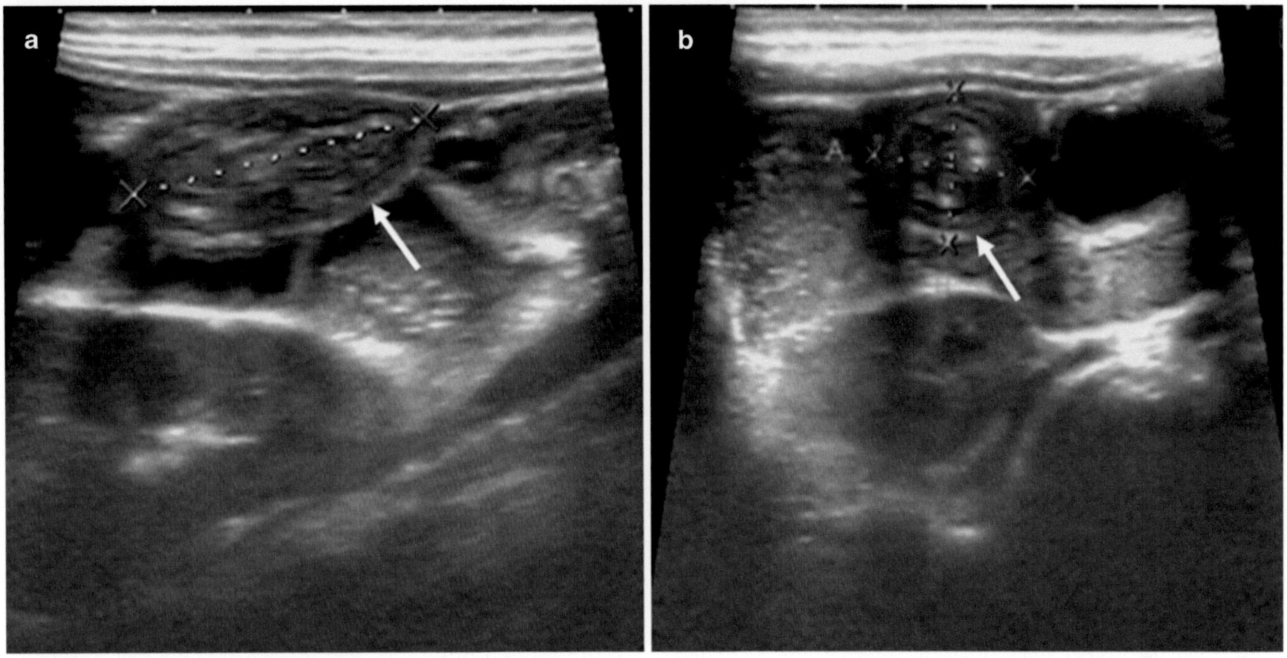

Fig. 4.28 On Day 18 of illness, emergency abdominal ultrasound detected a 1.8 cm × 3.2 cm × 1.7 cm mass, which presented "sleeve sign" (**a**) on longitudinal section and "target sign" (**b**) on transverse section

On Day 17, all the symptoms and signs disappeared but desquamation. Tests revealed WBC 7.5 × 10^9/L, NE 27.0%, HGB 96 g/L, PLT 799 × 10^9/L. CRP 5.84 mg/L. ALB 44.7 g/L, ALT 91 U/L, AST 114 U/L. ESR 71 mm/h. Compound glycyrrhizin, polyene phosphatidyl choline were infused to protect hepatocyte. Oral ferralia and vitamin C were applied. On Day 18, she vomited stomach content suddenly, with paroxysmal crying. Beside several lymphadenectasis (1.5 cm × 0.6 cm) with clear boundary, emergency abdominal ultrasound detected a 1.8 cm × 3.2 cm × 1.7 cm mass, which presented "sleeve sign" on longitudinal section and "target sign" on transverse section (Fig. 4.28a, b). The patient was immediately transferred to pediatric surgery ward and underwent, under the guidance of ultrasound, intussusception reduction procedure using an enema with warm saline. After taking oral carbon power, she was returned to our ward, with fever (38.5 °C) and nausea. Retested results revealed WBC 7.2 × 10^9/L, NE 76.9%, HGB 85 g/L, PLT 640 × 10^9/L. CRP 6.03 mg/L. Serum and urine amylase, and serum lipase were normal.

On Day 19, the fever regressed gradually; the girl vomited and had dark green diluted defecation, with normal urine volume. Examination showed abdominal distension and slight tenderness around belly button, bowel sound was active. Tests revealed positive stool rotavirus titer; ALT 65 U/L, ALB 44.9 g/L; serum K^+ 2.9 mmol/L. Oral probiotics and potassium ion infusion were applied. On Day 20, she was afebrile and retested serum K^+ was 3.3 mmol/L. On Day 21, all the symptoms were settled, repeated echo revealed bicuspid valve mono-wave (Fig. 4.29), coronary artery was normal. She was discharged.

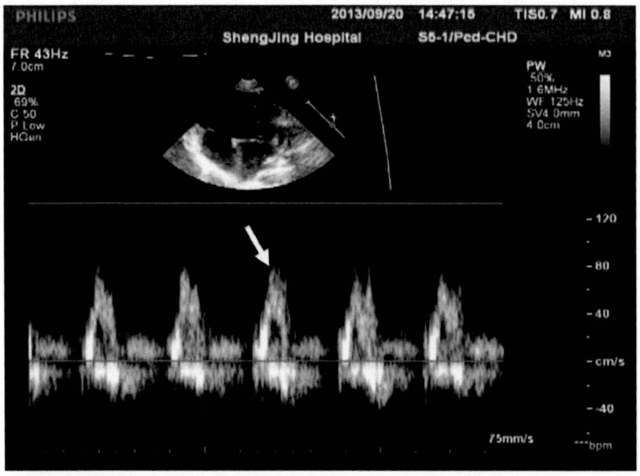

Fig. 4.29 On Day 21 of illness, repeat echo revealed bicuspid valve mono-wave

4.5.1 Clinical Course of this Patient

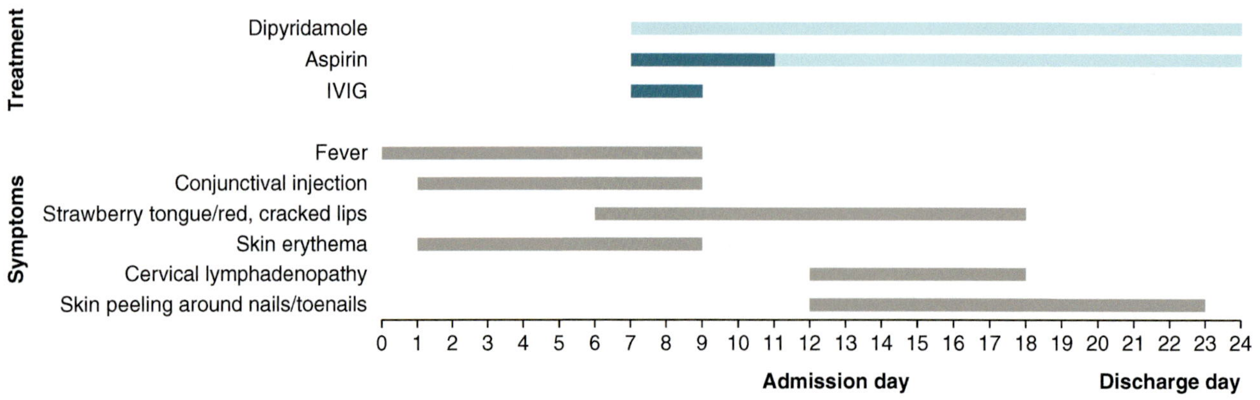

4.5.2 Follow Up

Besides routine medication, oral compound glycyrrhizin was prescribed to protect liver function, until Retested hepatic function 1 week later.

One month later test results revealed HGB 110 g/L, PLT 436 × 10^9/L, while echo performed at 1 month and 2 months later showed normal coronary artery. Echo performed 1 year later revealed normal coronary artery.

4.5.3 Diagnosis

1. KD.
2. Intussusception.
3. Liver dysfunction.
4. Hypoalbuminemia.
5. Moderate anemia.
6. Thrombocytosis.
7. Hypokalemia.
8. Acute bronchopneumonia.
9. MP infection.
10. CP infection.
11. Rotavirus infection.

4.5.4 Discussion

This patient met all the criteria of KD. She had persistent fever over 5 days, unresponsive to antibiotics infusion, along with (1) bilateral conjunctivitis without purulent excretion; (2) cervical lympha nodes were larger than 1.5 cm detected in ultrasound; (3) red fissuring lips, strawberry tongue; (4) red and edema extremities. Additional WBC 18.9 × 10^9/L, NE 73.5%, HGB 98 g/L, PLT 977 × 10^9/L. CRP 52 mg/L. KD accompany with intussusception made this case special.

4.5.5 The Special Features of the Patient

1. Intussusception is the most common cause of intestinal obstruction in infants; its etiology was unclear, probably associated with polyposis intestinalis, lymphadenopathy, and diverticulum. However, in most cases the cause is unknown and is thought to be due to enlarged Peyer's patches. Enlarged intestinal lymph nodes have been described in those requiring surgical intervention [21]. Intestinal lymphadenectasis are usually accompanied with a series of diseases including Crohn's disease, tumors, gastrointestinal infections or medicine reactions. Nevertheless, enlarged Peyer's patches occur most often in young children as a reaction following viral infections in upper respiratory tract or gastrointestinal system [22]. Thus, intussusception emerged mostly in spring and autumn. About 40% KD patients have cervical lymphadenopathy, possible have lymph nodes at other place involved. It could be the same infection that provoked KD as well as intestinal lymphadenopathy and consequently intussusception. But in this case, rotavirus infection during hospitalization was mostly likely causing mesenteric lymphadenectasis and secondary intussusception.
2. Most intussusception happened in infants, especially infants less than 2 years old with obesity. The typical clinical manifestations include: (1) paroxysmal cry (The interval was in accord with peristalsis, accompanied with agony and apastia. Patients could play normally during the interval); (2) vomiting stomach content or subsequent bile-like substance and intestinal content; (3) abdominal mass (can be palpable at ileocecal junction in patients with low-muscle-tension); (4) jam-like blood stool, diluted mucus or jam stool, caused by intestinal injury; (5) systemic syndromes at late stage, dehydration, ion disorder, fatigue, sleepiness, blunt reflection. Toxic shock could be presented while intestinal necrosis.

3. In this case, the 14-month-female vomited stomach content, and had paroxysmal crying, on Day 19 of illness. The preferred exam was abdominal ultrasound, which presented target sign on transverse section and sleeve sign on longitudinal section. Once diagnosis identified, ultrasound guided reduction of hydrostatic enema was performed, which was more convenient and radiation-free compared with traditional X-ray guided air enema reduction.
4. Surgical indications of intussusception include (1) ultrasound guided reduction of hydrostatic enema failed; (2) persistent intussusception for 24–48 hours, intestinal necrosis accompanied; (3) recurrent intussusception, especially child patients; (4) adult cases. In this case, we were concerned about intussusception when KD patients developed paroxysmal abdominal pain, vomiting, and unappeasable crying. For the characteristic signs shown in ultrasound, diagnosis of intussusception was easy. Moreover, once intussusception patients develop high fever, are unresponsive to antibiotics, have bilateral conjunctivitis, red and cracked lips, and rashes, clinicians should be aware of the possibility of KD.
5. IVIG was administrated on Day 12 of illness, out of the best period (5th–7th day) for IVIG treatment. Thrombocytosis had presented, and the large dose of IVIG within 24 hours might increase PLT, too. The parents were fully informed the risk of thrombocytosis and thrombosis. Thus, they were very cooperative in the following treatment schedule for oral aspirin and dipyridamole. Following the improvement of KD, PLT was back to safe range 1 week later. Therefore, it is very important for patients to have regular blood routine tests, oral aspirin, and dipyridamole.
6. Hypokalemia may be a result of not enough intake, vomiting, diarrhea, and possible oral compound glycyrrhizin. It is notable extra K^+ supplement was necessary when using oral compound glycyrrhizin in long term.
7. Doppler mode of echo indirectly measures LV diastolic function through changes that occur in the pressure gradients between the LA and LV. E and A waves represent peak early mitral inflow velocity and peak late mitral inflow velocity separately. Normal filling occurs predominantly early in diastole because of rapid LV relaxation that "suck" blood from the LA; represented by $E > A$. Impairment of myocardial relaxation leads to a reliance on filling during late diastole; represented by $E < A$. In more severe stages of diastolic dysfunction as LA pressure rises in response to ineffective filling, this ratio may be "normalized." LA blood is "pushed" into the LV; that is, $E > A$ (pseudo-normal) or $E >> A$ (restrictive) [23]. The mono-wave appeared in heart function insufficiency, atrial fibrillation, atrioventricular dis-synchronization, complete left bundle branch block. Those with a history of coronary artery aneurysms have prolonged deceleration time of the transmitral E wave, compared with patients without history of coronary artery aneurysms.
8. Vessel relaxation is impaired in patients who are in the early phases of KD and who had coronary artery dilation during the disease course. The diastolic dysfunction may contribute to the increased BNP levels seen in these patients [24]. There are two patterns of serum BNP changes before and after IVIG: the serum BNP level decreased after IVIG; and the serum BNP level increased after IVIG even if LVEF was improved after IVIG. If IVIG is effective, cardiac muscle contraction itself should be improved and then the serum BNP levels would decrease after IVIG [25, 26]. On the other hand, high-dose IVIG administration increases circulating blood volume, and the resulting LV volume overload may increase the LV wall stress, which promotes BNP secretion from cardiac muscle cells even though LV function is preserved [27]. These different effects of IVIG on LV wall stress affect the relationship between LVEF and the serum BNP level, and in turn may have caused the loss in correlation between the LVEF and Log BNP after IVIG administration. In conclusion, serum BNP level reflects LV contraction before IVIG administration, but does not reflect LV contraction after IVIG administration [28].

Xue-xin Yu

References

1. Zulian F, Falcini F, Zancan L, et al. Acute surgical abdomen as presenting manifestation of Kawasaki disease. J Pediatr. 2003;142(6):731–5.
2. Valentini P, Ausili E, Schiavino A, et al. Acute cholestasis: atypical onset of Kawasaki disease. Dig Liver Dis. 2008;40(7):582–4.
3. Uehara R, Yashiro M, Hayasaka S, et al. Serum alanine aminotransferase concentrations in patients with Kawasaki disease. Pediatr Infect Dis J. 2003;22(9):839–42 PMID: 14515833 https://doi.org/10.1097/01.inf.0000086388.74930.0d.
4. Eladawy M, Dominguez SR, Anderson MS, et al. Abnormal liver panel in acute Kawasaki disease. Pediatr Infect Dis J. 2011;30(2):141–4 PMID: 20861758 https://doi.org/10.1097/INF.0b013e3181f6fe2a.
5. Nicholson JP, Wolmarans MR, Park GR. The role of albumin in critical illness. Br J Anaesth. 2000;85(4):599–610.
6. Ballmer P. Causes and mechanisms of hypoalbuminemia. Clin Nutr. 2001;20(3):271–3.
7. Franch-Arcas G. The meaning of hypoalbuminemia in clinical practice. Clin Nutr. 2001;20(3):265–9.
8. Nemeth E, Ganz T. Anemia of inflammation. Hematol Oncol Clin N Am. 2014;28(4):671–81.
9. Keel SB, Abkowitz JL. The microcytic red cell and the anemia of inflammation. N Engl J Med. 2009;361(19):1904–6.
10. Kawasaki T. Kawasaki disease. Proc Jpn Acad Ser B Phys Biol Sci. 2006;82(2):59–71.

11. Yilmaz M, Akbulut S, Kutluturk K, et al. Unusual histopathological findings in appendectomy specimens from patients with suspected acute appendicitis. World J Gastroenterol. 2013;19(25):4015–22.
12. Taddio A, Pellegrin MC, Centenari C, et al. Acute febrile cholestatic jaundice in children: keep in mind Kawasaki disease. J Pediatr Gastroenterol Nutr. 2012;55(4):380–3.
13. Kimura A, Inoue O, Kato H. Serum concentrations of total bile acids in patients with acute Kawasaki disease. Arch Pediatr Adolesc Med. 1996;150(3):289–92.
14. Sánchez-Ramírez CA, Larrosa-Haro A, Flores-Martínez S, et al. Acute and recurrent pancreatitis in children: etiological factors. Acta Paediatr. 2007;96(4):534–7.
15. Cherry R, Naon H, Cohen H, et al. Common bile duct stenosis and pancreatitis in Kawasaki disease. Pediatr Infect Dis J. 2010;29(6):571–3.
16. Brown TJ, Crawford SE, Cornwall ML, et al. CD8 T lymphocytes and macrophages infiltrate coronary artery aneurysms in acute Kawasaki disease. J Infect Dis. 2001;184(7):940–3.
17. Falcini F, Resti M, Azzan C, et al. Acute, febrile cholestasis as an inaugural manifestation of Kawasaki disease. Clin Exp Rheumatol. 2000;18(6):779–80.
18. Amano S, Hazama F, Kubagawa H, et al. General pathology of Kawasaki disease. On the morphological alterations corresponding to the clinical manifestations. Acta Pathol Jpn. 1980;30(5):681–94.
19. Spiegel R, Miron D, Sakran W, et al. Acute neonatal suppurative parotitis: case reports and review. Pediatr Infect Dis J. 2004;23(1):76–8.
20. Chiu CH, Lin TY. Clinical and microbiological analysis of six children with acute suppurative parotitis. Acta Paediatr. 1996;85(1):106–8.
21. Hussain RN, Ruiz G. Kawasaki disease presenting with intussusception: a case report. Ital J Pediatr. 2010;36:7.
22. Eschel G, Barr J, Heyman E, et al. Intussusception: a 9-year survey (1986-1995). J Pediatr Gastroenterol Nutr. 1997;24(3):253–6.
23. Ravi R, Majesh M, Julio E. The Washington manual of echocardiography. Philadelphia: Lippincott Williams & Wilkins; 2012. p. 52.
24. Kawamura T, Wago M. Brain natriuretic peptide can be a useful biochemical marker for myocarditis in patients with Kawasaki disease. Cardiol Young. 2002;12(2):153–8.
25. Kawamura T, Wago M, Kawaguchi H, et al. Plasma brain natriuretic peptide concentrations in patients with Kawasaki disease. Pediatr Int. 2000;42(3):241–8.
26. Takeuchi D, Saji T, Takatsuki S, et al. Abnormal tissue doppler images are associated with elevated plasma brain natriuretic peptide and increased oxidative stress in acute Kawasaki disease. Circ J. 2007;71(3):357–62.
27. Maeder MT, Mariani JA, Kaye DM. Hemodynamic determinants of myocardial B-type natriuretic peptide release: relative contributions of systolic and diastolic wall stress. Hypertension. 2010;56(4):682–9.
28. Hashimoto I, Saitou Y, Sakata N, et al. Evaluation of longitudinal and radial left ventricular functions on 2-D and 3-D echocardiography before and after intravenous immunoglobulin in acute Kawasaki disease. Pediatr Int. 2017;59(12):1229–35.

Five-Blood System Involvement-Case 26_MAS

5

Hong Wang and Xuan Liu

Abstract

KD is recognized as a systemic vasculitis. Although the most common and serious complication of KD is CAA, changes in the blood system can also threaten the life of children in the acute phase, such as significant decrease in granulocytes (agranulocytosis), significant decrease and increase in platelets (thrombopenia) and (thrombocytosis), severe anemia, coagulation mechanism disorders and so on. At beginning of the disease, routine blood test results may be normal, but one week after the onset, they may change dramatically, the WBC is usually more than 15×10^9, more than 75% NE, PLT, more than 450×10^9. One week later, whether treated or not, platelet can increase over 700×10^9 (thrombopenia) one week later, and lasts about 2–3 weeks. It will gradually decline, back to normal in 4–6 weeks [Dumont et al., Arch Pediatr. 24(7):640–6, 2017]. If there is IVIG resistance, repeated application of IVIG and high dose glucocorticoids (GCs) may significantly increase PLT. In our center, the highest PLT number reached 1470×10^9. Therefore, treatment with oral aspirin and dipyridamole on time is particularly important. Because it usually takes place in patients with IVIG resistance, and the patients likely develop CAA and have coronary artery thrombosis at acute phase (case 11). However, in the acute phase, if thrombocytopenia is developed, it may also indicate an onset of CAA [Dumont et al., Arch Pediatr. 24(7):640–6, 2017]. In acute phase, neutrophil may be normal or significantly increased. However, in the subacute stage, agranulocytopenia ($<1.0 \times 10^9$) or even agranulocytosis ($<0.5 \times 10^9$) occur in some cases. The mechanism is not clear. In the absence of MAS, both can be restored to normal by treating with intramuscular injection of granulocyte colony stimulating factor (agranulocytosis) or with oral medication (agranulocytopenia). As to the anemia, the causes include bone marrow suppression due to infection; decreased iron intake due to lost appetite; decreased iron absorption due to diarrhea; increased blood loss due to repeated blood drawings; and, more importantly, the presence of hepcidin in the acute phase [Doğan et al., Balkan Med J 33(4):470–2, 2016].

In numerous blood system complications of KD, macrophage activation syndrome (MAS) is the most serious [Han et al., Ann Rheum Dis. 75(7):e44, 2016; Islam, et al., Mymensingh Med J. 26(2):356–63, 2017], but as long as timely diagnosis, early high-dose GCs application [Wang, Case analysis of pediatric Kawasaki Disease. [M] People's Medical Publishing House. Beijing. 2017, 218–24], most of them can recover. Even if the GC can't control, tumor necrosis factor inhibitor (infliximab) [Kinjo et al., J Clin Apher. 33(1):117–20, 2018] and plasma exchange [Itamura et al., Pediatr Cardiol 32(5):696–9, 2011] can be controlled, and the prognosis was well. As to increase of D-dimer, the meaning is associated with tissue disrupt, though without literature report it. In our center, it most happed in cases with multi organ damages.

In this chapter, we presented 4 cases. Because they were associated with multiple organs damage, they were arranged in different chapters according to the severity of organ damage. Thrombocytopenia was seen in case 20, and granulocytopenia was seen in case 9 and case 20. Thrombocythemia and acute coronary thrombosis were found in case 11. Severe anemia, MAS and leukemia-like reactions were seen in case 26.

H. Wang (✉)
Department of Pediatric Cardiology,
Shengjing Hospital of China Medical University, Shenyang, China

X. Liu
Department of Hematology laboratory,
Shengjing Hospital of China Medical University, Shenyang, China

H. Wang (ed.), *Paediatric Kawasaki Disease*, https://doi.org/10.1007/978-981-15-0038-1_5

A 3-year-old healthy girl presented with unremarkable past medical history and family history.

She presented on Day 10 of illness. At beginning, she had headache. On the following days she had remittent fever (peak to 40.7°C) for 9 days. She was given ibuprofen, which did not reduce her fever. She received infusion of clindamycin for one day, mezlocillin for 3 days, and first-generation cephalosporin for 2 days. The fever did not subside and she developed rashes all over the body, edema hands and feet, along with vomiting and diarrhea on Day 4 of illness. Furthermore, bilateral conjunctivitis, red lips, dry and rhagadia were developed on Day 6. She was diagnosed as KD. After treatment with IV antibiotics, IVIG 15 g/day for 2 days, and methylprednisolone 3 mg/day for 2 days, her vomiting and conjunctivitis improved. But fever was only under control for one day, then came back, along with sleepiness and conjunctivitis recurrence. After infusion of dexamethasone 5mg and fourth-generation cephalosporin, both fever and rashes were aggravated, accompanied by pain all over the body and motion restriction. She was transferred to our pediatric cardiology ward. Examination showed T37.3°C, PR 90bpm, RR 26bpm, BP 95/55 mmHg. WT18 kg. She was listless but conscious, breathes smoothly. Rashes were all over the body with fusion, majorly at her thigh. Cervical lymph nodes were enlarged with tenderness, the largest one was 2.5 cm × 2 cm. Examination also found conjunctival congestion without pus secretion and abdominal distention with slight tenderness. Liver was enlarged 8 cm below the right costal margin, medium texture. Spleen was enlarged 4 cm below the left costal margin, medium texture. Peeling skin occurred around anus. Neck rigidity was positive, while Babinski sign was negative. Others were normal. Blood test on Day 6 showed significantly elevated WBC and CRP (showed in Table 5.1). K^+3.2 mmol/L. Echo showed normal coronary artery, mild MI/TI. Cervical ultrasound showed cervical lymphadenectasis, the largest one was 2.4 cm × 1.2 cm. Admission liver ultrasound showed pervade liver damage (Fig. 5.1a). The wall of gallbladder was rough and enlarged (Fig. 5.1b). There were some small stones in both kidneys. There was a little abdominal cavity effusion (Fig. 5.1c). Hepatic venous was dilated (Fig. 5.1d). She had met all criteria for KD. Patient was treated with (1) oral aspirin and dipyridamole; (2) 20 gram albumen infusion; (3) infusion of potassium chloride.

Table 5.1 The dynamic changes of lab parameters

Day of illness	6 day	11 day	14 day	17 day	22 day
WBC ($\times 10^9$/L)	32.01	30	42.3	21.3	7.8
NE (%)	77.2	84.3	68	83.4	71.5
Premature cell (%)	5	5	14	0	0
RBC ($\times 10^{12}$/L)	3.42	3.2	2.4	3.5	2.9
HGB (g/L)	89	85	69	105	92
PLT ($\times 10^9$/L)	427	412	818	667	497
CRP (mg/L)	196	129	32.3		12.3
ESR (mm)	55	63			23
Ferritin (ng/ml)		678.3	827		603.5

On Day 11 of the illness, she still had fever (38.6°C), sleepy, moaning, irritable, without appetite. Examination found she had swelling face and lower limbs. CBC and CRP results were shown in the Table 5.1. DIC parameters revealed PT 13.8s, FDP 17.7mg/L, D-dimer 1368μg/L. Urobilinogen +1. ALT 43(<40U/L), T Bil 35.8(<21μmol/L), D Bil 23.5(<4μmol/L). ASO 73.3(<200U/L). NT pro-BNP 1516(<300pg/ml). BUN, Cr, CK, CK-MB, MYO, and cTnI were normal. CP-IgM was mildly positive. MP-IgM(+). MP-IgG 1:1280. Ferritin was 678.3 (NR 11-336.2ng/ml). She had met the criteria of IVIG resistance and was highly suspected to have MAS. She was treated with second dose of IVIG 2g/kg/day, total over 12 hours under ECG and BP monitoring at the same time. She started to take oral aspirin and dipyridamole, and meanwhile continued on sulbenicillin sodium plus azithromycin infusion. Mannitol (20%) infusion was given at the dose of 2.5ml/kg. Without consent from her parents, we did not perform bone marrow puncture and lumbar puncture. She received infusion of methylprednisolone 15mg/kg/day for 3 days. This girl was in critical condition and her condition might continue to deteriorate. On Day 12, she developed nausea and vomited undigested food. Body temperature was 38.1°C to 37.2°C. RR 30bpm, SaO_2 97%, HR 95bpm, BP was 91/53 mmHg. Her general state was impotent and irritated. She had normal defecate and urine. The rashes disappeared only left pigmentation behind. Face and feet were mild edematous. Lips were still dried, bleeding, and cracked. Liver enlarged 7 cm and spleen was 4 cm under costal margin. Echo showed normal LCA (Fig. 5.2a) and RCA (Fig. 5.2b). LVED was enlarged to 39.1 mm and LVEF was normal (Fig. 5.2c). On Day 13, she had vomit once during azithromycin infusion azithromycin infusion and had discomfort at the site of puncture. Her body temperature was down to 37.3°C. She had better appetite and slept. Dry lips were relieved but still with strawberry tongue. Oral mucosa was found with white floccus, and it was difficult to get it out. She had enlarged cervical lymph nodes and hepatosplenomegaly. Her neck was stiff. A neurologist was consulted, and she suggested to perform lumbar puncture test as soon as possible. But patient's parents refused to give consent again. They only allowed EEG and head MR being performed. Blood test showed normal K^+, Na^+, Cl^-, and glucose contents. Chest CT scan showed inflammation on both lungs (Fig. 5.3a) with pleural effusion (Fig. 5.3b). She received infusion of antibiotics over 10 days and methylprednisolone for 3 days. Then, she had developed thrush. Oral fluconazole was given for antifungal purpose. On the following days, everything got better. She was afebrile. Examination showed the thrush disappeared. There was no tenderness at sternum, and no tapping pain at long bone. Skin peeled off around fingernails. Retested blood work results were shown in Table 5.1. Ferritin, GTP, T-bile, and D-bile were

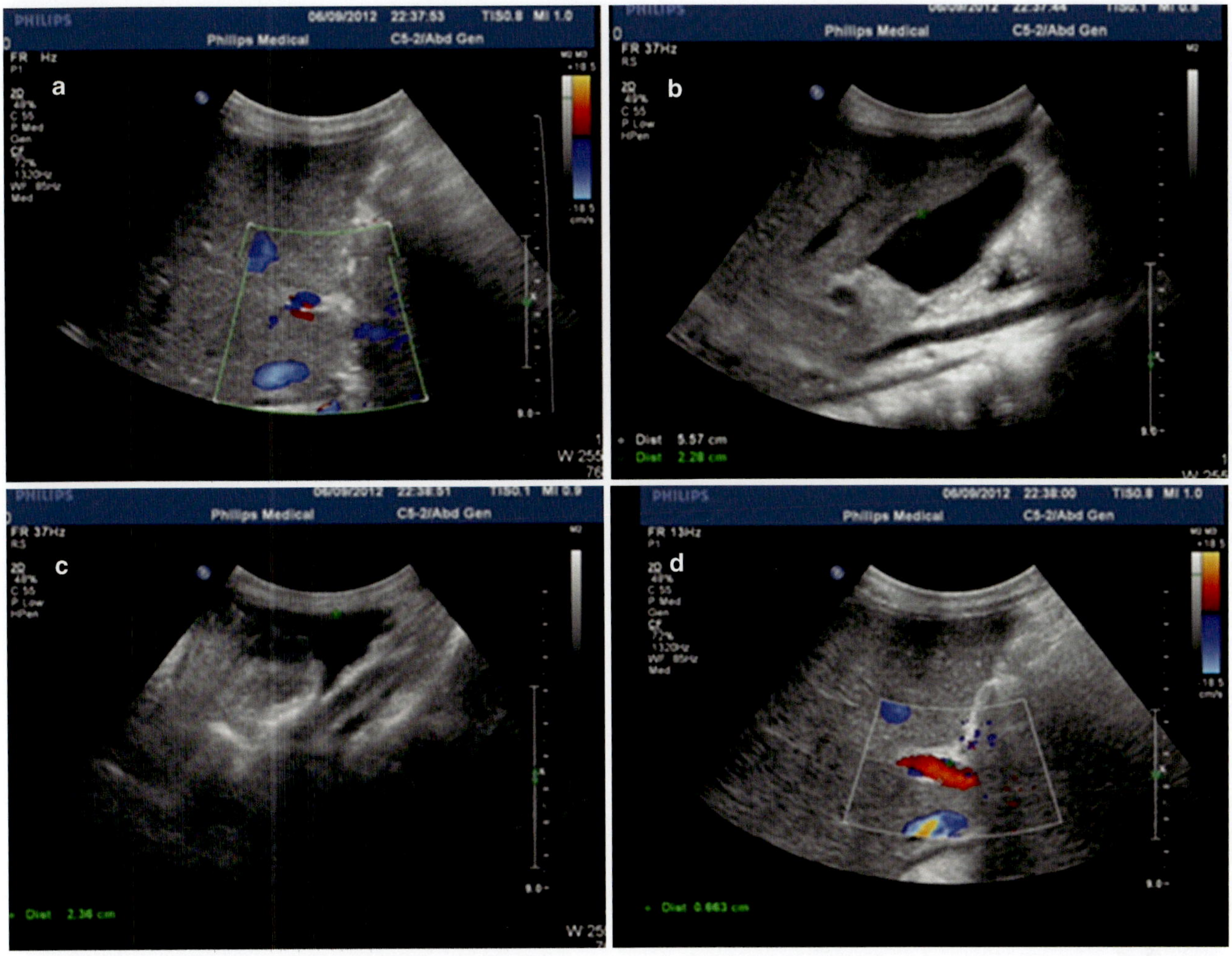

Fig. 5.1 On Day 10 of illness, liver ultrasound showed pervade liver damage (**a**). The wall of gallbladder was rough and enlarged (**b**). There were some small stones in both kidneys. There was a little abdominal cavity effusion (**c**). Hepatic venous was dilated (**d**)

normal. Albumin 31.2 g/L. NT pro-BNP 594.2 (<300 pg/ml). She was treated with: (1) oral prednisone instead of methylprednisolone infusion; (2) aspirin reduced to one dose 5mg/kg/d; (3) bone morrow puncture test performed; (4) received erythrocytes (1U) (filtered out white blood cells) for her progressing anemia. On Day 15, all symptoms disappeared. Bone morrow puncture revealed: leukemoid reaction, macrophage phagocytosis of reticulocytes, pigment granules neutral red cell, and neutrophils (Fig. 5.4a, b, c). She was treated with (1) additional filter white blood cells 1U; (2) staying on taking oral glucocorticoid recommended by consulting hematologist. Mannitol had been given intravenously for 5 days and was stopped. EEG showed there were more slow waves on both cerebrum with 4–7 Hz θ wave and 2–3 Hz δ wave (Image could not be saved). Her parents still refused to have lumbar puncture performed. Head MR was ordered.

On Day 17, she developed cough with a little sputum, without asthma. Liver regressed to 6 cm below right costal margin, spleen to 3 cm. She received infusion of ambroxol. On Day 18, she was afebrile. Head MRI scan showed her cortical signal was extended (Fig. 5.5a) and there was an occipital cyst (Fig. 5.5b). Possibilities of encephalanalosis and meningitis were not excluded. Repeated echo showed normal LCA (Fig. 5.6a) and RCA (Fig. 5.6b). Both LVED and LVEF were normal (Fig. 5.6c, d). She was given half dose of methylprednisolone. Pediatric neurologist suggested performing lumbar puncture but was denied again by her parents. On Day 19, cough got better, but auscultation found wheeze on both lungs. Liver regressed to 4 cm below the right costal margin and spleen was 2 cm below left. She was treated with (1) azithromycin infusion again for another 3 days; (2) budesonide and combivent inhalers. Two days later, ferritin was retested and was still high (Fig. 5.7). On Day 22 of illness, her body temperature was 37.1°C, cough was improved. Retest blood results were shown in Table 5.1. GPT, albumen, K^+, Na^+, and Cl^- were normal. Chest CT scan showed inflammation improved (Fig. 5.8a), pleural effusion absorbed (Fig. 5.8b). EEG was normal (Fig. 5.9). She was discharged.

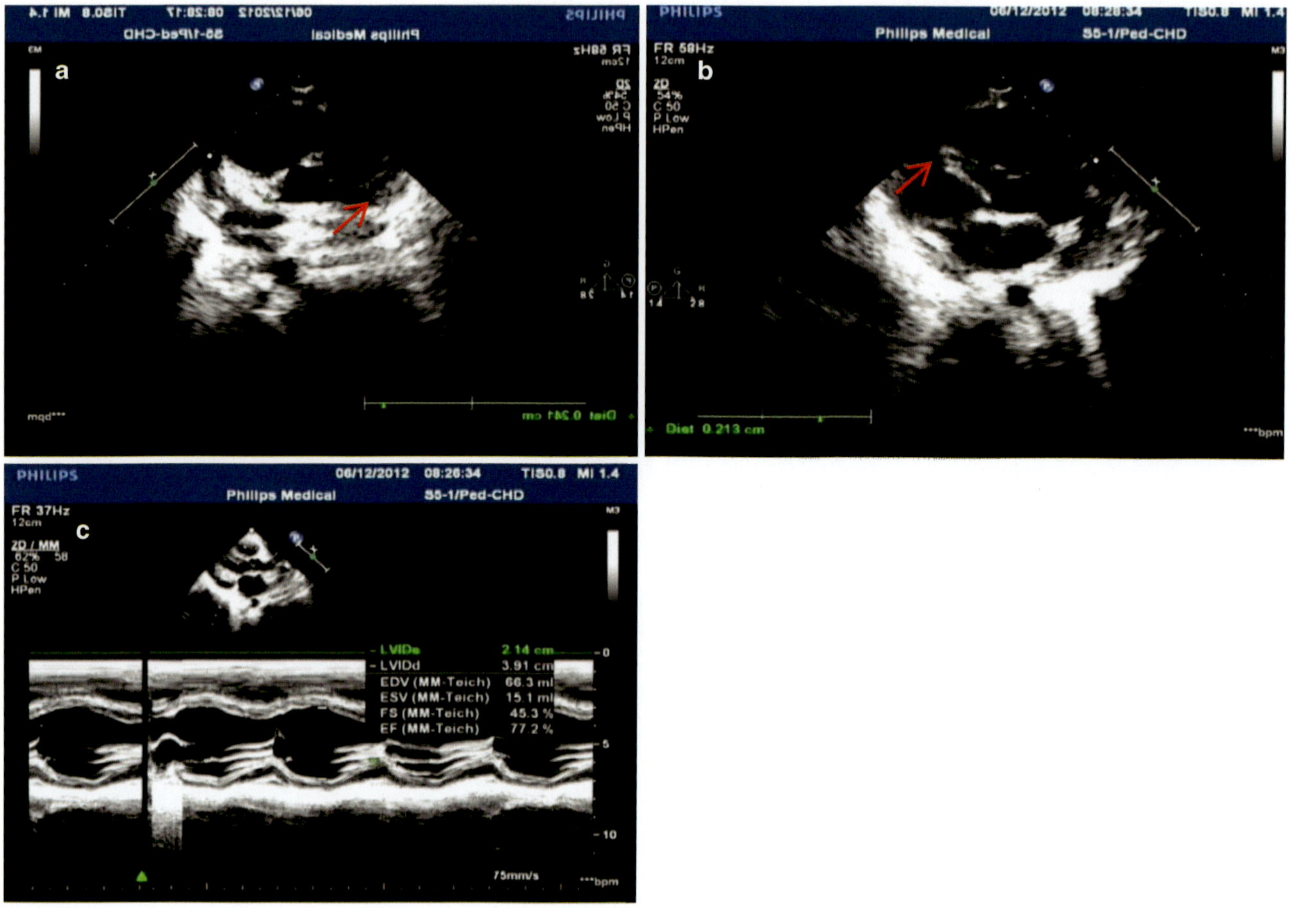

Fig. 5.2 On Day 12 of illness, echo showed normal LCA (**a**). RCA (**b**). LVED enlarged 39.1 mm, but LVEF was normal (**c**)

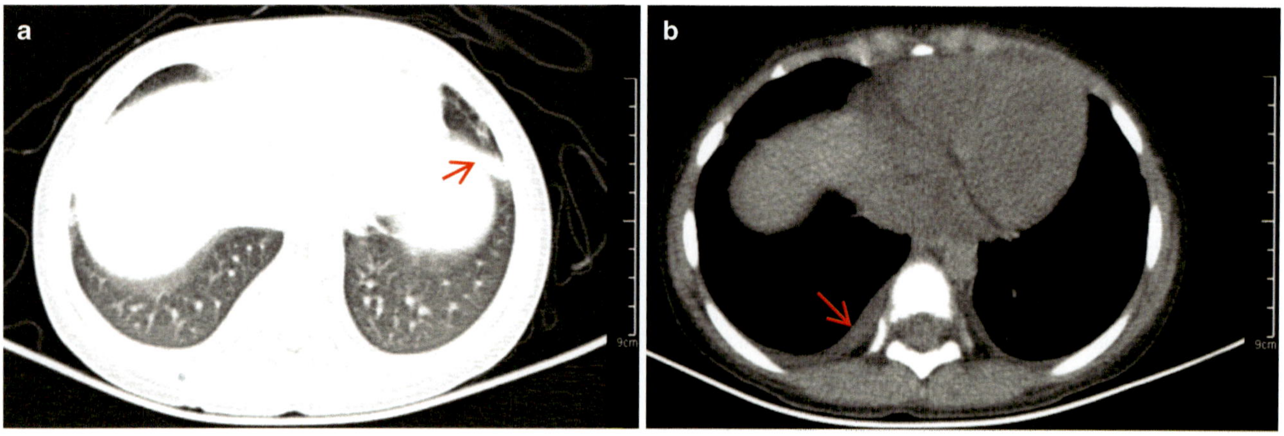

Fig. 5.3 On Day 13 of illness, chest CT scan showed inflammation on both lungs (**a**) and with pleural effusion (**b**)

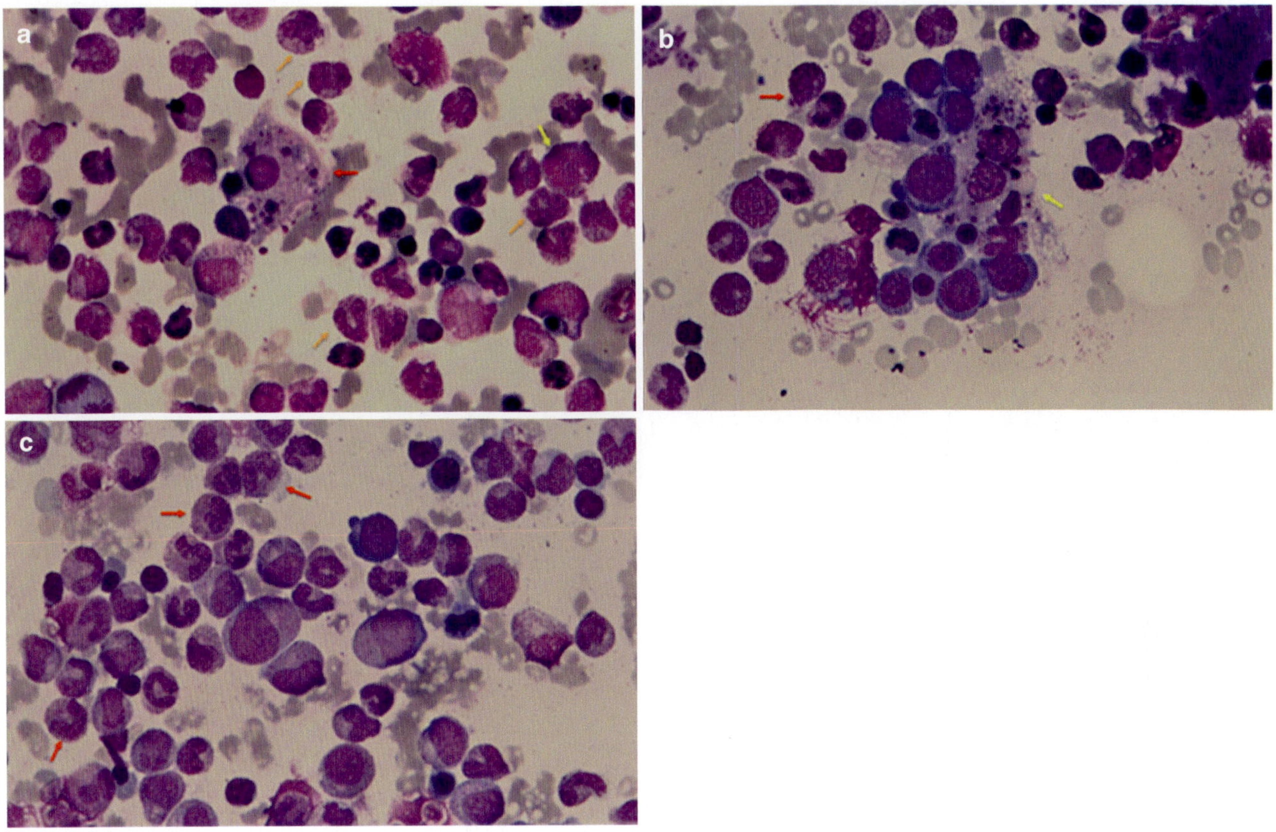

Fig. 5.4 On Day 15 of illness, bone marrow smear: Wright-Giemsa ×1000. Phagocytes phagocyte platelets and pigment granules (red arrow). The cytoplasmic granules of immature granulocytes were increased (yellow arrow). Toxic granules are seen in mature neutrophil cytoplasm (orange arrow)

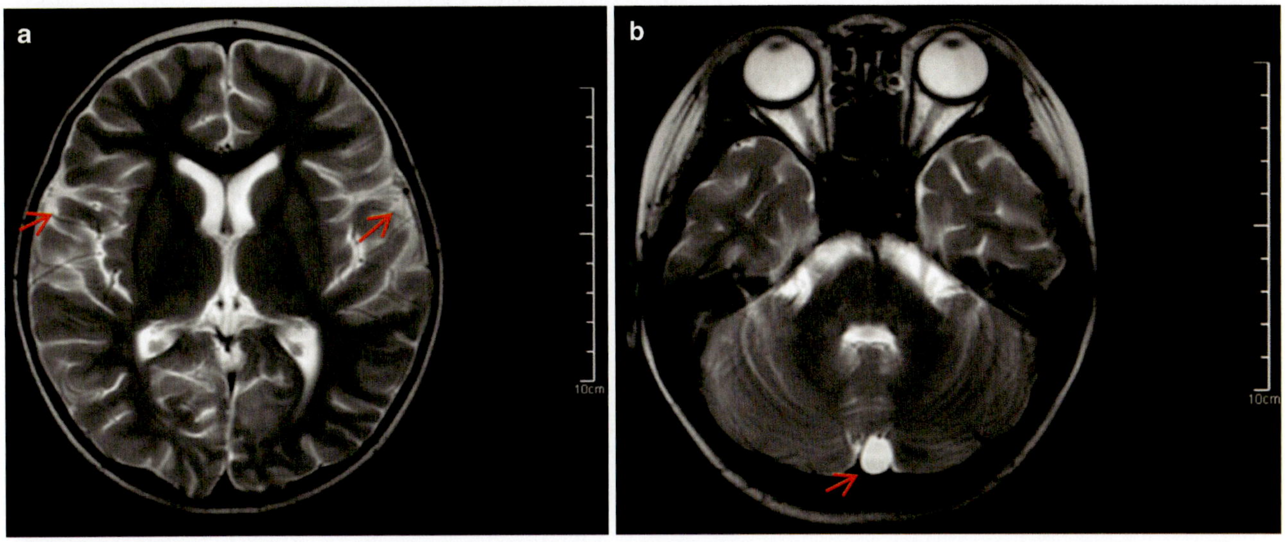

Fig. 5.5 On Day 18, head MRI scan showed her cortical signal was extended (**a**) and there was an occipital cyst (**b**)

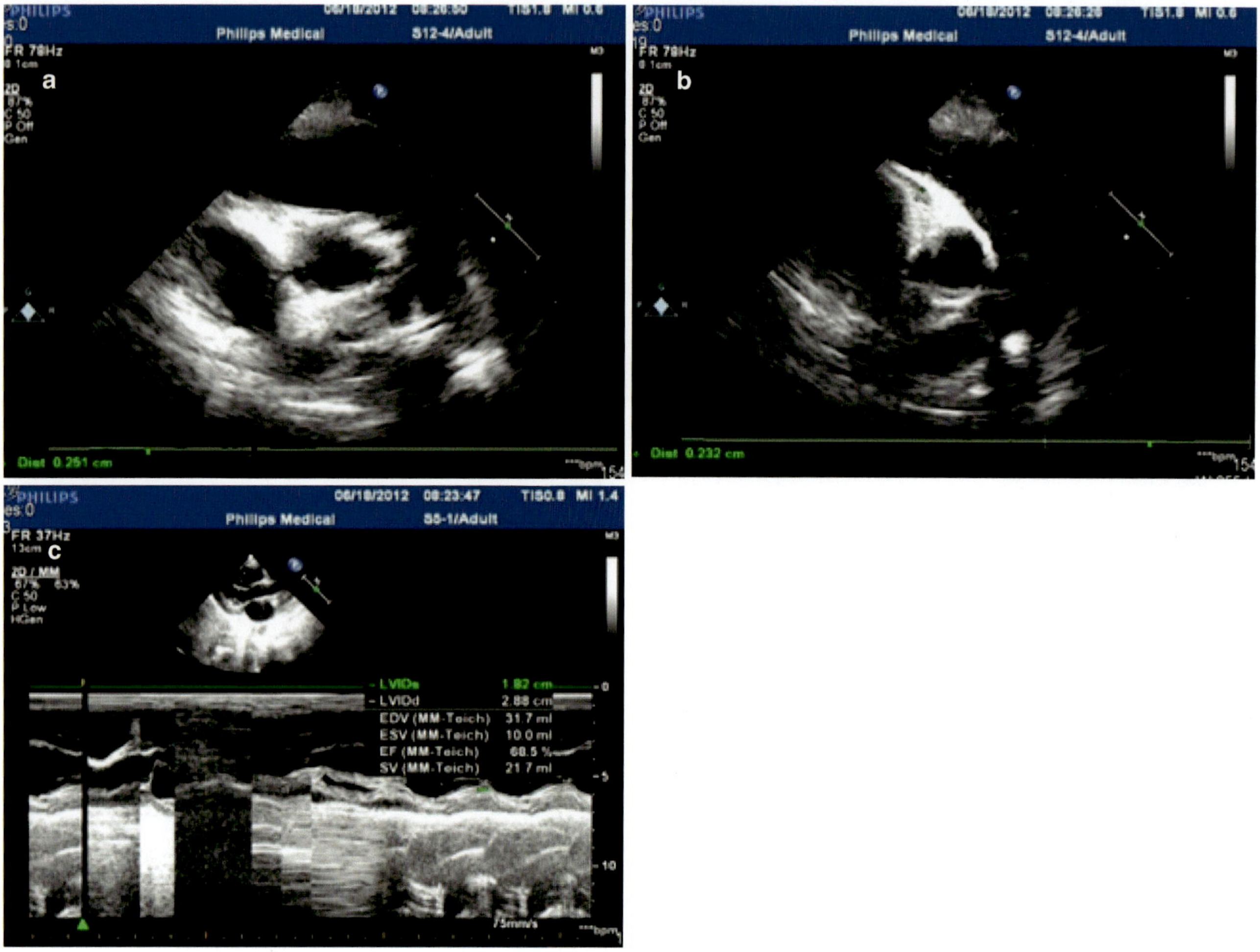

Fig. 5.6. On Day 19 of illness, echo showed normal LCA (**a**) and RCA (**b**). Normal LVED (28.8mm) and LVEF (68.5%) (**c**)

Fig. 5.7 The dynamic changes of ferritin

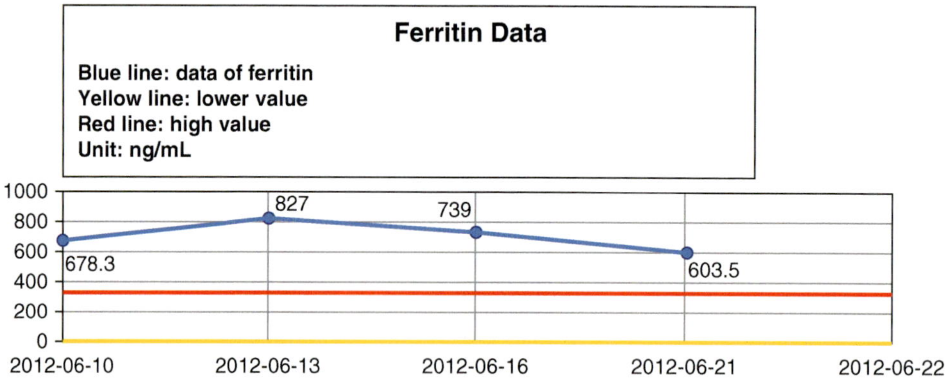

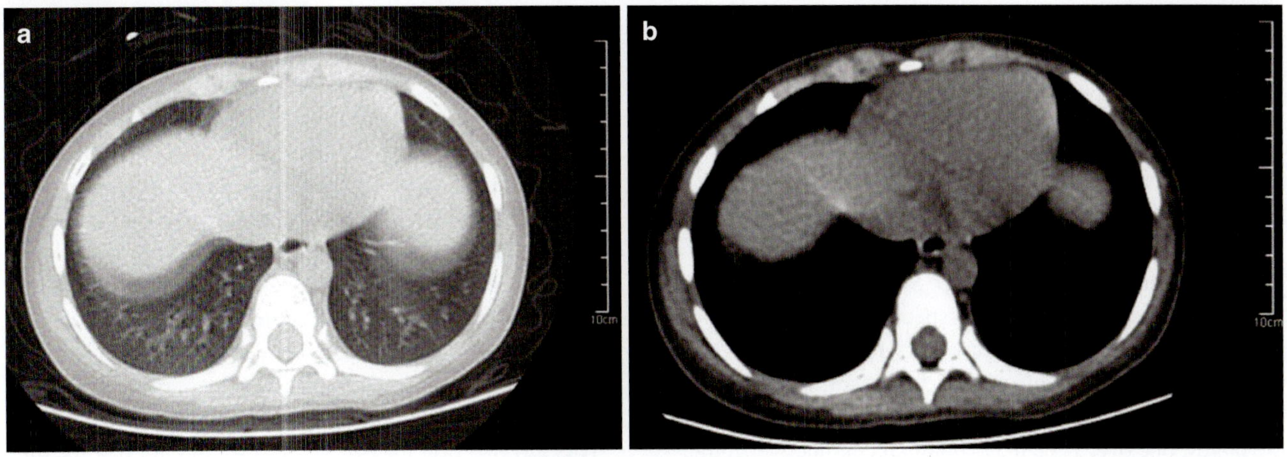

Fig. 5.8 On Day 22 of illness, chest CT scan showed inflammation improved (**a**) and pleural effusion absorbed (**b**)

5.1.1 Clinical Course of the Patient

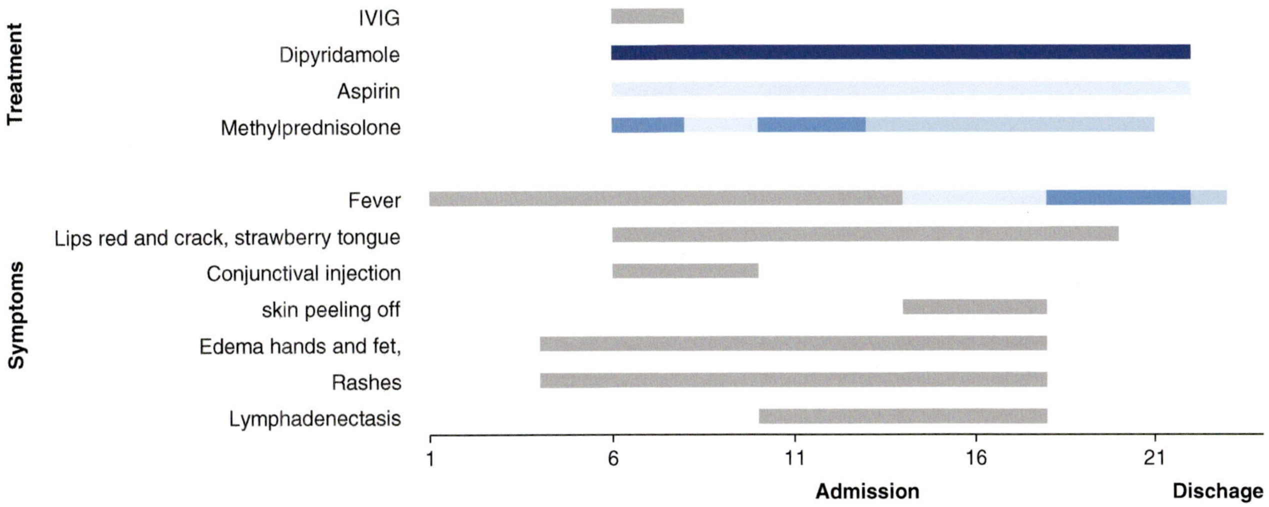

5.1.2 Follow-up

Since discharge, she took (1) oral methylprednisolone 8 mg for 3 days, 4 mg for next 3 days, and 2 mg for another 3 days in the morning; (2) oral aspirin 75 mg once a day and dipyridamole 25 mg, three times a day; (3) oral azithromycin 180mg three days later, once a day for 3 days; (4) oral vitamin B_{12} 5 ml, three times a day for 2 weeks. One week later, CRP and ferritin subsided. Echo was performed at one and two months, and it showed that coronary artery was normal. Result from liver ultrasound was normal. Then all medications were stopped. She never had follow-up with us.

5.1.3 Diagnosis

1. KD, IVIG resistance
2. MAS
3. Liver dysfunction
4. Leukemoid reaction
5. Middle to severe anemia
6. Pneumonia
7. Hypoalbuminemia
8. Pleural effusions
9. Hypokalemia
10. Seroperitoneum
11. Sterility Meningitis should be excluded

12. MPI
13. CPI
14. White mouth
15. Cisterna hydatoncus

5.1.4 Discussion

The patient met all criteria for KD. She had continuous fever that was unresponsive to broad-spectrum antibiotics, along with (1) strikingly dry lips, strawberry tongue; (2) red palms and later skin peeling off around fingernail; (3) congestive rashes all over the body; (4) cervical lymphadenectasis, with the largest one over 1.5 cm; (5) bilateral conjunctival congestion without pus secretion. She also met the criteria for IVIG resistance: her fever remained (>38.5°C) after IVIG treatment at 2 g/kg in the first 48 hours, with all aforementioned KD symptoms.

This girl met the criteria of MAS which include (1) continuous high fever; (2) hepatosplenomegaly; (3) anemia; (4) continuously increased ferritin; (5) increased FDP in DIC; (6) macrophage phagocytosis of red blood cells in bone marrow sample; (7) the immature cells seen in routine blood test [1, 2].

Differential diagnosis of sepsis, acute leukemia, pediatric rheumatic diseases, and acute meningitis should be considered.

5.1.5 Case Specific Clinical Features

1. Up to now, of the pathogenesis of KD is still unknown. Generally it is accepted it is inflammation resulting in vessel injury. This is similar to JID and therefore it can also induce MAS [3, 4]. Some literature described quick progression, and multiple organ damages. The fatality rate is very high [2]. But, they usually do not have coronary artery lesions [1].
2. The MAS resulted from inflammation. Thus, glucocorticoid is the first choice in treatment [1]. The dose of glucocorticoid depends on severity of illness. For this girl, 15–30 mg/kg/day was needed and the results demonstrated it was a proper dose. Otherwise, CTX, Cyclosporine A, VP_{16} [5], and serum replacement [6] can be used too.
3. This girl had symptoms including abdomen ache and vomiting. Liver function test revealed increased T Bil and D Bil. If without bilateral conjunctival congestion, conjunctiva jaundice maybe found earlier. The jaundice indicated inflammation in liver. Abdomen ultrasound showed her gallbladder wall was rough. Thus, cholecystitis was suspected. Cholecystitis is common in KD (see Chap. 4). It is one of the symptoms of KD and usually recovered after IVIG and oral aspirin.
4. In our center, the most affected system in all the KD complications is digestive system, including stomach, duodenal mucosa, cholecystitis, and hypoalbuminemia. Like in this case, complications include toxicosis hepatitis, cholestatic hepatitis, pancreatitis, and intestinal indigitation involved serous coat of ileocecal junction. Among these complications observed in our center, the top one is liver disease. Usually liver is enlarged after hypoalbuminemia, less than 5 cm under costal margin. In most cases hepatomegaly occurs without spleen enlargement but with possible thickening [7]. Most cases have even ultrasonic echo in livers. But this girl had hepatomegaly over 8 cm, and echo was enhanced locally. Otherwise, the echo of gallbladder wall was enhanced. Meanwhile the routine blood work showed sustained anemia and increased ferritin. All these together suggested that she had MAS [2].
5. This girl had oral thrush. Though we did not test for fungus infection, she received infusion of antibiotics over two weeks and glucocorticoid (high doses for 3 days) over one week. This highly indicated that she had a complication with fungus infection. After treatment with oral fluconazole for three days, the thrush disappeared. It in turn supported our interpretation.
6. Sterility meningitis was also common in KD [8]. It is usually transient and reversible. Cisterna hydatoncus might be the original changes or result from meningitis. Definite diagnosis depends on follow-up. If they disappeared soon, it suggested meningitis. Without lumbar puncture, we could not present CSF evidence. Since she had headache before fever and IVIG treatment, we speculated that it was not from IVIG [9] but from KD disease itself.

References

1. Dumont B, Jeannoel P, Trapes L, et al. Macrophage activation syndrome and Kawasaki disease: Four new cases. Arch Pediatr. 2017;24(7):640–6.
2. Doğan V, Karaaslan E, Özer S, et al. Hemophagocytosis in the Acute Phase of Fatal Kawasaki Disease in a 4 Month-Old Girl. Balkan Med J. 2016;33(4):470–2.
3. Han SB, Lee SY, Jeong DC, et al. Should 2016 Criteria for Macrophage Activation Syndrome be applied in children with Kawasaki disease, as well as with systemic-onset juvenile idiopathic arthritis? Ann Rheum Dis. 2016;75(7):e44.
4. Islam MI, Talukder MK, Islam MM, et al. Macrophage Activation Syndrome in Paediatric Rheumatic Diseases. Mymensingh Med J. 2017;26(2):356–63.
5. Wang H. Case analysis of pediatric Kawasaki Disease. [M] People's Medical Publishing House. Beijing. 2017, 218–24.
6. Kinjo N, Hamada K, Hirayama C, et al. Role of plasma exchange, leukocytapheresis, and plasma diafiltration in management of refractory macrophage activation syndrome. J Clin Apher. 2018;33(1):117–20.
7. Itamura S, Kamada M, Nakagawa N. Kawasaki disease complicated with reversible splenial lesion and acute myocarditis. Pediatr Cardiol. 2011;32(5):696–9.
8. Okanishi T, Enoki H. Transient subcortical high-signal lesions in Kawasaki syndrome. Pediatr Neurol. 2012;47(4):295–8.
9. Kemmotsu Y, Nakayama T, Matsuura H, et al. Clinical characteristics of aseptic meningitis induced by intravenous immunoglobulin in patients with Kawasaki disease. Pediatr Rheumatol Online J. 2011;9:28.

6 KD with Respiratory System Involvement

Hong Wang, Yali Zhang, and Jing Dong

Abstract

KD can cause systemic vasculitis, usually with minor respiratory complications. Both bronchopneumonia and a mild to moderate amount of pleural effusion associated with Mycoplasma pneumoniae were recovered by routine IVIG, oral aspirin and macrolides (Tang et al., Ital J Pediatr 42(1):83, 2016). But once a patient developed necrotizing pneumonia, it is possible to lead to bullae, pneumothorax and even life-threatening (Chatha et al., Can Respir J 21(4):239–245, 2014; Sakamoto et al., Respir Investig 56(2):189–194, 2018). As neutrophil changes in KD patients, combined with necrotizing pneumonia, their CRP may sharp deterioration, accompanied by remittent fever, poor mental state, lack of appetite, and anemia. In the presence of necrotic cavities, although there is extensive consolidation in lungs, the back knocking should not be used to prevent pneumothorax. This type of pneumonia is often caused by a G+ coccal infection (Alhammadi and Hendaus, Int J Gen Med 6:613–616, 2013; Leahy et al., Can J Infect Dis Med Microbiol 23(3):137–139, 2012); so the antibiotic dose should be high enough and the course of treatment should be long enough. Vancomycin is the preferred antibiotic, but acoustic monitoring is necessary. Owing to the diagnosis of KD is often delayed in children who have a predominantly pulmonary presentation, which can have adverse clinical consequences (Singh et al., Pediatr Pulmonol 53(1):103–107, 2018). Interestingly, the prognosis of children with KD was independent of the type of associated pneumonia.

This chapter introduces three cases. Case 27 describes a 4 months boy with mild bronchial pneumonia. He was diagnosed with KD at 7 days of the onset, and was treated with IVIG as soon as KD diagnosis confirmed. But he developed CAA, which may be related to infusion of glucocorticoid at early disease phase (Zhao et al., Chin Med J (Engl) 129(8):922–928, 2016). Case 28 reported an 11 year-old girl, with mild bronchial pneumonia and pleural effusion. She was also diagnosed with KD at 11 days of illness. CAA was developed eventually Case 29 describes a 14 months boy with necrotizing pneumonia. He was diagnosed with KD at 14 days of onset, and had remittent fever more than 20 days. But CAA wasn't developed in this patient. This may be due to the early (around 10 days of onset) use of IVIG in accordance with sepsis.

6.1 Case 27 KD with CAA and Pneumonia

A 4-month-old male was presented with an unremarkable past medical and family history.

He presented on Day 7 of illness with a history of intermittent fevers with poor appetite and diarrhea for 7 days, rashes and red conjunctiva for 2 days. He had remittent fever and was treated with dexamethasone for 2 days and first-generation antibiotics for 1 day on Day 2 and 3 of illness at a local hospital. Diarrhea was improved, but his fever only regressed about one and half days and recurred. He had rashes and red conjunctival congestion on Day 6 of illness. He was admitted to our pediatric cardiology ward. From the onset of illness, he slept well. Examination revealed his mental stage was nice, had mild fever (37.5 °C) and smooth breathe (HR 104 bpm, RR 26 bpm). His weighed 6.9 Kg Ht 60 cm. Rashes were all over the body, along with bilateral conjunctiva hyperemia. Others were normal. Investigation revealed on Day 6, CBC: WBC 13.2 × 10^9/L, NE 41.4%. CRP 25.5 mg/L. CP-IgM(+/−),

H. Wang (✉)
Department of Pediatric Cardiology, Shengjing Hospital of China Medical University, Shenyang, China

Y. Zhang
Department of PICU, The First Affliated Hospital of Zhengzhou University, Zhengzhou, China

J. Dong
Department of Cardiology Function, Shengjing Hospital of China Medical University, Shenyang, China
e-mail: dongj@sj-hospital.org

H. Wang (ed.), *Paediatric Kawasaki Disease*, https://doi.org/10.1007/978-981-15-0038-1_6

MP-IgM, rotavirus, HSV, and EBV-IgM(−). Chest DR showed double lung texture enhanced. Admission cervical ultrasound showed bilateral cervical lymphadenectasis. The larger one was 1.3 cm × 0.4 cm on the left and about 1.1 cm × 0.4 cm on the right side. He had met the diagnostic criteria for atypical KD, and was treated with (1) aspirin, 30–50 mg/kg/day, in 3 divided doses and dipyridamole 3–5 mg/kg/day oral; (2) infusion of erythromycin and second-generation antibiotics after blood sample drawn for culture; (3) IVIG 1 g/kg/day for 2 days.

On Day 8, he had fever up to 38.5 °C, and coughed occasionally. Rashes and red conjunctiva were reduced. Liver function, myocardial enzyme, renal function, NT-pro BNP, and DIC were all normal. ESR 42 mm/h. IgM and IgA were normal. IgG 2.72 g/L was lower than normal. Random blood sugar was 2.99 mmol/L. On Day 9, his fever and rashes settled, and red conjunctiva was significantly improved. Chest CT showed inflammation in multi-lobed segments at both lungs (Fig. 6.1). Echo showed LAC aneurysm dilation, with LCA 3.2–5.4 mm (Fig. 6.2a), LAD about 7.5 mm (Fig. 6.2b). RCA dilated about 3.2–3.9 mm (Fig. 6.2c). There was no thrombus in the

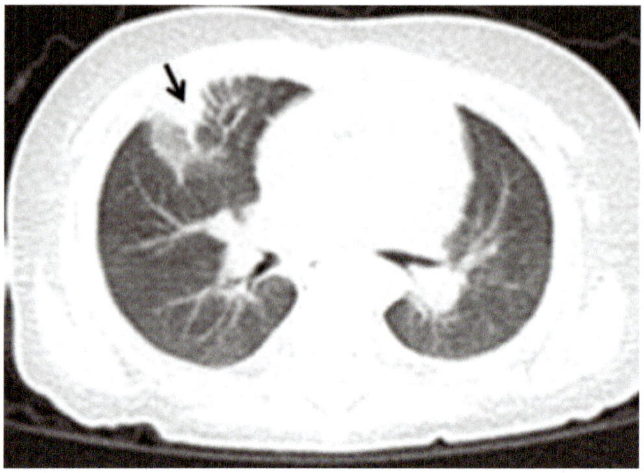

Fig. 6.1 On Day 9, chest CT showed inflammation on multi-lobed segments in both lungs

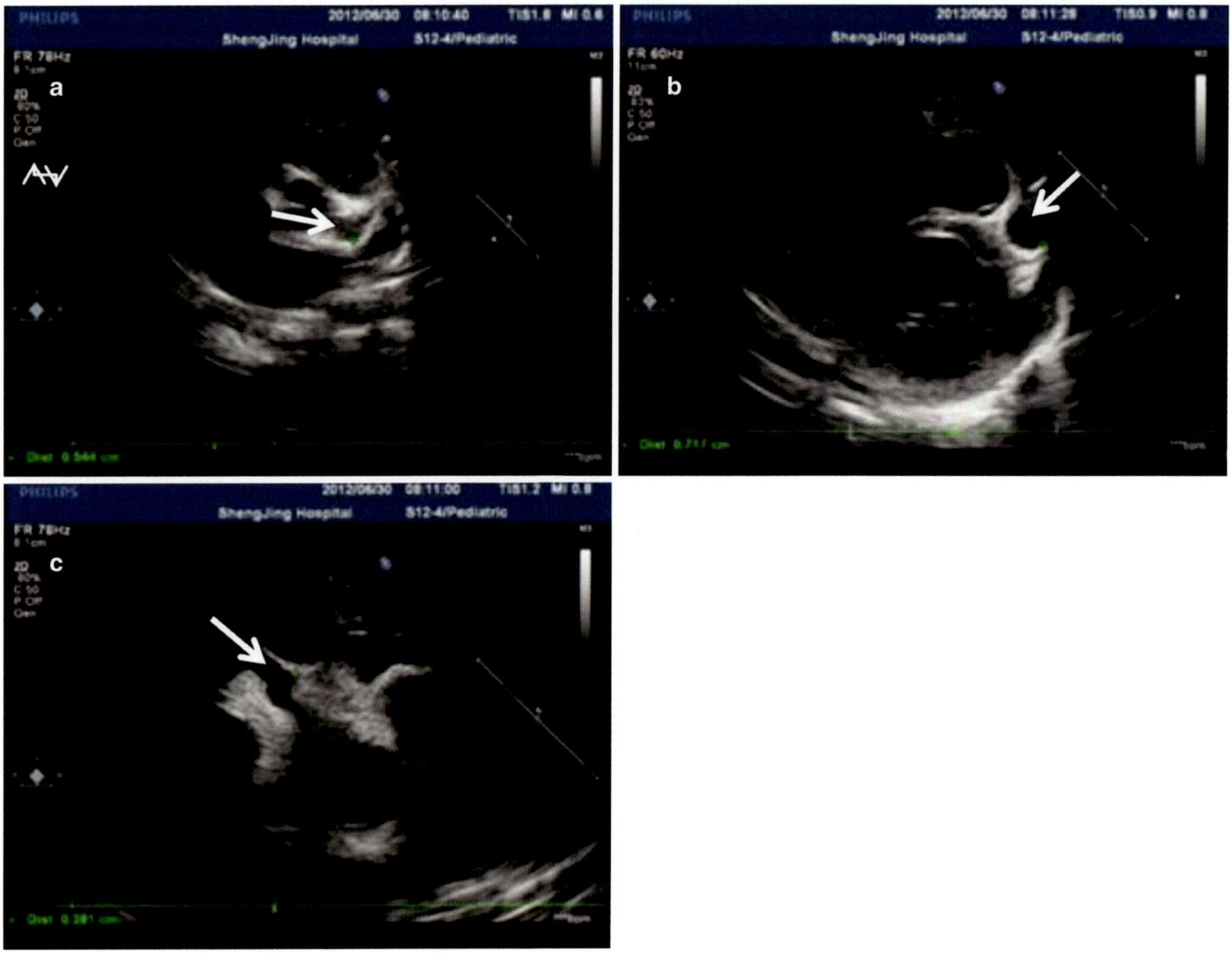

Fig. 6.2 On Day 9 of illness, echocardiography showed LCA dilated to 5.4 mm (**a**), LAD dilated to 7.5 mm (**b**), RCA dilated to 3.9 mm (**c**)

expanded coronary artery. ASD was 4.5 mm. Warfarin in 0.1 mg/kg/day was applied. On Day 10, after 48 hours afebrile, red conjunctiva regressed. Aspirin was reduced to one dosage 3–5 mg/kg/day. On Day 12, investigation revealed CBC as following: WBC 5.9 × 10^9/L, NE 0.62 × 10^9/L, HGB 97 g/L, PLT 620 × 10^9/L. ESR 41 mm/h. normal CRP. ALB 31.7 g/L, TP, ALT, and AST were normal. INR 2.1, PT 30.8 s, APTT 45 s, D-dimer 889 μg/L. Repeated echo showed LCA dilated about 3.1–6.3 mm (Fig. 6.3a), LAD about 7.5 mm (Fig. 6.3b). RCA dilated about 3.1–3.9 mm (Fig. 6.3c). Due to clotting time was significantly prolonged, aspirin, dipyridamole, and warfarin were discontinued. Vit-K1 was injected once. Blood routine showed small cell hypochromic anemia and granulocyte were reduced significantly. Iron and traditional Chinese medicine were added in treatment. On Day 15, diarrhea was improved. Repeated DIC test revealed PT 15.7 s, INR1.2, D-dimer 502 μg/L. Clotting time was normal. Aspirin and dipyridamole were resumed. On Day 18, he had no diarrhea. Echocardiography showed aneurismal dilatation in LCA and LAD, LCA was about 3.1–6.3 mm, and LAD about 7.6 mm. RCA dilated about 3.0–3.7 mm. ECG was normal. He was discharged.

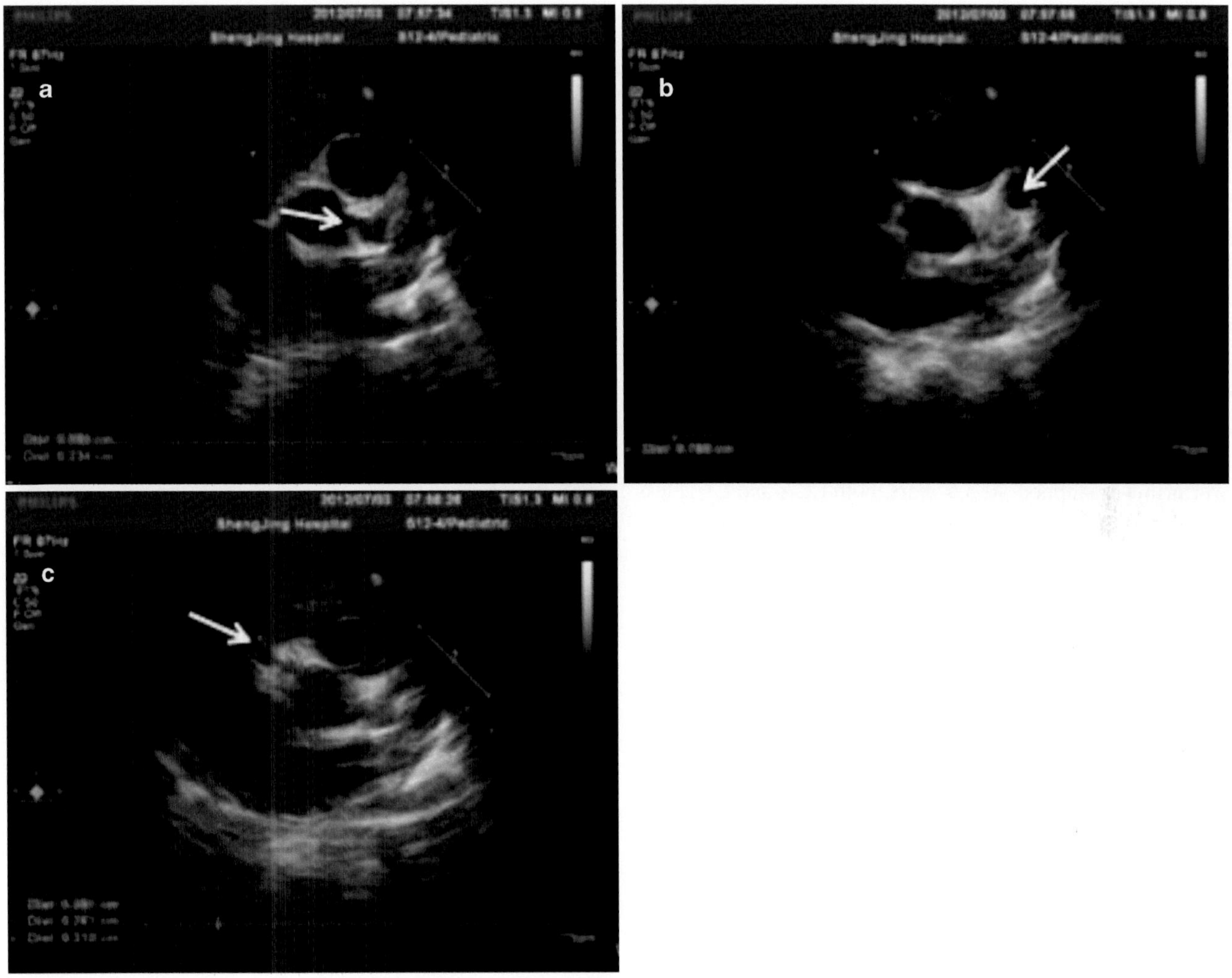

Fig. 6.3 On Day 12 of illness, echocardiography showed LCA dilated to 3.1–6.3 mm (**a**), LAD dilated to 7.5 mm (**b**), RCA dilated to 3.1–3.9 mm (**c**)

6.1.1 Clinical Course of the Patient

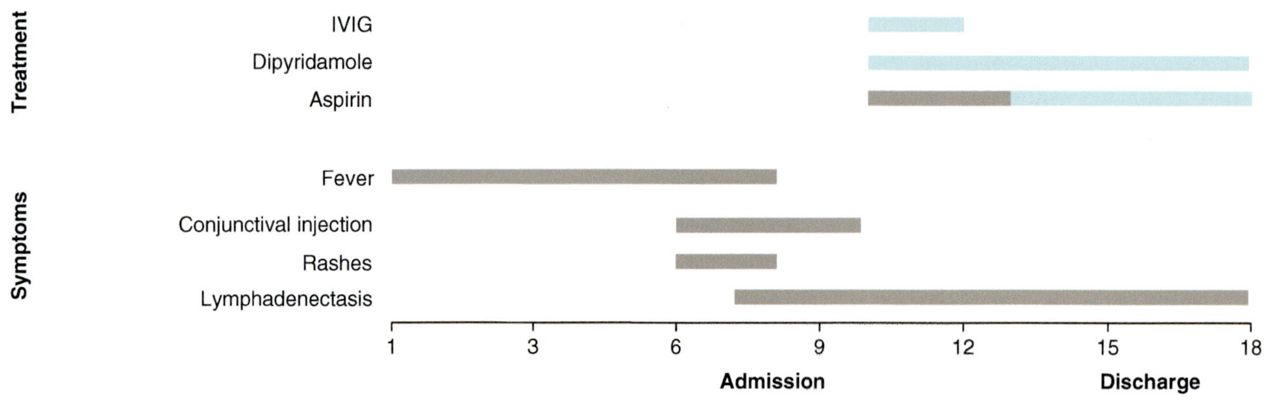

6.1.2 Follow-Up

He was followed up over 3.5 years after diagnosis (Table 6.1). Echo was performed at 1 month, 2 months (Fig. 6.4a), 6 months (Fig. 6.4b), 11 months (Fig. 6.5a), 21 months (Fig. 6.5b), 28 months, 33 months (Fig. 6.6a), and 3.5 years (Fig. 6.6b). LVED and LVEF% were always normal. There was no detectable thrombus in LCA and LAD. At 2 months of illness, he continued to take oral aspirin and warfarin, while dipyridamole was stopped. At 6 months of illness, echocardiography showed that was RCA recovered. Meanwhile, Both LCA and LAD were improved, too. Warfarin was stopped. At 3.5 years, both LCA and LAD less than 4 mm. At 4 years of illness, LCA (Fig. 6.7a) was almost normal and LAD was mildly dilated 3.6 mm (Fig. 6.7b). ECG was normal (Fig. 6.8).

6.1.3 Diagnosis

1. KD.
2. Giant CAA.
3. Acute bronchopneumonia.
4. CP infection.
5. Neutropenia.
6. Acute diarrhea.
7. CHD: second ASD.

6.1.4 Discussion

He had met the criteria of KD: he had fever over 5 days (after treated with dexamethasone in the course of the disease, body temperature was normal for 1.5 days), and did not respond to broad-spectrum antibiotics, along with (1) red lips; (2) bilateral conjunctival congestion; (3) cervical lymphadenectasis; (4) LAD aneurysm dilatation tested in echo. Differential diagnosis of sepsis should be included.

6.1.5 Case Specific Clinical Features

1. It has been reported in the literature that, even with IVIG treatment on time, there is still about 10% coronary artery lesion occurring in patients [1]. He was given IVIG during the optimal treatment period (on Day 7–8), but still had an aneurysm formed in coronary artery. In addition to pathological types, risk factors for coronary aneurysm include: boys, less than 1 year old, and early use of glucocorticoid alone [2]. This maybe related with glucocorticoid infusion at early phase.
2. It is not uncommon to have pneumonia in KD patients. There were few cases of severe pneumonia in our center. In terms of pathogenic bacteria, some literature reported that streptococcal pneumonia [3] and fatal desquamate pneumonia [4] can occur in KD. Although this boy had a severe lung changes, the prognosis was well after timely treatment.

Table 6.1 The dynamic changes of coronary artery

Time of diagnosis	9 days	12 days	18 days	1 month	2 months	6 months	11 months	21 months	28 months	33 months	3.5 years
LVED (mm)	22.9	23	23	23.5	23.9	26	27	31	32	33	35
LVE F (%)	68.7	75	75	78	50	62	62	75	75	65	59
LCA (mm)	3.2–5.4	3.1–6.3	3.1–6.3	3.4–6.4	3.5–6.2	2.1–5.4	2.3–4.8	2.4–4.7	2.9–4.3	1.9–2.6	2.1–3.5
LAD (mm)	7.5	7.5	7.6	7.4	8.0	6.6	6	6.4	4.6	3.5–4.0	3.9
RCA (mm)	3.2–3.9	3.1–3.9	3.0–3.7	2.9–3.1	2.4–2.6	N	N	N	N	N	N

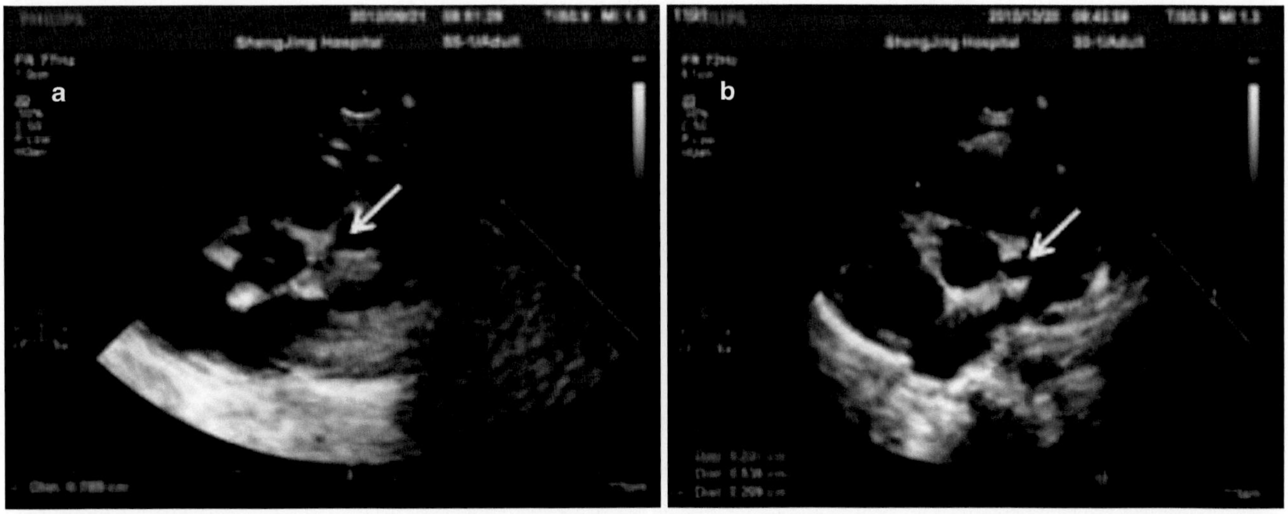

Fig. 6.4 Echocardiography showed LAD was about 8 mm at 2 months of illness (**a**), LCA was about 5.4 mm at 6 months of illness (**b**)

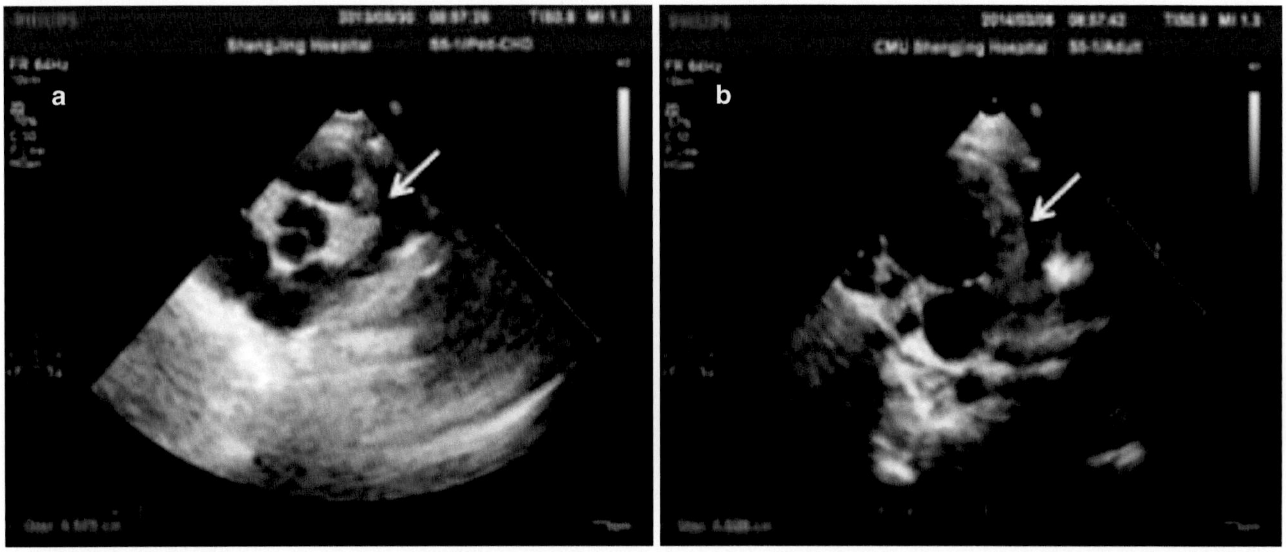

Fig. 6.5 Echocardiography showed LAD was about 5.8 mm at 11 months of illness (**a**), while 6.1 mm at 21 months of illness (**b**)

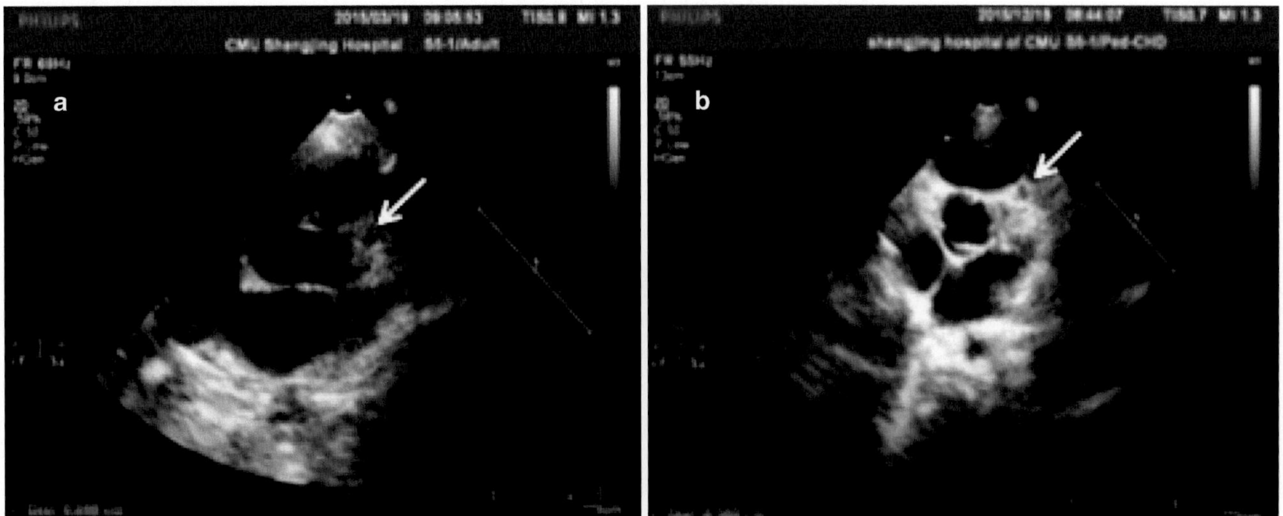

Fig. 6.6 Echocardiography showed LAD was about 4.1 mm at 33 months of illness (**a**), while 3.9 mm at 3.5 years of illness (**b**)

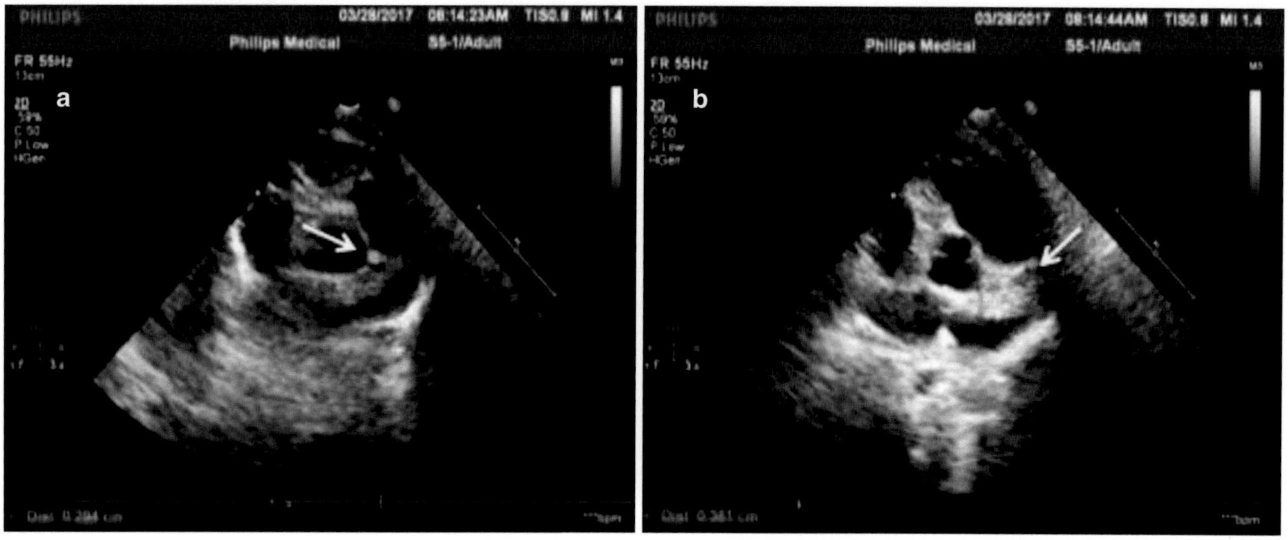

Fig. 6.7 At 4 years of illness, echocardiography showed LAD about 3.6 mm (**a**), LAD 3.0 mm (**b**)

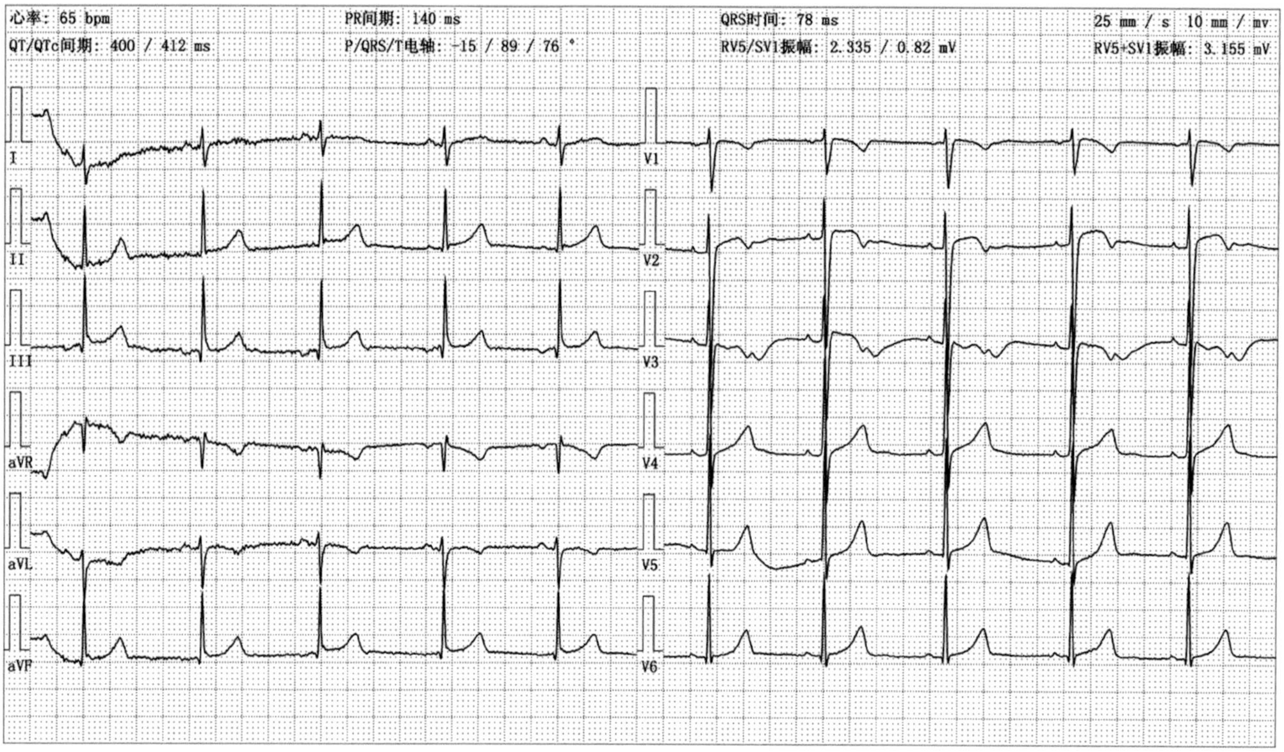

Fig. 6.8 At 4 years of illness, ECG was normal

3. Warfarin is an antagonist to vitamin K. It inhibits the synthesis of coagulation factors II, VII, IX, and X involved in vitamin K in the liver. The production of vitamin K is derived from intestinal E. coli. There are less intestinal bacteria in infants and young children. After application of broad-spectrum antibiotics, intestinal flora imbalance is common. If diarrhea present, reduced amount of E. coli result in less vitamin K synthesis accordingly. Warfarin is an indirect anticoagulant with a long half-life and is stable after 5–7 days after administration. Therefore, it is necessary to observe the patient for 5–7 days to determine if the dose is safe. In adults, if the coagulation function is normal before taking oral warfarin, coagulation function is retested 5–7 days after warfarin application [4]. However, in children, especially those with diarrhea, it is necessary to review the coagulation function 2–3 days after treatment. If the prothrombin time (PT) is extended over 2.5 times than normal, or there is a tendency to develop hemorrhage, warfarin should be reduced or discontinued, and bleeding disorder should be checked and reviewed. Once bleeding starts, vitamin K_1 should be injection immediately [5].

4. Giant coronary artery is an absolute indication for the application of warfarin (if there is no bleeding). However, when coronary aneurysms is close to 8 mm, especially at stages I and II of the disease, with significantly elevated platelets, the application of warfarin remains as a question and need to be verified by large sample data. When hospitalized at the first time, he was given warfarin, because LAD was 7.1 mm as shown in imaging. When he had diarrhea and developed hypocoagulation, warfarin treatment was stopped immediately. Repeated echo showed improvement in coronary artery, under 8 mm. Warfarin was discontinued. Two months later, test showed that coronary aneurysm dilated to 8 mm, and warfarin was resumed. After taking warfarin for half a year, coronary arteries recovered significantly, and warfarin was stopped.
5. The guidelines recommend discontinuation of dipyridamole when applying aspirin and warfarin for giant tubular aneurysms, [5]. We reasoned that although both warfarin and dipyridamole have antithrombotic effects, the underline mechanisms are different. In the acute phase, if the platelets are significantly elevated, we recommend to use these three medicines together (monitoring coagulation function). Warfarin is discontinued, once the giant coronary aneurysm is improved. Dipyridamole was stopped after platelets recovered to normal and giant CAA reduced to mild dilation.

Hong Wang

6.2 Case 28 KD with CAA and Pleural Effusion

A 10-year-old girl presented with an unremarkable past medical, personal, allergy, and family history.

She presented on Day 11 of illness with a history of continuous fever for 11 days, along with lymphadenectasis for 10 days, red conjunctiva for 4 days. On Day 2 of illness, a painful mass was developed on her right neck. She was treated with azithromycin for 1 day at a local clinic and the infusion was stopped for uncomfortable abdomen. Next day, fever went up to 41 °C, with the neck mass aggravated. She was treated with second-generation cephalosporin for 1 day, but symptoms did not improve. She was transferred to our outpatient care center. She was diagnosed with acute cervical lymphadenectasis based on echo findings, and was given antibiotics infusion for another day at the local clinics. Her fever did not regress and she developed severe cough. She was admitted in a local hospital. MP-IgG(+). She received infusion of second-generation cephalosporin and erythromycin for 5 days. On Day 7, her cough was significantly improved but she developed red conjunctiva along with dry and red lips. On Day 8, her hands and feet started to be swollen. She was admitted to our pediatric cardiology ward as KD patient. Examination revealed that her mental stage was stable, she had conjunctiva hyperemia, hemorrhage spot about 2 mm × 4 mm on the left eye, dry and red lips, strawberry tongue, and cervical lymphadenectasis. Axillary temperature was 38.6 °C, HR102bpm, RR 25 bpm. Weight 45 kg. Auscultation on heart found 2–3/6 mild systolic murmurs on the apex, with normal P_2. Hepatomegaly was about 3 cm below the right costal margin and medium degree of hard. Others were normal. Cervical ultrasound showed lymphadenectasis on Day 3, the largest one was about 1.5 cm × 1.1 cm on the left and was about 2.5 cm × 1.3 cm on the right one. Admission blood test revealed WBC 25.5 × 10^9/L, NE 84.8%, HGB 102 g/L, PLT 463 × 10^9/L. CRP 115 mg/L. CK, CK-MB mass, cTnI, and NT-pro BNP were normal. ALT 87 U/L, AST 45 U/L, ALB 24.4 g/L. She had met the diagnostic criteria for KD. She received (1) oral aspirin 30–50 mg/kg/day, dipyridamole 3–5 mg/kg/day, both in three divided doses; (2) IVIG 1 g/kg/day for 2 days; (3) second-generation cephalosporin infusion 0.1 g/day in two divided doses, after blood drawn for culturing.

On Day 12, she continued to have fever and had pain at bilateral knee joints, especially when standing. Investigation revealed ASO <25 IU/ml. ESR 55 mm/h. MP-IgG 1:320. MP-IgM(−). CP-IgM(+). She rested on bed and was given (1) third-generation cephalosporin and azithromycin 10 mg/kg/day for 3 days; (2) albumin infusion at 1 g/kg/day for 2 days; (3) polyene phosphatidylcholine 5 ml/day for protecting liver. She should have a MR for knee joints, but her parents will not give consents. On Day 13, she was afebrile, and her limb swollen was significantly reduced. The knee joint pain was relieved. Test results showed: Ferritin 422.2 ng/ml. RF 20.8 IU/ml. ANA series: weakly positive Anti-SS-A, Anti-Ro-52, and anti-mitochondrial antibody M_2; ANA was little 1:100 positive; ANCA was negative. The chest CT scan showed inflammations in lungs at both sides (Fig. 6.9a), little effusion in bilateral pleural (Fig. 6.9b), and a small amount of interstitial fluid on the right side (Fig. 6.10a). Liver ultrasound showed hepatomegaly about 3.3 cm below right costal margin. Echocardiography showed pericardial effusion 3–5 mm (Fig. 6.10b), LCA 3.9 mm, LAD widened about 6 mm (Fig. 6.11a), RCA 7 mm and 20 mm in length (Fig. 6.11b). ECG was normal. On Day 15, her swollen limbs and ankles regressed, pain at knee joint subsided. Investigation revealed WBC 18.2 × 10^9/L, NE 59.9%, HGB 104 g/L, PLT 653 × 10^9/L. CRP 26 mg/L. After 48 hours afebrile, aspirin was reduced to one dose 3–5 mg/kg/day. On Day 17, physical examination found cervical lymphadenectasis regressed. Investigation revealed ALB 35.3 g/L, ALT 59 U/L, AST 53 U/L.

On Day 19, investigation revealed WBC 5.7 × 10^9/L, NE 39.6%, HGB 96 g/L, PLT 608 × 10^9/L. MPV 6.0 fL. CRP 6.72 mg/L. Repeated echo showed LVED 41 mm, LVEF 68%, LM 3.9 mm (Fig. 6.13a), LAD 6.3 mm (Fig. 6.13b), LCX 2.89mm (Fig. 6.13c), RCA 8.3 mm (Fig. 6.13d), and absence of pericardial effusion. ECG was normal. Liver ultrasound showed the liver regressed to 2.3 cm below right costal margin. Chest CT showed bilateral pleural effusions were almost absorbed (Fig. 6.14a). Lung inflammation was reduced (Fig. 6.14b). We advised her to take warfarin, but her parents refused. She was discharged.

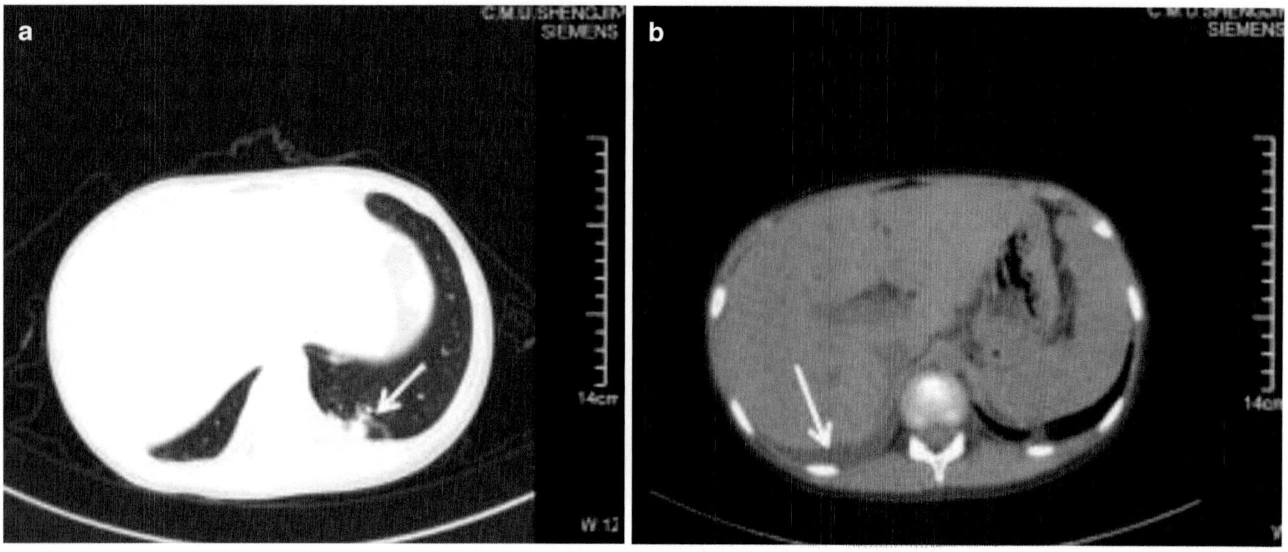

Fig. 6.9 On Day 13, chest CT showed inflammation on the left lung (**a**) and pleuro effusion on the right (**b**)

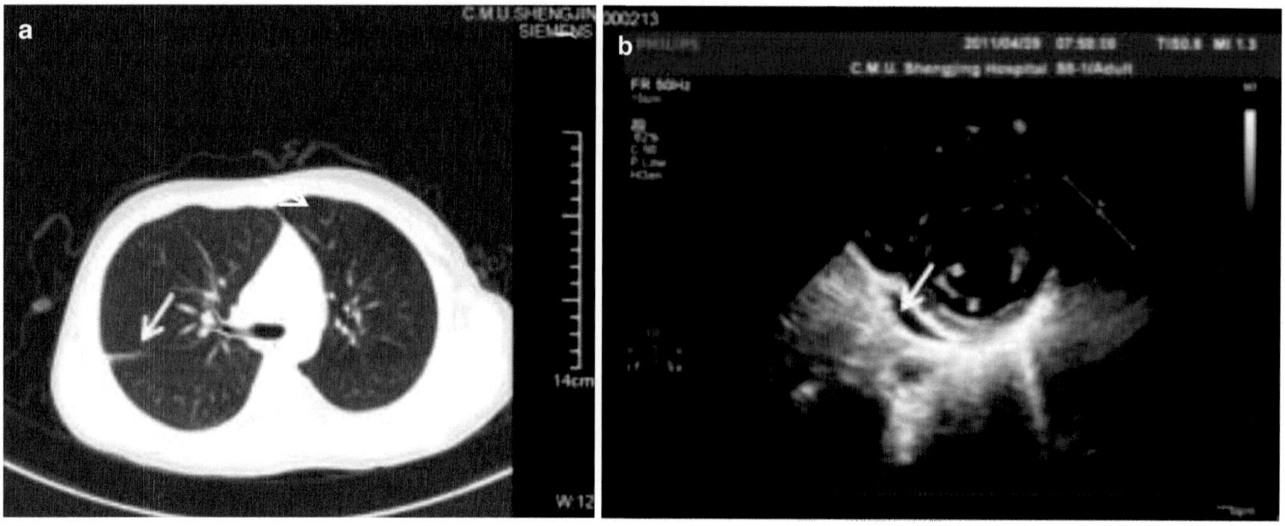

Fig. 6.10 On Day 13, chest CT showed a little interlobular pleural effusion on the right (**a**), echo showed mild pericardial effusion 3–5 mm (**b**)

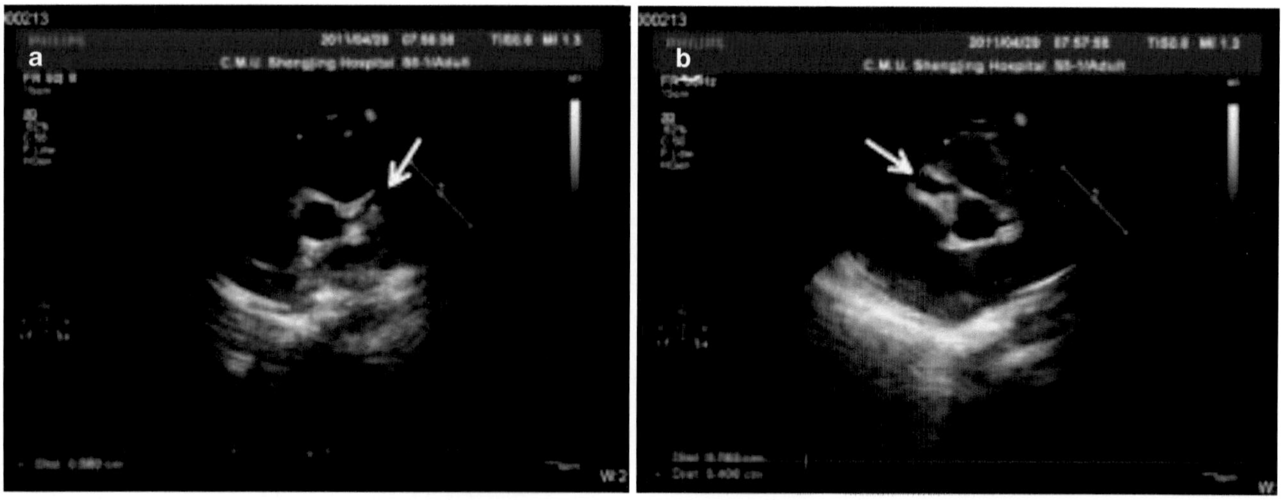

Fig. 6.11 On Day 13, echo showed LAD dilated about 5.8 mm (**a**) and RCA aneurysm dilated 4.1–7.6 mm (**b**)

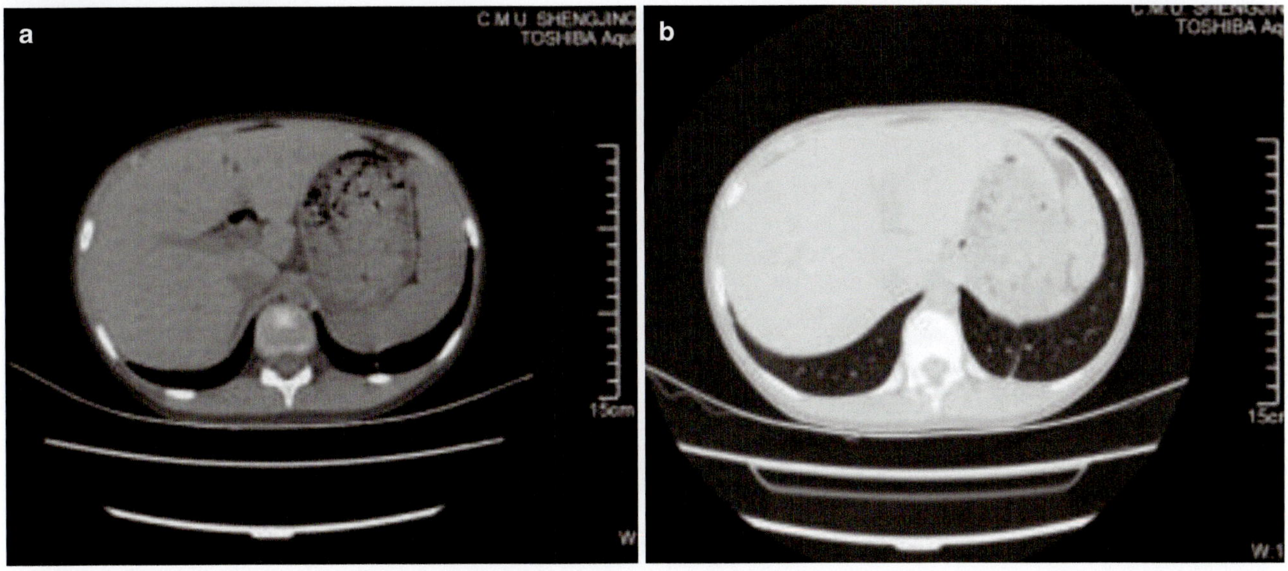

Fig. 6.12 On Day 19 of illness, chest CT showed both pleural effusion (**a**) and inflamation of lung (**b**) absorbed

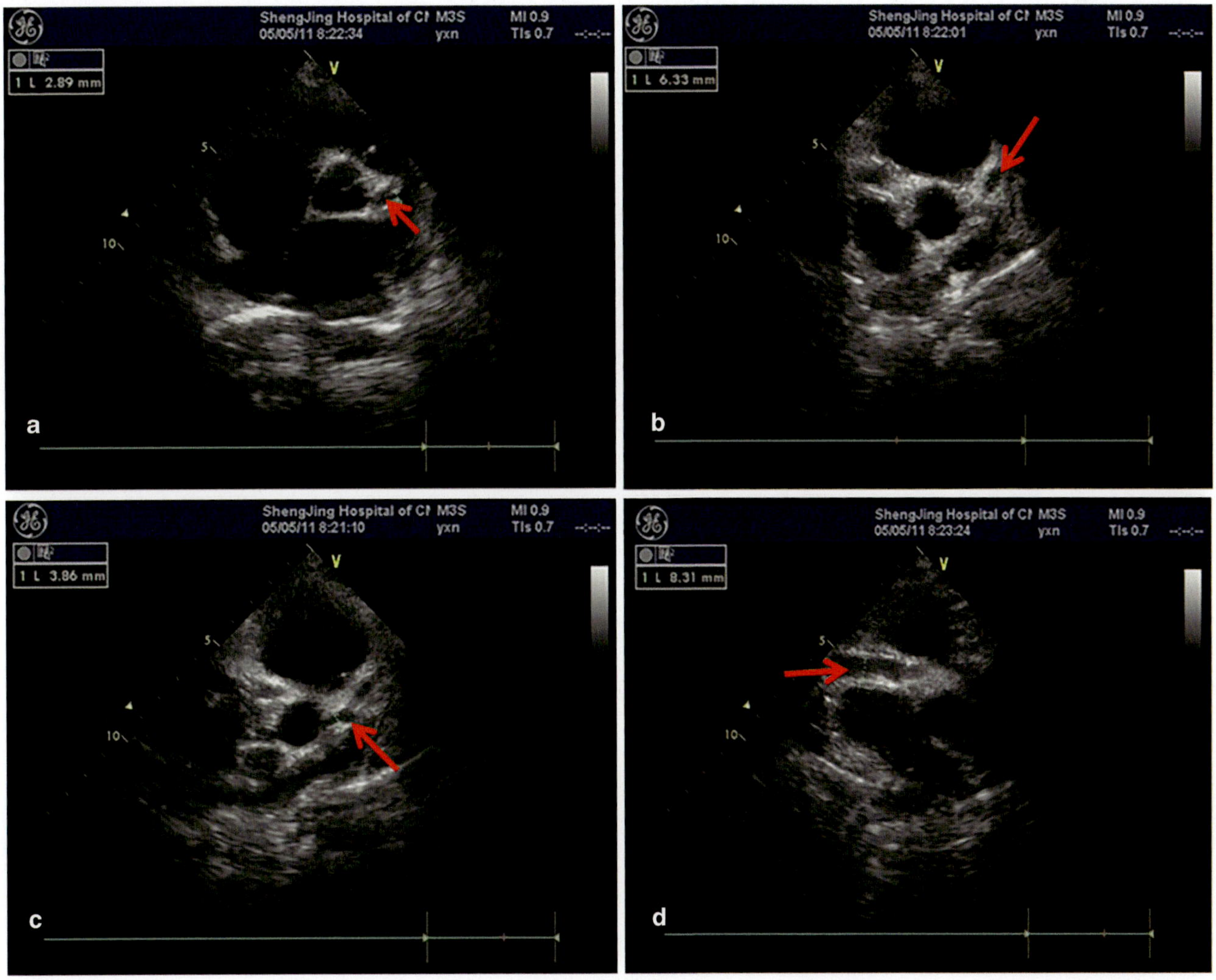

Fig. 6.13 On Day 19 of illness, echocardiography showed LM dilated to 3.9 mm (**a**), LAD 6.3 mm (**b**), LCX 2.89mm (**c**), RCA 8.3 mm (**d**)

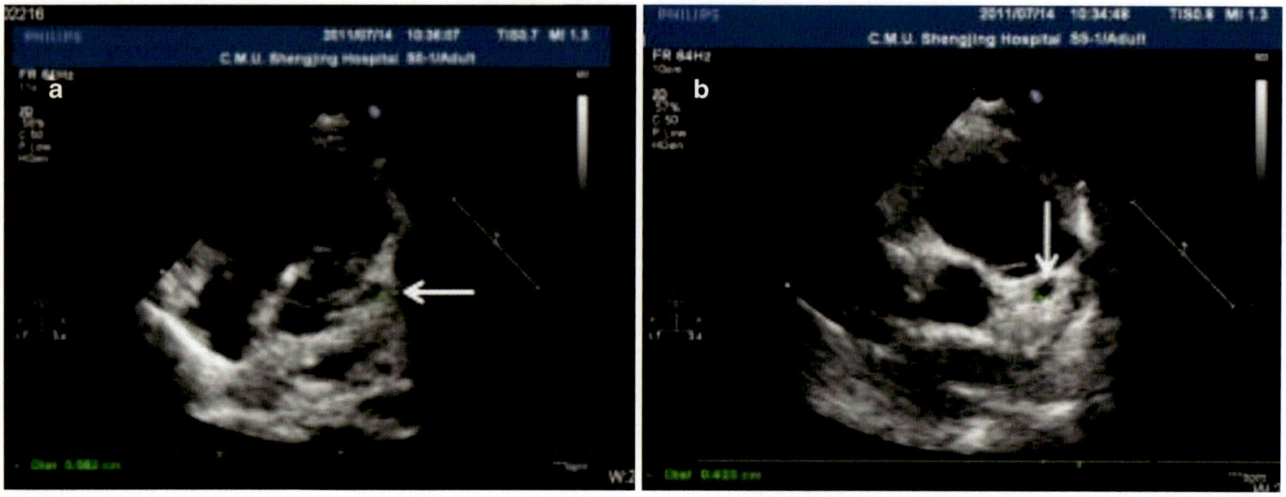

Fig. 6.14 At 3 months of illness, echocardiography showed LCA dilated to 5.8 mm (**a**), LAD was about 4.3 mm (**b**)

6.2.1 Clinical Course of the Patient

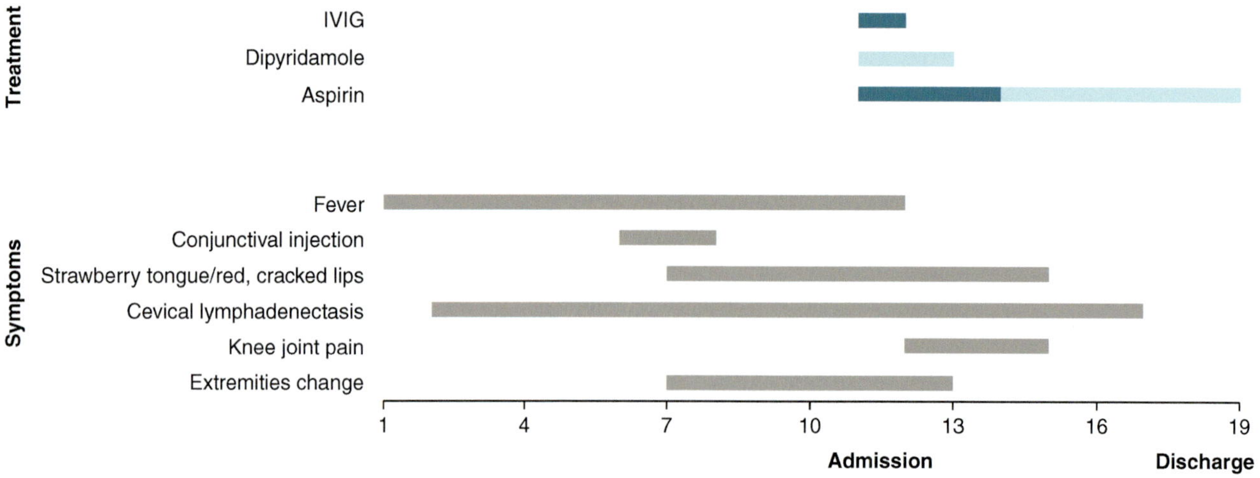

6.2.2 Follow-Up

On Day 81, investigation revealed WBC 7×10^9/L, NE 54.3%, HGB125g/L, PLT 254×10^9/L. DIC was normal. Repeated echo showed LVED 43mm, LVEF 67%, LCA 3.5mm (Fig. 6.14a), LAD 5.4mm (Fig. 6.14b), RCA 9.2mm (Fig. 6.15a). Coronary CTA showed LAD was bead-like changes were seen in the proximal part of the LAD. The aneurysm was about 5.5 mm. The aortic wall was thickened, with local fibrous plaque formation, slightly narrow. There was a fusiform aneurysm dilated to 10.0 mm (Fig. 6.15b), at the proximal and middle segment of the RCA, and 53.9 mm in length. She was given oral warfarin at 2.5mg/d to maintain INR between 1.5 and 2.5. At 4 years of illness, echo showed the RCA was diffusely widen about 10.9mm (Fig. 6.16a), LAD 4.6mm (Fig. 6.16b). Since then, she had not followed up with us.

6.2.3 Diagnosis

1. KD.
2. Bilateral CAA.
3. Joint involvement.
4. Acute bronchopneumonia.
5. Pleural effusion (small amount).
6. Liver dysfunction.
7. Hypoproteinemia.
8. Pericardial effusion (a very small amount).
9. MP infection.
10. CP infection.

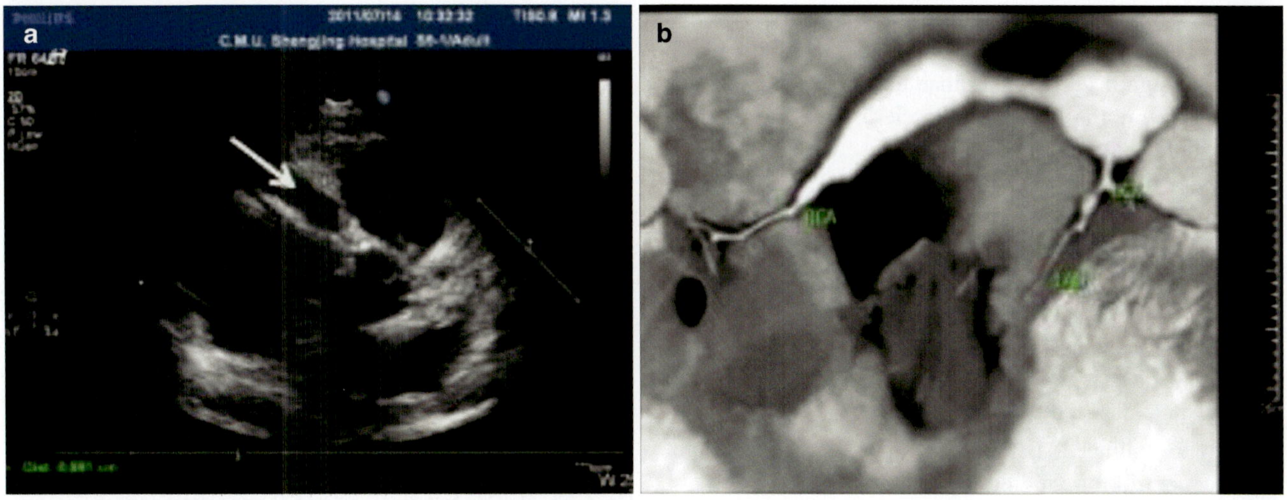

Fig. 6.15 At 3 months of illness, echo showed RCA aneurysm dilated 7.9 mm (**a**); coronary artery CTA showed LAD was bead like dilated and RCA proximal-middle fusiform aneurysm dilated 10.0 mm (**b**)

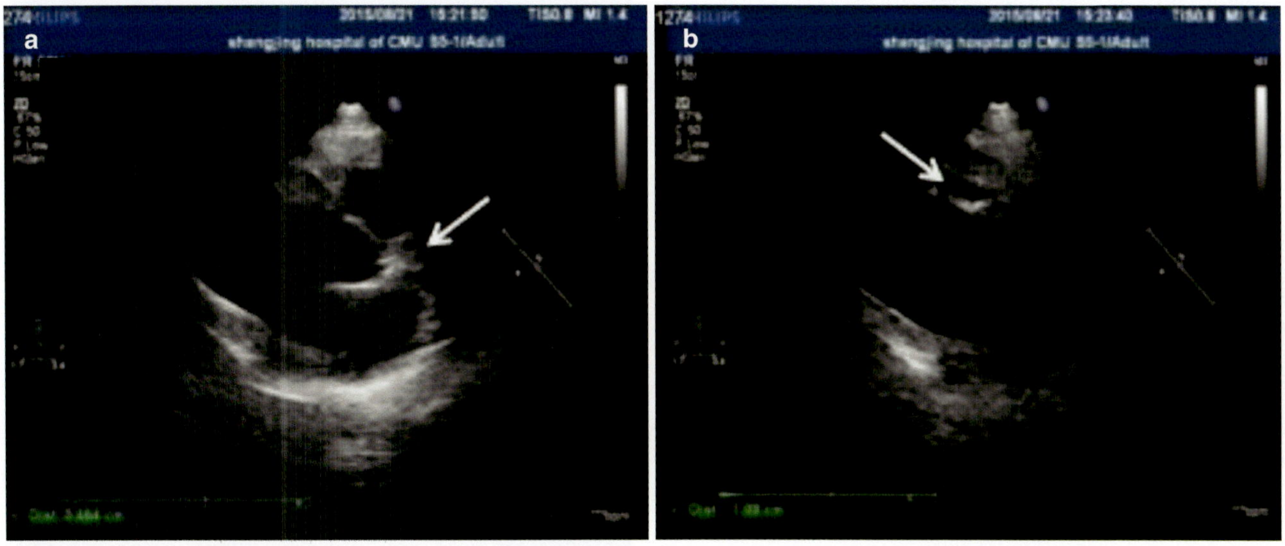

Fig. 6.16 At 4 years of illness, echo showed LCA aneurysm dilated 4.6 mm (**a**); RCA diffuse broadening about 10.9 mm (**b**)

6.2.4 Discussion

She had met the criteria of KD for she had persistent fever for more than 5 days, along with (1) cervical lymphadenectasis; (2) bilateral conjunctiva hyperemia without purulent discharge; (3) red lips; (4) swollen hands and feet; (5) bilateral CAA. Others factors included elevated WBC with majority of neutrophils and CRP > 30 mg/L. Differential diagnosis of infective endocarditis should be considered and excluded.

6.2.5 Case Specific Clinical Features

1. KD is a self-limited febrile disease with immune system involved. The etiology of KD is unknown. It mainly affects medium and small arteries, mostly coronary arteries, resulting cardiac-related complications [6]. KD often occurs in many Asian countries, especially in Japan. It is more common in children under 5 years of age, and occasionally occurs in adults [7, 8].
2. In untreated patients, the incidence of CAA is 15–25%, of which 2–3% die of coronary vasculitis [9]. The risk of coronary artery injury is the same in patients with atypical and as with KD. Therefore, in patients with IKD, IVIG should be administered similarly [6]. Twenty percentage of patients do not respond to IVIG, and they have higher risk in developing coronary complications [9]. The rupture of coronary arteries is associated with early mortality. Subacute vasculitis can last from months to years, which explains why the patient symptom was still

progressing after 2 months [10]. It has been reported that triglyceride and low-density lipoprotein in children with KD are significantly higher than those in normal people, and therefore the risk of atherosclerosis will increase in the future [11].

3. In the acute phase of KD, ESR and CRP are increased significantly during the first 10 days of disease [12]. The persistent increase in CRP is a risk factor for arterial intimal thickening and endothelial dysfunction in adults with KD [13]. Sustained elevation of CRP is one of the factors associated with cardiovascular accidents, but not an indicator for severity of coronary artery injuries [14, 15]. The hs-CRP in obese individuals with a history of KD is more likely to continue to rise, so it is important to have weight under control for children who have had KD [16].
4. KD can have multiple systems involved, digestive, respiratory, cardiovascular, hematological, and nervous systems. Her pleural effusion was not only associated with an increase in albumin leakage, but also associated with more leakage from pneumonia. Her fever was accompanied with weakly positive ANA and weakly positive indicators of inflammation associated with connective tissue diseases. However, the duration of joint swelling was very short, which did not support rheumatoid arthritis.

Ya-li Zhang

6.3 Case 29 KD with Necrotizing Pneumonia

A previous healthy 13-month-old boy without tuberculosis contact, or foreign-body inhaled history. He was vaccinated timely, without remarkable antenatal or family asthma history. His father and grandmother were reported allergic to sulfa antibiotics.

He presented on Day 14 of illness with interval fevers, coughing for 14 days, along with bilateral conjunctivitis for 9 days, peeling skin around fingernails for 3 days. He had moderate fever at about 38.6 °C for 14 days. He had mild cough and severe diarrhea with loose watery stool 7–8 times per day, nausea, and hypourocrinia, but had no vomiting. On Day 2, WBC and CRP were normal. On Day 4, his fever subsided and diarrhea improved, but cough was recurrent after catching a cold, along with sputum and running nose. On Day 6, he had recurrent fever to 38.5 °C and developed polymorphic rashes all over the body, along with bilateral conjunctivitis and edema feet. The repeated test results from CBC and chest DR (Fig. 6.17) were within normal range. On Day 8, the rashes regressed but fever increased up to 40.2 °C. His cough got worse and he developed dyspnea, occasionally vomit ted after persistent coughing. He was admitted in a local hospital as a pneumonia patient. Blood test showed his CRP was elevated significantly. He was given infusion of erythromycin and vancomycin. After vancomycin infusion, a different kind of rash appeared on his face (Fig. 6.18), and then he was treated with intramuscular injection of phenergan. Rashes disappeared, but conjunctivitis and edema feet had no improvement. Mepem was used to replace vancomycin for 6 days, Zyvox for 2 days, and IVIG for 4 days, 200 mg/kg for 1 day and 400 mg/kg for 3 days. Ganciclovir infusion was given for 3 days. On Day 11, his conjunctiva subsided, but fever and edema feet had not

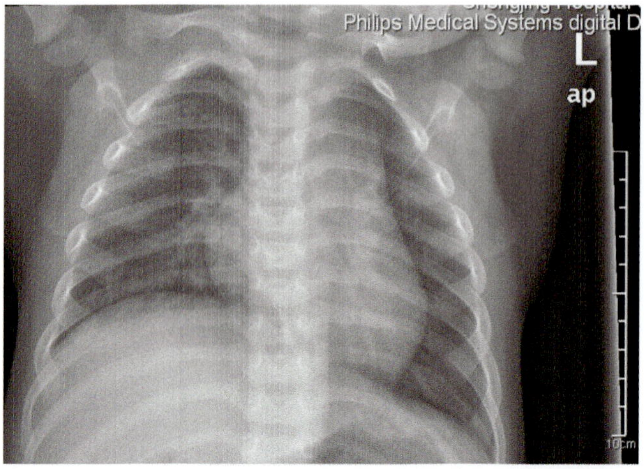

Fig. 6.17 On Day 6 of illness, chest DR was almost normal

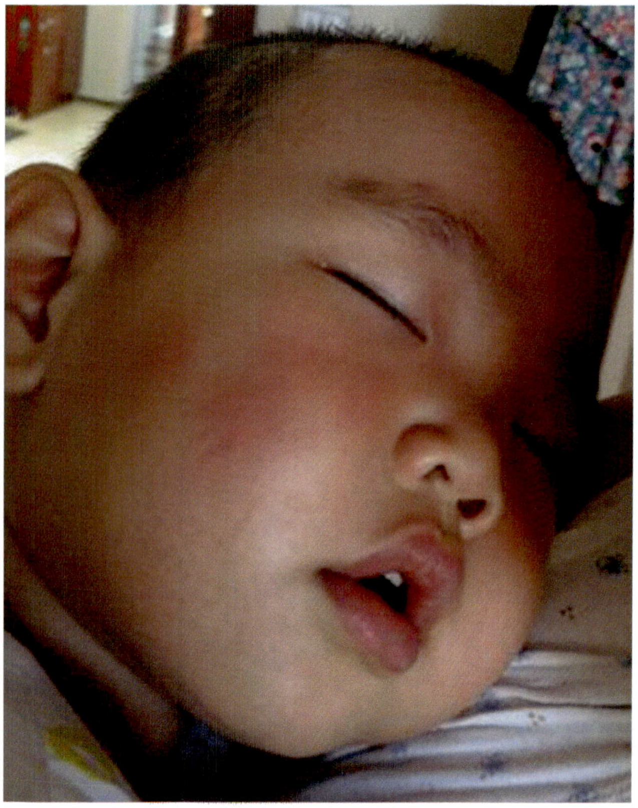

Fig. 6.18 On Day 8 of illness, after infusing vancomycin, there was a new type rash on his face

changed. Furthermore, he developed red lips, had peeling skin around right fingernails, lost appetite, and had dysthesia and ventosity. Results from bone marrow puncture suggested an infected bone marrow appearance. Lumbar puncture results showed normal CSF. Abdominal CT showed a thickening gallbladder wall. One day before admission, he developed wheeze. GC (methylprednisolone) infusion was given for 2 days, and his fever subsided. Cough, mental state, and appetite improved. In the afternoon on the admission day, fever recurred. Then he was transferred to our pediatric respiratory ward as pneumonia patient. Physical examination included red lips and desquamation of fingernails. After consulting with pediatric cardiologist, he was diagnosed with KD, severe pneumonia, and he was transferred to pediatric cardiology ward. Since the onset of illness, he had no night sweet, but was fatigued with weight loss. *Examination* showed general state was stable, and he had no dyspnea; T 38.8 °C, HR 152 bpm, RR 28 bpm. Weight 9.5 kg. Trachea was in the middle without rashes or conjunctivitis. Cervical lymphadenectasis was 2 cm on the left side. Lips were red and cracked. Auscultation found a weak respiratory sound at the right, without wheeze, bubbling sound or pleural friction sound. He presented edema feet and peeling skin around right fingernails. Others were normal. CBC at admission revealed elevated WBC and CRP, and hypoalbuminemia; PCT 0.738 ng/ml, IL6 37.52 pg/ml. On Day 12, chest CT showed atelectasis at the right inferior lobe and pleural effusion on both sides. Chest ultrasound showed pleural effusion, 1.5 cm on the right, 0.45 cm on the left. Abdominal ultrasound showed lymphadenectasis in enterocoelia. Cervical ultrasound showed lymphadenectasis about 2.0 cm × 0.7 cm on the left, about 1.8 cm × 0.7 cm on the right. He had met the criteria of KD and IVIG resistance, and he was treated with (1) blood sample drawn for culture test; (2) infusion of second-generation cephalosporin; (3) IVIG 2 g/kg (total 3.4 g/kg), within 24 hours; (4) oral aspirin 30–50 mg/kg, in three divided doses, dipyridamole 3–5 mg/kg, in two divided doses.

On Day 15, he had fever again, spiked up to 39.9 °C. Diarrhea regressed to 3–4 times a day and with decreased watery stool. Examination revealed there was no significant improvement. Investigation revealed IgG 14.40 g/L, IgA 0.708 g/L, IgM 1.79 g/L. ASO 48.7 IU/ml. CRP 28.40 mg/L. MP-IgM(−), MP-IgG(+/−). CP-IgM(−), CP-IgG(+). ALB 27.5 g/L. GPT, AST, CK, and CKMB were normal. LDH 318 U/L. HSV (I + II)-IgM(+). EB-IgM(+)(107)AU/ml, EB NA-IgG(+)(523); EB VCA-IgG(+)(199), EB-DNA < 10^3Copies/ml. ECG showed sinus arrhythmia (Fig. 6.19). Chest CT showed inflammation getting worse vacuolar lesions appearing (Fig. 6.20a) and pleural effusion on right (Fig. 6.20b). He was treated with (1) infusion of albumin 10 g for 2 days; (2) third-generation cephalosporin (sulperazone) to replace second generation; (3) infusion of ganciclovir for another 3 days;

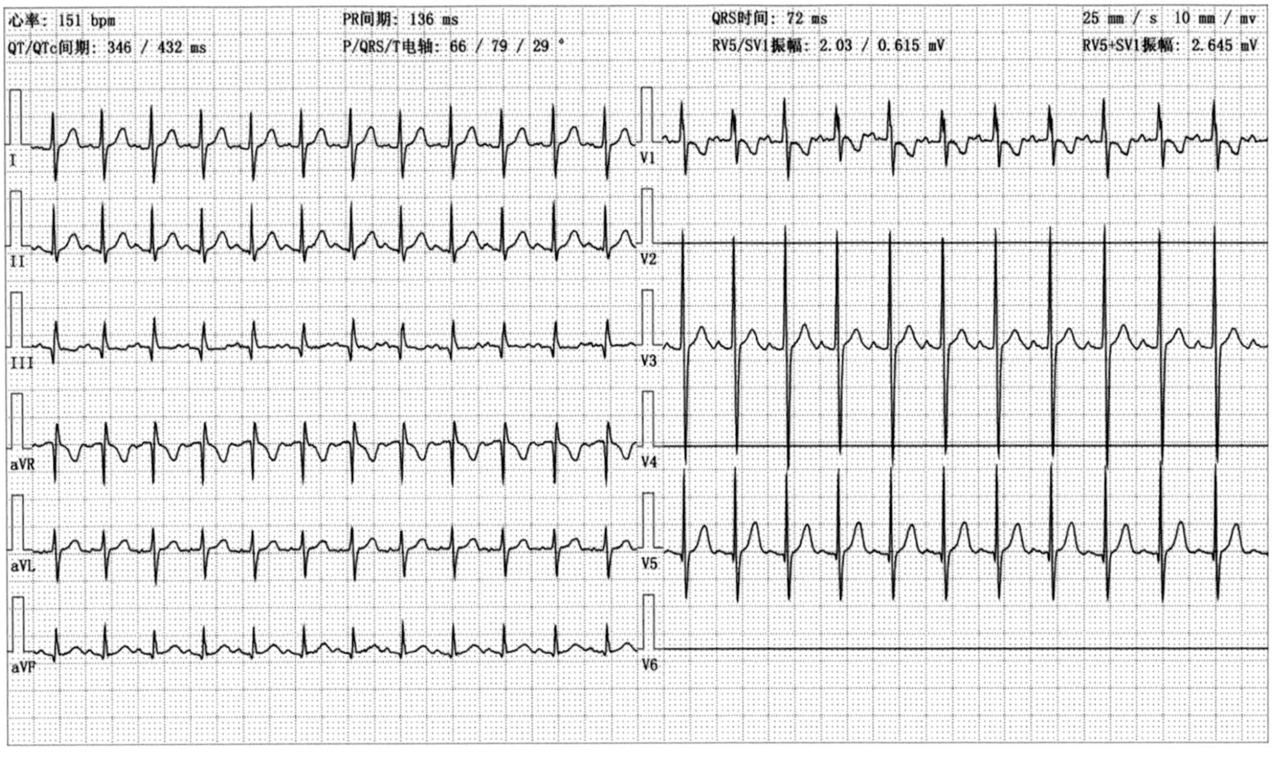

Fig. 6.19 On Day 15 of illness, ECG showed nodal tachycardia

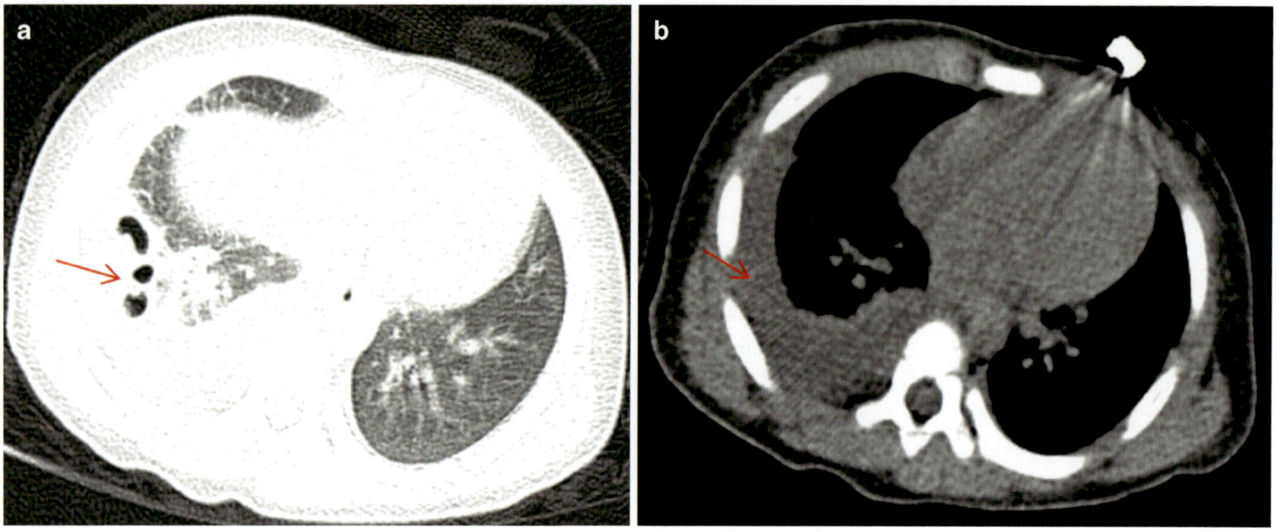

Fig. 6.20 On Day 15 of illness, chest CT showed inflammation on the right lower lobe (**a**), pleural effusion on the right (**b**)

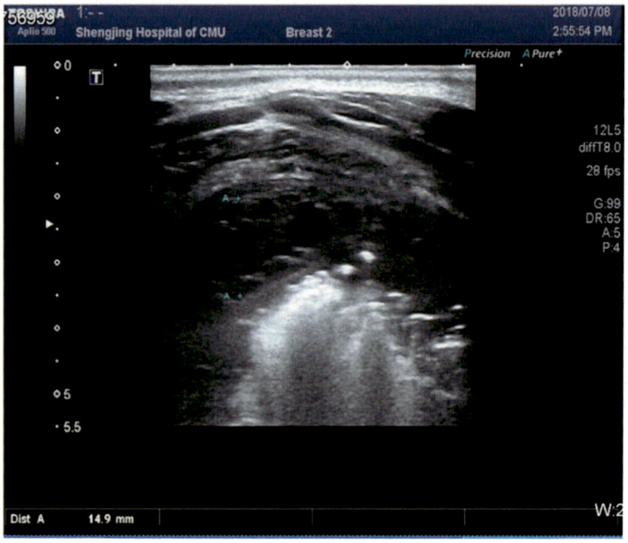

Fig. 6.21 On Day 16 of illness, chest ultrasound showed right pleural effusion about 1.5 cm

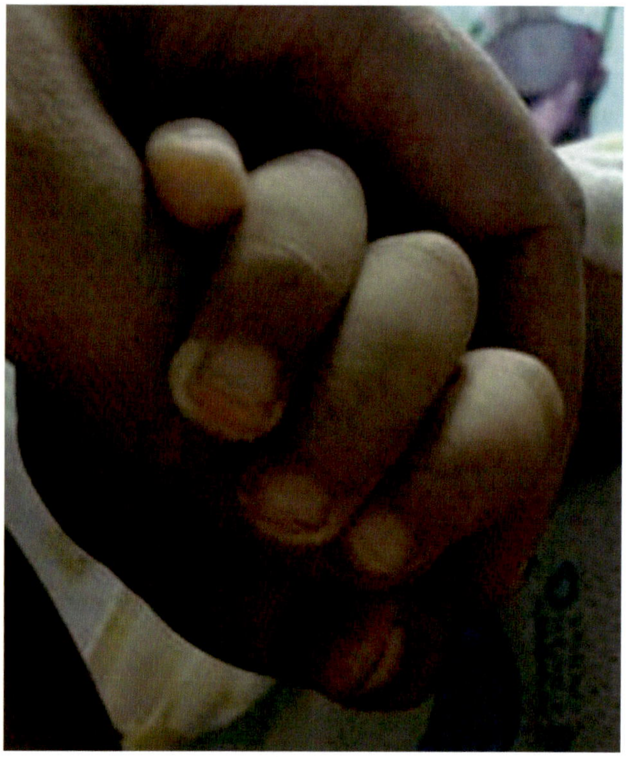

Fig. 6.22 On Day 17 of illness, skin peeling around fingernails

(4) azithromycin infusion for 4 days; (5) mucosolvan infusion. On Day 16, he was given IVIG within 24 hours, but his fever was still at 38.9 °C. Diarrhea was regressed to 2–3 times a day. Red lips and edema feet subsided. Left fingernails also had desquamation. Auscultation found gurgling with sputum at the right lung. Chest ultrasound showed pulmonary consolidation in the lower lobe of right lung, and pleural effusion about 1.5 cm in the right thorax (Fig. 6.21). On the 17 day of illness, 48 hours after 2 g/kg IVIG ends, his fever was not regressed, spiking up to 39.6 °C. More finger nails with desquamation were presented (Fig. 6.22). Retested blood work showed WBC 32.59 × 10^9/L, NE 65.0%, RBC 2.6 × 10^{12}/L, HGB 70 g/L, PLT 741 × 10^9/L. CRP 189 mg/L. ESR 29 mm/h. PCT 2.20 ng/ml. IL_6 155.4 pg/ml. D-Dimer 3836ug/L. CK, CKMB, ALB, GPT, AST, BUN, and Cr were normal. CRP was elevated again, he was treated with (1) vancomycin together with sulperazone for anti-inflammations purpose; (2) GC (methylprednisolone 2 mg/kg/day) infusion; (3) retesting anemia the next day due to worsening condition. His fever remained high after the second round of IVIG treatment. Pediatric respiratory specialist was consulted with. Retested CBC revealed elevated WBC,

CRP, and PCT, significantly decreased HBG. Lung abscess was not excluded. The following treatment and procedures were recommended: (1) remaining on antibiotics and GC; (2) infusion of erythrocytes; (3) dynamic reexamination of infection indicators; (4) performing chest ultrasound, if pleural effusion increased, thoracic puncture and drainage might be needed for analysis of hydrothorax. His conditions were complicated, pneumonia was serious, and he may have worse prognosis and his parents were informed. His fever was settled on Day 18. He had more sweat and coughed occasionally. In the absence of diarrhea, his appetite was not improved. Auscultation revealed a few rales on lung. Repeated blood work revealed WBC 24.77 × 10^9/L, NE 76.3%, RBC 2.4 × 10^{12}/L, HGB 64 g/L, PLT 362 × 10^9/L. ABO blood type was B, while RH(D) blood type was positive. CRP 153 mg/L. Echo showed normal LVED, LVEF (Fig.6.23), and coronary artery (Fig. 6.24a, b). Results from brain stem auditory were abnormal. For he had developed moderate to severe anemia, he was given infusion of B-type RBC 1 U and tapping on the back to help drain phlegm. On Day 19, chest ultrasound showed consolidation in right lower lobe (Fig. 6.25), pleural effusion on both side, right depth about 1.0 cm, densely divided interior, left depth about 0.3 cm. On Day 20, he was afebrile over 48 hours, had mild cough with a little sputum. Retested blood results: WBC 17.94 × 10^9/L, NE 33.7%, RBC 3.3 × 10^{12}/L, HBG 98 g/L, PLT 711 × 10^9/L. CRP 29.50 mg/L. IL_6 7.38 pg/ml. GPT 69 U/L, AST 37 U/L, and normal ALB and blood glucose (free). He was treated with (1) reduced dose aspirin at 3–5 mg/kg; (2) reduced dose of methylprednisolone; (3) infusion of polyene phosphatidylcholine to protect hepatocyte. On Day 21, he had fever at 38.0 and vomited 3 times but without diarrhea, after exposed to his dad who had mild cold symptoms. Examination found peeling skin around toenails. Retested blood results showed: WBC 13.71 × 10^9/L, NE 57.1%, RBC 3.2 × 10^{12}/L, HBG 93 g/L, PLT 724 × 10^9/L. CRP 22.1 mg/L. ALB, GTP, AST, and blood glucose (free) were normal. Chest CT showed the lesion cavity and wall of right inferior lobe were larger and thinner than before (Fig. 6.26a), and pleural effusion was reduced (Fig. 6.26b). Tapping on the back was stopped and he was given polyene phosphatidylcholine infusion.

On the Day 22 of illness, he was afebrile and had diarrhea 3 times with watery stool. Stool sample analysis showed positive norovirus antibody titer. Liver ultrasound showed normal gallbladder (Fig. 6.27). We consulted with pediatric respiratory specialist again, and he pointed out that: (1) after

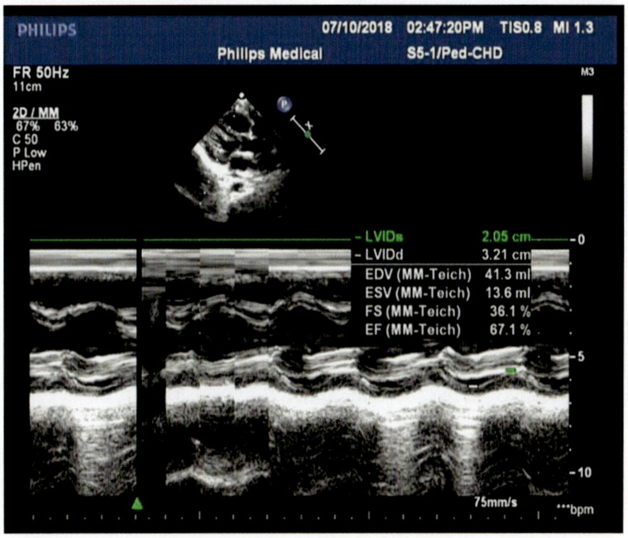

Fig. 6.23 On Day 18 of illness, echo showed normal LVED/LVEF

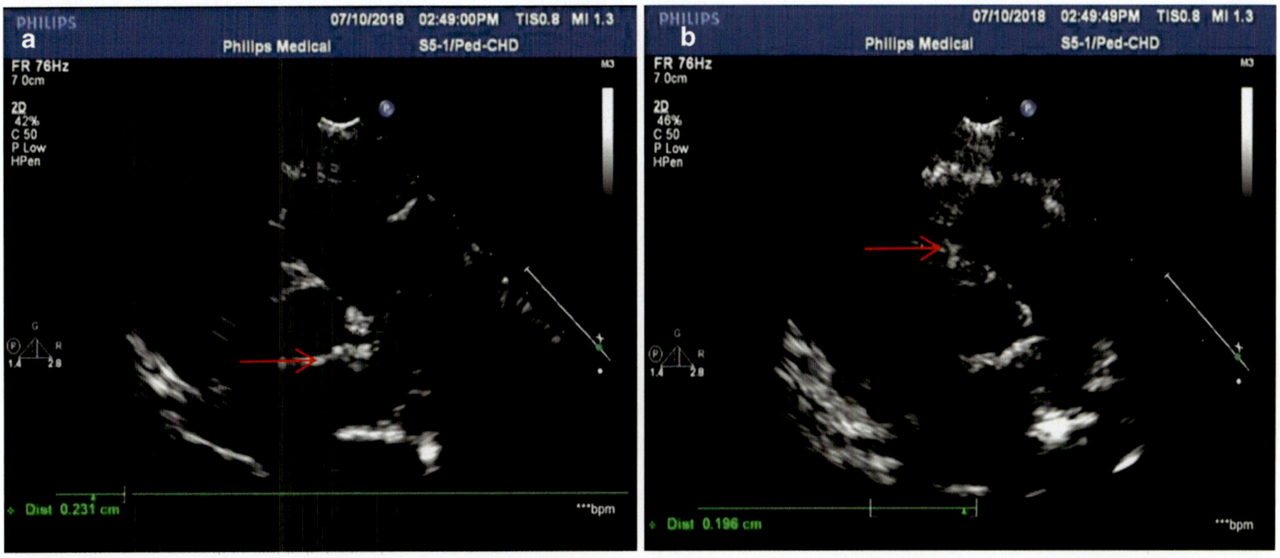

Fig. 6.24 On Day 18 of illness, echo showed normal LCA (**a**) and RCA (**b**)

treated with antibiotics and GCs, his symptoms had improved; (2) the transient fever he had 2 days ago might be a result of nosocomial infection: (3) he was convalescing from pneumonia with local necrotic confluence. (4) However, since both routine blood test and CRP were still abnormal, the patient should continue to take antibiotics. By now, the etiology of the boy's syndromes was not clear. MP antibody, CP antibody, MP-DNA, and CP-DNA should be retested, which would be helpful to predict the prognosis and to direct following treatments. Pneumonia with necrotic confluence be expose to pleural cavity, forming bronchial pleural fistula, leading to pneumothorax, which is a serious complication of necrotic pneumonia. Therefore, his parents should be informed, and surgeon should be consulted with to determine whether thoracic surgery was needed. Regarding norovirus infection, he was treated with (1) oral rehydration salts; (2) oral quadruple live bacterium; (3) oral montmorillonite powder; (4) reduced dose of GC. On Day 25, he was still afebrile with diarrhea 3–4 times. Retested blood work results were showing: WBC 20.11 × 10^9/L, NE 30.2%, RBC 3.5 × 10^{12}/L, HGB 102 g/L, PLT 695 × 10^9/L, normal free glucose and CRP. MP-IgM(−), MP-IgG(+/−), CP-IgM(−), CP-IgG(+). Chest CT showed a larger lesion cavity and thinner wall of right inferior lobe compared to previous results (Fig. 6.28a), and reduced pleural effusion (Fig. 6.28b). Thoracic surgery specialist suggested that necrotic cavity in the right lower lobe had been wrapped/covered; thus, there was no need for him undergoing surgical treatment; patient should be followed up at clinic 1 month later. Patient was informed to see doctor immediately if pneumothorax would occur during observation, and follow-up with clinics if there were any changes in symptoms. He was treated with (1) intramuscular injection of vitamin K_1 for 3 days; (2) withdrawal of vancomycin but staying on sulperazone; (3) second round of azithromycin infusion; (4) reduced dose of GC. On Day 27, the boy could run on the ground without any discomfort. There was no peeling skin around the toenail.

On Day 28, after the boy finished the second round of azithromycin infusion, and was discharged.

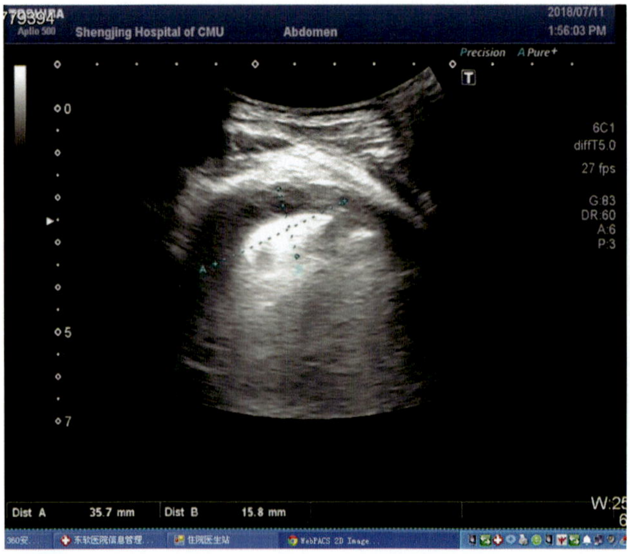

Fig. 6.25 On Day 19 of illness, chest ultrasound showed consolidation on right lower lobe

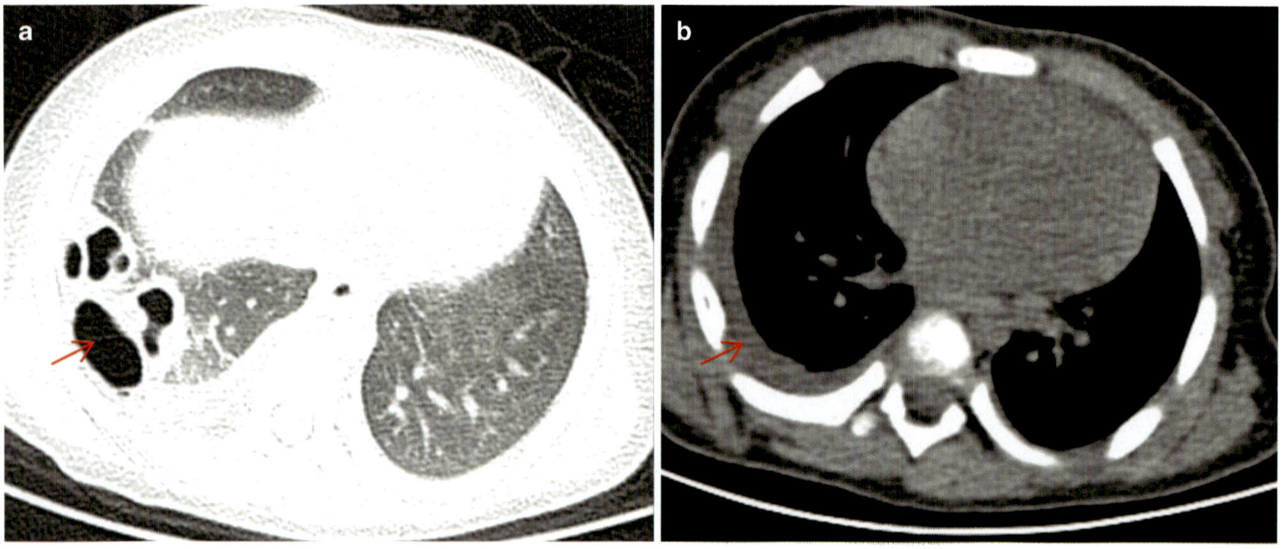

Fig. 6.26 On Day 21 of illness, chest CT showed bullae of right lung (**a**), and right pleural effusion improved (**b**)

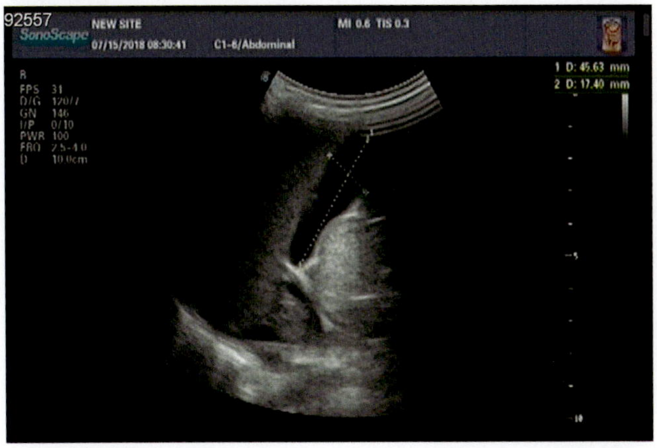

Fig. 6.27 On Day 21 of illness, liver ultrasound showed gallbladder was normal

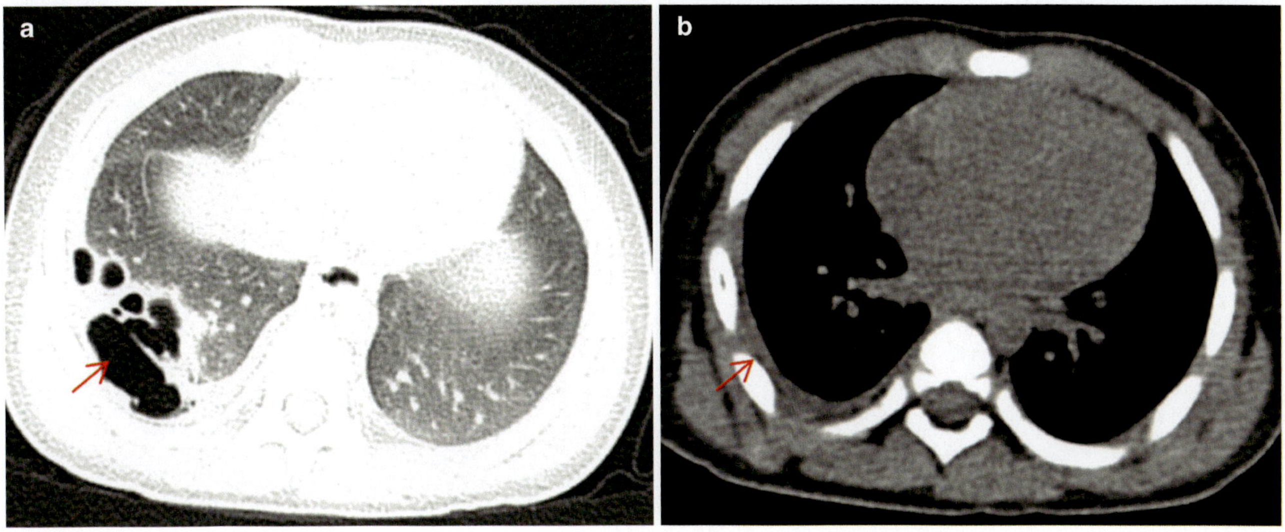

Fig. 6.28 On Day 25 of illness, chest CT showed bullae enlarged of right lung (**a**), and right pleural effusion was less (**b**)

6.3.1 Clinic Course of the Patient

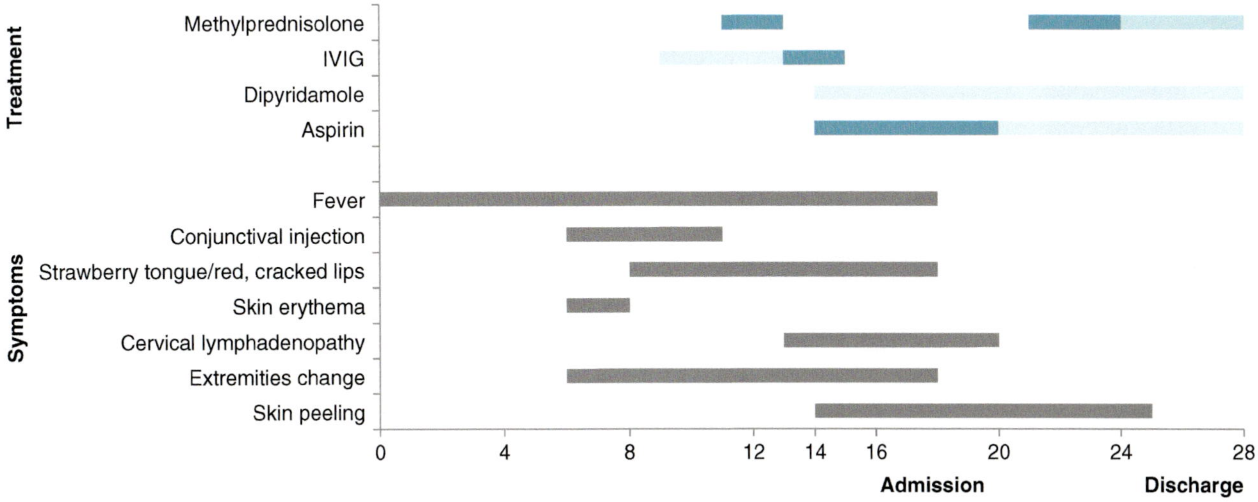

6.3.2 Follow-Up

Since discharged, he was treated with (1) oral aspirin and dipyridamole; (2) oral third-generation cephalosporin for 1 week; (3) oral intestinal probiotics; (4) ferralia and vitamin C.

On Day 56, retested blood results showed normal CBC, ESR, CRP, ACTH, cortisol. Echo showed normal results (Fig. 6.29a, b). Repeated chest CT showed the pneumonia was improved (Fig. 6.30a) significantly, the cavity in the lower lobe of the right lung was diminished (Fig. 6.30b). All medications were stopped.

At 3 months, chest CT showed reduced lesion at the right lower lobe and absence of necrotic cavity (Fig. 6.31a). The density shadow of the fluid in the right thoracic arc was slightly less than before (Fig. 6.31b). The rest was the same as before (Table 6.2).

6.3.3 Diagnosis

1. KD.
2. IVIG resistance.
3. Severe necrotic pneumonia.
4. Pleural effusion.
5. Hypoalbuminemia.
6. Liver dysfunction.
7. Moderate to severe anemia.
8. Acute cholecystitis.
9. Virus infection (HSV/EBV/Norovirus).

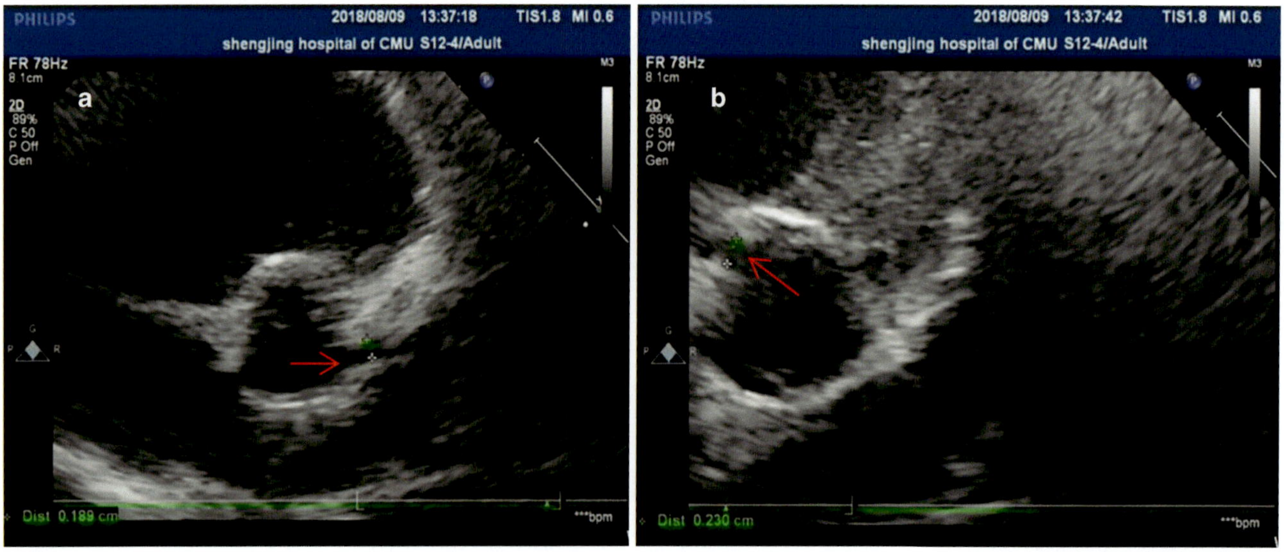

Fig. 6.29 On Day 56 of illness, echo showed normal LCA (**a**) and RCA (**b**)

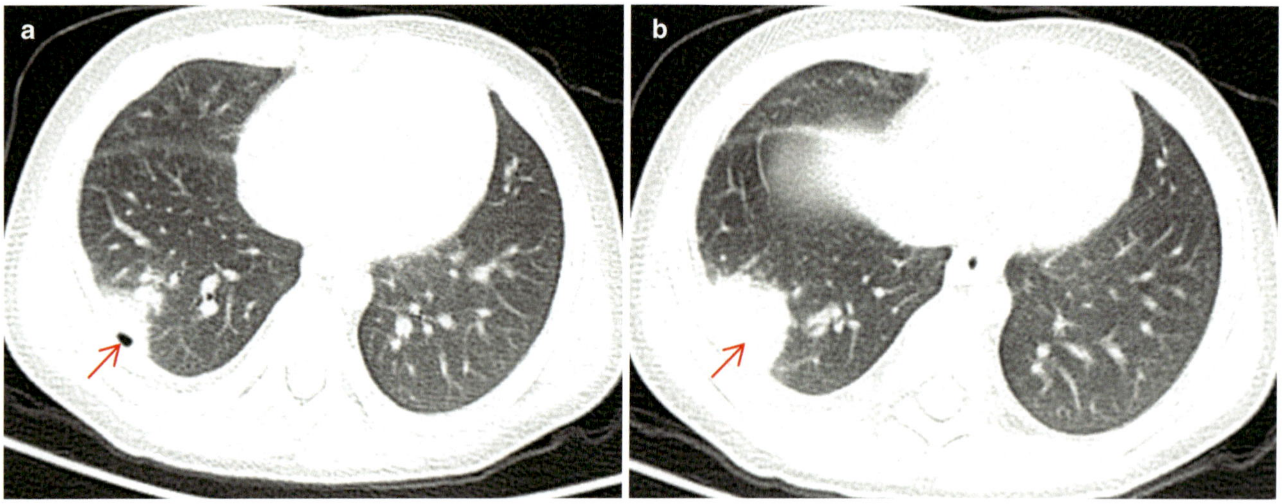

Fig. 6.30 On Day 56 of illness, chest CT showed the bullae of right lung minimized obviously (**a**), and right lung consolidation improved (**b**)

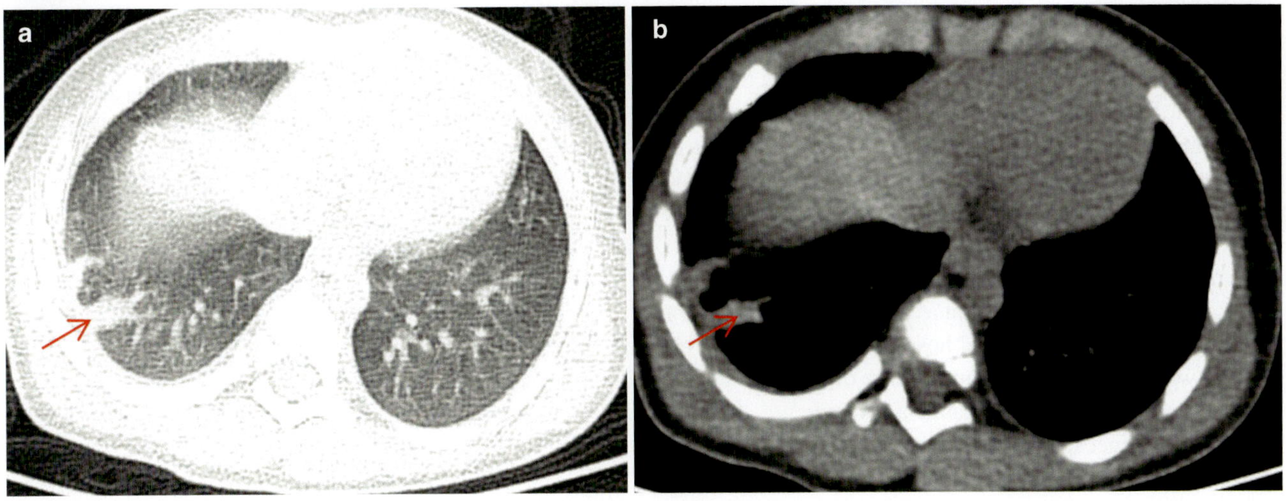

Fig. 6.31 At 3 months of illness, chest CT showed both the bullae (**a**) and pleural effusion (**b**) of right lung disappeared

Table 6.2 The dynamic changes of laboratory parameters

Time of illness	2 days	6 days	8 days	9 days	11 days	13 days	14 days	17 days	18 days	20 days	22 days	25 days	56 days
WBC ($\times10^9$/L)	9.6	6.5	14.6	14.5	15.3	20.4	20.27	32.59	24.77	17.94	13.7	20.11	5.73
NE (%)	56.2	50.3	86	81	63	41	26.9	65	76.3	33.7	57.1	30.2	67.4
HGB (g/L)	110	114	108	90	104	91	80	70	64	98	93	102	117
PLT ($\times10^9$/L)	191	164	116	97	85	111	491	741	362	711	724	695	171
CRP (mg/L)	5.6	3.3	212	149	56.6	48.2	28.4	189	153	29.5	22.1	4.55	8.61
ESR (mm/L)								29					5
ALB (g/L)							27.5	38.9		38.2	38.7		45.5
GTP(U/L)							34	Ok		69	33		33

6.3.4 Diagnosis

1. He had met the criteria of KD for he had prolong remittent fevers over 5 days, along with (1) bilateral conjunctivitis; (2) strikingly red lips; (3) edema feet; (4) polymorphic erythematous rashes; (5) bilateral lymphadenopathy over 1.5 cm.
2. He had also met the criteria of KD/IVIG resistance for he had prolonged remittent fevers over 38.5 °C 48 hours after IVIG, along with strikingly red lips and edema in feet. He was given another infusion of 2 g/kg IVIG, but had no response to the drug. Then he was given infusion of methylprednisolone [16].
3. He had met the criteria of infant necrotic pneumonia for he had prolonged remittent fevers along with severe coughing. Auscultation detected some sputum sounds. Laboratory parameters revealed WBC and NE were significant increased. CRP was elevated to 212 mg/L. Chest CT showed consolidation in the right lower lobe containing intermediate necrotic bullous, with pleural effusion.
4. He also met the criteria of acute cholecystitis, he had KD, remittent fevers along with lack of appetite, ventosity and significantly elevated WBC and CRP. Abdominal CT at the local hospital showed thickened gallbladder wall. Fortunately he recovered after local anti-inflammation treatment.
5. Differential diagnosis of purulent meningitis, monocytic angina should be considerated.

6.3.5 Case Specific Clinical Features

1. Compared to acute bronchopneumonia, necrotic pneumonia is very rare. But, it is a severe complication of bacterial pneumonia, with high mortality. Currently, available information regarding management of necrotizing pneumonia is limited to case reports and small cohort studies from retrospective observations [17]. Therefore, appropriate management for these patients remains unclear, especially for infants or toddlers. Necrotic pneumonia is commonly resulted from Gram positive cocci, such as streptococcus pneumonia, *staphylococcus aureus* [17]. Thus, the first choice of antibiotics is vancomycin. Due to its ototoxicity, we were very careful when we used this drug to treat patients. Once the inflammation was under control, we immediately withdraw this drug. Meanwhile, the BSAEP

was monitored. Necrotic pneumonia can also be caused by *pseudomonas aeruginosa* [18]. So the broad-spectrum antibiotics infusion was also given to the patient at the same time. In addition, MP/CP infection can result in necrotic pneumonia, too. Therefore, we gave the patient 2 rounds of azithromycin infusion. When he was given Mepem and Zyvox infusion at local hospital, though his fever was not under control, his cholecystitis, ventosity, and mental state were improved. Right after he was transferred to our ward, we did not choose vancomycin as a treatment selection, for his had "allergy" in the local hospital. However, when his fever was unresponsive to another dose of 2 g/kg IVIG, we used vancomycin, and the treatment worked.

2. For a long time, speculated factors associated with severe anemia developed in KD kids include high dose of aspirin [19], physical exhaustion caused by infection, lack of appetite, repeated blood sample drawn, and so on. Recently, one literature reports that, in children with KD, a peptide, named hepcidin, is increased in the acute stage of KD and this is associated with the progressively deteriorating anemia [20]. It is usually reduced after IVIG treatment along with fever subsides. In the presence of IVIG resistance, body temperature remains high, and hepcidin also stays at high levels.
3. His CRP on Day 6 was 3.3 mg/L. Two days later it was drastically elevated to 212 mg/L. Nine days later the level was 189 mg/L. To suppress excessive inflammation, inhibit pleural effusion and pleural adhesion, glucocorticoid infusion was given to this patient.
4. It has been reported that risk factors for KD patients to develop CAA include the following: male, WBC > 15 × 10^9/L, NE > 75%, CRP > 100 mg/L, decreased PLT at early stage, and hypoalbuminemia. Though KD diagnosis was delayed, this patient was treated with IVIG timely on the Day 10 of illness. As he developed severe pneumonia, additional infusion of 2 g/kg IVIG and methylprednisolone would ensure a good prognosis. Patients with severe complications, similar to MAS, rarely had coronary sequela after the episode [21].

Hong Wang

References

1. Agarwal S, Agrawal DK. Kawasaki disease: etiopathogenesis and novel treatment strategies. Expert Rev Clin Immunol. 2017;13(3):247–58.
2. Zhao CN, Du ZD, Gao LL. Corticosteroid therapy might be associated with the development of coronary aneurysm in children with Kawasaki disease. Chin Med J. 2016;129(8):922–8.
3. Leahy TR, Cohen E, Allen UD. Incomplete Kawasaki disease associated with complicated Streptococcus pyogenes pneumonia: a case report. Can J Infect Dis Med Microbiol. 2012;23(3):137–9.
4. Orenstein JM. Kawasaki disease has so much to teach us! Ultrastruct Pathol. 2014;38(2):83–5.
5. Qilu Pharmaceutical. The instructions of warfarin; 2012.
6. Soriano-Ramos M, Martínez-Del Val E, Negreira Cepeda S, et al.Risk of coronary artery involvement in Kawasaki disease. Arch Argent Pediatr. 2016;114(2):107–13.
7. Fraison JB, Sève P, Dauphin C, et al. Kawasaki disease in adults: observations in France and literature review. Autoimmun Rev. 2016;15(3):242–9.
8. Watanabe H, Kato M, Ayusawa M. Potentially fatal arrhythmias in two cases of adult Kawasaki disease. Cardiol Young. 2016;26(3):602–4.
9. Eleftheriou D, Levin M, Shingadia D, et al. Management of Kawasaki disease. Arch Dis Child. 2014;99(1):74–83.
10. Orenstein JM, Shulman ST, Fox LM, et al. Three linked vasculopathic processes characterize Kawasaki disease: a light and transmission electron microscopic study. PLoS One. 2012;7(6):e38998.
11. Zhang H, Xu MG, Xie LJ, et al. Meta-analysis of risk factors associated with atherosclerosis in patients with Kawasaki disease. World J Pediatr. 2016;12(3):308–13.
12. Anderson MS, Burns J, Treadwell TA, et al. Erythrocyte sedimentation rate and C-reactive protein discrepancy and high prevalence of coronary artery abnormalities in Kawasaki disease. Pediatr Infect Dis J. 2001;20(7):698–702.
13. Nakagama Y, Inuzuka R, Hayashi T, et al. Fever pattern and C-reactive protein predict response to rescue therapy in Kawasaki disease. Pediatr Int. 2016;58(3):180–4.
14. Shah V, Christov G, Mukasa T, et al. Cardiovascular status after Kawasaki disease in the UK. Heart. 2015;101(20):1646–55.
15. Chen YC, Shen CT, Wang NK, et al. High sensitivity C reactive protein (hs-CRP) in adolescent and young adult patients with history of Kawasaki disease. Acta Cardiol Sin. 2015;31(6):473–7.
16. Rowley AH. The complexities of the diagnosis and management of Kawasaki disease. Infect Dis Clin N Am. 2015;29(3):525–37.
17. Chatha N, Fortin D, Bosma KJ. Management of necrotizing pneumonia and pulmonary gangrene: a case series and review of the literature. Can Respir J. 2014;21(4):239–45.
18. Sakamoto N, Tsuchiya K, Hikone M. Community-acquired necrotizing pneumonia with bacteremia caused by Pseudomonas aeruginosa in a patient with emphysema: an autopsy case report. Respir Investig. 2018;56(2):189–94.
19. Kuo HC, Lo MH, Hsieh KS, et al. High-dose aspirin is associated with anemia and does not confer benefit to disease outcomes in Kawasaki disease. PLoS One. 2015;10(12):e0144603.
20. Huang YH, Kuo HC, Huang FC, et al. Hepcidin-induced iron deficiency is related to transient anemia and hypoferremia in Kawasaki disease patients. Int J Mol Sci. 2016;17(5):E715.
21. Dumont B, Jeannoel P, Trapes L, et al. Macrophage activation syndrome and Kawasaki disease: four new cases. Arch Pediatr. 2017;24(7):640–6.

7 KD with Urinary System Involvement

Hong Wang and Xuemei Li

Abstract

KD is an acute febrile exanthematous illness and the diagnosis is made based on clinical signs and symptoms; KD is also vasculitis of medium-sized vessels and commonly seen in children. Multi-system organs are involved, including coronary artery lesions, myocarditis, arthritis, hepatitis, central nervous system disease, kidney and urinary tract abnormalities, hyponatremia [Watanabe et al., Pediatr Nephrol., 21(6):778-81, 2006]. The involvement of the genitourinary tract in KD manifests itself clinically in various forms. The most common presentations are sterile pyuria and proteinuria. Fewer patients have transient microscopic hematuria. Although they are rare, severe complications such as renovascular hypertension, hemolytic uremic syndrome, interstitial nephritis, and acute renal failure [Bonany et al., Pediatr Nephrol, 17(5):329–31, 2002] have been reported. And pathological findings in percutaneous biopsy included tubulointerstitial nephropathy with mild mesangial expansion, without vessel involvement or deposits in basal membrane [Watanabe et al., Pediatr Nephrol., 21(6):778-81, 2006]. But cases presentation of hematuria with massive proteinuria is very rare. Usually, aseptic urethritis does not require special treatment and can be cured by conventional IVIG and oral aspirin.

In this chapter, we presented 2 cases of KD with hematuria and massive proteinuria. Another case with sterile pyuria (case 12) is listed in chapter one.

H. Wang (✉) · X. Li
Department of Pediatric Cardiology, Shengjing Hospital of China Medical University, Shenyang, China

7.1 Case 30: KD with Large Proteinuria

A 3-year-old boy had measles 2 years ago but had no significant family history.

He presented on Day 5 of illness with fever lasting for 5 days, along with rashes and non-suppurative bilateral conjunctivitis for one day. He was treated with broad-spectrum antibiotics for 5 days in local clinic, but the treatment was ineffective. Congest rashes on the back and non-suppurative bilateral conjunctivitis developed on Day 4. *Examination* revealed afebrile. His mental stage was stable, had nonsuppurative bilateral conjunctivitis, strawberry tongue, and cervical lymphadenopathy. Examination did not find rashes. His systemic examination was otherwise unremarkable. *Admission blood* test revealed a normal complete blood count, with slightly elevated CRP (19.1 mg/L). The ultrasonography revealed cervical lymphadenopathy with the biggest one measured about 2.9 cm × 1.1 cm. Based on these findings, KD treatment was initiated: (1) IVIG 1g/kg/day for 2 days; (2) oral aspirin 30–50 mg/kg/day, and dipyridamole 3–5 mg/kg/day, divided into three doses.

On Day 6, investigation revealed normal ALT, and ALB was 25.3 g/L. Both protein and erythrocyte were positive in urine test. Serological studies for viral agents were negative. He was treated with albumin 1 g/kg for 2 days. On Day 8, after IVIG treatment, his fever settled over 48h. The bilateral conjunctivitis and strawberry tongue subsided. Aspirin was reduced to 3–5 mg/kg/day. Erythrocyte was negative but the urine protein was positive in urine samples.

On Day 10, his liver function panel was normal. Total protein in urine was 3.73 g/day; Echocardiography demonstrated that the size of the coronary artery was within the normal range (Fig. 7.1a, b). Parents refused to give consent for further examinations on the massive proteinuria. Patient was discharged.

H. Wang (ed.), *Paediatric Kawasaki Disease*, https://doi.org/10.1007/978-981-15-0038-1_7

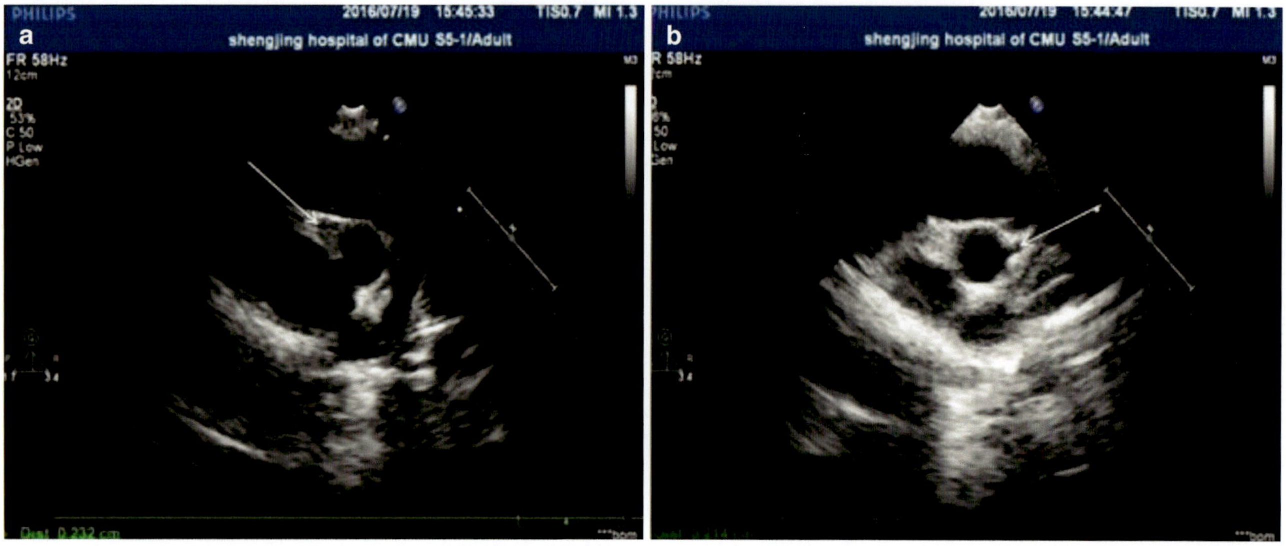

Fig. 7.1 On Day 10 of illness, echocardiography showed the normal RCA (**a**) and LCA (**b**)

7.1.1 Clinical Course of the Patient

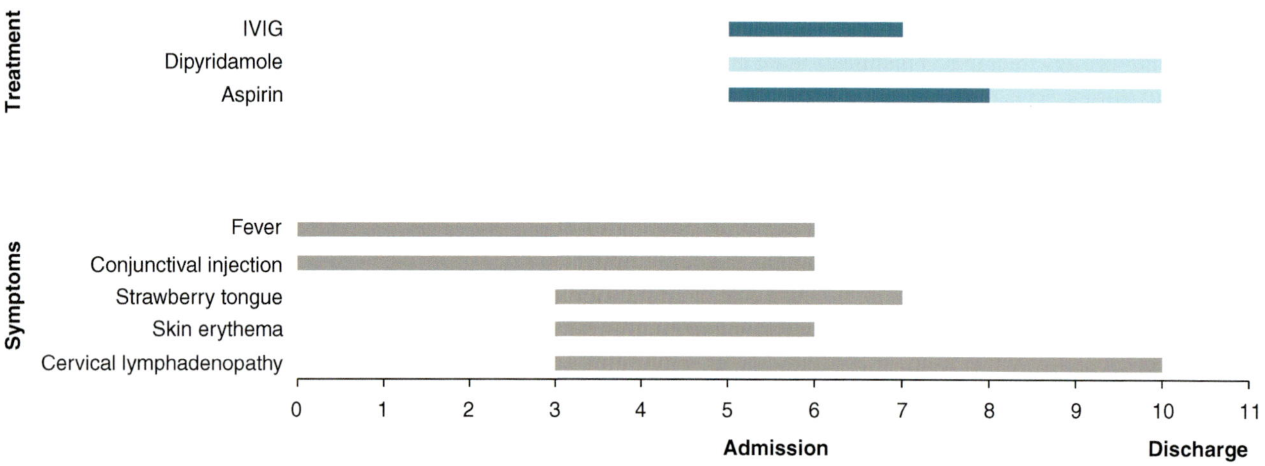

7.1.2 Follow up

Since discharged, he took oral: (1) aspirin and dipyridamole; (2) FDP and levocarnitine. After 8 weeks at clinic follow-up, echo showed normal coronary artery. All medications were stopped. His ALB was recovered but proteinuria was not improved.

7.1.3 Diagnosis

1. KD
2. Hypoalbuminemia
3. Proteinuria

7.1.4 Discussion

He had met the criteria of Kawasaki disease: (1) fever for more than 5 days; (2) conjunctival congestion without exudation; (3) generalized rashes; (4) strawberry tongue; (5) cervical lymphadenopathy.

7.1.5 Case Specific Clinic Features

1. KD (also known as mucocutaneous lymph node syndrome) is an infants' and children's illness. The most common pathologic findings are systemic vasculitis and a high incidence of inflammatory lesions affecting various organs, including liver,

kidney, lungs, and nervous system. The most serious and life-threatening aspect of KD is the development of angitis and aneurysmal dilation of the coronary arteries accompanied by thrombosis and, in some cases, death. The mechanism of kidney injury may be related to a cell-mediated immune response or antibodies directed against the tubular basement membrane [1]. The biopsy showed a patchy interstitial infiltrate of plasma cells and eosinophils [2]. Histological findings included normal glomerulus or mild expansion of mesangial matrix, interstitial infiltration with lymphocytes, plasmocyte, and eosinophils, focus of tubular necrosis, normal vessels, and normal immunofluorescence. Immunofluorescence showed IgM and C3 within the mesangium. However the involvement of the genitourinary tract in KD manifests itself clinically in various forms. The most common presentations are sterile pyuria and proteinuria; fewer patients have transient microscopic hematuria [3]. Cases of Kawasaki disease with acute renal failure or multiple organ dysfunction syndromes have been reported [4, 5]. Therefore, the renal function and urine routine should be monitored in patients with KD.

2. In this case, the diagnosis of KD was certain, and he had a good response to the IVIG treatment. Echocardiography demonstrated that the size of the coronary artery was within the normal range. He had hematuria and proteinuria when admitted. The hematuria disappeared after the IVIG treatment. But he still had a significant proteinuria (3.37 g/day), which reached the criterion of nephrotic syndrome. But the others were normal. The transient hematuria in this case was consistent with literature report, but the persistent massive proteinuria could not be explained. Perhaps this child had a certain type of nephropathy. Unfortunately, the child's parents refused to give consent for further examinations on the massive proteinuria. Long-term follow-up was still necessary.

Xue-mei Li

7.2 Case 31: Recurrent KD with Hematuria

A previously healthy one-year-old boy had an unremarkable past medical and family history.

He presented on Day 5 of illness with fever for 5 days, along with nonsuppurative bilateral conjunctivitis for 3 days and congestive rashes for 2 days. He was treated with cefmenoxime and vidarabine monophosphate for 4 days in clinic, but the treatment was ineffective. He was admitted in pediatric cardiology ward as KD. *Examination* revealed he still was febrile but in good spirits. There were some congestive rashes all over the body. The laterocervical lymph nodes were swollen. He had nonsuppurative bilateral conjunctivitis, red lips, and strawberry tongue. Neurological system was normal. Others were normal. *Admission blood* test revealed WBC 17.6×10^9/L. CRP 16.3 mg/L. Cervical ultrasonic showed lymphadenopathy on both sides, the bigger one was 2.0 cm × 0.6 cm. He was diagnosed with KD and treated with (1) IVIG 1 g/kg/day for 2 days; (2) oral aspirin 30–50 mg/kg/day and dipyridamole 3–5 mg/kg/day, in three divided doses.

On Day 6, test results showed negative MP-IgM and CP-IgM, MP IgG 1:160, ESR 66 mm/h, urinary protein (+), RBC 7.0/HP, WBC 11.03/HP. He was given oral azithromycin 10 mg/kg/day for 3 days. On Day 8, his fever settled over 48 h and urine routine test result was normal. The dosage of aspirin was reduced to 3–5 mg/kg/day. On Day 10, he was in good condition. Retested results showed WBC 8.29×10^9/L, Hb 106 g/L, PLT 649×10^9/L. CRP 7.11 mg/L; Liver function ALB 31.8 g/L, ALT 12 U/L, AST 33 U/L. Echo showed normal coronary artery (Fig. 7.2a, b). He was discharged.

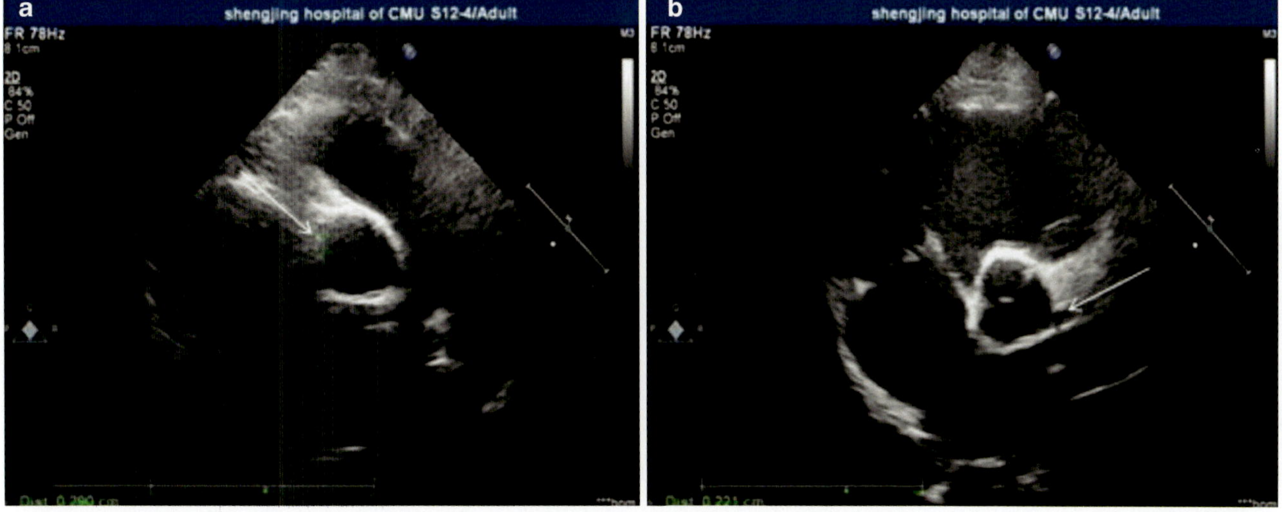

Fig. 7.2 On Day 10 of illness, echocardiography showed the normal RCA (**a**) and LCA (**b**)

7.2.1 Clinical Course of the Patient

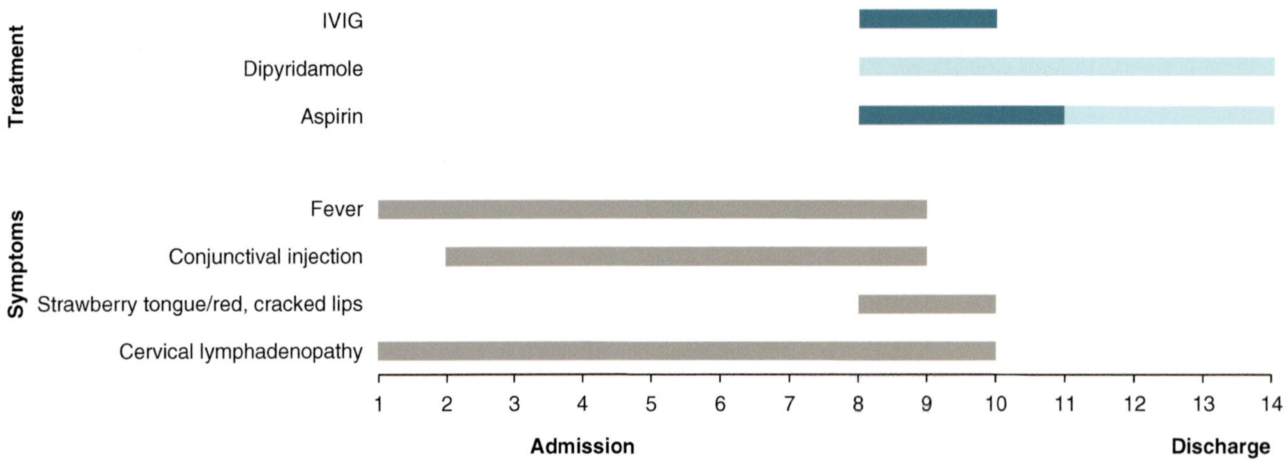

7.2.2 Follow Up

Since discharged, he took aspirin and dipyridamole. Echo was performed 1 week later. Followed-up tests after 2 months showed normal PLT, ESR, and echo. All medications were stopped.

Fourteen months after diagnosis, he presented again with a 4-day history of fever, along with bilateral conjunctival congestion for 3 days. He took oral erythromycin for 3 days, but still had a fever. Then he was admitted in pediatric cardiology ward. *Examination*: He was febrile without irritability, auscultation revealed lung and heart normal. Abdominal examination was normal. There was no rash. The laterocervical lymph nodes were swollen. There were nonsuppurative bilateral conjunctivitis. Neurological system was normal. Admission blood test revealed WBC 13.46 × 10^9/L. CRP 19.1 mg/L. Cervical ultrasonic showed lymphadenopathy on both sides, the bigger one about 1.3 cm × 0.8 cm. He was treated with (1) cefuroxime sodium infusion at 100 mg/kg/day; (2) vidarabine monophosphate infusion at 5 mg/kg/day; (3) azithromycin infusion at 10 mg/kg/day.

On Day 8, he continued to have fever and bilateral conjunctivitis, and developed red lips. Retested results showed CRP 26.3 mg/L. NT-pro BNP 1430 pg/ml. ALB 31.4 g/L. Renal function was normal. Urine routine test showed urinary protein (+++), RBC 491.35/HP, WBC 10.4/HP. Renal ultrasound showed increased cortical echogenicity (Fig. 7.3a, b). MP-IgM was positive. Virus

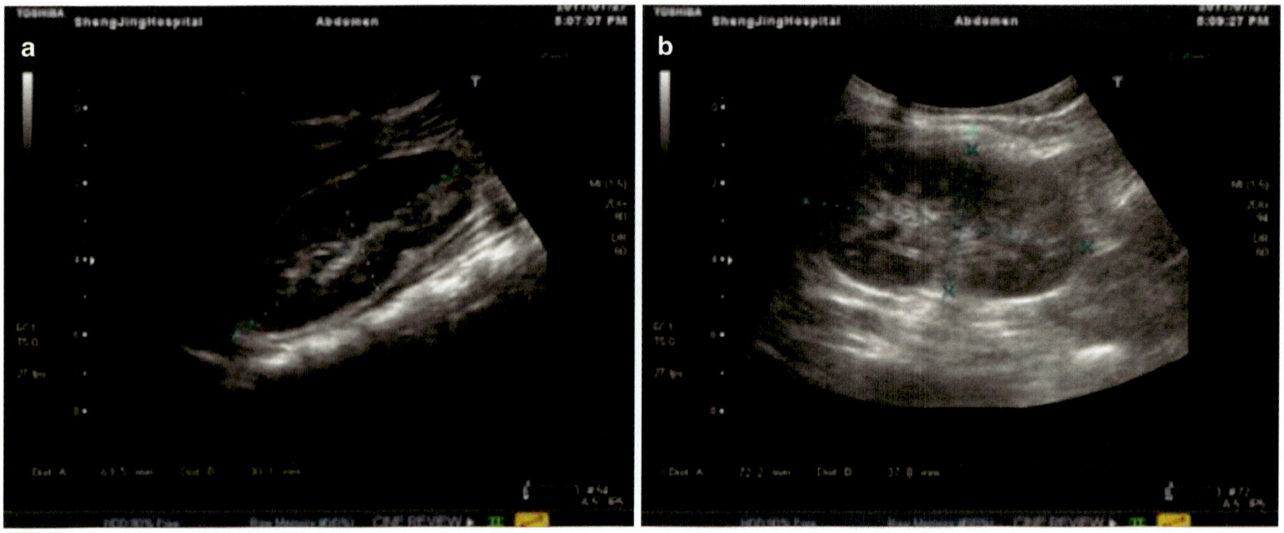

Fig. 7.3 On Day 8 of the second time KD, renal ultrasound showed the increased cortical echogenicity in longitudinal section (**a** and **b**)

antibodies was negative. He was diagnosed with recurrent KD and treated with (1) IVIG 1 g/kg/day for 2 days; (2) oral aspirin 30–50 mg/kg/day and dipyridamole 3–5 mg/kg/day, in three divided doses; (3) monitoring urine routine. On Day 11, he was afebrile over 48 h, aspirin was reduced to 3–5 mg/kg/day. Echo showed coronary artery was normal (Fig. 7.4a, b). Retested results were as the following: WBC 4.46 × 10^9/L, HGB 104 g/L, PLT 559 × 10^9/L. CRP 14.6 mg/L. NT-pro BNP 786.3 pg/ml. Liver function ALB 27.3 g/L, ALT and AST were normal. Renal function was normal. Urine routine test showed urinary protein (++), RBC 222.55/HP, WBC 2.2/HP, RBC deformity rate 70%. Urine β_2 microglobulin determination was further detected 0.277 mg/L (<0.24). Renal tubule function test showed urinary microglobulin 6.63 mg/dl (0–1.9), urinary transferrin 0.393 mg/dl, urinary α1-microglobulin and urinary IgG were normal. Total protein level in urine was normal. The BP of the child was normal, and there was no edema around the body. He was treated with albumin 1 g/kg/day for 2 days. Further examination showed that ceruloplasmin, antinuclear antibody series, and ANCA were normal. Fundus photography was normal. On Day 14, he was afebrile for 5 days. Retested renal ultrasound was normal (Fig. 7.5). Urine routine

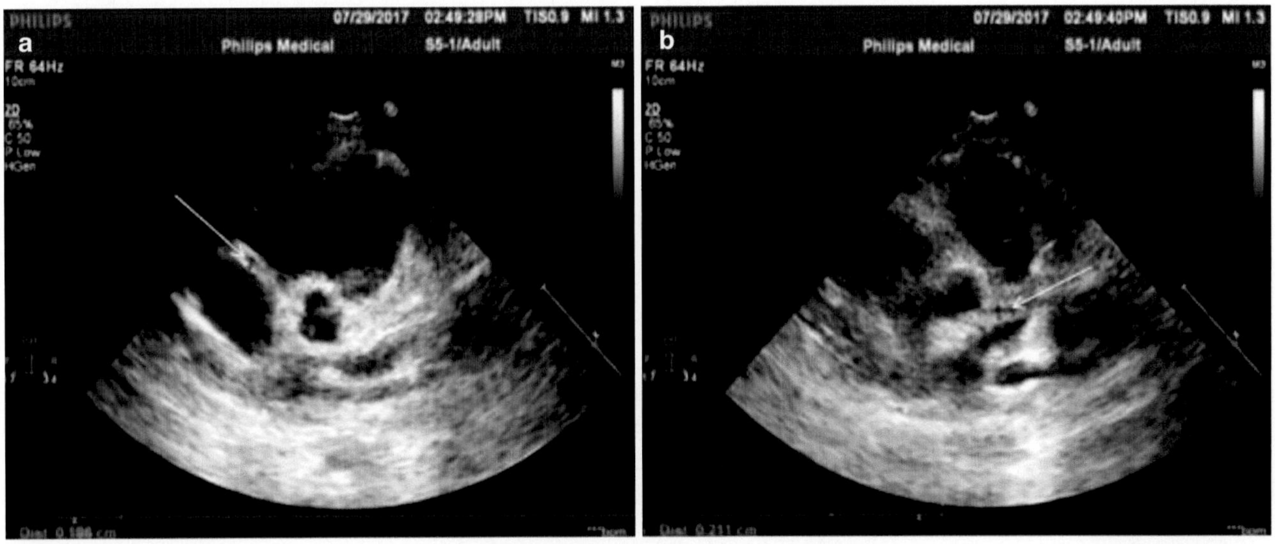

Fig. 7.4 On Day 11 of the second time KD, echocardiography showed the normal RCA (**a**) and LCA (**b**)

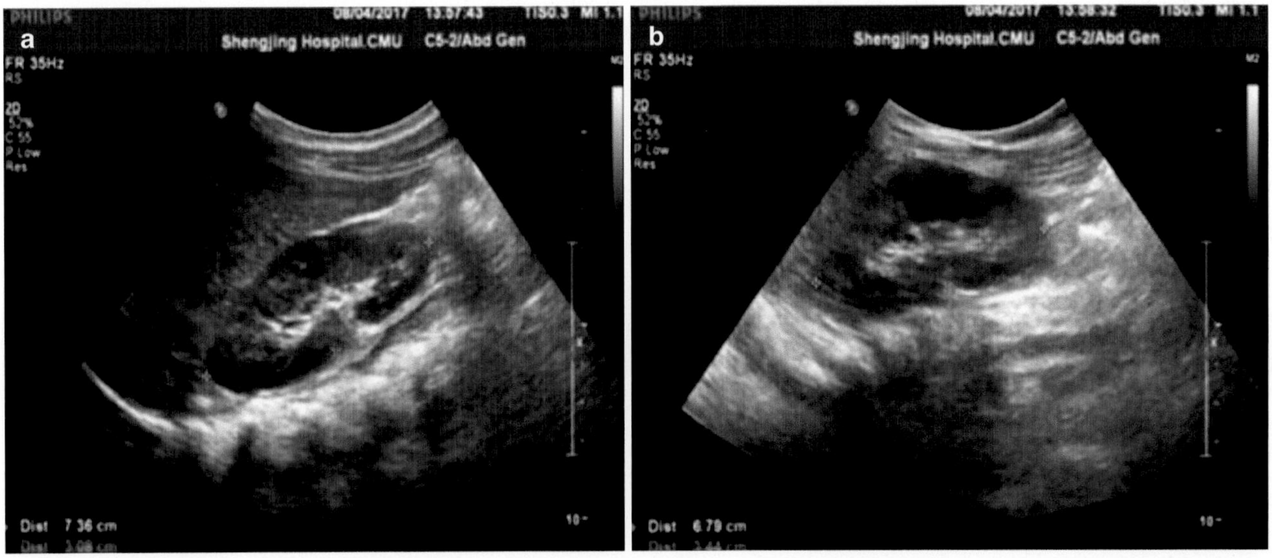

Fig. 7.5 On Day 14 of the second time KD, echocardiography showed the normal cortical echogenicity in longitudinal section (**a** and **b**)

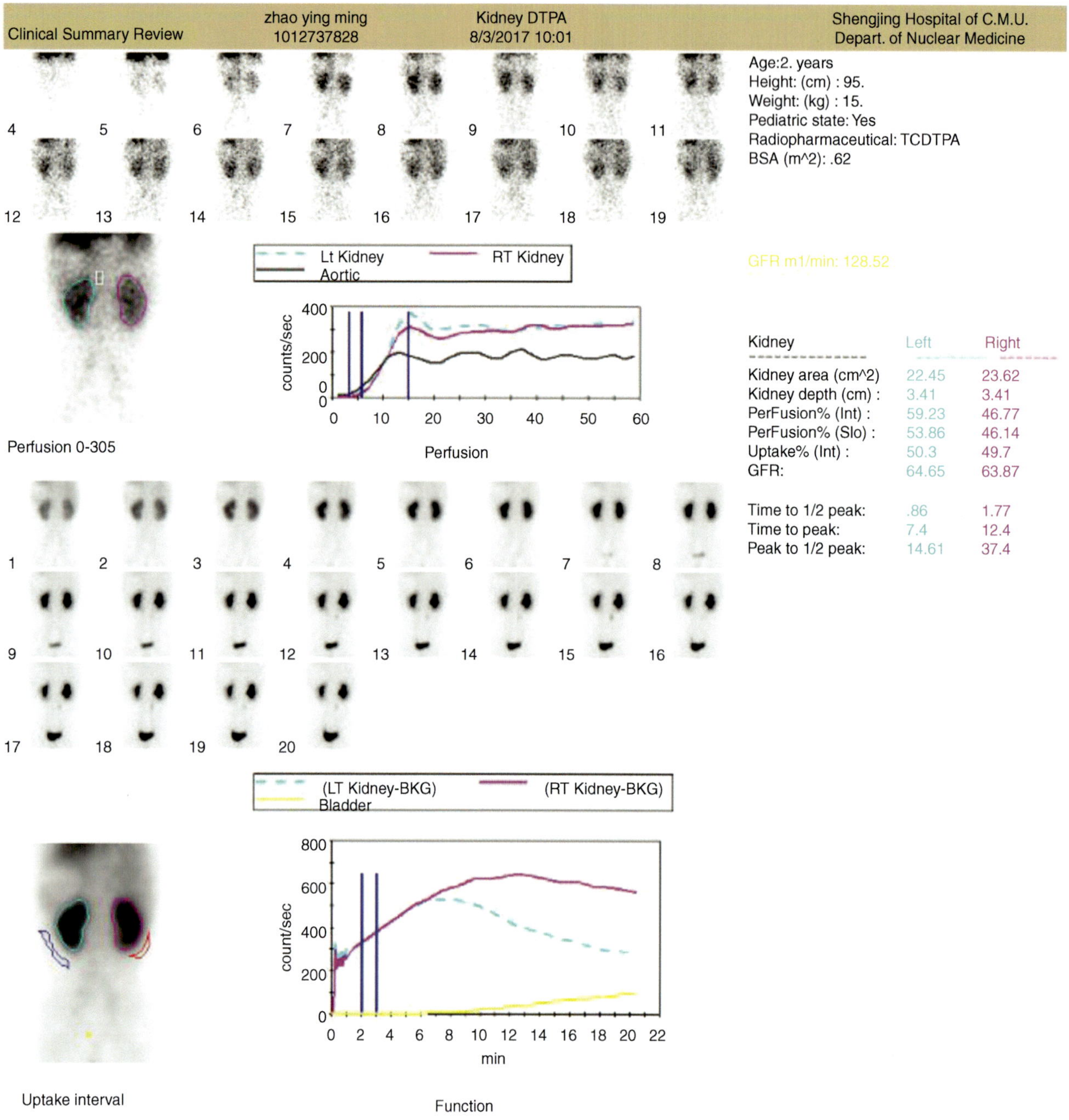

Fig. 7.6 On Day 14 of second KD, GFR of both were normal, but slow excretion in renal ECT

showed urinary protein (+), RBC 26.75/HP, WBC 00.63/HP, RBC deformity rate 70%. Urine β_2 micro-globulin determination was normal. Renal tubule function test results showed urinary micro-albumin 195 mg/dl (0–1.9), urinary transferrin 8.94 mg/dl, urinary IgG 21.5 mg/dl (0–0.8), urinary α1-micro-globulin was normal. Total urine protein was 0.82 g/day (0–0.15). Renal ECT revealed GFR of both kidneys were normal, but slow excretion (Fig. 7.6). The parents refused to give consent for further examinations on the massive proteinuria, and the patient was discharged.

7.2.3 Diagnosis

1. Recurrent KD
2. Hematuria and Proteinuria
3. Mp infection.

7.2.4 Discussion

He had met the criteria of KD: (1) fever for 5 days and oral antibiotics were not effective; (2) conjunctival injection without exudation; (3) generalized rash; (4) red lips; (5) cervical lymphadenopathy about 2.0 × 0.6 cm.

He had met the criteria of recurrent KD: (1) had fever for 5 days and intravenous antibiotics were not effective; (2) had been diagnosed with KD 14 months ago; (3) had conjunctival congestion without exudation; (4) had red lips; (5) had left cervical lymphadenopathy about 1.3 cm × 0.8 cm.

7.2.5 Case Specific Clinic Features

1. KD has syndromes with unknown causes. It typically affects infants and toddlers, and causes systemic vasculitis. The most common pathologic findings include systemic vasculitis and a high incidence of inflammatory lesions affecting various organs, such as liver, kidney, lungs, and nervous system. More and more attentions had been paid to KD complicated with kidney injury in recent years. The involvement of the genitourinary tract in KD manifests itself clinically in various forms. The most common presentations are sterile pyuria and proteinuria; fewer patients have transient microscopic hematuria. Although they are rare, severe complications such as renovascular hypertension, hemolytic uremic syndrome, interstitial nephritis, and acute renal failure have been reported [6, 7].
2. Histological findings included a normal glomerulus or mild expansion of the mesangial matrix; interstitial infiltration of lymphocytes, plasmocytes, and eosinophils; and a focus of tubular necrosis [8]. There are also a few literatures suggesting that KD may affect renal parenchyma. Renal scar formation was found about half a year after KD diagnosis [3].
3. In this case, when the patient was diagnosed with KD at first time, urine routine test indicated urinary protein (+), RBC 7.0/HP, WBC 11.03/HP. The second time he was diagnosed with KD, urine routine test showed that protein level was increased (+++), RBC 491.35/HP, and WBC 10.4/HP. Urologic ultrasonography revealed diffuse injury on both kidneys, but with normal Cr and BUN. RBC malformation rate was 70% indicating RBC coming from glomerular. After IVIG treatment, urine protein was regressed to (+), RBC was reduced to 26.75/HP, WBC was normal. In addition, urine β_2 micro-globulin was slightly increased, which suggest impaired renal tubular function. The increased urine transferrin suggested impaired renal glomerular function, too. But, normal Cr and BUN implied there were no severe renal function damages. Furthermore, kidney ultrasound showed they were recovered to normal, and urine β_2 micro-globulin was recovered, which suggested that the impaired renal tubular function may be transient and reversible. Further increased urinary transferrin suggested unrecovered glomerular function. Normal GRF but slow excretion indicated the injury was there for some time. This may be the reason to keep hematuria, and requires dynamic follow-up.
4. To determine the causes of hematuria proteinuria whether by KD-related vasculitis or by other immune-related diseases prior to KD, we test ANCA and antinuclear antibody serial examinations, but we did not find abnormalities. His parents refused to give consent on further tests including immunodeficiency screening, abdominal CT, lipid, scleral ciliary body, and nephrodialysis.
5. This was the first time for us to see KD children with both hematuria and proteinuria diagnosed in our center. With the improvement of the disease, the urine routine test results returned to normal at his first time KD, which was consistent with the literature reports. After the recurrence of KD, obvious hematuria and proteinuria were found in the acute phase, and the 24-h urine protein quantification reached the nephropathy standard. Although the urine routine was slightly improved at convalescence period at 2 months of illness, his conditions met the guideline standard for stopping all drugs. The urine routine was still abnormal. The long-term prognosis for this patient is unknown because we have not been given a chance to follow up with him.

Xue-mei Li

References

1. Veiga PA, Pieroui C, Baier W. Association of Kawasaki disease and interstial nephritis. Pediatrics Nephrol. 1992;6(5):421–3.
2. Grunebaum E, Blank M, Gohen S, et al. The role of antiendothelial cell antibodies in Kawasaki disease in vitro and in vivo studies. Clin Exp Immunol. 2002;130(2):233–40.
3. Wang JN, Chiou YY, Chiu NT, et al. Renal scarring sequelae in childhood Kawasaki disease. Pediatr Nephrol. 2006;22(5):684–9.
4. Bonany PJ, Bilkis MD, Gallo G, et al. Acute renal failure in typical Kawasaki disease. Pediatr Nephrol. 2002;17(5):329–31.
5. Gatterre P, Oualha M, Dupic L, et al. Kawasaki disease: an unexpected etiology of shock and multiple organ dysfunction syndrome. Intensive Care Med. 2012;38(5):872–8.
6. Foster BJ, Bernard C, Drummond KN. Kawasaki disease complicated by renal artery stenosis. Arch Dis Child. 2000;83(3):253–5.
7. Bonany PJ, Bilkis MD, Gallo G, et al. Acute renal failure in typical Kawasaki disease. Pediatr Nephrol. 2002;17(5):329–31.
8. Grunebaum E, Blank M, Cohen S, et al. The role of anti-endothelial cell antibodies in Kawasaki disease-in vitro and in vivo studies. Clin Exp Immunol. 2002;130(2):233–40.

KD with Bone and Joins Injury

8

Hong Wang, Yanxia Yang, Man Xu, Yang Hou, and Yunlong Huo

Abstract

The criteria of KD does not include arthritis, but arthritis is not rare in KD [Sahin et al., Clin Exp Rheumatol, 35 Suppl 104 (2):10, 2017]. For the good prognosis, we won't be concerned about it, and treatment was also not difficult. The incidence of KD with arthritis is from 16% [Sahin et al., Clin Exp Rheumatol, 35 Suppl 104 (2):10, 2017] to 15–45% [Shaikh et al., Cases J, 26962, 2009]. It may occur earlier at interphalangeal joint, cervical spine and temporo-mandibular [Jen et al., Pediatr, 118(5):e1569–71, 2006], usually along with high-grade fever that would subside after IVIG treatment. However it mostly take place at both knees and hip joints after IVIG treatment, around 10 days of illness. Some patients develop arthritis right after discharge [Lee et al., Eur J Pediatr, 164 (7): 451–2, 2005]. Differential diagnosis of juvenile rheumatoid arthritis, leukaemia, and neuroblastoma is necessary, if fever persists combined with swollen and painful joints [Martins et al., J Paediatr Child Health, doi: 10.1111/jpc.14102, 2018]. The common image changes in KD with arthritis were liquid effusion (see case 33). By now, the treatment guideline for KD with arthritis is to use IVIG at first [Rodriguez and Wagner-Weiner, Pediatr Ann., 46 (1):e19–24, 2017], and then glucocorticoid combined with oral aspirin [Okubo et al., Arthritis Care Res (Hoboken), 70 (7):1052–7, 2018]. For those in mild cases simple aspirin may also work. Fortunately, once treated with either aspirin or glucocorticoid, patient's prognosis was very good, without sequelae [Sahin et al., Clin Exp Rheumatol, 35 Suppl 104 (2):10, 2017].

To author's best understand, no literature has reported complication of bone marrow in KD. The prognosis for bone/joint injury of KD is different from that for acute suppurative osteomyelitis. Therefore it has been a hot topic to use imaging in distinguish these two at disease early stage. We have less knowledge in CT imaging of bone injuries in KD, compared to that of bone marrow inflammation, though we deduce the prognosis would be better, like arthritis [Álvarez et al., Reumatol Clin., 13 (3):145–9, 2017], than osteomyelitis. It need to be confirmed by further clinical practice.

H. Wang (✉) · Y. Yang · M. Xu
Department of Pediatric Cardiology, Shengjing Hospital of China Medical University, Shenyang, China

Y. Hou
Department of Radiology, Shengjing Hospital of China Medical University, Shenyang, China

Y. Huo
Department of Pathology, Shengjing Hospital of China Medical University, Shenyang, China

8.1 Case 32: KD with Bone Injury

A previously healthy 3-year-old boy had an unremarkable antenatal history. His grandfather was diagnosed with tuberculosis 6 months ago and took oral medication. The patient seldom had dinner with his grandfather.

He presented on Day 12 of illness with prolonged fever for 9 days, along with rashes and left leg pain for one week. On Day 1 of illness, he had fever at 39.8°C, along with abdominal pain and vomiting. On Day 2, his fever continued and he developed rashes on his face with itchy, and gradually developed rashes all over body; he also developed bilateral conjunctival congestion. He was given infusion of erythromycin for 2 days and intramuscular injection of acetaminophen (unknown name) once. His fever persisted and red and crack lips developed, and he had numbness on his left lower limb and could not walk on Day 6. He was admitted in local hospital as KD on Day 7, was given IVIG 22.5g for two days and infusion of azithromycin for 5 days and second-generation cephalosporin for 3 days. Pharyngeal brush culture results revealed he had positive streptococcal infection, and antibiotics was changed to penicillin for 2 days according to the drug susceptibility test. On Day 9, both his fever and bilateral conjunctivitis settled down. On Day 11, leg MR indicated pyogenic osteomyelitis

H. Wang (ed.), *Paediatric Kawasaki Disease*, https://doi.org/10.1007/978-981-15-0038-1_8

that could not be excluded. He was transferred to our pediatric cardiology ward. Examination found his lips were red and cracked with strawberry tongue. Liver was enlarged about 3 cm below right coastal margin. Peeling skin occurred around fingernails. Left knee joint and leg presented normal color and temperature with motion difficulties. Others were normal. Before admission, blood test in local hospital on Day 3 revealed WBC 8.9×10^9/L, NE 91.2%, HGB 107g/L, PLT 245×10^9/L. CRP 12.3 mg/L. ESR 65 mm/h. MP-IgM mild positive. MP-Ab IgG 1:320. Swallow brush bacterial culture was streptococcus growth. PCT 0.726 ng/ml. DIC, RF, IgG, IgA, IgM, C_3 and C_4 were normal. Echo showed mitral and tricuspid waves with mild regurgitation. Chest CT scan showed local emphysema at lower lobes of bilateral lungs. Cervical ultrasound showed bilateral lymphadenectasis, the bigger one about 2.5 cm on the right and 2.3 cm on the left. Hips MR scan showed mild fluid signal at right inguinal region. Left knee MR showed abnormal signal on the near side of left tibia and surrounding soft tissue with edema-like signal. Impression diagnosis indicated skeleton system injuries associated with infectious lesion? Admission blood test revealed WBC 7.1×10^9/L, NE 33.7%, HGB 107g/L, PLT 285×10^9/L. CRP 22.4mg/L. cTnI, hs-cTnT, MYO, and NT pro-BNP were normal. ECG was normal (Fig. 8.1). He was tested positive for strep throat. Meanwhile, MRI showed abnormalities in his left proximal tibia (information obtained from the local hospital where he had these tests done), prompting us to suspect a possible pyogenic osteomyelitis. He was given infusion of vancomycin, and BAEP test was ordered. After consultation with pediatric orthopedist, we were informed that bone density of the left tibia near side was not uneven based on previous left leg MR. Infection was suspected. But physical examination revealed normal local skin. CT and 3D reconstruction for left tibia and on left inner side of knee were performed. Because of elevated CRP, he continued to take vancomycin infusion.

On Day 13, everything went well except limited left knee motion. Investigation revealed ALB 32.4g/l. CK, CKMB, and CK-MB were normal. ASO 74.0IU/ml. MP-IgM, MP-IgG, and CP-IgG were positive. BAEP was normal. Limb ultrasound showed a low density echo mass about 11.9mm (Fig.8.2a) on the surface of left tibia; there was lymphadenectasis about 0.8 × 0.6 cm on the left popliteal space (Fig. 8.2b); distal section blood flow was sufficient (Fig. 8.2c). Left leg DR was normal (Fig. 8.2d). Left knee MR showed a mass-like with high and low mixed signals, about 1.2 cm × 0.8cm × 2.0 cm (Fig. 8.3a, b). There were detected long T_1 and long T_2 signal at peripheral bone marrow, and mild fluid signal on the left knee. Soft tissue surrounding the near side of left tibia showed edema. Acute purulent osteomyelitis needed to be excluded. After consultation with pediatric orthopedist again, we were recommended to perform left leg CT and monitor body temperature for 3 days. In the absence of fever the patient could be transferred to pediatric orthopedic ward for operation. Left leg CT scan and 3D reconstruction showed an

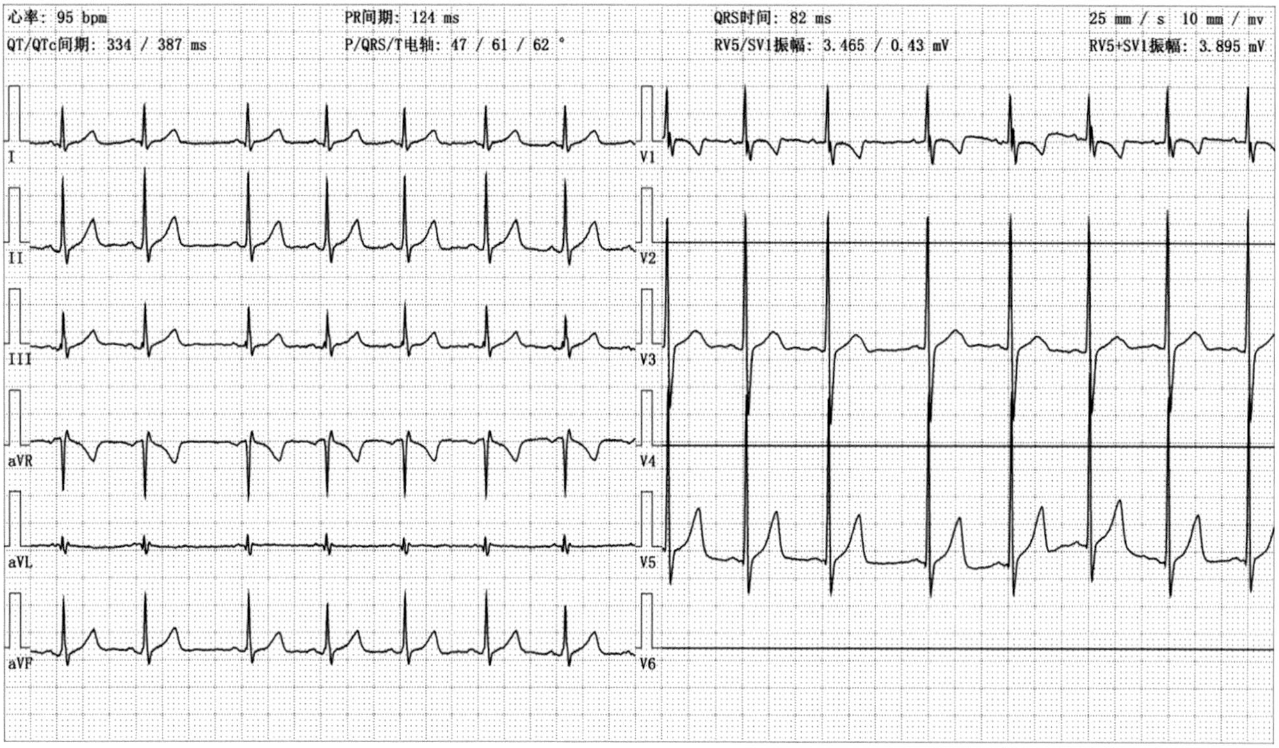

Fig. 8.1 On Day 12 of illness, ECG was normal

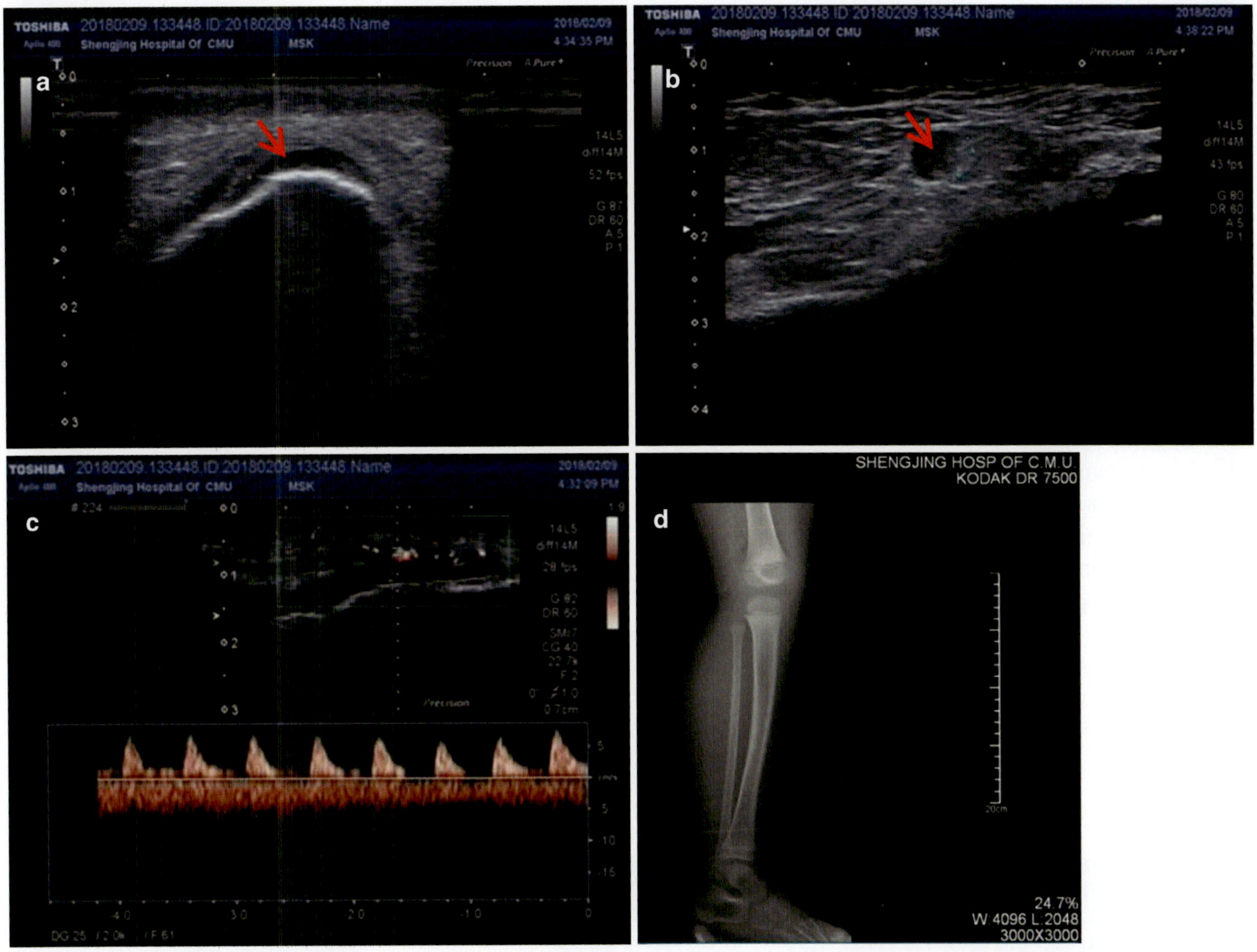

Fig. 8.2 On Day 13 of illness, leg ultrasound showed on the left tibia surface there was a low echo mass about 11.9 mm (**a**), lymphadenopathy on the left popliteal space (**b**), the blood flow was abundant in the left knee joint (**c**), left leg DR was normal (**d**)

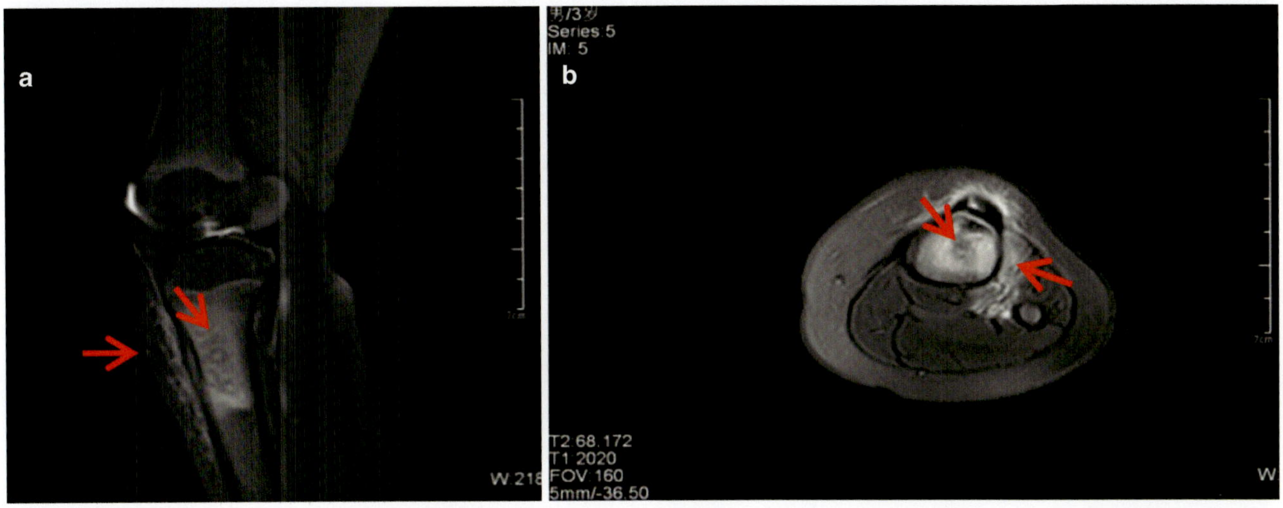

Fig. 8.3 On Day 13 of illness, MR PDW-SPAIR showed a mass-like high and low mixed signals, about1.2 cm × 0.8 cm × 2.0 cm (**a**), peripheral bone marrow showed a long T1 and long T2 signal. There was mild fluid signal on the left knee. Soft tissue surrounding the near side of left tibia was edema (**b**)

inhomogeneous increase in density of the medullary cavity at the proximal end of tibia (Fig. 8.4a, b), surrounding soft tissue were with edema and effusion. The far side of left tibia was normal. Malignant could not be excluded. On Day 14, he was afebrile for 5 days. Lab findings revealed cox virus 1–6 IgM, virus IgM, EB virus EA/NA/VCA-IgG, and Parainfluenza virus IgM were positive. Echo showed LCA, RCA, and LVEF (Fig. 8.5a, b, c) were normal. Chest DR was normal (Fig. 8.5d). Left knee MR scan suggested acute purulent osteomyelitis (Fig. 8.6a, b). On Day 15, ECT scan was performed. Radioactivity imaging of 99Mtc- MDP showed all bone imaging were normal except for there was abnormal nuclide concentration at proximal end of left tibia (Fig. 8.7). He was given infusion of ganciclovir 7.5mg/kg/day for 5 days. We recommended a test for tumor-related antibody, but the recommendation was turned down by his parents. Parents insisted on surgical treatment first since it was close to Chinese spring festival holidays. Then he was transferred to pediatric orthopedic ward.

On Day 16, incision operation and drainage were performed on the left lower leg under general anesthesia, and there was no pus found in marrow of left leg. Some bone marrow sample was taken for immunohistochemistry test. Three hours later, he was transferred to our pediatric cardiology. On Day 17, the first day after the operation, he was afebrile and mental stage was stable. Incision site was covered by elastic bandage without errhysis. Left toes were warm and had normal color. Peeling skin occurred around toenails. Pulse at left dorsal foot artery was normal. There was about 3 ml of bloody fluid in the drainage tube. First-generation cephalosporin was injected in drainage tube. Two days later, everything went well. Investigation revealed WBC 7.12×10^9/L, NE 44.9%, HGB 98 g/L, PLT 435×10^9/L. CRP 11.2 mg/L. CK and CK-MB were normal. ASO 56.2 IU/ml. Repeated BAEP was normal. Vancomycin infusion was given for one week and stopped. On Day 21, there was total about 4 ml of bloody liquid in the drainage tube. The drainage tube was removed, and a new elastic bandage was replaced. On the following day, left toes had normal color and temperature. Blood test revealed ALP was normal. Left knee MR was performed and showed postoperative change on the left lower limb (Fig. 8.8a, b), the surrounding soft tissue was edema.

On Day 24, no more peeling skin occurred around toenails. Repeated echo was normal. He was discharged next day. On Day 30, pathohistology result of bone marrow came back and revealed inflammatory reactive hyperplasia (Fig. 8.9).

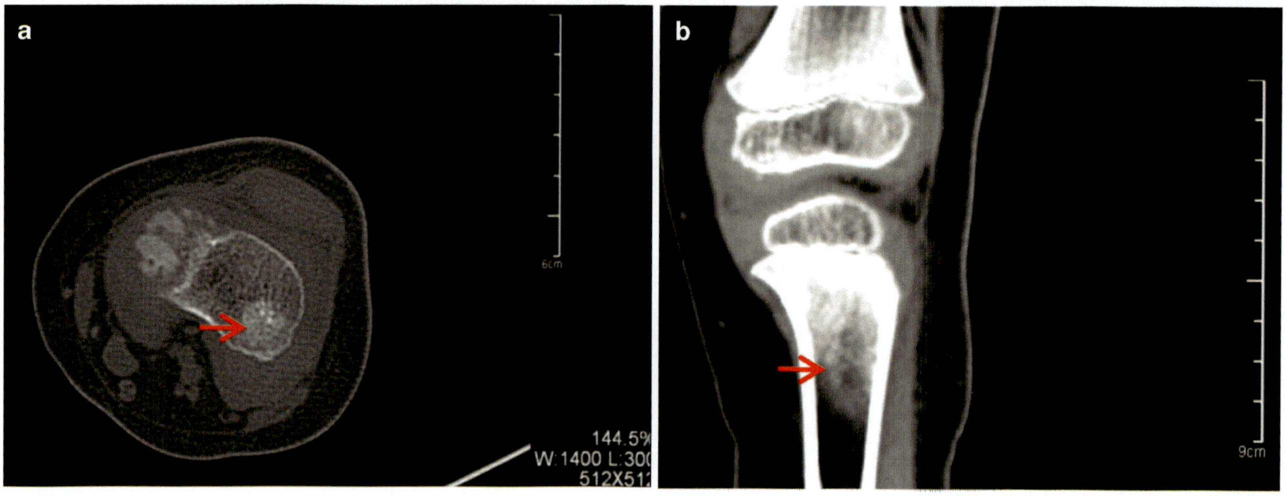

Fig. 8.4 On Day 13 of illness, CT showed the density of the medullary cavity was inhomogeneous increased (a-cross section) (b-vertical section), and the surrounding soft tissue with edema and effusion. On the far side of left tibia was normal

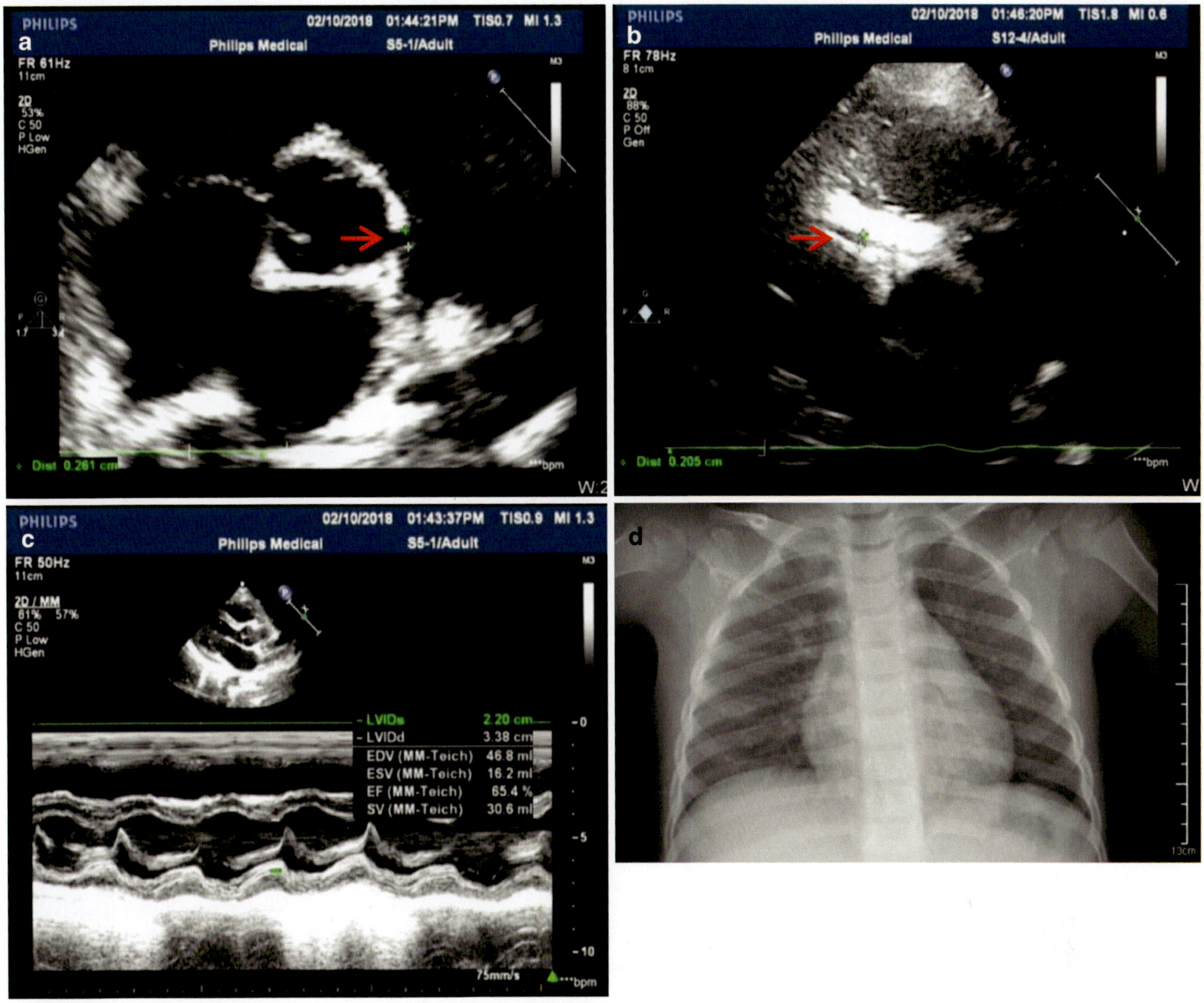

Fig. 8.5 On Day 14 of illness, echo showed normal LCA (**a**), RCA (**b**), and LVEF (**c**). Chest DR was normal (**d**)

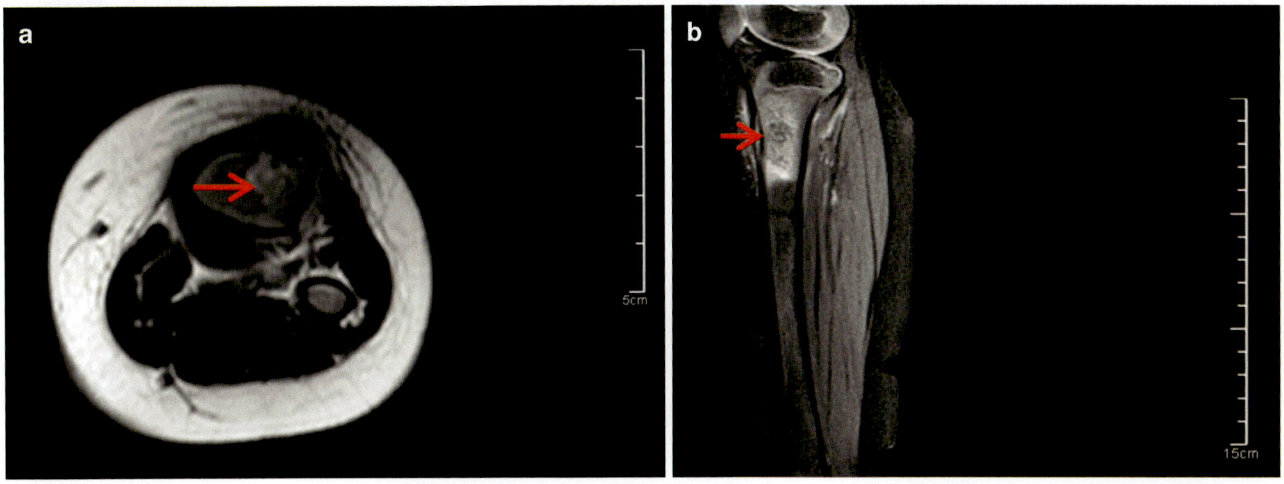

Fig. 8.6 On Day 14 of illness, MR T1W1 showed that mainly low signal with a mainly high signal patch mixed with low signal on T2W1 at the near side of left tibia (a-cross section,) (b-vertical section)

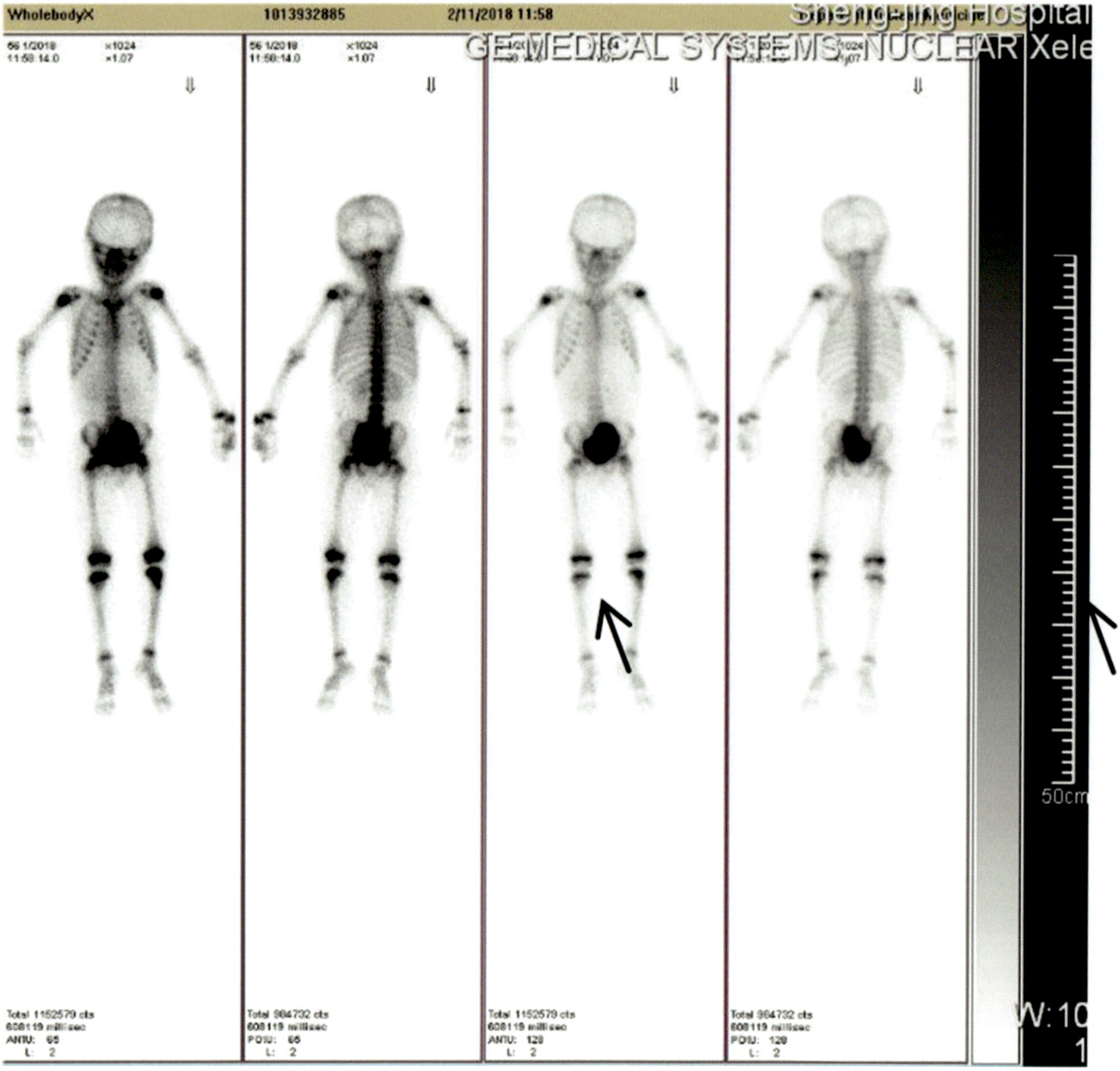

Fig. 8.7 On Day 16 of illness, ECT showed there was abnormal nuclide concentration of proximal end of left tibia (black arrow)

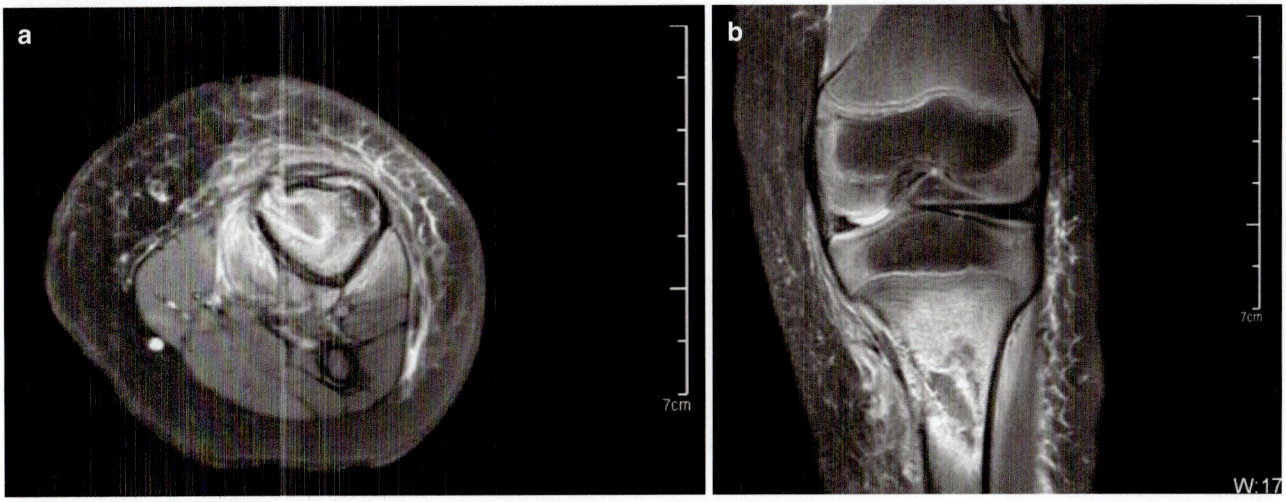

Fig. 8.8 On Day 22 of illness, MR T1W1 showed that after bone marrow drainage, left leg MR showed the T1W1 was more low signal, while high signal-dominated mixed signal shadow on T2W1 at the near side of left tibia (a-cross section) (b-vertical section), and edema was evidence in surrounding soft tissue

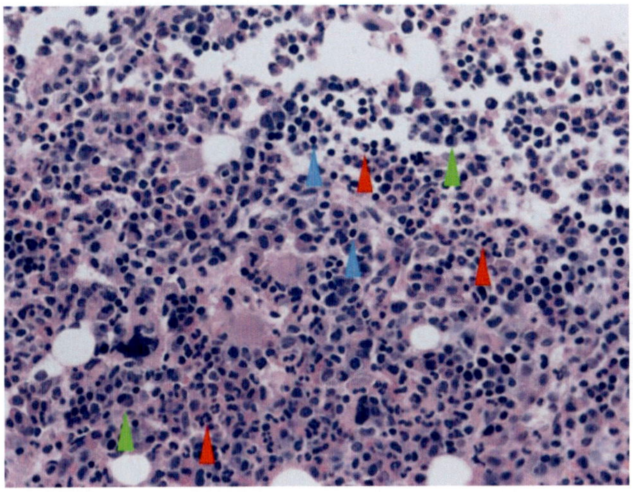

Fig. 8.9 On Day 30 of illness, pathology of bone marrow showed inflammatory reactive hyperplasia (red arrow-neutrophile granulocyte, blue arrow-lymphocyte, green arrow-plasmocyte)

8.1.1 Clinical Course of the Patient

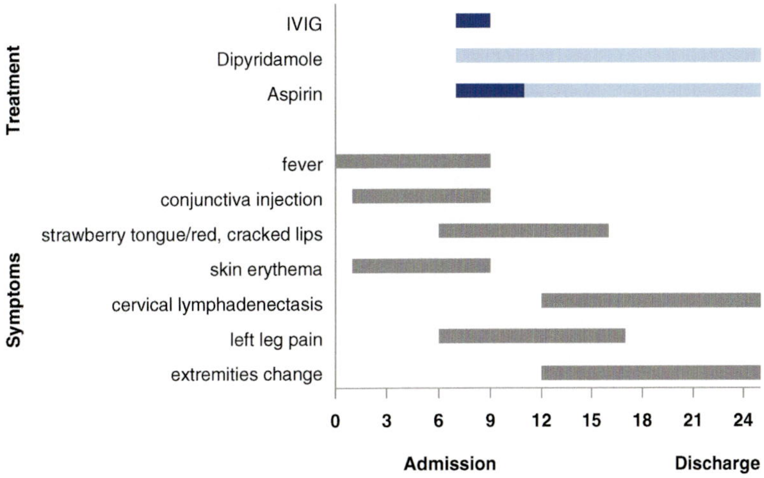

8.1.2 Follow-Up

ECG and echo were performed at 2, 4, 9, and 13 months of illness, all in normal range. Left knee MR at 2 months showed regressed peripheral soft tissue edema (Fig. 8.10a), and improved abnormal density of bone marrow cavity compared to previous result (Fig. 8.10b). Left leg CT performed at 4 (DR also performed), 9, and 13 months showed the bone marrow cavity was not uniform, and swollen soft tissue around the left knee joint was improved (Figs. 8.11a, b, 8.12a, b, 8.13a, b, 8.14a, b). Aspirin was discontinued after ESR recovered to normal at 4 months of illness.

8.1.3 Diagnosis

1. KD, bone injury
2. Mycoplasma infection
3. Viral infection (EB, COX, ECHO, PINE).

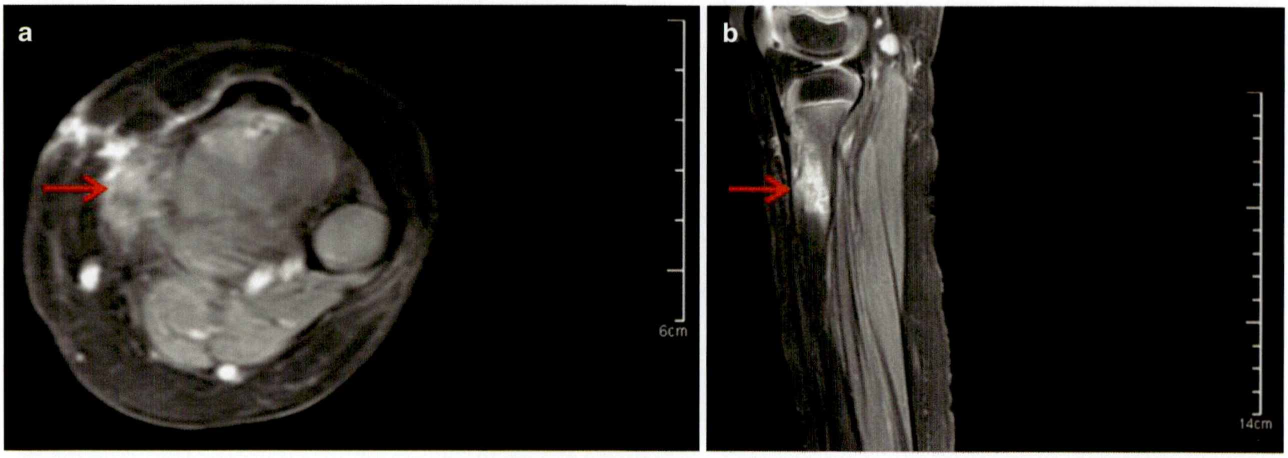

Fig. 8.10 At 2 months of illness, MR T1W1 showed the T1W1 was more low signal, while low signal-dominated mixed signal shadow on T2W1 at the near side of left tibia (a-cross section) (b-vertical section), and edema was improved in surrounding soft tissue

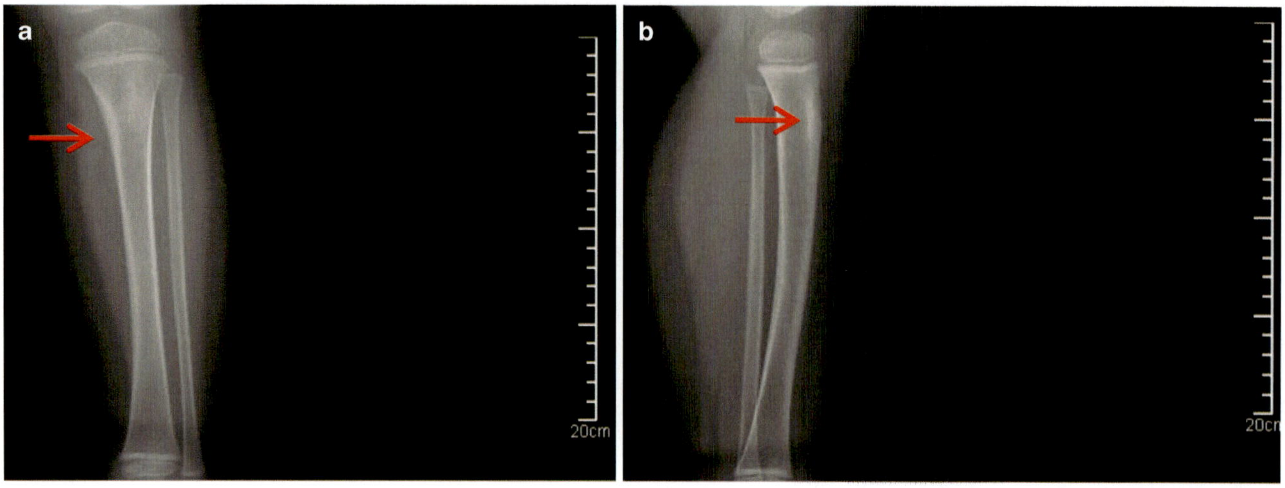

Fig. 8.11 At 4 months of illness, leg DR showed the mixed signal shadow at the near side of left tibia (a-position, b-side position), and slight edema in surrounding soft tissue

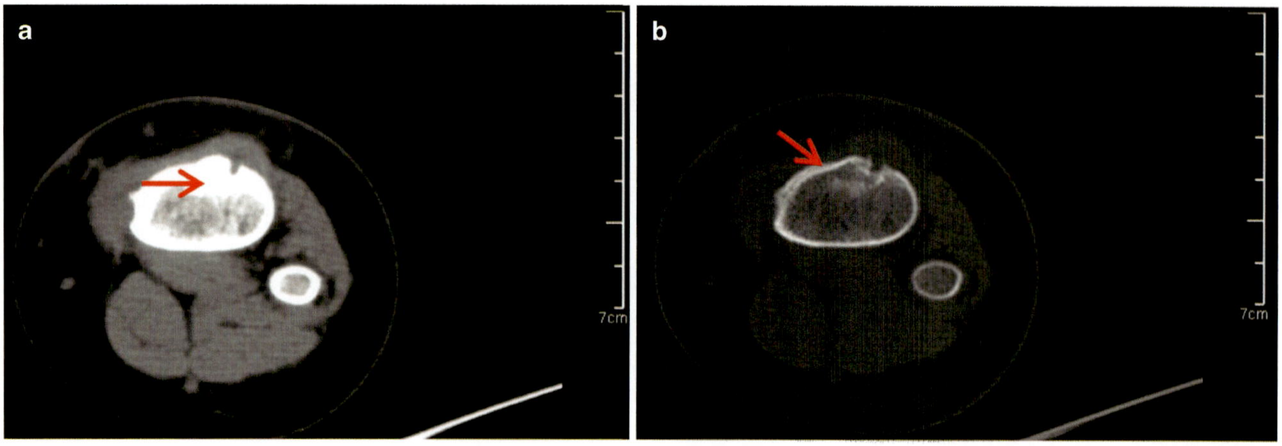

Fig. 8.12 At 4 months of illness, CT showed the mixed signal shadow at the near side of left tibia (**a**, **b**), and slight edema in surrounding soft tissue

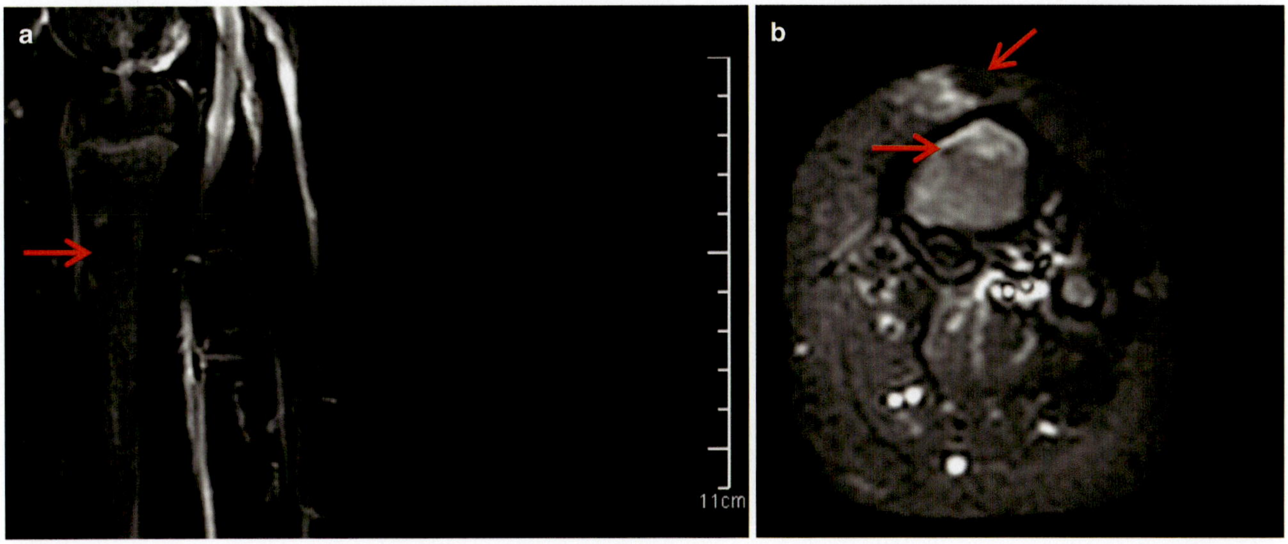

Fig. 8.13 At 9 months of illness, MR showed the mixed signal shadow at the near-end of left tibia (**a**), (b-down arrow), and slight edema in surrounding soft tissue. Mild pneumatosis (b-top arrow)

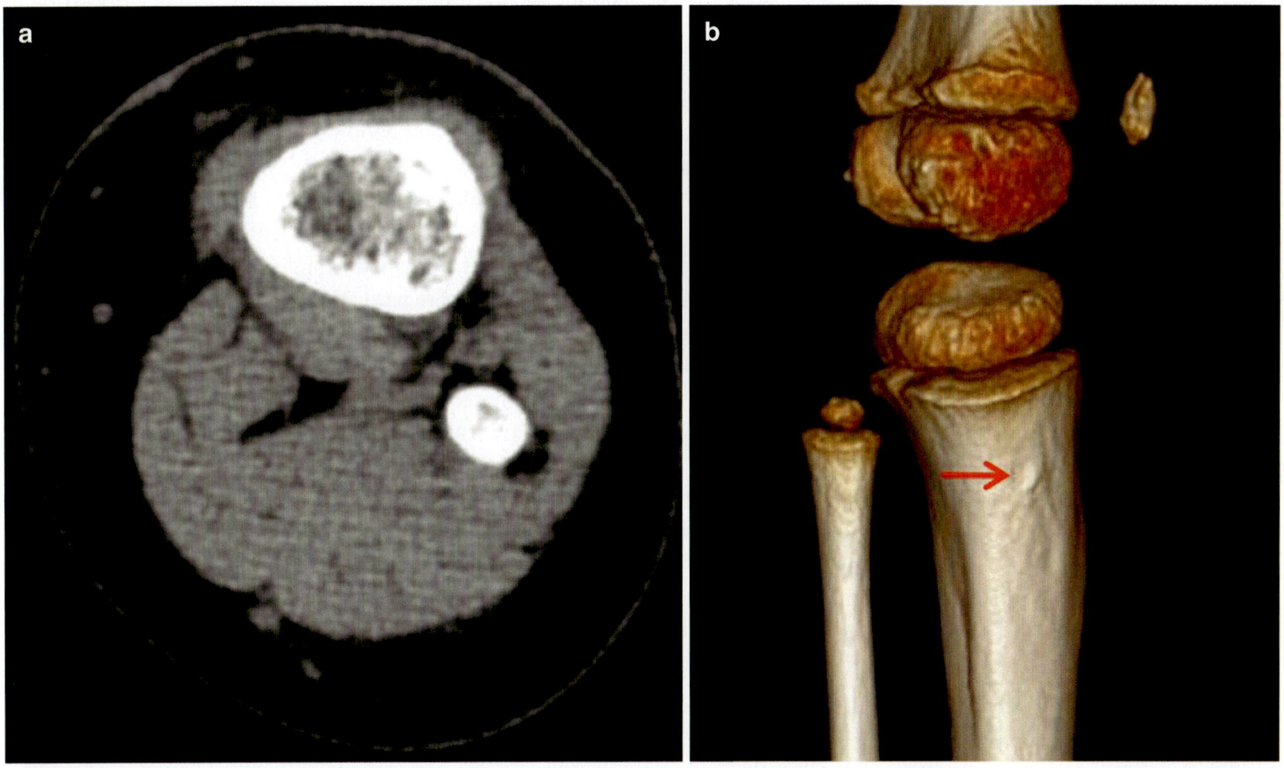

Fig. 8.14 At 13 months of illness, CT showed rounding soft tissue was slightly swollen and exuded. No definite showed the bone morphology of the proximal left tibia was irregular, abnormality was found in the morphology and density of left fibula the density of bone marrow cavity was increased unevenly, and the surrounding soft tissue was slightly swollen and exuded. No definite abnormality was found in the morphology and density of left fibula

8.1.4 Discussion

He met the criteria of KD for he had persistent fever for 9 days, antibiotic treatment was ineffective, along with (1) red and cracked lips with strawberry tongue, the course of the disease has perianal red, desquamate; (2) bilateral cervical lymphadenopathy over 1.5cm; (3) in the course of the disease, there was rashes all over body; (4) peering skin around fingernails.

The incidence of KD with arthritis was ranged from 16% [1] to 15–45% [2]. It may occur earlier at interphalangeal joint, cervical spine, and temporomandibular joints [3], usually accompanied with high-grade fever and subsequently subsided after IVIG. While arthritis mostly occurs at both knee and hip joints after IVIG around 10 day of illness (like this case), someone developed arthritis right after being discharged. The common changes shown in images were liquid effusion (see case 33). By now, the guideline for treating KD with arthritis was to use IVIG at first [4], followed by glucocorticoid combined with oral aspirin. In cases with mild arthritis, simple aspirin may also work. The prognosis was well after being treated with either aspirin or glucocorticoid, without sequelae [1].

8.1.5 The Specific Features of This Patient

1. He had fever, left knee pain and motion limit, positive streptococcus pneumonia growth from swallow brush culture, increased WBC with NE dominant, and elevated CRP. Both left knee CT permeability and MR signals showed periosteal hyperplasia and edema at surrounding soft tissue. Taken together, differential diagnosis of acute pyogenic osteomyelitis should be considered. But in the absence of pus in tibia marrow, acute purulent osteomyelitis could be excluded thoroughly. Pain symptoms are not severe, inactivity is not painful. Thus, we speculate that the lesion in the bone marrow may be a kind of aseptic necrosis.
2. Prior to this case, we usually perform DR, CT, or MR but not bone MR on joints (it was common seen on knee or hip) when patients complained about limb pain, and We have no experience with bone damage image initially, especially after his pharyngeal brush culture was positive with streptococcus growth, we could not sure definitely this image was bone damage rather than pyogenic osteomyelitis, of cause, his limb pain was happened only after fever, local skin and bone CT did not support osteosarcoma. Thus, once ECT scan did not found other lesions, incision and drainage operation were performed, the pathological examination confirmed it was inflammation other than tumor.
3. In order to determine bone injury before operation, both CT and MR were used and showed uneven density in bone marrow cavity; DR was normal. Therefore, we recommended to use CT or MR first rather than DR when suspecting bone damages.
4. After all, he was only a 3-year-old boy and the destruction of bone near the knee joint, the long-term prognosis was terrible if missed the optical treatment time. He was afebrile and local skin was normal when he was admitted in our ward. Based on gold standard, suppurative osteomyelitis was excluded, since there was no pup found in operation. Thus, we stop giving him antibiotics infusion as soon as CRP was subsided. At 1, 4, and 9 months of illness, rechecked CT of left knee joint also confirmed it.

Yan-xia Yang

8.2 Case 33: KD with Arthritis

A 5-year-old healthy girl was presented without significant past medical history or family immunology disease history.

She presented on Day 10 with intermittent fever for 10 days, along with red conjunctiva and red lips for 4 days. She received intramuscular injection of antifebrile medication, and intravenous injection of azithromycin and cefodizime in the local hospital for 3 days. Her fever was not reduced and she developed bilateral non-suppurative conjunctival congestion and red lips, along with watery stools, lack of appetite, and poor sleep. Examination found her mental state was stable, T 38.8°C, HR 138bpm, RR 28 bpm. Lymph nodes were significantly enlarged in both neck areas. Bilateral conjunctiva was congested without purulent secretion. She had red and cracked lips, strawberry tongue, and pharyngeal congestion. Her palms were hard and swollen, with the most serious edema at the right index finger. Others were normal. Auxiliary inspection was performed. On Day 8, WBC and CRP were elevated. Chest CT showed mild pneumonia. Admission blood test revealed WBC 30.19×10^9/L, NE 80.8%, HGB 10^9g/L, PLT 384×10^9/L. CRP 111mg/L. Troponin I, MYO, CKMB-Mass, and hs-cTnT were normal. NT-pro BNP 592.2pg/ml. Total 25 hydroxy vitamin D 18.67ng/ml. Na^+ 127mmol/L. DIC: PT 13.5s, PT activity 68%, INR 1.2, APTT 32s, D-dimer 666μg/L, FDP 10.1 mg/L, anti-thrombin activity assay 84%. IgG, IgA, and IgM were normal. ASO 45.2 IU/ml. Cervical ultrasound showed lymphadenectasis, the bigger one 1.3 cm×0.8 m on the left and 1.3 cm×1.0 m on the right. Liver ultrasound was normal. She had met the KD criteria four out of five, she was treated with (1) IVIG 2g/kg/day inner 24 hours; (2) oral aspirin 30–50mg/kg/day, dipyridamole 3–5mg/kg/day, in 3 divided doses; (3) third-generation cephalosporin infusion after blood sample drawn for culture test; (4) intravenous infusion of saline solution.

On Day 11, she had fever up to 38.6°C. Lab findings showed WBC 17.38×10^9/L, NE 71.6%, RBC 3.8×10^{12}/L, HGB 102g/L. CRP 145mg/L. K^+ 3.39mmol/L, Na^+ 134 mmol/L, Cl^- 99mmol/L. Fever was settled down on Day 12,

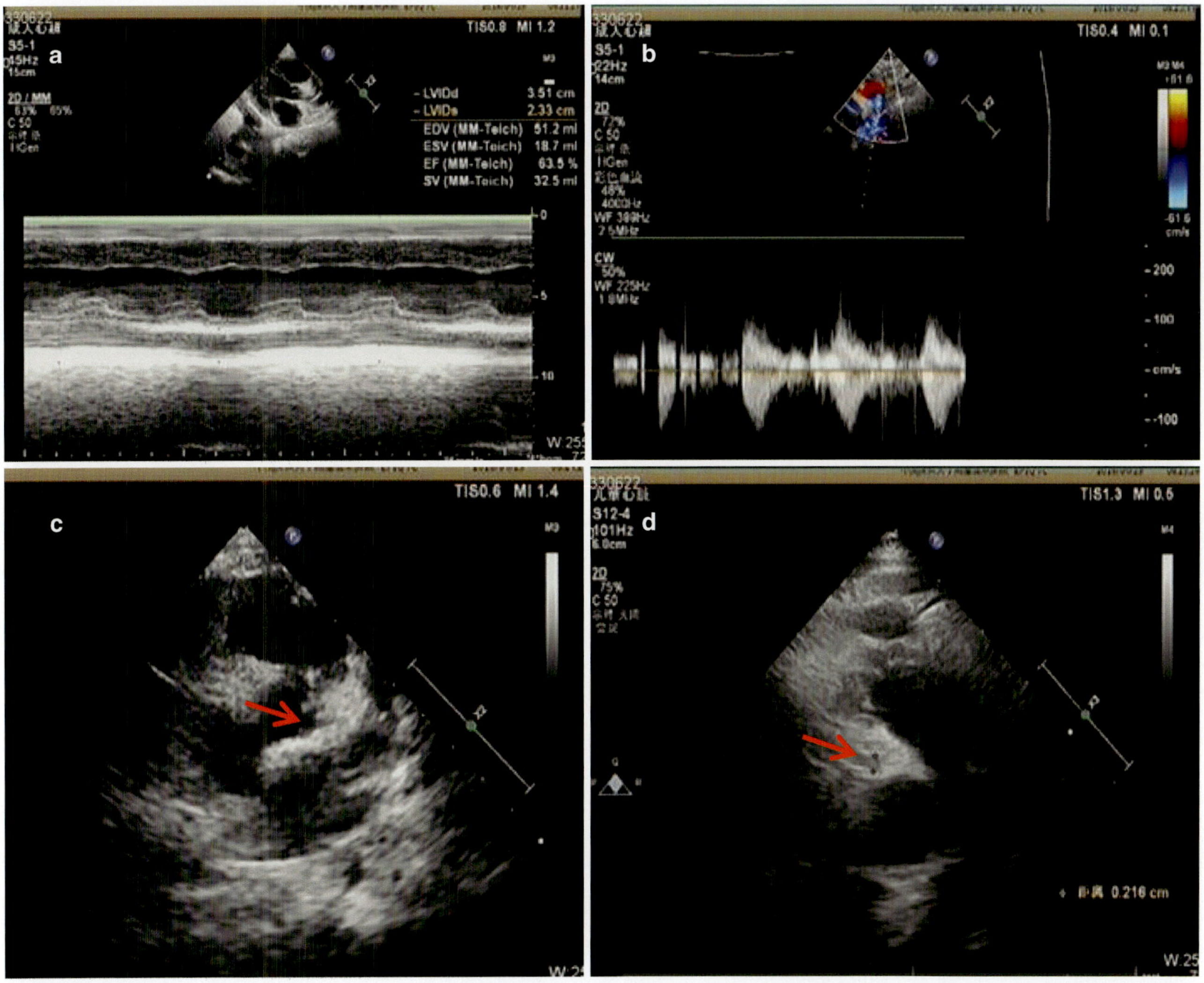

Fig. 8.15 On Day 12 of illness, echo showed LVED 33mm, LVEF 64% (**a**), mitral valve single peak (**b**), LCA 2.6mm (**c**), RCA 2.2mm (**d**)

the mental state was well. Physical examination results showed the same as when admitted. Echo showed normal LVED and LVEF (Fig. 8.15a). Mitral valve was single peak (Fig. 8.15b), normal LCA (Fig. 8.15c) and RCA (Fig. 8.15d). On Day 13, conjunctiva hyperemia improved. The skin peeled around right ring nail, edema hands were relieved. PPD 48–72 h was negative. Afebrile kept over 48 hours, aspirin was reduced to one dose 3–5mg/kg/day. On Day 15, bilateral conjunctiva disappeared. Strawberry tongue was regressed. CBC revealed WBC 11.13×10^9/L, NE 62.7%, RBC 4.6×10^{12}/L, HGB 121g/L, PLT 412×10^9/L. CRP 17.4mg/L. NT pro-BNP 669.6pg/ml. On Day 16, she was in good condition. Infusion medication was replaced with oral second-generation cephalosporin and then she was discharged. On Day 17, she felt numbness at both knee joints. On Day 18, the pain at knee joints was progressively aggravated. She limped around and her fever was up to 38.5°C 2 times. On Day 19, she still felt numbness at both knee joints, and was admitted again. Examination showed she had fever (T 38°C), bilateral knee joints showed normal skin and temperature, but had limited motion range. Retested CBC showed WBC15.0×10^9/L, NE 72.3%, HGB 98g/L, PLT 400×10^9/L. CRP 53.3mg/L. ESR 72mm/h. PCT 0.147ng/ml. Liver and kidney function, myocardial enzyme, glucose, and NT pro-BNP were normal. The bilateral knee DR result was normal (Fig. 8.16a, b). She was treated to continue to take oral aspirin and dipyridamole.

On Day 20, she had fever up to 38.5°C with occasionally painful knee joints and limited motion range, but had no swelling, redness, or heat on the skin. The ultrasound of right knee joint showed hydrops articuli, and the depth of effusion in suprapatellar sac was about 4.3 mm (Fig. 8.17a), while in suprapatellar sac was about 1.6 mm (Fig. 8.17b). The depth of effusion in suprapatellar sac on the left was about 7.3mm (Fig. 8.17b). She was given GCs (methylprednisolone 2mg/kg/day) infusion, aspirin was resume to 30–50mg/kg/day. On

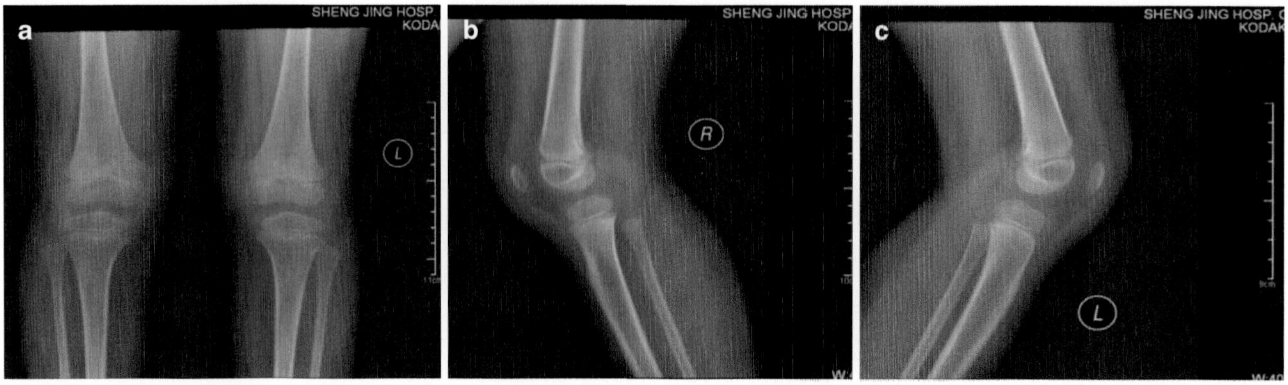

Fig. 8.16 On Day 19 of illness, bilateral knee showed normal joints DR anteroposterior position (**a**), right knee joint side position (**b**), and left knee joint side position (**c**) were normal

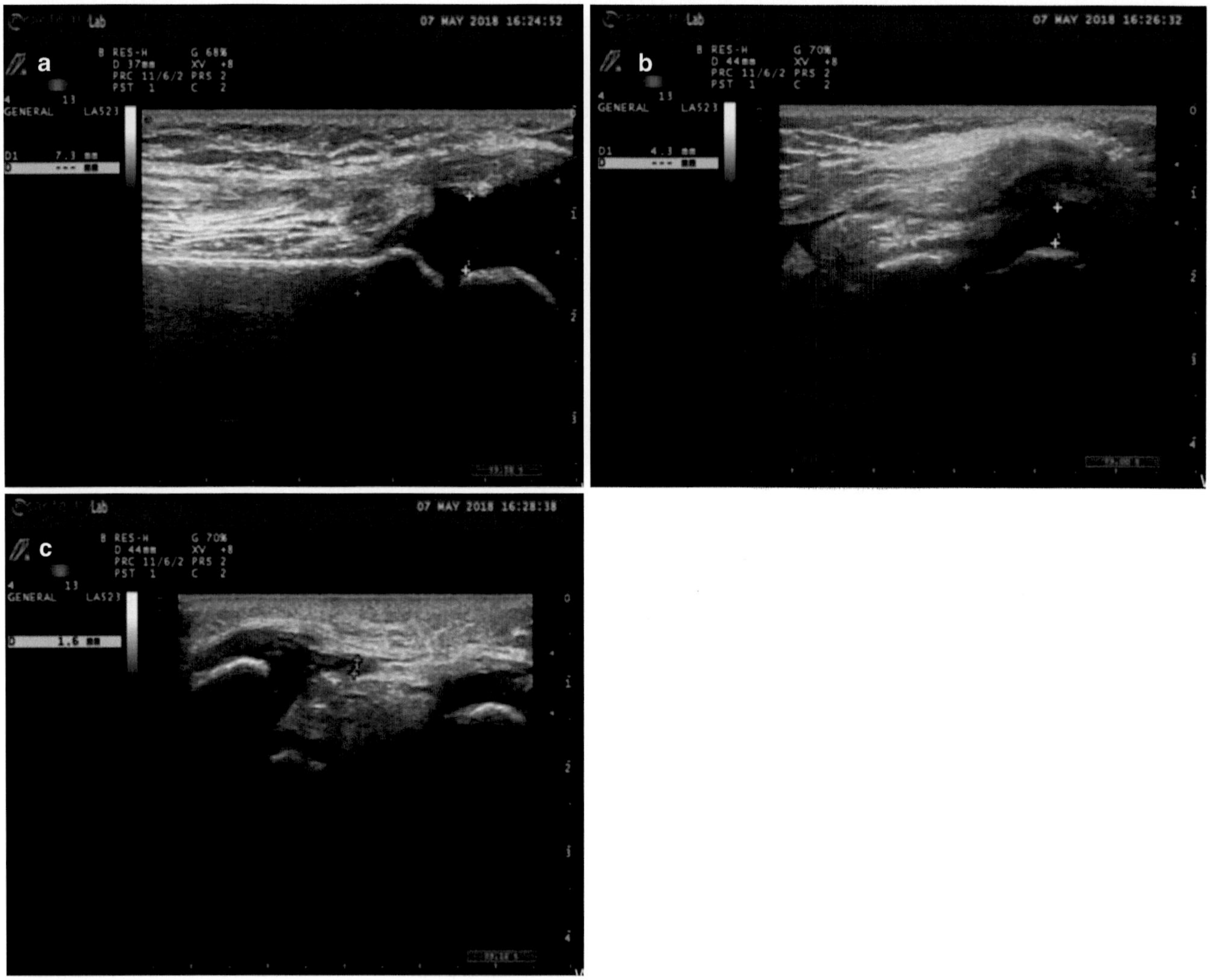

Fig. 8.17 On Day 20, sacral fluid of left knee was 7.3mm (**a**), right knee suprapatellar sac effusion was 4.3mm (**b**), infrapatellar sac effusion of right knee was 1.6mm (**c**)

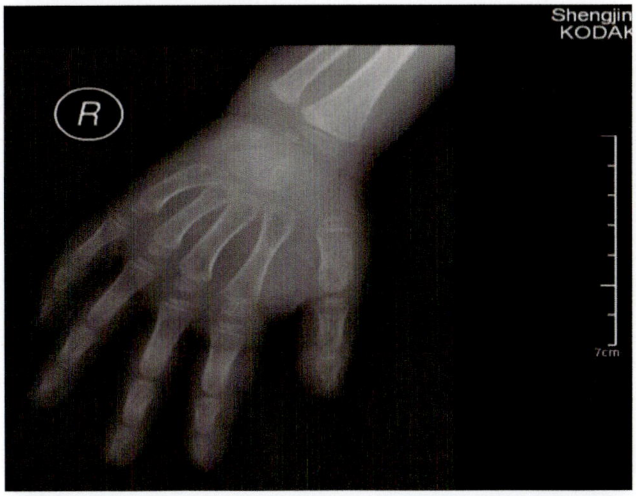

Fig. 8.18 On Day 20 of illness, right hand DR was normal

Day 21, her fever settled, the knee joints moved freely, but she felt numb on right hand and could not clench her fist. Examination found her right hand was swollen without redness, but DR of the right hand was normal (Fig. 8.18). On Day 22, the child walked freely. The right hand was tender, unable to make a fist, but swollen improved. The enlarged cervical lymphadenopathy regressed. Blood test revealed WBC 13.87×10^9/L, NE 60.2%, HGB 104g/L, PLT 424×10^9/L. PCT 0.095ng/ml. Liver function and glucose level were normal. On Day 23, her swollen right hand was obviously alleviated and could clench. After 3 days of low-dose methylprednisolone infusion, her fever and joins numbness were settled and her knees showed free range of motion. Her medication was switched to oral GC (prednisone 1mg/kg/day). Aspirin was reduced to one dose 3–5mg/kg/day and oral dipyridamole was continued. She was discharged on Day 24.

8.2.1 Clinic Course of the Patient

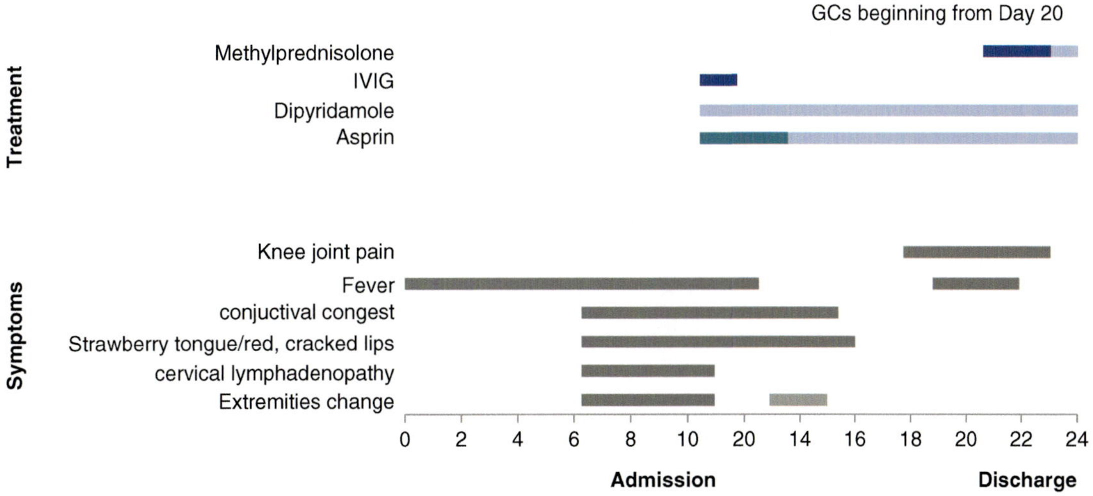

8.2.2 Follow-up

Since discharged, she took oral aspirin and dipyridamole 5mg/kg/day. Her joint symptoms disappeared one week after discharged. GC (prednisone) was tapered off within 15 days. At 2 months, ESR and PLT recovered to normal. Echo performed at 1 and 2 months of illness showed normal results. She stopped taking any medications. By now, she had followed up for 6 months, without uncomfortable and coronary artery was always normal (Table 8.1).

8.2.3 Diagnosis

1. KD
2. Bilateral knee arthritis
3. Acute bronchopneumonia
4. Vitamin D deficiency.

8.2.4 Discussion

This girl met the criteria of KD for she had persistent fever for 10 days, which was unresponsive to broad-spectrum antibiotic, along with (1) bilateral conjunctival hyperemia without purulent secretions; (2) red lips and cracked, strawberry tongue; (3) swollen hands and later peeling skin around fingernails; (4) cervical lymphadenectasis, lymphadenopathy on the first day 3–5 of illness followed by gradual regression, measured 1.3cm on Day 10 of illness. She had not met the criteria of IVIG resistance for she had no major KD symptoms except fever when she was admitted second time.

KD with joint symptom and recurrent fevers usually make diagnosis process difficult [5]. Differential diagnosis of juvenile rheumatoid arthritis (JRA) [6] should be considered.

Table 8.1 The dynamic changes of lab parameters

Days of illness	8 days	10 days	11 days	16 days	19 days	22 days	60 days
WBC (×10⁹/L)	33.1	30.19	17.38	11.13	15.0	13.87	
NE (%)		80.8	71.6	62.7	72.3	60.2	
HGB (g/L)		109	102	121	98	104	
PLT (×10⁹/L)		384		412	400	424	320
CRP (mg/L)	99.7	111	145	17.4	53.3		
ESR (mm)					72		14
PCT (ng/ml)					0.147	0.095	
NT pro-BNP (pg/ml)		592.2		669.6			
Sodium (mmol/L)		127	134				

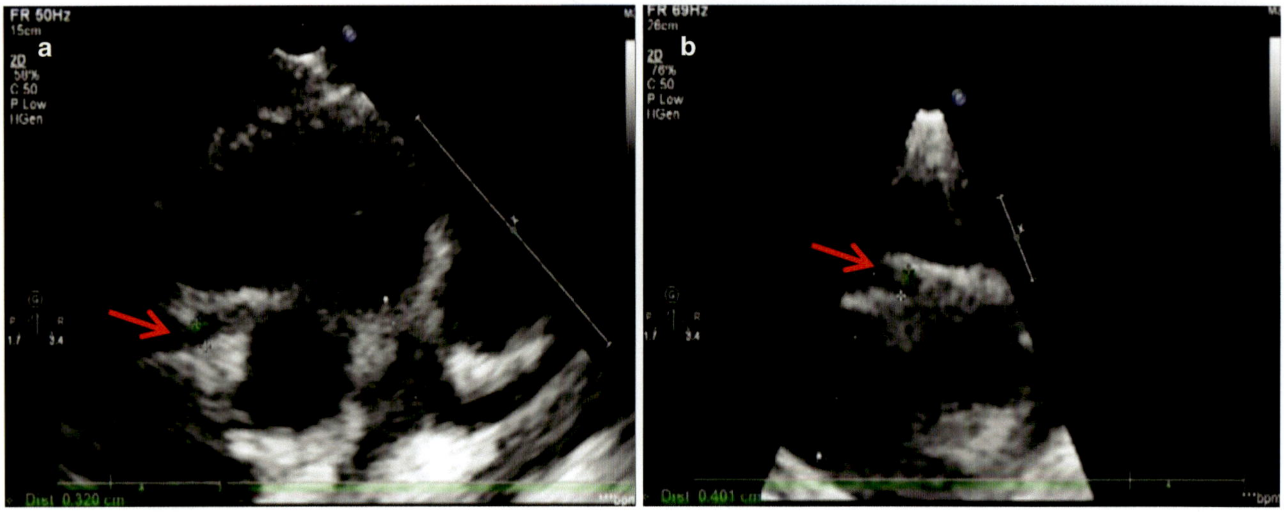

Fig. 8.19 Another 5-year-old KD girl, her RCA was 3.2mm on Day 7(**a**), and 4.0mm on Day 21(**b**) of illness

8.2.5 Case Specific Clinical Features

1. She had almost all KD phenotype, especially her joint symptoms were transient. She was treated with 2mg/kg/day of methylprednisolone for nearly 3 weeks until tapered down. At 6 months of illness, she did not have any of the following symptoms: fever, joint pain, swelling, or limited motion range, thus, JRA was excluded. KD with arthritis is not rare in clinic, but KD involved with joints is relatively rare compared to digestive and nervous systems [7].
2. For KD with arthritis, the first line treatment is to use non-steroidal anti-inflammatory drugs, such as aspirin at 30–50mg/kg/day. If it is ineffective, the alternative treatment is to use GCs. Based on the literature reports, different dosage of GCs has the same impact on CALs but has different effects on hospitalization duration [8]. Even in the absence of arthritis, GCs has been a popular treatment used in those IVIG resistance cases [9].
3. In our center, multiple small interphalangeal erythema and swollen during the first week of illness, and predominantly large weight-bearing joints, especially knees and ankles, which usually occurs after fever settled and mainly involving the lower limbs supporting weight joints in the second to third week of illness, The main symptoms include limited motion range, normal skin temperature at the affected joint, and rare floating patellar sign. This is basically consistent with the literature reports [10, 11]. KD joint involvement mainly include the joint cavity effusion without articular surface damage. Therefore, the prognosis is well, and no joint deformity or dysfunction would be formed. However, it is difficult to find hydrops articuli in DR test, but it would be seen clearly when using ultrasound, CT, and MR scan.
4. Most of the children with arthritis had no complication in coronary arteries. But in our center, we treated a 5-year-old girl with mild RCA dilation 4mm who had hydrops articuli at the same time (Figs. 8.19, 8.20, 8.21, 8.22). The joint symptoms recovered at 3 weeks and the coronary artery recovered at 3 months of illness. She took aspirin for total 6 months. By now, she has followed up with us almost 4 years, and both coronary arteries and joints are normal.

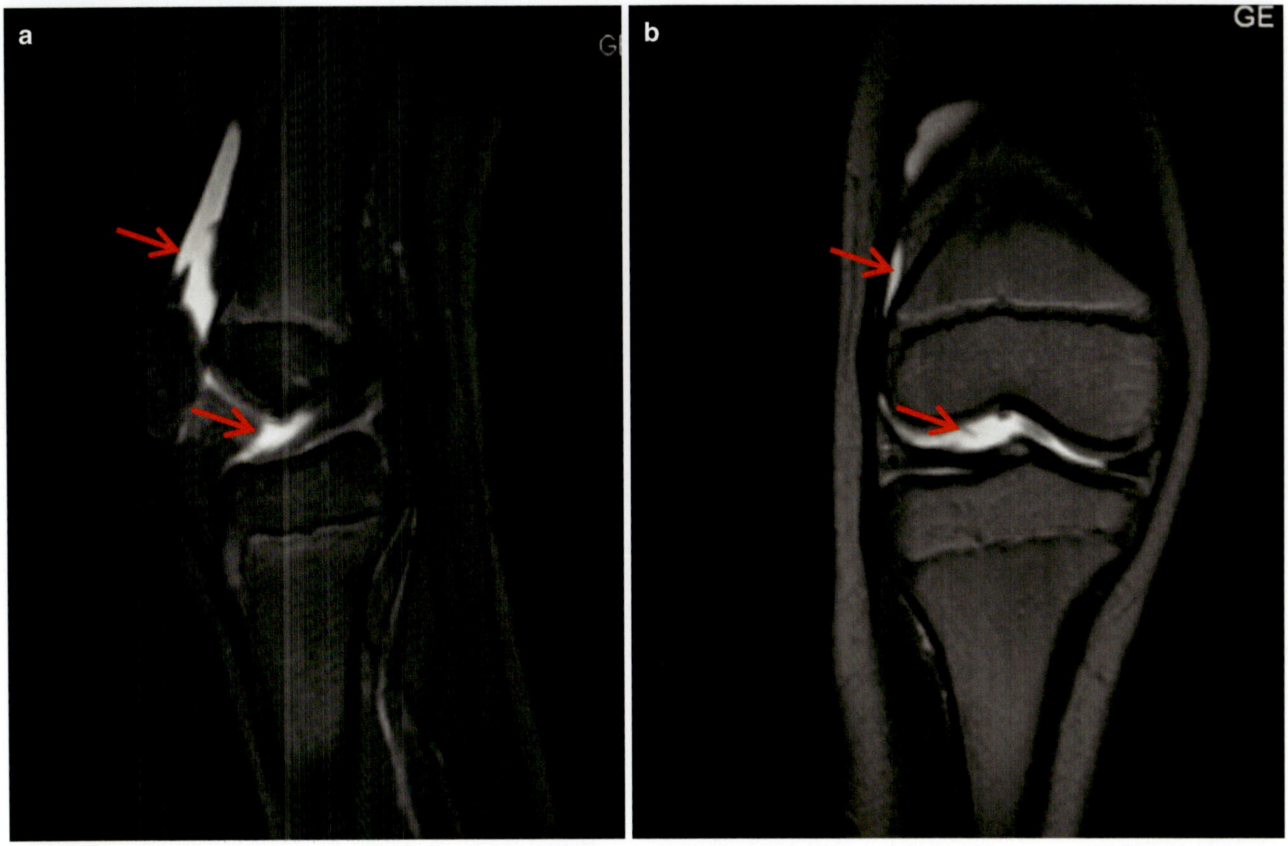

Fig. 8.20 Another 5-year-old KD girl, on Day 20, her right knee MR showed mild hydrops articuli (a-side position) (b-anteroposter)

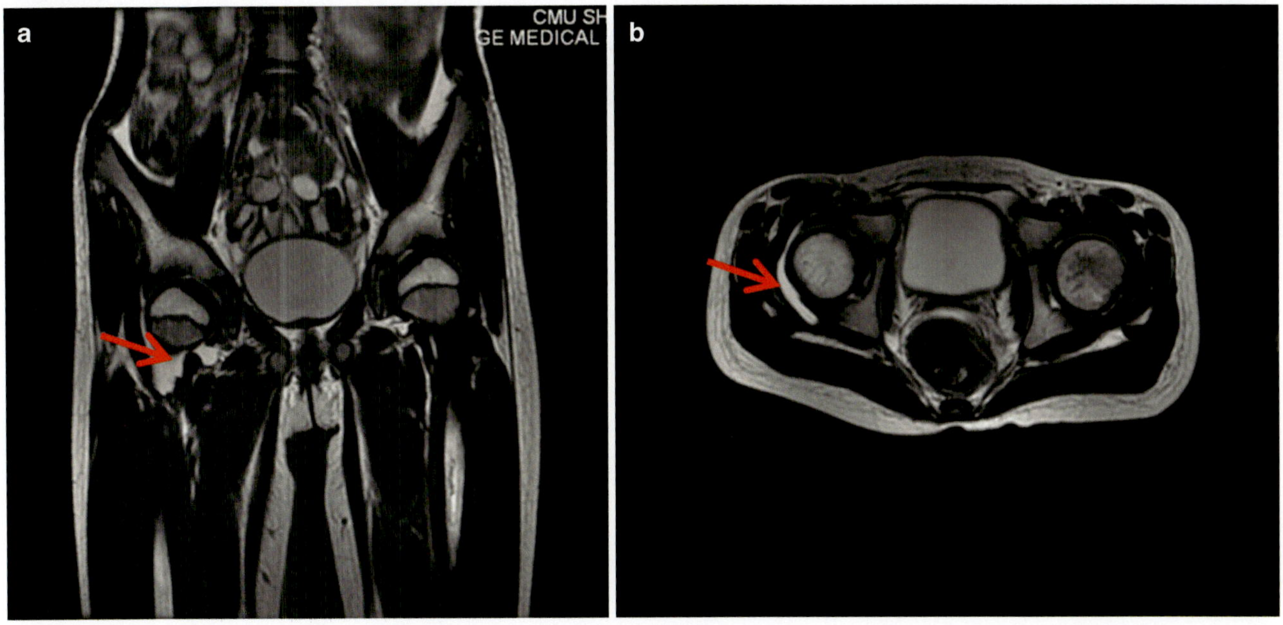

Fig. 8.21 Another 5-year-old KD girl, on Day 21, MR showed mild fluid effusion (a-longitudinal section) (b-cross section) on her right hip

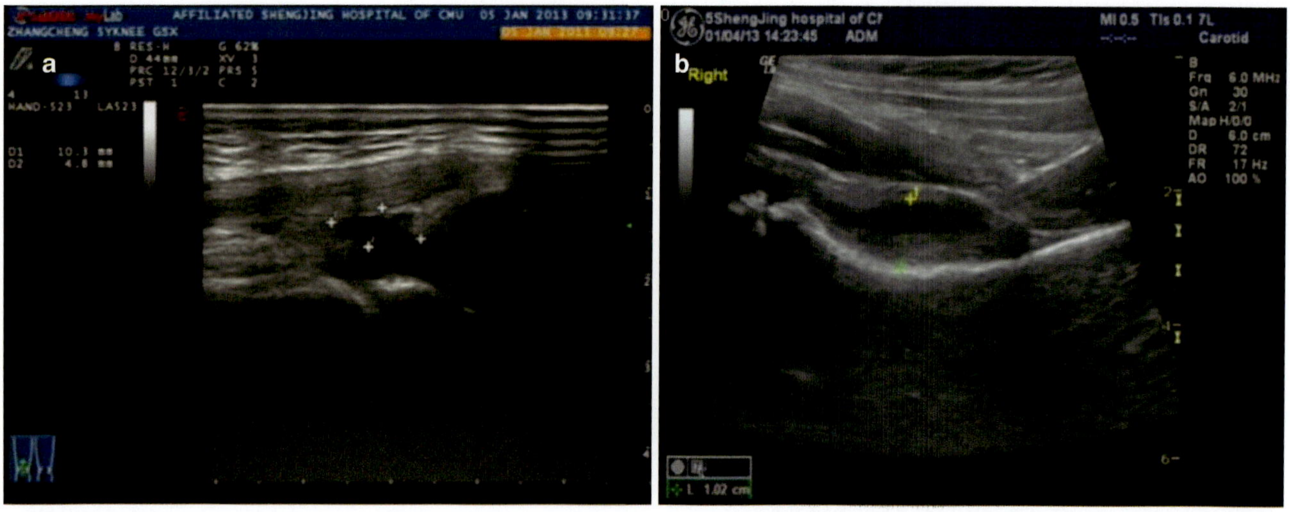

Fig. 8.22 Another 5-year-old KD girl, on Day 21, ultrasound showed mild knee fluid on her right knee join (**a**), and right hip joint (**b**)

Man Xu

References

1. Álvarez EP, Rey F, Peña SC, et al. Has joint involvement lessened in Kawasaki disease? Reumatol Clin. 2017, 13 (3):145-9.
2. Lee KY, Oh JH, Han JW, et al. Arthritis in disease after responding to intravenous immunoglobulin treatment. Eur J Pediatr. 2005;164(7):451–2.
3. Jen M, Brucia LA, Pollock AN, et al. Cervical spine and temporomandibular joint arthritis in a child with Kawasaki disease. Pediatr, 2006, 118(5):e1569-71.
4. Rodriguez MM, Wagner-Weiner L. Intravenous immunoglobulin in pediatric rheumatology: when to use it and what is the evidence. Pediatr Ann. 2017, 46 (1):e19-24.
5. Sahin S, Adrovic A, Barut K, et al. Systemic-onset juvenile idiopathic arthritis or incomplete Kawasaki disease: a diagnostic challenge. Clin Exp Rheumatol, 2017 May-Jun 35 Suppl 104 (2):10.
6. Shaikh S, Ishaque S, Saleem T. Incomplete, atypical Kawasaki disease or evolving systemic juvenile idiopathic arthritis: a case report. Cases J, 2009 Aug; 26962.
7. Martins A, Conde M, Brito M, et al. Arthritis in Kawasaki disease: A poorly recognised manifestation. J Paediatr Child Health. 2018, 54(12):1371-4.
8. Okubo Y, Michihata N, Morisaki N, et al. Association between dose of glucocorticoids and coronary artery lesions in Kawasaki disease. Arthritis Care Res (Hoboken).2018, 70 (7):1052-7.
9. Sundel RP, Burns JC, Baker A, et al. Gamma globulin re-treatment in Kawasaki disease. J Pediatr.1993, 123(4):657-9.
10. Gong GW, McCrindle BW, Ching JC, et al. Arthritis presenting during the acute phase of Kawasaki disease. J Pediatr.2006, 148:800-5.
11. Baker AL, Lu M, Minich LL, et al. Associated symptoms in the ten days before diagnosis of Kawasaki disease. J Pediatr.2009, 154:592-5.

KD with Adrenal Calcification

9

Hong Wang

Abstract

KD is a systemic vasculitis of unknown etiology that accumulates throughout the entire body, including the adrenal glands. It has been reported that KD may results in necrosis of adrenal medulla for inflammatory mediators [Orenstein and Kawasaki, Ultrastruct Pathol. 38(2):83-5, 2014]. However, we had no information how the patient develop calcification without a history of TB infection, and whether this calcification occurred this time. At least we hadn't found related literature to describe it. It's also not clear why this calcification shrinks. The adrenal medulla is the center of the adrenal gland. Under the innervation of sympathetic nerve, it can secrete adrenalin. It's most important function is to create the internal conditions for flight or fight through the sympathetic nerves in an emergency. Adrenomedullary chromaffin cell secrete the catecholamine hormones (including adrenal and norepinephrine). According to this inference, once the adrenal calcification occurs, the catecholamine secretion is reduced and the stress ability is reduced, which may be related to the shock and severe complications. The child had gastrointestinal and urinary tract involvement, but did not go into shock. Adrenal calcification may occur at the acute phase or before the onset of KD. In our center, there was a 4-year-old girl with KD complicated with shock (case 2). Chest CT and abdomen CT examination were performed during the acute phase, but we couldn't found adrenal abnormality. So it seems to suggest that the adrenal lesions at KD are not associated with shock.

In this chapter, we presented one case. She was a 16-month old girl with first time KD. Adrenal calcification was found by chance on chest CT when she had her first KD. Two years later when she got KD again, this calcification was is regression. The mechanism was still unclear and future research needs to be done to understand the mechanism.

H. Wang (✉)
Department of Pediatric Cardiology, Shengjing Hospital of China Medical University, Shenyang, Liaoning, P. R. China

9.1 Case 34: KD with Adrenal Calcification

A previous healthy 16-month-old girl presented with unremarkable past medical history and family history.

She presented on Day one of illness, with fever for one day and dyspnea for 4 h. One day prior, she had a fever 39.0 °C, with cold hands and feet, took ibuprofen but fever did not subside, and rashes developed on her trunk. Early this morning she had fever at 38.5 °C again, lost appetite, and came to our emergency room. After intravenous aspirin 0.12 treatment, fever did not regress, dyspnea was developed, and general condition was deteriorating. Thus, she was admitted in PICU. Examination revealed the following results: T 39.8 °C, PR 148 bpm, RR 37 bpm, BP 95/50 mmHg. Wt. 12 kg. SO_2 was 98% after oxygen inhalation by nasal catheter. Her spirits were drooping. Cervical lymphadenectasis was 1.5 cm. Auscultation findings included phlegm in both Lungs. She had Cold hands and feed, capillary refilling time (CRT) was 4 s. Others were normal. Admission blood test revealed WBC 12.4×10^9/L, NE 80.18%, RBC 3.917×10^{12}/L, HBG 113.9 g/L, PLT 250×10^9/L. CRP 30.90 mg/L. Blood ammonia 41.6 μmol/L. DIC: FIB 5.3 g/L, D-Dimer 748 μg/L. ALT 472U/L, AST 1447U/L. CK-MB 38U/L. CK, CKMB-M, cTnI, and blood gas analysis were normal. She was treated with (1) infusion of erythromycin and liver protectant; (2) oral paracetamol; (3) planned chest CT scan but turned down by her parents.

On the Day 3, she was febrile, 38–39 °C. Examination found cervical lymphadenectasis. Lips were red and cracked. She had strawberry tongue, and congested pharynx. Perianal redness occurred but no peeling. Investigation revealed MP-IgM mild positive, MP-IgG 1:80. Ultrasound showed left cervical lymphadenopathy, the bigger one 1.9 cm × 0.7 cm on the left, 2.3 cm × 0.7 cm on the right.

H. Wang (ed.), *Paediatric Kawasaki Disease*, https://doi.org/10.1007/978-981-15-0038-1_9

Abdominal ultrasound showed there was a mass on the left lower ventral (Fig. 9.1). Indigitation was suspected. Chest DR showed texture enhancement on both lungs. She had following disorders: (1) MP infection; (2) liver dysfunction; and (3) suspected intestinal intussusceptions. She was treated with (1) third-generation cephalosporin to replace current antibiotics; (2) pediatric surgeon suggested fasting water transiently, taking carbon powder, observing her vomiting and abdominal signs. If carbon dust was found in stool, it indicated there was no ileac obstruction, and she would be allowed to intake liquid food. Then she was followed up.

On the Day 4, she had fever at 39 °C. Carbon powder was found in stool and she took some liquid without ventosity. She was transferred to respiratory ward as "severe pneumonia," and the resident found she had bilateral conjunctival congestion, red and cracked lips, lymphadenectasis, and erythema palms. KD was highly suspected. Consultation with cardiologist concluded that she had met the criteria 4 out of 5 for KD. Then she was transferred to cardiology ward and treated with (1) oral aspirin and dipyridamole; (2) IVIG 1 g/kg/day for 2 days.

On the Day 5, her fever (38.6 °C) could subside with physical therapy and she developed a little dysesthesia. Otherwise, there was a band of itching rash about 3 cm on her hands, back, and pygal. We stopped to give her third-generation cephalosporin infusion and oral aspirin. Investigation revealed WBC 18.3 × 10^9/L, NE 68.6%, RBC 3.8 × 10^{12}/L, HGB 110 g/L, PLT 330 × 10^9/L. ESR 45 mm/h. NT pro-BNP 484 (<300 pg/ml). Liver function showed: ALB 38.9 g/L, ALT 534 (<40 U/L), AST 114 U/L. CK 190 U/L, CKMB 167 U/L. DIC PT 12.3 s, APTT 31 s, INR 1.2, D-dimer 688 μg/L. Abdominal CT scan showed more air accumulated in the middle and upper abdominal intestine accompanied with ventosity. There was some gas-liquid level in the intestine located at the left lower abdomen (Fig. 9.2). We were concerned about partial intestinal obstruction. On the Day 8, fever continued to stay up to 39.6 °C. She started to cough and there was a laryngeal stridor when breathing in. She was treated with (1) oral paracetamol; (2) continued on IVIG 1 g/kg/day (total 3 g/kg/day); (2) infusion of azithromycin; (4) dexamethasone inhale.

On the Day 10, she was afebrile over 48 h but mild cough. Rashes regressed. Lips were still red and dry with strawberry tongue. There occurred peeling skin around left fingernails. Investigation revealed WBC 7.9 × 10^9/L, NE 39.4%, RBC 3.6 × 10^{12}/L, HGB 101 g/L, PLT 578 × 10^9/L. CRP 8.34 mg/L. TP 81.9 g/L, ALB 28.40 g/L, ALT 71 U/L. AST, CK, and CKMB were normal. Chest CT scan showed mild pneumonia on the right lung (Fig. 9.3a) and there were multiple calcifications in the right adrenal gland (Fig. 9.3b). She was treated with (1) reduced dose of aspirin at one dose 3–5 mg/kg; (2) infusion of medication for liver protection; (3) infusion of albumin 1 g/kg/day for 2 days. Consultation with dermatologist concluded she had drug related rash. Abdominal ultrasound revealed no concentric circle sign. She stopped taking liver protection medication but continued to take oral aspirin and clarityne.

On the Day 14, everything went well. Rash settled though with itching. Cough improved. Strawberry tongue symptom disappeared. Peeling skin occurred around multiple fingernails. The patient was discharged next day.

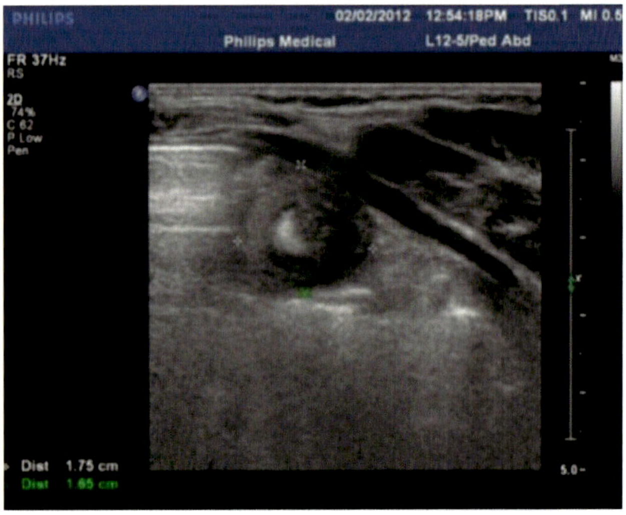

Fig. 9.1 On Day 2 of illness, abdominal ultrasonic showed there was a mass on the left lower ventral. Indigitation was suspected

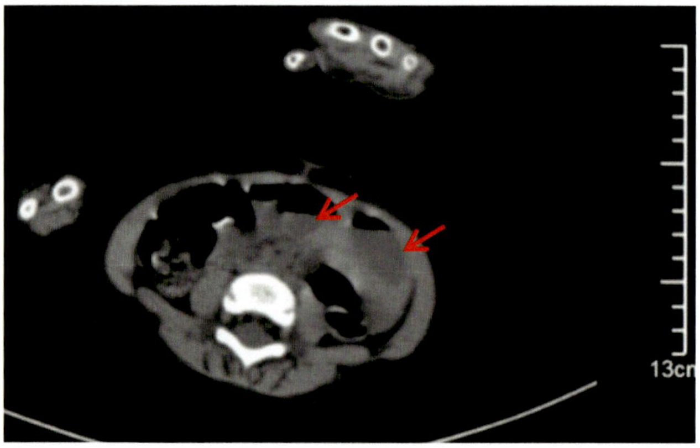

Fig. 9.2 On Day 5 of illness, abdominal CT showed there was more accumulation of air in the middle and upper abdominal intestine accompanied by expansion, there was some gas-liquid level in the intestine on the left lower abdomen

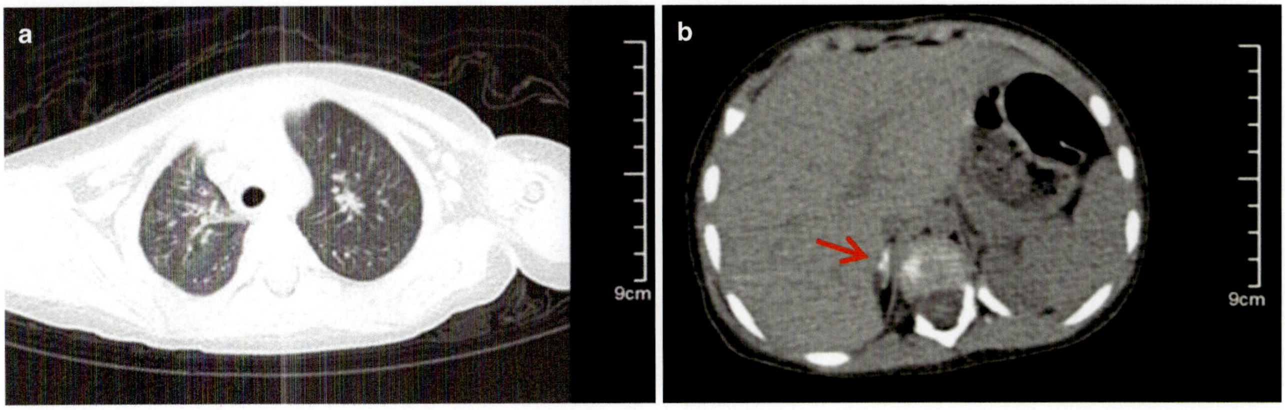

Fig. 9.3 On Day 10 of illness, chest CT showed there was mild pneumonia on the right lung (**a**). There were calcifications in the right adrenal gland (**b**)

9.1.1 Clinical Course of the Patient—First Admission

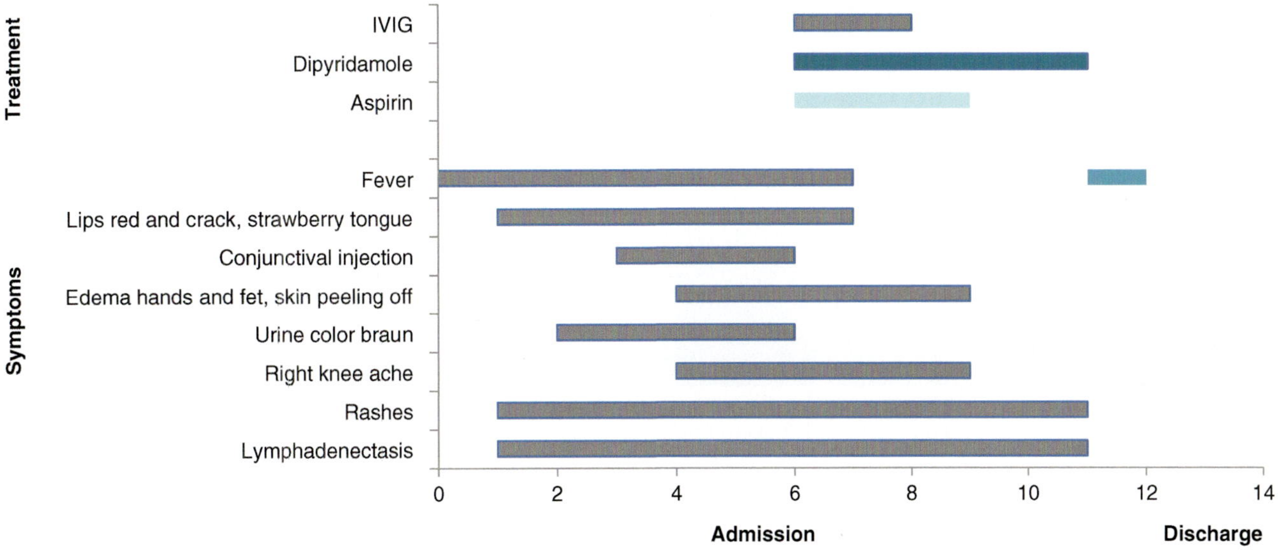

9.1.2 Follow-Up

Since discharge, her parents stopped to give her any medications about one week later. She did not have follow-up at out-patient clinic until recurrent KD.

Twenty months later, she presented again on Day 4 with constant fever at 40–38.3 °C, along with dry and red lips for 3 days, bilateral conjunctive congestion for one day. On Day 2 of illness, she developed abdomen ache and diarrhea. Her abdomen ache was not subsided after watery stool. At a local hospital, she received infusion of fourth-generation cephalosporin for 3 days in local, but her fever did not subside. On Day 2, her urine was dark like bean oil, and she lost appetite significantly and slept lightly. Urine account was normal. On Day 3, she was given dexamethasone 3 mg infusion, fever was under control for only 10 h, and she developed bilateral conjunctiva congestion. On Day 4 she developed rashes all over the body along with ache and numbness at right knee and had difficulty when walking. Examination revealed the following results: T 38.9 °C, PR 144 bpm, RR 36 bpm, BP 116/69 mmHg. Wt. 16 kg. Mental state was bad. There were scattered rashes on the trunk, without jaundice and bleeding. She had fast breathe rate, bilateral conjunctiva congestion, red and cracked lips with strawberry tongue. Left leg had free range of motion, right knee presented limited range of motion, and local skin and temperature were normal. Others were normal. Investigation revealed on Day 3 of illness, WBC 30.3 × 10^9/L, NE 84.8%, RBC 4.32 × 10^{12}/L, HBG 122 g/L, PLT 207 × 10^9/L. Urobilinogen+, bilirubin+. No occult blood and erythrocyte. Chest CT scan showed pneumonia regress and smaller adrenal calcification (Fig. 9.4). On Day of 5, she had persistent fever with significant malaise. The urine color was still dark brown but lighter than that at admission. Investigation revealed Bil T 28.8 μmol/L, Bil D 18.7 μmol/L. She had met the criteria for recurrent KD and liver dysfunction. She was treated with IVIG 1 g/kg/day for two days and oral aspirin and dipyridamole. Reticulocyte (1.7%) was normal, though dark brown urine color, which was not consistent with hemolysis. There was no need to perform Coombs test. On Day 6 of recurrence of illness, her fever regressed to 37.4 °C and she had a little cough and her urine color was normal. Extremity showed edema feet and hands and erythema of the palms. Echo was performed and showed coronary artery was normal. Civiler ultrasound showed right cervical lymphadenectasis 2.1 cm × 0.8 cm.

On Day 7, fever was settled. Blood test revealed ALT 306 U/L, AST 28 U/L, γ-GT 175 U/L, T Bil 20.8 μmol/L, D Bil 13.7 μmol/L. TBA 12.5 μmol/L. EBV-IgM negative (3.6) AU/ml. EBV EA-IgG positive (41.6), both EBV NA-IgG (3.0) and EBV VCA-IgG (10.0) were negative. Additional diagnosis of EBV infection was made, and she was given infusion of ganciclovir 7.5 mg/kg/day for 5 days and oral ursodeoxycholic acid. On Day 9, she had afebrile over 48 h, edema hand and feet were settled. Aspirin dose was reduced. On Day 11, she had epistaxis once, but it stopped when nasal cavity pressed. Investigation showed CKMB-M, CRP, and TB antibody were normal. ALT 51 (<40 U/L), blood culture was negative and she was discharged. After discharge from second admission, she had never followed up with us at outpatient clinic (Table 9.1).

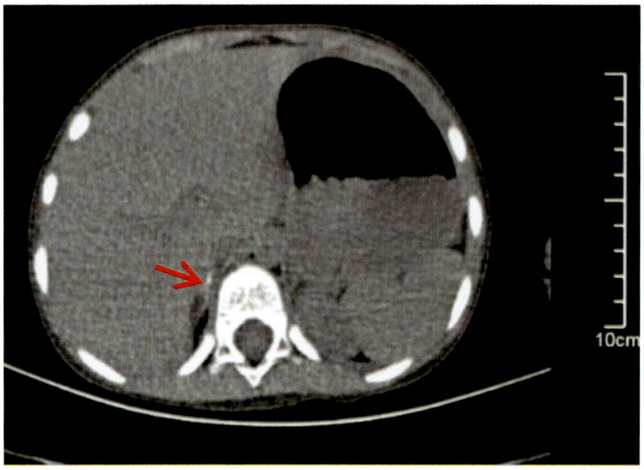

Fig. 9.4 At 20 months of illness, chest CT showed calcification of right adrenal gland improved

Table 9.1 The dynamic changes of lab parameters

	First admission				Second admission			
Days	2 days	5 days	10 days	14 days	3 days	4 days	5 days	11 days
WBC ($\times10^9$/L)	12.4	18.3	7.9	6.25	30.3	15.3	19.5	9.9
N (%)	80.2	68.6	39.4	45.8	84.8	80	88.2	31.2
RBC ($\times10^{12}$/L)	3.92	3.8	3.6	3.82	4.32	4.4	4.4	4.3
HGB (g/L)	113	110	101	106.9	122	119	117	114
PLT ($\times10^9$/L)	250	330	578	492	207	348	344	594
RC (%)						1.7	1.7	
CRP (mg/L)	30.9		8.34	2.82		33.9		4.23
ESR (mm)		45					60	
ALT (U/L)	472	534	71	26		487	306	51
ALB (g/L)		38.9	28.4	31.5		39.5	35.2	30
NT pro-BNP (pg/ml)		484					109.7	
TBA (μmol/L)							12	9.1
GGT (U/L)							175	73

9.1.3 Clinical Course of the Patient—Second Admission

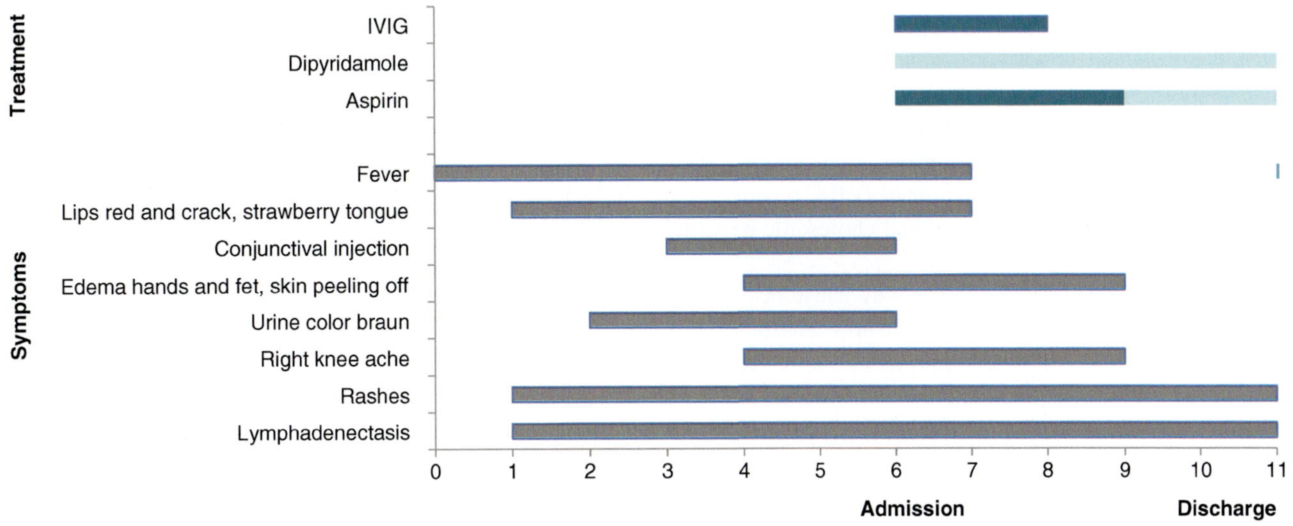

9.1.4 Diagnosis

1. KD recurrence
2. Adrenal Calcification
3. Liver Dysfunction
4. Hypoalbuminemia
5. Intussusception, incomplete ileus
6. Acute bronchopneumonia
7. EBV infection.

9.1.5 Discussion

She had met all KD criteria at both first and second time when presented at hospitals [1]. Differential diagnosis of sepsis and viral conjunctivitis should be considered.

9.1.6 Case Special Clinical Features

1. This girl was taken to hospital at first illness, on Day 2–3 she developed rashes all over body and cervical lymphadenectasis, and investigation revealed WBC and CRP increased significantly. A resident on duty considered she had KD and requested tests on the NT pro-BNP and ESR. But she was in PICU, where residents shift frequently and are very busy in PICU of China. The next resident on duty neglected the note and missed her red conjunctiva, and transferred the patient to respiratory ward as severe pneumonia patient. If he reviewed her chest CT scan results with care, he would have found her pneumonia was not so severe, but her ALT was up to 437 U/L and she had hands/feet edema (on Day 5 of illness her albumen was normal). Thanks to the resident of respiratory ward who found her symptoms met criteria of KD and requested consultation with. Luckily she was treated on time.
2. Aspirin has been the first choice to treat KD. This girl developed rashes after taking aspirin when she had recurrent KD. Considering she had taken aspirin before and did not have itch, we continued to give her aspirin and monitored the dynamic changes in rashes at the same time. Eventually, rashes regressed. We concluded that she was not allergic to aspirin [2].
3. It has been reported that about 1–2% KD patients will have recurrent KD within 2 years [1]. During the treatment for her first KD, aspirin was stopped earlier, and there was no record showing when she stopped taking aspirin during recurrent KD. Coronary dilation was not found until on Day11 of recurred KD.
4. KD vasculitis can present all over the body, which can cause inflammation in intestinal arteries, leading to edema in intestinal wall. As a result of this edema, indigitation is developed and will need warm saline clysis to be relieved (case 25). However, if it is not identified on time, the complication can lead to intesti-

nal obstruction, and then the necrosis segment need to be surgically removed. This girl had incomplete indigitation, and the inflammation regressed after IVIG and oral aspirin treatment, and then edema in intestine settled subsequently.

5. The most common complication in KD is digestive system symptoms. When this patient had recurrence of KD, she had black stool and dark brown urine. Investigation revealed higher T Bil and major in D Bil, positive urobilirubin, which supported she had cholestatic hepatitis (case 17).
6. In KD, inflammatory mediators may cause necrosis of adrenal medulla [3]. It is not clear how calcification is developed in acute stage and there is no literature reporting this. The calcification was found by chance in chest CT performed in her first KD diagnosis. It was regressed two years later when she had recurrent KD. The mechanism is not clear and further researches need to be done.

Hong Wang

References

1. Newburger JW, Takahashi M, Gerber MA, et al. Diagnosis, treatment, and long-term management of Kawasaki disease: a statement for health professionals from the Committee on Rheumatic Fever, Endocarditis and Kawasaki Disease, Council on Cardiovascular Disease in the Young, American Heart Association. Circulation. 2004;110(17):2747–71.
2. Jiao LP. A case repot of Aspirin allergy in child. Clin J Med Officer. 2004;32(4):9.
3. Orenstein JM. Kawasaki Disease has so much to teach us! Ultrastruct Pathol. 2014;38(2):83–5.

KD with IVIG Resistance

10

Yanqiu Chu, Xuexin Yu, Hong Wang, Ce Wang, and Xuan Liu

Abstract

The IVIG resistance defines that patients with KD develop recrudescent or persistent fever at least 36 h after the end of IVIG infusion [McCrindle et al., Circulation 135(17):e927–99, 2017]. Although IVIG was administered as soon as KD was established within 10 days of illness, approximately 10–20% patients developed IVIG resistance. These patients have an increased risk of CAA compared to those IVIG responders (15% vs. 5%) [Tremoulet et al. J Pediatr. 153(1):117–21, 2008]. Thus, identification of children who are likely to be IVIG resistant would allow utilizing additional therapies early in the course of their illness, and thus it would be possible to prevent coronary artery lesions. In 2006, Kobayashi et al designed scoring systems to predict IVIG resistance, risk factors include sodium≤133 mmol/L; days of illness at initial treatment≤4; ALT≥100 IU/L; neutrophils≥80%; CRP≥100 mg/L; age ≤12 months; platelet count ≤300 × 10^9/L[Kobayashi et al., Circulation 113:2606–12, 2006]. In 2007, Kuo et al reported that post-IVIG eosinophilia (peripheral blood eosinophils ≥4%) had an inverse correlation to IVIG resistance and pre-IVIG hypoalbuminemia (albumin≤3.0 g/dL) was positively correlated with IVIG resistance[Kuo et al., Pediatr Allergy Immunol. 18:354–9, 2007]. In 2013, Fu PP et al established scoring systems especially to predict IVIG resistance in Chinese Children with KD, plus clinical characteristics (polymorphous exanthema, changes around the anus) compared with the previous system [Fu et al. Pediatr Infect Dis J. 32:e319–23, 2013].

It is reasonable to administer a second dose of IVIG (2 g/kg) to IVIG-resistant patients [Sundel et al., J Pediatr. 123(4):657–9, 1993], high-dose pulse steroids (usually methylprednisolone 20–30 mg/kg intravenously for 3 days, with or without a subsequent course and taper of oral prednisone) may be considered as an alternative to a second infusion of IVIG or for retreatment of patients with KD who have had recurrent or recrudescent fever after additional IVIG [Kobayashi et al. J Pediatr. 163(2):521–6, 2013]. Administration of infliximab (5 mg/kg) may be considered as an alternative to a second infusion of IVIG or corticosteroids for IVIG-resistant patients, cyclosporine may be considered in patients with refractory KD in whom a second IVIG infusion, infliximab, or a course of steroids has failed, immunomodulatory monoclonal antibody therapy (except TNF-α blockers), cytotoxic agents, or (rarely) plasma exchange may be considered in highly refractory patients who have failed to respond to a second infusion of IVIG, an extended course of steroids, or infliximab [McCrindle et al., Circulation 135(17):e927–99, 2017].

Y. Chu · X. Yu · H. Wang (✉) · C. Wang
Department of Pediatric Cardiology, Shengjing Hospital of China Medical University, Shenyang, Liaoning, P. R. China

X. Liu
Department of Hematology Laboratory, Shengjing Hospital of China Medical University, Shenyang, Liaoning, P. R. China

10.1 Case 35: KD with IVIG Resistance-IVIG too Early

A previously healthy 2-year-old male presented with unremarkable past medical history and family history.

He presented on Day 5 of illness with a 5-day history of persistent high fever along with rashes and 4-day history of bilateral conjunctivitis. Edema showed on hands and feet after cephalosporin infusion once. On Day 3 of illness he was admitted to local hospital as KD where he received IVIG (1 g/kg/day), furosemide, and methylprednisolone. Rashes were settled down but not fever. On the Day 5, he was transferred to our pediatric cardiology ward. *Examination* revealed fever (39.9 °C), poor mental state, and delayed response to surroundings. Cervical lymphadenectasis (1.5 cm), bilateral conjunctivitis, red cracked lips with strawberry tongue, and red and edematous palms and soles were

H. Wang (ed.), *Paediatric Kawasaki Disease*, https://doi.org/10.1007/978-981-15-0038-1_10

Table 10.1 The dynamic changes of Laboratory parameters

Time	3 days	5 days	6 days	9 days	13 days	16 days	19 days	22 days	6 months
WBC (×10^9)		9.6		21.67	22.1	14.94	7.11		7.4
NE (%)		79.5		75.7	77.2	55.1	36.5		38.1
HGB (mg/L)		100		99	90	104	108		127
PLT (×10^9)		252		799	799	600	363		305
CRP (mg/L)	74	35.6		91	18.8	11.4	13.3	6.58	3.76
NT pro- BNP (pg/ml)	2580	962.9		846.9		80.42			305
ALT (U/L)	103		75						
ALB (U/L)			30.2						

present. There were rashes on his face, skin around BCG site, and crissum was red without desquamation. Others were normal. *Admission blood* test results were listed in Table 10.1. Echo in local hospital showed bilateral dilation at initial part of coronary artery (LCA 4.1 mm, RCA 4.6 mm). For the boy met all the criteria of KD, he was given oral aspirin (30–50 mg/kg/day), dipyridamole (3–5 mg/kg/day), erythromycin, and third-generation cephalosporin, also polyene phosphorus ester acid radical choline (0.5 g/day) and compound glycyrrhizin (20 ml/day, to protect liver).

On the Day 6, he was still febrile (>38.5 °C) and dispirited. The neck stiffness was positive. Liver function showed Alb 30.2 g/L, ALT 75 U/L, AST 63 U/L. MP-IgG (+), CP-IgG (+). ESR 60 mm/h. Neck ultrasound revealed bilateral cervical lymphadenectasis, with the biggest one about 2.3 cm × 1.0 cm. IVIG (2 g/kg) infusion was given within 24 h/over 12 h. Mannitol and furosemide were administrated after half of IVIG infusion. On Day 7, the high fever was persistent (39.5 °C) and he was in significant malaise. The lumbar puncture showed CSF pressure was 72 drops/min and CSF was lightly yellow and transparent, Pandy test(+), total cell 238 × 10^6/L, WBC 238 × 10^6/L, NE 17.6%. Serum pInf-IgM(+). He was treated with (1) mannitol (20%, 2.5 ml/kg, Qd) and furosemidum (1 mg/kg, 30 min after mannitol) infusion; (2) deproteinized calf blood extract 0.4 g/day, once per day; (3) human serum albumin 10 g/day infusion for 2 days. On Day 8, his body temperature regressed to 38 °C, and the bilateral conjunctivitis was partly relieved. There were rashes left on the arms and legs. The skin peeled around crissum. Neck was stiff. On Day 9, he developed sleepiness, poor appetite, cough with sputum. The body temperature reached 38.5 °C over 48 h after repeated IVIG. Chest auscultation presented wheezy phlegm. His neck was still stiff and the right scrotum had edema. Laboratory parameters were shown in Table 10.1, both urine and CSF cultures were negative. NT pro-BNP 846.9 pg/ml. Echo showed PDA (Fig. 10.1) while coronary artery was normal, LCA 2.1 mm, RCA

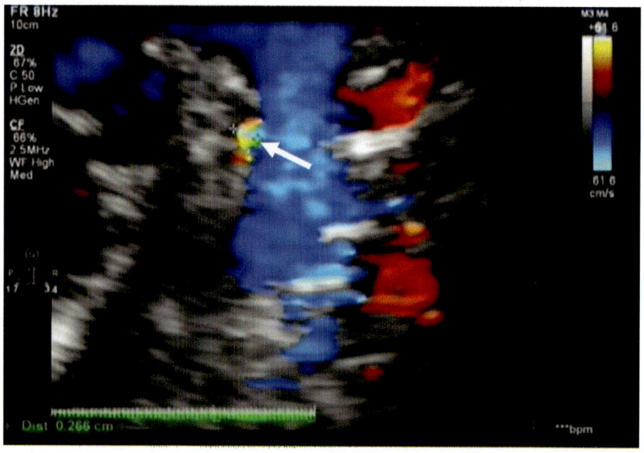

Fig. 10.1 On the Day 9 of illness, echo showed PDA 2.66 mm

2.0 mm (Fig. 10.2). No restricted dilation was detected. Brain MR showed slight dilation in the extracranial space around frontal, parietal, and temporal lobes (Fig. 10.3), and external cerebral fluid accumulation. He was treated with (1) additional IVIG 2 g/kg (6 g/kg in total); (2) oral methylprednisolone 6 mg/kg/day, Qd; (3) second generation of cephalosporin to replace the first generation.

On Day 10, his temperature was settled down, spiritual state was slightly improved, too, thus mannitol was added to the treatment every 12 h. On Day 11, for the persistent dispirited state, lumbar puncture was repeated and results were shown as followings: the CSF pressure 40–50 drops/min, light yellow transparent CSF, Pandy's test (+), total cells 24 × 10^6/L, WBC 24 × 10^6/L, NE 8.3%, glucose 2.86 mmol/L, Cl^- 114.3 mmol/L, protein 0.62 g/L. On Day 13, his body temperature was 37.7 °C, then regressed voluntarily. There were condensed red rashes in variable sizes showing on his trunk and hip skins, neck stiffness (+), bilateral Babinski sign (+). CSF culture test revealed negative bacterial colony after 48 h. Blood routine test revealed WBC 22.10 × 10^9/L, NE 77.2%, HGB 90 g/L, PLT 799 × 10^9/L. CRP

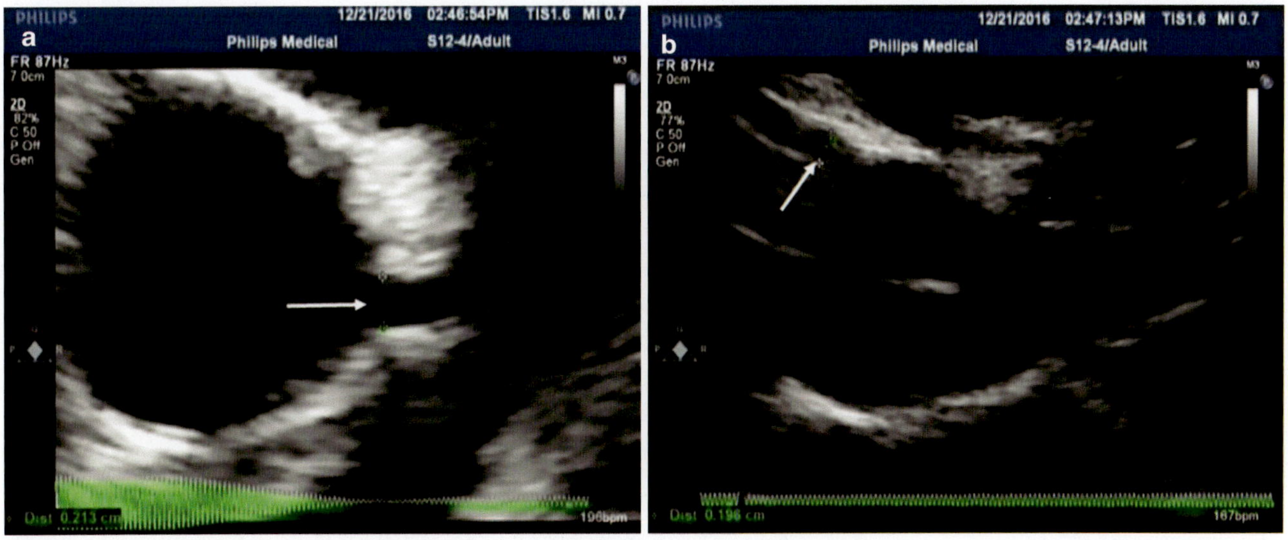

Fig. 10.2 Echo showed LCA 2.13 mm (**a**) and RCA 2.0 mm (**b**) on the Day 9 of illness

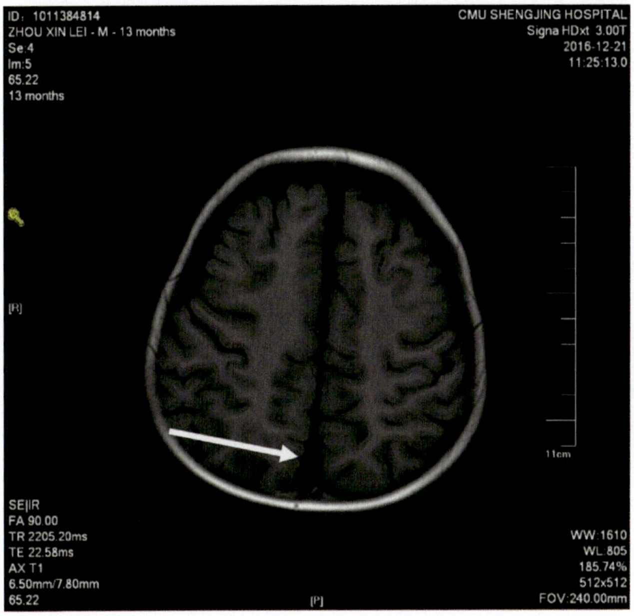

Fig. 10.3 MR showed dilation of extra-cerebral space on the Day 9 of illness

18.80 mg/L. Consultation with dermatologist concluded that the symptoms were drug eruption related. All the antibiotics were stopped, compound glycyrrhizin and Claritin plus hydrocortisone emulsifiable paste were used to relieve rashes.

On Day 14, he had cracked lips, and he coughed only once a while but with thick sputum, accompanied with the wheezy phlegm auscultated. He had watery stools twice, rotavirus was tested positive in stool. Oral aspirin and infusion of zithromax were prescribed. Probiotics and bismuth subsalicylate were administrated orally as anti-diarrhea measures.

On Day 15, he excreted yellow thin stools (three times a day), while the appetite loss trivially, urine volume remained adequate. The skin on knees was scratched broken from itching. 1:1 (Glucose: NS) solution was infused to replenish body fluid. On Day 17, his cough subsided but sputum increased with normal body temperature. His stool texture was almost normal. Lumbar puncture was performed again, the CSF pressure turned out to be 60 drops/min, CSF routine revealed total cell 11.00×10^6/L, WBC 11×10^6/L, NE 9.1%.

On Day 18, he got fever again (38.5 °C), with running nose. Sporadic red rashes appeared on bilateral opisthenar, with pruritus. Membranoid peeling skin appeared around nails. There was white yogurt-like substance in his mouth. He was given interferon inhaled. On Day 19, rechecked brain MRI revealed slight dilation of bilateral paraceles, which make us suspecting he had bilateral mastoiditis. Echo showed normal coronary arteries. On Day 21, his diarrhea was settled down, while the rashes stay unchanged. We reduced methylprednisone to 2 mg/kg/day. On Day 22, he was discharged.

10.1.1 Clinical Course of This Patient

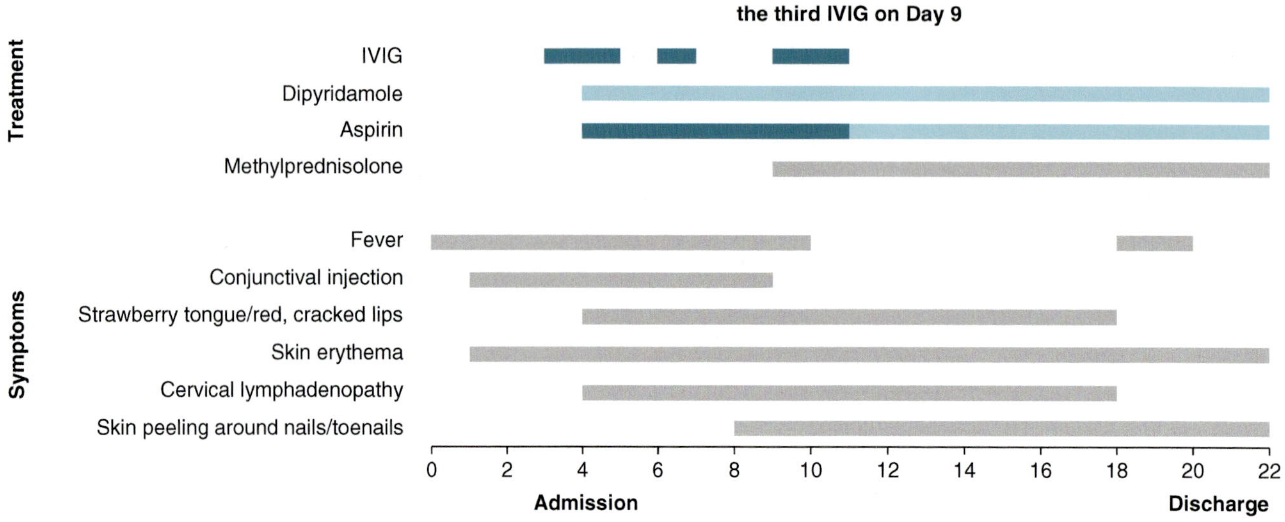

10.1.2 Follow-Up

At 4 weeks of fever onset, echo revealed LCA 2.0 mm, RCA 2.2 mm. Six months later, echo revealed LCA 2.3 mm, RCA2.1 mm (Table 10.2). NT pro-BNP 69.11 pg/ml. CRP 3.76 mg/L; WBC 7.4 × 10^9/L, N%38.1%, HGB 127 g/L, PLT 305 × 10^9/L. Oral aspirin and dipyridamole were given for 3 months. Methylprednisolone 1 mg/day was gradually stopped in 1–2 weeks after disappearance of meningeal and normal EEG. He had taken oral cerebroprotein hydrolysate tablets until EEG was normal when rechecked. He also had taken oral lysine inositol vitamin B12 liquid for 2 months. Head MRI was performed after 2 months (Table 10.2).

10.1.3 Diagnosis

1. KD, IVIG resistance
2. Aseptic meningitis
3. Liver dysfunction
4. Parainfluenza virus infection
5. Acute bronchopneumonia
6. MP infection
7. CP infection
8. CHD: PDA
9. Bilateral lateral ventricles dilatation
10. Bilateral mastoiditis?
11. Acute severe diarrhea: rotavirus infection
12. Decompensated metabolic acidosis

Table 10.2 The dynamic changes of echo parameters

Time	3 days	9 days	19 days	28 days	6 months
LCA (mm)	4.1	2.1	1.9	2	2.3
RCA (mm)	4.6	2	2.3	2.2	2.1

10.1.4 Discussion

The boy met all the criteria of Kawasaki disease, high fever more than 5 days combined with (1) bilateral conjunctivitis; (2) red and cracked lips and strawberry tongue; (3) rashes; (4) cervical lymphadenectasis; (5) swelling of extremities and followed by typical peeling skin; additional laboratory parameters: WBC ≥ 15 × 10^9/L, CRP ≥ 30 mg/L, NT pro-BNP extremely high.

On Day 3 of illness, considering the typical symptoms, the boy was given infusion of IVIG 1 mg/kg/day, for 2 days, but his fever was not improved. After transferred to our ward, high dosage IVIG infusion was given twice (totally IVIG 6 g/kg), followed by oral methylprednisolone (5 mg/kg/day). Then his symptoms were gradually settled down.

10.1.5 The Special Features of the Patient

1. The peak temperature in KD patients is usually >39 °C, even >40 °C. With timely and adequate medications (aspirin and IVIG), fever is usually improved within 36 h. Without appropriate medical treatment, the fever may last 3–4 weeks, 11 days on average. Approximately 10–20% of patients with KD are refractory to IVIG therapy, and these "non-responders" are at higher risk of developing coronary artery abnormalities. This is generally thought to be the result of failure to halt the inflammatory process and is commonly referred to as refractory or resistant KD. The differential activation of monocytes from T cells involves endothelial activation and systemic vascular inflammation [1]. The effects of IVIG treatment could arise from FcγRIIB-mediated immune-regulation [2] and regulatory T cell functions [3]. The standard treatment protocol for IVIG-resistant KD has not yet been estab-

lished. Corticosteroids are the second most commonly used medication used to treat KD patients who have recurrent or persistent fevers after IVIG treatment. Additional second-line drugs for IVIG-resistant KD including methylprednisolone (high-dose pulse methylprednisolone 20–30 mg/kg intravenously for 3 days [4]), infliximab, cyclosporine, and methotrexate have been reported.

2. The best timing to give IVIG infusion is Day 5–9 after fever onset. Application of IVIG earlier than that may be one of the reasons causing IVIG non-response, possibly that IVIG disturbs the varying balance and recovery of inflammatory factors/mediators at different stages of the disease course. Timing of IVIG administration is important, as a very early treatment of KD within 4 days presents an additional risk factor for IVIG non-responsiveness [5].
3. A multicenter study indicates that IVIG non-responders are prone to develop CAA (18.6%), though initial sufficient IVIG therapy decreases the risk of IVIG nonresponse. Recent studies have focused on determining the predictive factors for initial IVIG-resistance [6] and adjunctive anti-cytokine therapies to reduce the risk of cardiac sequelae [7]. Clinical trials and meta-analyses demonstrated that treatment with addition of corticosteroids to IVIG is beneficial for the prevention of coronary artery aneurysms in severe cases with the highest risk of IVIG-resistance [8]. Disease susceptibility genes could affect the incidence of KD as well as the response to IVIG [9]. According to the critical assessment of risk scoring systems (Egami score, Kobayashi score, and Sano score) for Kawasaki syndrome, high CRP level is globally considered a risk factor for non-responsiveness to IVIG and the subsequent risk of CAA in all systems, probably as a result of stronger systemic inflammation driving endothelial abnormalities and final development of cardiovascular complications [10]. In addition, most scores have considered thrombocytopenia and patient's age less than 6–12 months as individual risk factors for the occurrence of CAA. Damage to coronary arteries is still a substantial risk for a non-negligible percentage of children with KD, mostly in the cases showing resistance to IVIG [9]: the identification of this cohort of children at the time of first clinical assessment may help in discerning those who would benefit from a combined primary treatment with IVIG and corticosteroids.
4. At the acute stage of KD, 50% patients present WBC >15 × 10^9/L. As a result of increase of premature and mature neutrophil, leukopenia was rare. The convalescent stage was characterized by thrombocytosis (even more than 1000 × 10^9/L), which gradually peaked on the third week after illness, then dropped to normal during the fourth week. Thrombocytopenia at the acute stage should be concerned for it may be a sign of DIC, also a risk factor of aneurysm.
5. ESR and CRP are parameters to assess acute stage of KD. They were dropped to normal 6–10 weeks after onset of illness. For IVIG infusion can increase ESR, ESR alone can't be used to assess activation of inflammation [5]. In this case, after the first and second IVIG infusions, WBC and CRP were elevated persistently, indicating a persistent activation of immune-reaction. The slowly decreased tendency of WBC may partially attribute to methylprednisolone.
6. Hypoalbuminemia is common in severe or refractory KD patients, as the result of capillary and vessel leakage and frequent blood drawn. Albumin is vital in the course of vascular repair. In our ward, albumin dosage was 1 g/kg/day, for 2 days once ALB<30 mg/L.

Xue-xin Yu

10.2 Case 36: KD with IVIG Resistance-Oral Prednisone

A 3-year-old boy presented without significant past medical history or family history.

He presented on Day one with fever and cervical lymphadenectasis for 1 day. He was admitted in PICU. Examination revealed: T 38.2 °C, HR 120 bpm, RR 26 bpm, BP 85/56 mmHg. No rashes, bilateral cervical lymphadenectasis, with the largest one about 3 cm × 2 cm, with a little pain when touched. Others were normal. Admission blood test revealed WBC 25.6 × 10^9/L, NE 76.8%, HGB 126 g/L, PLT 195 × 10^9/L. CRP 50.7 mg/L. Liver function, myocardial enzyme, and amylase were normal. Cervical ultrasound showed a lymphadenectasis about 2.5 × 1.8 cm on left. He had been diagnosed with acute cervical lymphadenitis and treated with ceftriaxone tazobactam sodium. On Day 3 of illness, he had remittent fever along with neck pain and cervical lymphadenopathy. He was treated with (1) IVIG 1 g/kg/day; (2) infusion of dexamethasone 5 mg/day for 2 days. On Day 5 of illness, he still had fever 39.3 °C and developed red and cracked lips, bilateral conjunctival congestion, and erythema and edema on hands and feet erythema and edema. Consultation with pediatric cardiologist confirmed diagnosed of KD. He was treated with (1) 5 mg dexamethasone; (2) oral aspirin 200 mg/time, and dipyridamole 25 mg/time, three times a day. On Day 6, he had fever at T38 °C. But on Day 7, fever rised up to 39 °C again, along with conjunctival hyperemia. Considering IVIG resistance, he was given another IVIG 1 g/kg and dexamethasone 5 mg infusion.

On Day 8, he was transferred to pediatric cardiology ward. Retested blood results showed WBC 31.5 × 10^9/L, NE 78.3%, HGB 95 g/L, PLT 274 × 10^9/L. CRP 162 mg/L. NT-pro BNP 377.7 pg/ml. Albumin 23.9 g/L. Echo showed LCA dilated about 2.9–3.6 mm, RCA dilated about 3.9–4.2 mm (Fig. 10.4). He was treated with (1) another dose of IVIG 1 g/kg; (2) GC discontinued; (3) infusion of albumin 1 g/kg/day for 2 days. On Day 10, he still had fever at 38.5 °C, along with conjunctivitis, red and cracked lips. Retest blood showed WBC 26 × 10^9/L, HGB 95 g/L, PLT 373 × 10^9/L. CRP 111 mg/L. Albumin 37.4 g/L. Further treatment was given: (1) additional IVIG 2 g/kg within 24 h. On Day 11, his body temperature was 37.3 °C and he showed irritability. Examination found swollen left eyelid, and he could not open his eyes. This is a way to detect facial nerve damage movement was not cooperative, but without mouth skew when crying. Lumbar puncture was performed, and CSF Pandy's reaction was negative. The total number of cells was 22 × 10^6/L, WBC 22 × 10^6/L, RBC 0 × 10^6/L. Protein 0.93 g/L. CSF pathogens were negative. Retested WBC 15.9 × 10^9/L, NE 57.6%, HGB 83 g/L, PLT 632 × 10^9/L. CRP 65.9 mg/L. Consulted ophthalmologist suggested that he had infective conjunctivitis and was prescribed with eye drops. He was treated with (1) mannitol (20%) 2.5 ml/kg fast infusion, q12h, half an hour later furosemide 1 mg/kg infusion, q12h; (2) deproteinized calf serum 0.4 g infusion, once a day; (3) cefuroxime sodium 0.1 g/kg/day for 7 days; (4) methylprednisolone 1 mg/kg/day for 3 days; (5) erythromycin eye drops, three times per day.

On Day 14, he was afebrile for 2 days. After the eye drops, both eyes opened well. There were scattered hemorrhagic spots on his back and shoulders. Took oral aspirin and dipyridamole were discontinued. The following day, examination found periungual desquamation on left thumb. Head MR plus facial nerve scan showed no abnormality. On Day 16, he felt everything went better. Retested blood revealed WBC 10.52 × 10^9/L, NE 47.3%, HGB 82 g/L, PLT 530 × 10^9/L. CRP 10.6 mg/L. Albumin 34.4 g/L. DIC were normal. BVEP result was normal. BAEP showed right auditory hearing threshold increased to 50dBnHL. Repeated echo showed LCA about 4.0–5.0 mm, RCA about 3.5–4.5 mm (Fig. 10.5).

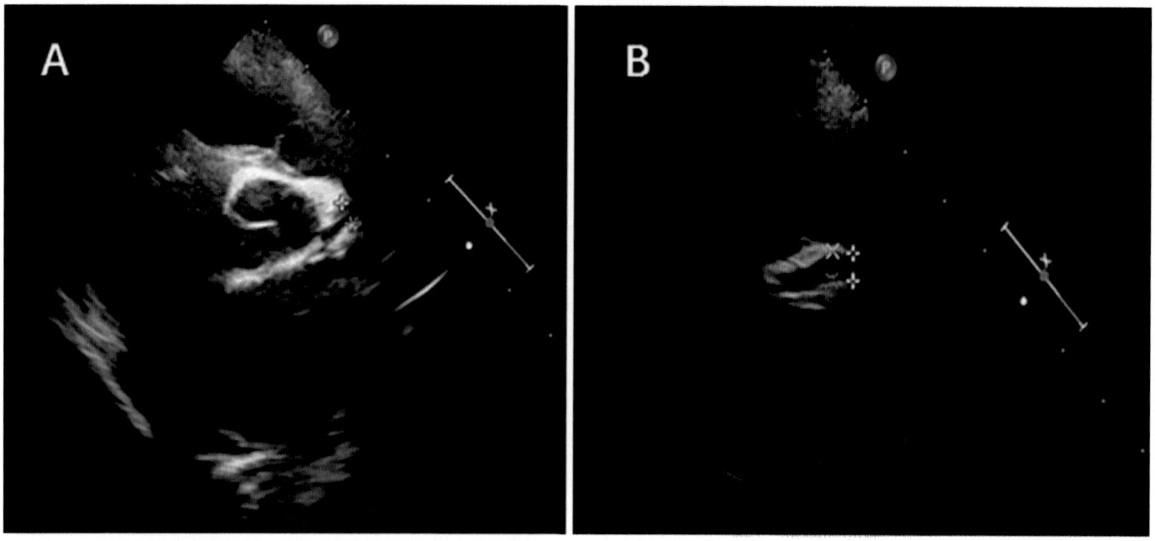

Fig. 10.4 On Day 8 of illness, LCA 3.6 mm (**a**), RCA 4.2 mm (**b**)

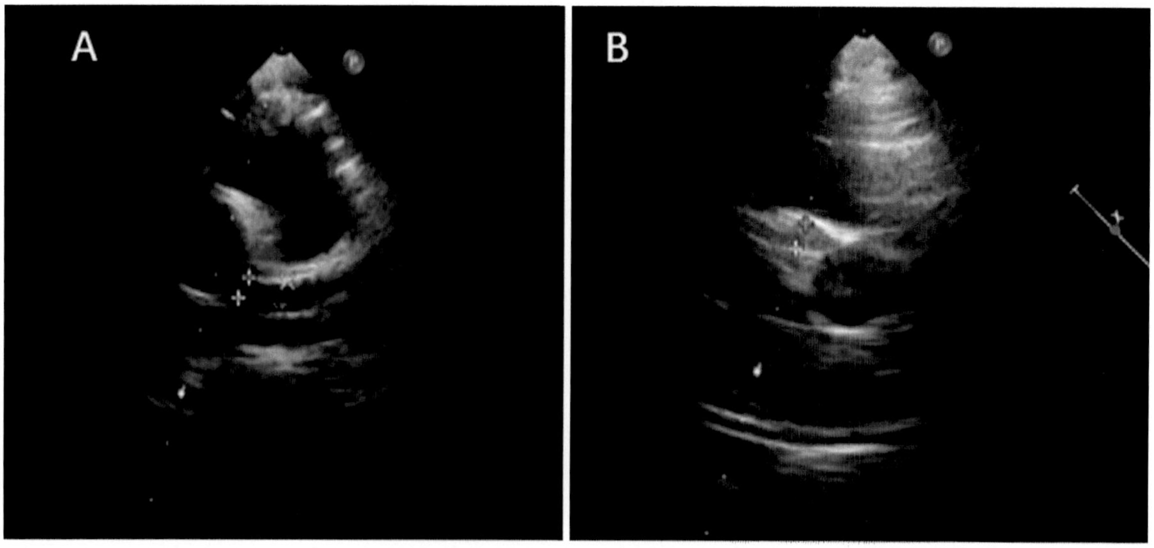

Fig. 10.5 On Day 16 of illness, LCA 5.0 mm (**a**), RCA 4.5 mm (**b**)

10.2.1 Clinical Course of the Patient

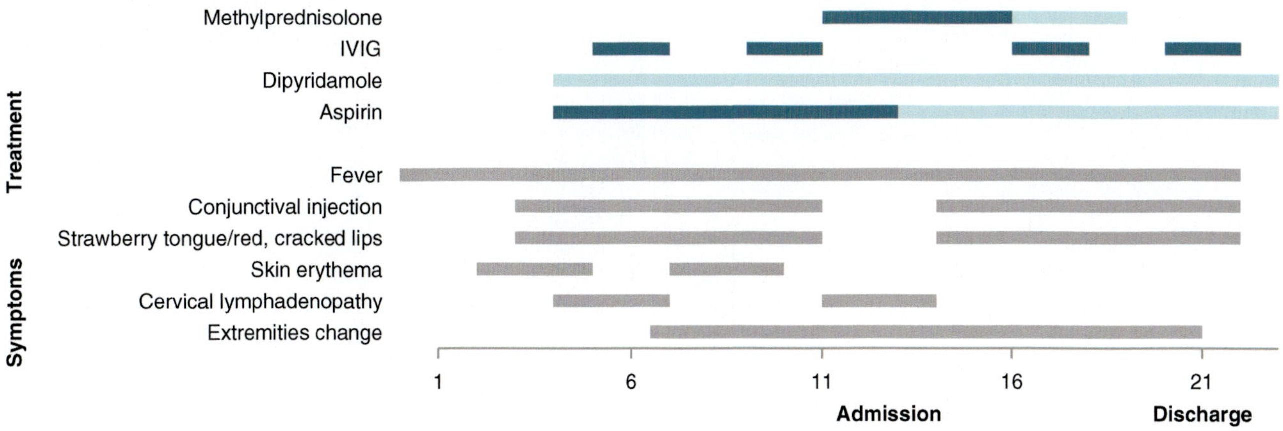

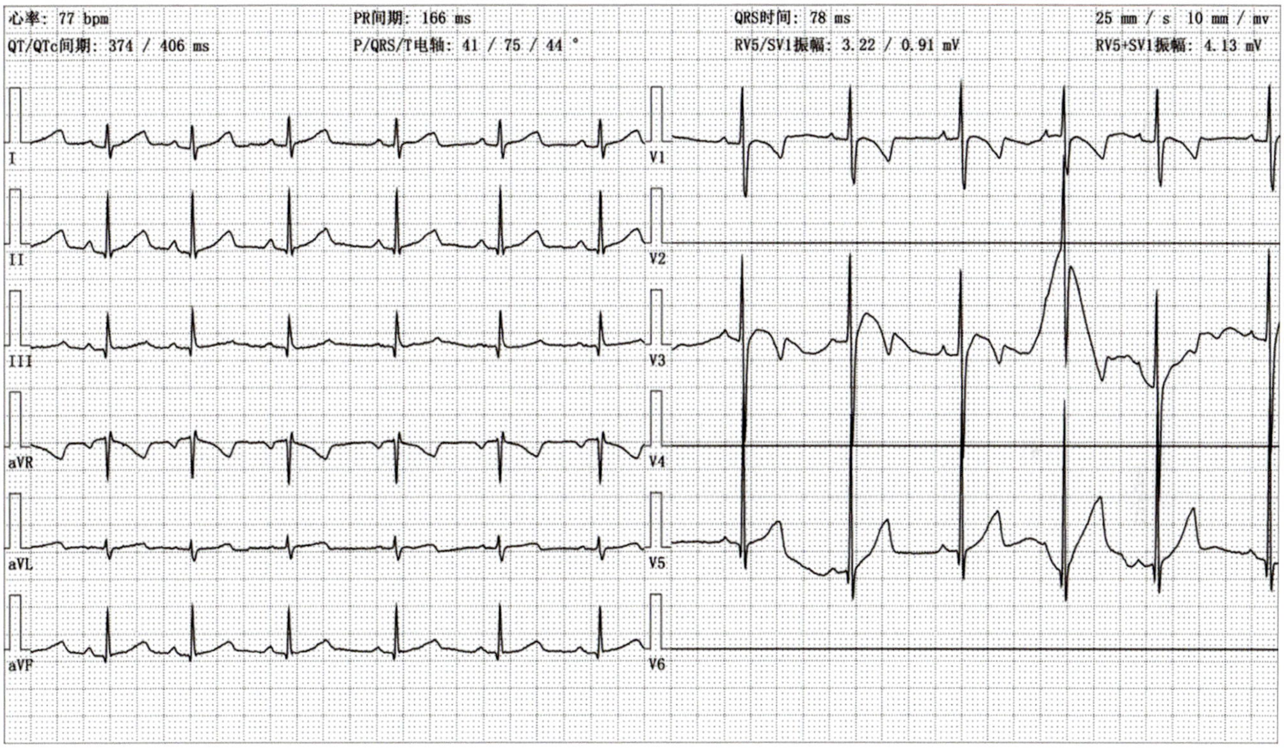

Fig. 10.6 Three months after onset, ECG was still normal

10.2.2 Follow-Up

One month after the illness, brain hydrolyzed tablets and vitamin B were stopped when BAEP recovered. Three months after onset, ECG was still normal (Fig. 10.6). Oral fructose was stopped.

Six months after the illness, the coronary artery was abnormal. L-carnitine was stopped. Nine months after onset, repeated echo showed coronary artery remaining normal (Fig. 10.7). All medications were stopped.

10.2.3 Diagnosis

1. KD, IVIG resistance
2. Bilateral CAA
3. Aseptic meningitis
4. Hypoalbuminemia
5. Conjunctivitis
6. Moderate anemia

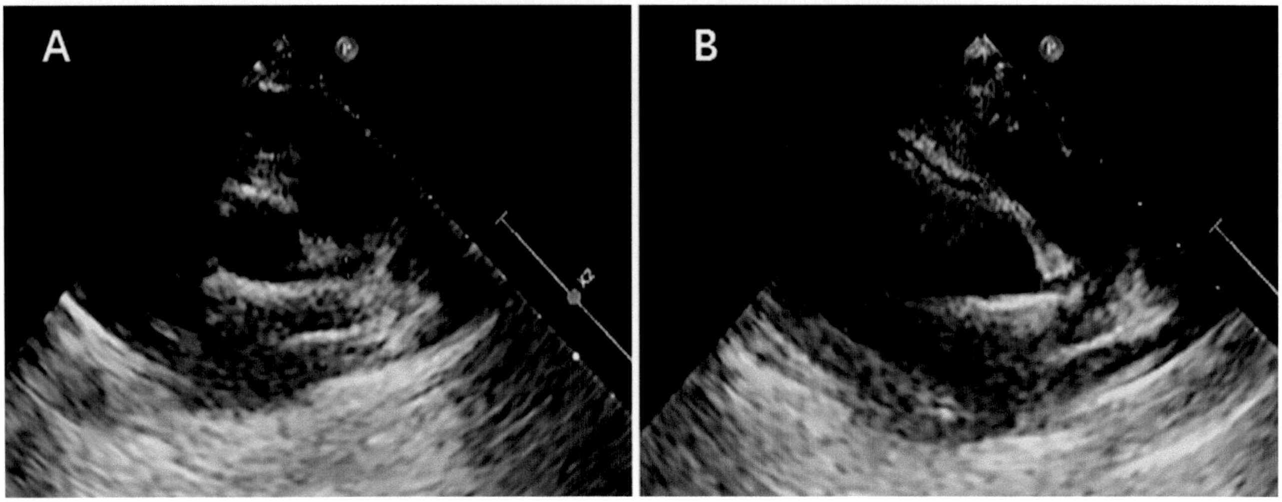

Fig. 10.7 Nine months after onset, repeated echo showed LCA was normal (**a**), RCA was normal (**b**)

10.2.4 Discussion

The diagnosis of KD was sufficient. The patient had persistent fever over 5 days and unresponsive to antibiotics infusion, along with (1) rash in the course of the disease; (2) bilateral bulbar conjunctival congestion without exudates; (3) erythema of the hands and skin peeling around fingernails on 13 days of the illness; (4) cervical lymphadenectasis; (5) echo showed bilateral CAA; additionally WBC 31.5×10^9/L, CRP 162 mg/L.

Differential diagnosis of sepsis and purulent meningitis should be considered. If the inflammatory parameters are significantly higher in child with fever, early diagnosis of KD and treatment with IVIG timely could significantly reduce the incidence of coronary artery dilatation. When the patient was admitted to the hospital, he was given IVIG 400 mg/kg/day because of the severity of the infection. When he was diagnosed with KD, the amount was increased to 2 g/kg.

GCs have been a controversial drug in treating children with KD [11], although GCs have been specifically used to treat children with KD once [12]. A randomized, double-blind, placebo-controlled trial has been initiated at the National Heart and Lung Institute Pediatric Heart Network to evaluate the efficacy of a single intravenous injection of methylprednisolone (30 mg/kg per dose), IVIG (2 g/kg for 1 day), and aspirin (80–100 mg/kg 1 day) [13]. Data analysis suggests that initial GC therapy may be beneficial for children with initial IVIG resistance, which may reduce the risk of coronary artery malformation in children. Another randomized controlled study group was conducted in a multicenter, prospective, randomized, open-label, blind-end point trial showed that IVIG and GCs therapy were good for KD, a similar conclusion was obtained [14].

After the patient had been applied with IVIG twice, the patient still had low fever. However the patient's physical signs and auxiliary tests were not enough for IVIG resistance, oral GCs were administered and fever was gradually reduced for 1 week, which might be better than the third round of 2 g/kg IVIG. Whether GCs should be applied depend on the results of different conditions.

10.2.5 Case Specific Clinic Features

1. In children with central nervous system involvement, we apply small doses of GCs on one hand to control inflammation, on the other hand to reduce cerebral edema. Infusion of second-generation cephalosporin that can pass through the blood–brain barrier was given for 1 week. Retested CSF was normal.
2. KD in children with nervous system involvement may be caused by small-vessel inflammation. Microvasculitis causes neuronal ischemia and cranial pressure elevation, which in turn aggravates neuronal damages. Some children with KD have symptoms of abducens nerve palsy [15].
3. Facial nerve damage results in palpebra unable to be closed. This child had his right eye closed all the time, which may be caused by conjunctivitis. In addition, head MR did not find abnormalities. Therefore possibility of facial nerve damage was excluded. All symptoms disappeared after eye drops were applied, which in turn supported our interpretation.

Table 10.3 The dynamic changes of lab parameters and treatment

Day of illness	5	6	8	9	10	15	17	19	23	27
CBC ($\times 10^9$/L)	19.1		27.6			34	23.2	28.1	23.7	9.7
NE (%)	94.5		89.1			71.7	67.4	69.3	70	33.3
HGB(g/L)	106		99			111	96	98	96	101
PLT($\times 10^9$/L)	178		164			550	636	866	733	651
Premature cells (%)						3				
CRP (mg/L)	122	159	177			36.3	30.3	58.4	52.3	13.6
ESR (mm/h)		43								
NT pro-BNP (pg/ml)	1472		1445			107.6				
IVIG (g/kg)	1	1		1	1				2	
Methylprednisolone (mg/kg)					1	1.5	2	1	0.5	0.2

Ce Wang

10.3 Case 37: KD with IVIG Resistance and Transient CAA

A previously healthy 3-year-old girl had no significant past medical or family history.

She presented on Day 5 of illness with fever and rashes for 4 days, red conjunctiva for 3 days. One day before fever onset, she had cervical mass and pain. *Examination* revealed fever (38.5 °C), smooth breath (HR 150 bpm, RR 28 bpm), warm hands and feet (BP113/80 mmHg), rashes distributed on the face and limbs, cervical lymphadenectasis, non-purulent bilateral conjunctival hyperemia, dry and cracked lips with strawberry tongue, hepatomegaly (the liver was 2 cm enlarged below right costal margin and 1 cm below the xiphoid), bilateral hand and feet edema, red palms. Others were normal. *Admission* blood test revealed CBC, CRP, and NT-pro BNP increased (see Table 10.3). Blood gas analysis was normal, K^+ 2.50 mmol/L, DIC PT 18.1 s, APTT 29 s, D-dimer 1471 (0–252)μg/L.CK-MB mass, cTnI, and hs-cTnT were normal. Abdominal ultrasound was normal. Chest CT scan showed pneumonia. She had met all criteria of KD, except fever lasting less than 5 days, she was treated with (1) oral aspirin 30–50 mg/kg/day, dipyridamole 3–5 mg/kg/day; (2) intravenous infusion of potassium; (3) second-generation cephalosporin infusion after blood drawn for culture test. On Day 5 of illness, she had persistent fever, physical examination did not show improvement. Investigation revealed K^+ 2.84 mmol/L. CRP 159 mg/L. ESR 43 mm/h. ALB 22.4 g/L, ALT 72 U/L, TSA 57.5μmol/L. MP IGG 1:40. Her fever had last over 5 days, she was treated with (1) IVIG 1 g/kg/day for 2 days; (2) infusion of albumin 1/kg/day for 2 days; (3) continuous infusion of potassium. On Day 7, she had constant fever and was irritable. Investigation revealed positive adenovirus antibody titer. EEG was normal. She received muscle injection of Alpha 1 beta interferon 10μg, qd, for 3 days. On Day 8, her fever persisted at 39 °C, her mental state was not improved along with red conjunctiva and cracked lips. Investigation revealed CBC, CRP, and NT-pro BNP unimproved (see Table 10.3).

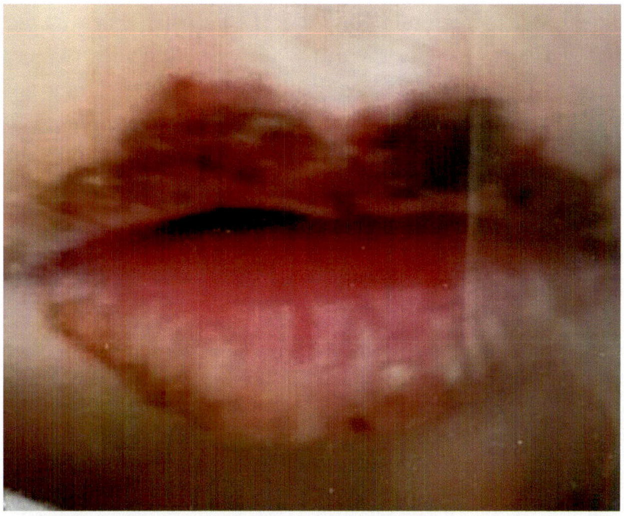

Fig. 10.8 On Day 11 of illness, her lips were dry and cracked

K^+ 3.20 mmol/L. ASO 50.1 IU/ml. Echo showed LCA 2.9 mm while RCA 2.5 mm. She had met the criteria of KD with IVIG resistance Thus, she was treated with IVIG 1 g/kg/day for 2 days (total IVIG 4 g/kg). On Day 9, her fever and mental state were not improved. She was treated with methylprednisolone 1 mg/kg/day infusion. On Day 10, she had fever at 38.1 °C and was irritable. Lips were red and cracked (Fig. 10.8). Interphalangeal joint had edema. Investigation revealed ALB 32.5 g/L. MP-IgG 1:160. Blood culture results were negative. She was treated with (1) third-generation cephalosporin; (2) infusion of azithromycin 10 mg/kg/day for 3 days.

On Day 12 of illness, she was afebrile, and her mental state was slightly improved. Repeated EEG was abnormal, most was θ wave. Lumbar puncture revealed the following results: CSF pressure 72 drops/min, cells count 112×10^6/L, WBC 12×10^6/L, RBC 100×10^6/L (bleeding at beginning). CSF biochemistry showed protein 0.48 g/L, etiology examination was negative. Head MR was normal. He was treated with (1) mannitol 2.5 ml/kg/day fast infusion and furosemidum 1 mg/kg/day infusion to reduce intracranial pressure;

(2) calf blood protein extract 0.4 g/day to nourish brain cells. On Day 15 of illness, the highest temperature that day was 37.7 °C. The mental state was better than before. Both body rashes and conjunctival congestion disappeared. Swelling on hands and feet improved slightly. Investigation revealed there was no improvement in CBC and 3.0% premature cells were found. CRP was 36.3 mg/L. The dosage of methylprednisolone was increased to 1.5 mg/kg/day.

On Day 17 of illness, her fever was up to 38.7 °C. Investigation revealed reduced WBC and CRP. Repeated echo showed LCA was 2.9 mm and the RCA was 2.6 mm. Treatment included: (1) infusion of azithromycin again for another 3 days; (2) the dosage of methylprednisolone increased to 2 mg/kg/day; (3) oral fluconazole 75 mg/day and vitamin C to correct anemia. On Day 19 of illness, her temperature was 37.7 °C. Perianal skin was red and started to peel, her vulva with white floccules plaque, difficult to rub away. Investigation revealed everything got better. The dosage of methylprednisolone was decreased to 1 mg/ kg/day. On Day22 of illness, she had persistent fever over 20 days, along with leg ache, and her blood routine showed immature cells. Thus, bone marrow puncture was performed and test showed marrow infection (Fig. 10.9), without macrophage system activation syndrome. On Day 23 of illness, she still had mild fever and the highest point was 37.4 °C. Investigation revealed no significant improvement in CBC and CRP. Repeated echo showed LCA was widened to 3.4–3.9 mm (Fig. 10.10a), and RCA was 2.8 mm. She was treated with (1) IVIG 2 g/kg (total 6 g/kg), infusion process over 12 h; (2) mannitol (20%) and furosemidum infusion after 1 g/kg IVIG; (3) oral prednisone 0.5 mg/kg/day to replace methylprednisolone.

On Day 25 of illness, she was afebrile for 32 h, rashes disappeared, swollen hands and feet obviously were regressed. Strawberry tongue disappeared. So aspirin was reduced to 3–5 mg/kg/day. On Day 27 of illness, she was afebrile for 3–4 days. Investigation revealed WBC 9.7×10^9/L, NE 33.3%, HGB 101 g/L, PLT 651×10^9/L. DIC D-dimer 531μg/L. ASO 88.6 IU/ml, CRP 13.60 mg/L. She was discharged.

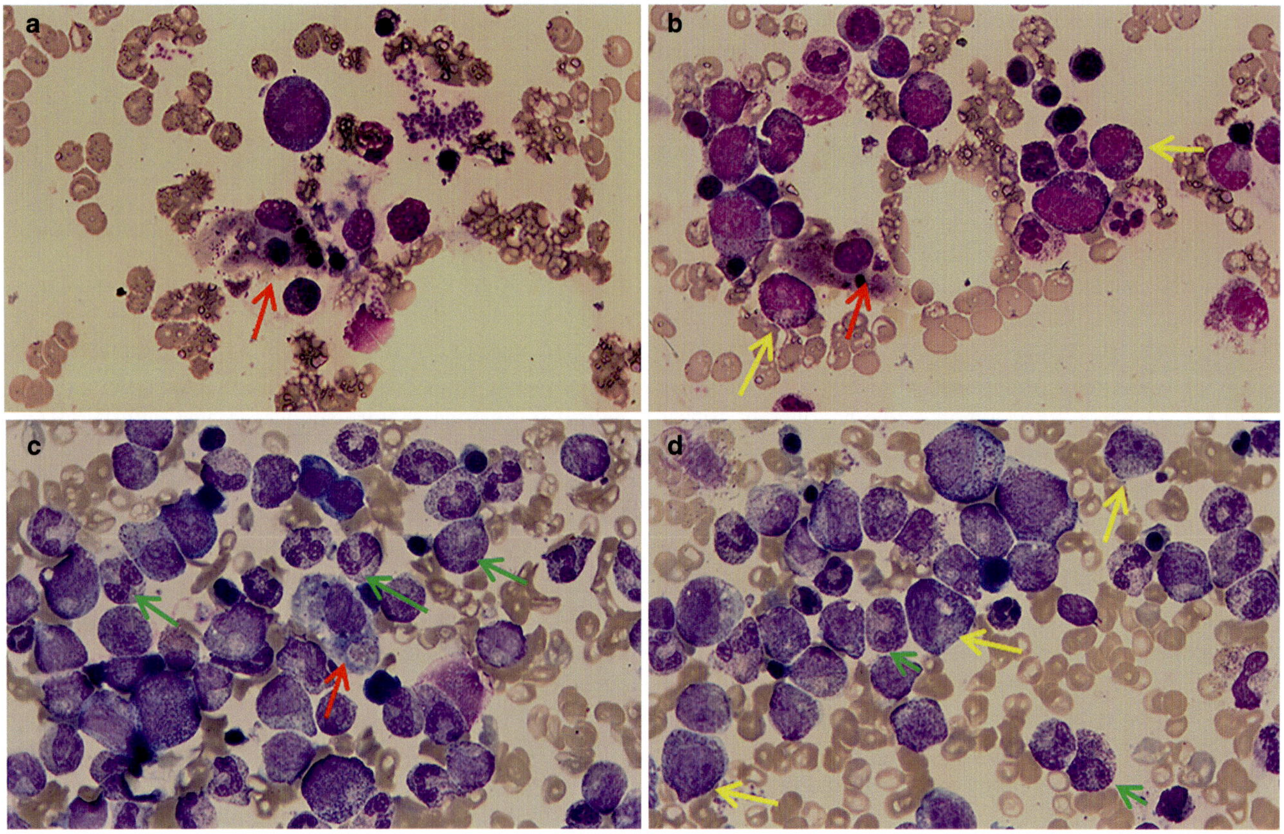

Fig. 10.9 On Day 20 of illness, bone marrow smear showed Wright-Giemsa×1000. Hypercellular marrow with high myeloid-to-erythroid ratio, phagocytes gobble up histiocytes of platelets, pigment granules, and degenerate cells ((**a**) and (**b**), red arrow). Neutrophil precursors showed increased granules ((**b**) and (**d**), yellow arrow). Mature neutrophils showed toxic granulation ((**c**) and (**d**), green arrow)

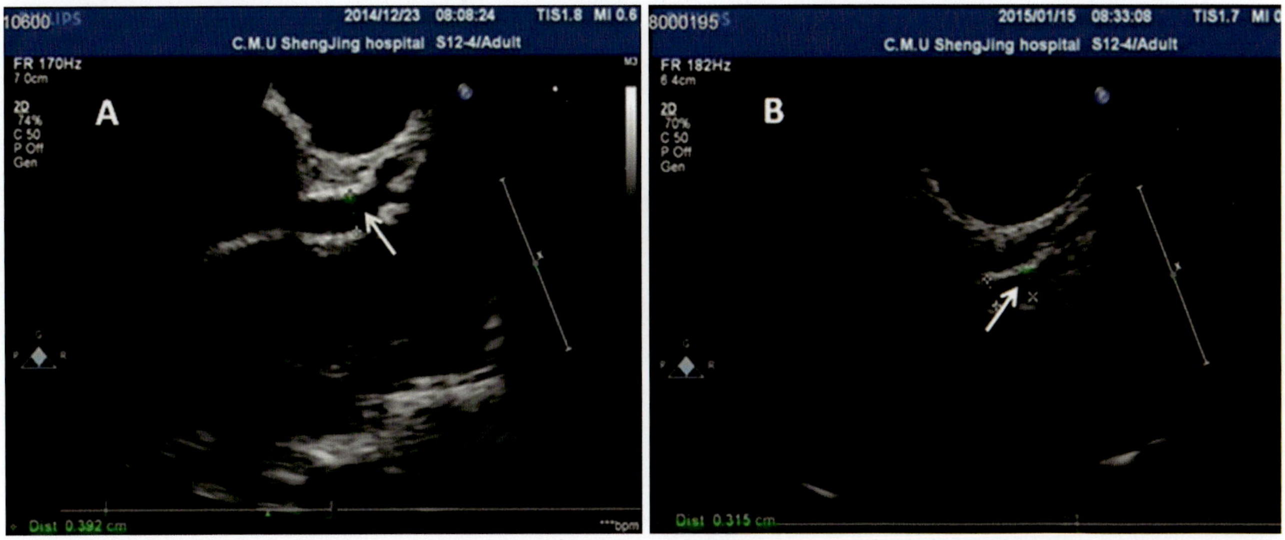

Fig. 10.10 Echo showed LCA dilatation about 3.9 mm on Day 23 (**a**), while regress to 3.1 mm on Day 45 of illness (**b**)

10.3.1 Clinical Course of the Patient

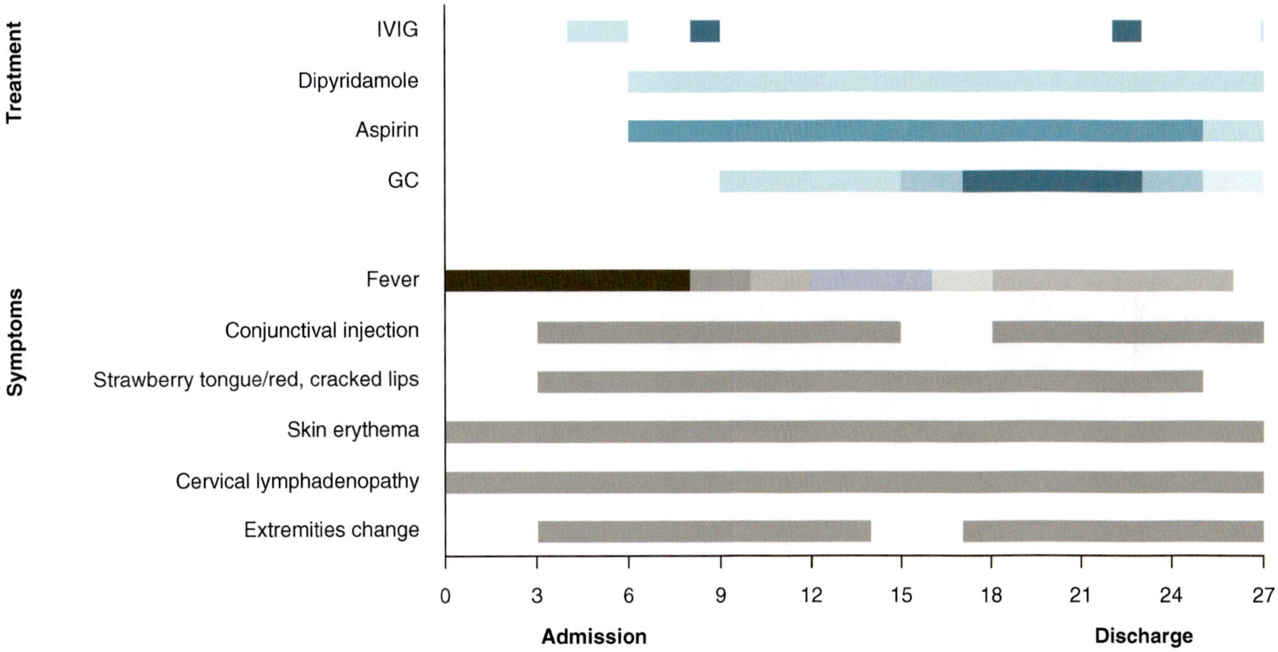

10.3.2 Follow-Up

Since discharged, she took (1) oral aspirin and dipyridamole 3–5 mg/kg/day about 2 months; (2) oral brain protein hydrolysate tablets and composite vitamin B for 1 month; (3) prednisone tapered off within a week.

On Day 45 of illness, LCA was 2.9–3.2 mm (Fig. 10.10b). At 2 months of illness, transverse sulci were found on her toenails (Fig. 10.11). At 3 months of illness, LCA was recovered to normal (Fig. 10.12). At 6 months of illness, LCA was still normal. All medications were stopped. By now, she had followed up with us for 3 years and her coronary arteries remained normal.

10.3.3 Diagnosis

1. KD, IVIG resistance
2. LCA dilation
3. Aseptic meningitis

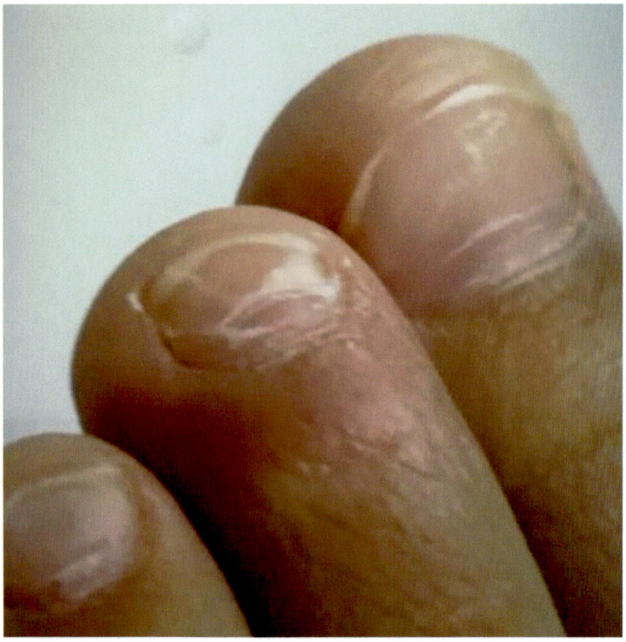

Fig. 10.11 On Day 60 of illness, transverse sulci on her toenails

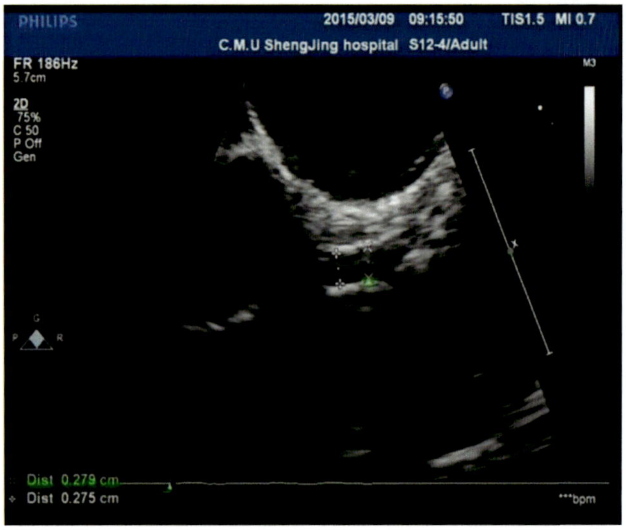

Fig. 10.12 On Day 90 of illness, echo showed LCA was normal

4. Liver dysfunction
5. Hypoproteinemia
6. Cholestatic hepatitis
7. Leukemoid response
8. Acute bronchial pneumonia
9. MP infection
10. Adenovirus infection
11. Hypokalemia

10.3.4 Discussion

She was diagnosed with KD on the basis of the presence of fever for more than 5 days, unresponsiveness to oral and antibiotics infusion, along with other clinical features: (1) congestive rashes all over body; (2) bilateral conjunctival congestion, without purulent secretions; (3) cracked or fissured lips with strawberry tongue; (4) edema feet and hands and later peeling skin around fingernails; (5) cervical lymphadenopathy over 1.5 cm; (6) coronary artery dilation. Additionally WBC, especially neutrophils increased, CRP and NT-pro BNP were significantly increased.

Differential diagnosis of purulent meningitis, pharyngeal conjunctival fever should be considered.

The girl was treated with IVIG total 6 g/kg. She still had high-grade fever after IVIG 2 g/kg treatment. It is necessary to treat the patient with another dose of IVIG [16] and/or glucocorticoid [17]. By now, it has been suggested that IVIG together with glucocorticoid is more effective in reducing risk of developing coronary artery dilation, compared to IVIG alone [17]. For patients who are IVIG resistant, adding glucocorticoid in the treatment is more effective in reducing fever than IVIG treatment alone. But it cannot effectively protect coronary arteries and prevent coronary artery dilatation [18].

In some severe KD cases, leukemoid response can occur. It is a compensatory response that immature cells appear in the peripheral blood. The ratio of immature cells in bone marrow examination was normal, and the immature cells will disappear with inflammation subsided.

The 2017 AHA KD Guideline proposed that aspirin is given at beginning of disease and is continued to be given until patients have no evidence of coronary changes 6–8 weeks after onset of illness. For children who develop coronary abnormalities, aspirin may be continued indefinitely [19]. We suggest her continue to take oral aspirin for another 3 months. Even so, in our center, there was a case whose coronary arteries injury had recovered but developed to coronary artery aneurysm half year later. Her LCA regressed to normal after 3 months, but the other patient (see case 10) developed giant CAA 1 year later.

10.3.5 Case Specific Clinical Features

1. The first dose of IVIG 2 g/kg was applied timely and within 10 days of illness, but it was ineffective to have fever under control. In a case like this, adenovirus infection and mycoplasma infection should be considered.

However, infusion of antiviral drugs and azithromycin was still ineffective, and WBC and CRP were still significantly high. These were consistent with IVIG resistance.

2. This girl had obvious hypoproteinemia at admission. If fever persisted, hypoproteinemia could result in coronary edema and exacerbate coronary artery injuries. Some patients have albumin between 30 and 35 g/L at admission. But if fevers continue, their albumin levels can be reduced below 30 g/L 2 days later. So it was important to repeat albumin test and supplement would be provided timely. Although the girl had continuous fever for more than 20 days, her coronary artery dilation was mild (less than 4 mm and regressed to normal after 3 months).
3. After long-term broad-spectrum antibiotic treatment, if abnormal signs in the oral cavity and vulva observed, possible fungal infections should be considered, and treatment to symptoms should be applied. Her fungal smear test was negative. However since she received infusion of second- and third-generation cephalosporin early 2 weeks 7 days and glucocorticoid for 8 days, fungal infection was highly suspected. Therefore she was given oral fluconazole 5 mg/kg/day for 3 days.
4. Neurological system symptoms associated with KD in children often occur during the time when body temperature was decreased to normal. Clinical symptoms include lethargy, headache; possible positive meningeal irritation and most of the EEG may be abnormal. Once suspected neurological system involvement, lumbar puncture should be performed; head CT or MR should be performed, so proper treatment to symptoms can be given to patient. The patient's EEG was normal before hospitalization. As the disease progressed, once she developed sleepiness and neck stiffness, neurological complication should be highly concerned and EEG needs to be repeated. Once meningitis diagnosis was validated it was enough to give 20% mannitol infusion for 1 week, intravenous drugs to nourish brain for 1–2 weeks. After discharged, she continued to take oral medications for about 4 weeks.

Yan-qiu Chu

References

1. Ikeda K, Yamaguchi K, Tanaka T, et al. Unique activation status of peripheral blood mononuclear cells at acute phase of Kawasaki disease. Clin Exp Immunol. 2010;160(2):246–55.
2. Samuelsson A, Towers TL, Ravetch JV. Anti-inflammatory activity of IVIG mediated through the inhibitory fc receptor. Science. 2001;291(5503):484–6.
3. Guo MM, Tseng WN, Ko CH, et al. Th17-and Treg-related cytokine and mRNA expression are associated with acute and resolving Kawasaki disease. Allergy. 2015;70(3):310–8.
4. McCrindle BW, Rowley AH, Newburger JW, et al. Diagnosis, treatment, and long-term management of Kawasaki disease: a scientific statement for health professionals from the American Heart Association. Circulation. 2017;135(17):927–99.
5. Muta H, Ishii M, Egami K, et al. Early intravenous γ-globulin treatment for Kawasaki disease: the nationwide surveys in Japan. J Pediatr. 2004;144(4):496–9.
6. Davies S, Sutton N, Blackstock S, et al. Predicting IVIG resistance in UK Kawasaki disease. Arch Dis Child. 2015;100(4):366–8.
7. Tremoulet AH, Jain S, Jaggi P, et al. Infliximab for intensification of primary therapy for Kawasaki disease: a phase 3 randomized, double-blind, placebo-controlled trial. Lancet. 2014;383(9930):1731–8.
8. Newburger JW, Sleeper LA, McCrindle BW, Pediatric Heart Network Investigators, et al. Randomized trial of pulsed corticosteroid therapy for primary treatment of Kawasaki disease. N Engl J Med. 2007;356(7):663–75.
9. Onouchi Y, Ozaki K, Burns JC, et al. A genome-wide association study identifies three new risk loci for Kawasaki disease. Nat Genet. 2012;44(5):517–21.
10. Kibata T, Suzuki Y, Hasegawa S, et al. Coronary artery lesions and the increasing incidence of Kawasaki disease resistant to initial immunoglobulin. Inte J Cardiol. 2016;214:209–15.
11. Shulman ST. Is there a role for corticosteroids in Kawasaki disease? J Pediatr. 2003;142(6):601–3.
12. Furusho K, Kamiya T, Nakano H, et al. High-dose intravenous gamma globulin for Kawasaki disease. Lancet. 1984;2(8411):1055–8.
13. Newburger JW, Sleeper LA, McCrindle BW, et al. Randomized trial of pulsed corticosteroid therapy for primary treatment of Kawasaki disease. N Engl J Med. 2007;356(7):663–5.
14. Kobayashi T, Saji T, Otani T, et al. Efficacy of immunoglobulin plus prednisolone for prevention of coronary artery abnormalities in severe Kawasaki disease (RAISE study): a randomized, open-label, blinded endpoints trial. Lancet. 2012;379(9826):1613–20.
15. Rodríguez-Lozano A, Juárez-Echenique JC, Rivas-Larrauri F, et al. VI nerve palsy after intravenous immunoglobulin in Kawasaki disease. Allergol Immunopathol (Madr). 2014;42(1):82–3.
16. Sundel RP, Burns JC, Baker A, et al. Gamma globulin re-treatment in Kawasaki disease. J Pediatr. 1993;123(4):657–9.
17. Kobayashi T, Saji T, Otani T, et al. Efficacy of immunoglobulin plus prednisolone for prevention of coronary artery abnormalities in severe Kawasaki disease (RAISE study): a randomised, open-label, blinded -endpoints trial. Lancet. 2012;379(9826):1613–20.
18. Yang X, Liu G, Huang Y, et al. A meta-analysis of re-treatment for intravenous immunoglobulin-resistant Kawasaki disease. Cardiol Young. 2015;25(6):1182–90.
19. McCrindle BW, Rowley AH, Newburger JW, et al. Diagnosis treatment and long-term management of Kawasaki disease: a scientific statement for health professionals from the American Heart Association. Circulation. 2017;135(17):e927–99.

Recurrent KD

11

Xuemei Li, Hong Wang, Xuexin Yu, Jing Dong, and Bai Gao

Abstract

Since the first description of KD in 1967, there have been case reports from more than 50 countries. The etiology of the disease is yet to be clarified. It is well known that the disease recurs in some children. The U.S. surveys showed that the proportion of recurrent KD among all of the patients was 1.7% and 3.5% in Japan [Maddox et al. Pediatr Int 57(6):1116–1120, 2015], while another literature reports recurrence of KD in Japan was 0.65–0.39% from 2000 to 2017 [Sudo and Nakamura. Acta Paediatr 106(5):796–800, 2017]. However, despite a considerable number of cases of disease recurrence, analysis of related factors such as document about the KD recurrence is limited. If the initial KD fever settled over 1 week and other clinical symptoms of KD (except swollen lymph nodes) regressed, when fever recurred for 5 days and anti-inflammatory therapies had no effect, along with other 4 out of 5 KD symptoms, the diagnosis of KD recurrence was established. Theoretically, recurrent KD is more likely to cause coronary artery damage [Goswami et al. Children 5(11):E155, 2018]. However, it has also been reported that recurrent KD tend to be mild and incomplete [Guleria et al. Int J Rheum Dis 22(7):1183–1187, 2019]. In our center, two children had KD three times, and none of them showed CAA.

In this chapter, we present four cases with recurrent KD. One of them, the second KD occurred within 8 weeks of the first KD onset before aspirin is discontinued. One of them had KD three times.

X. Li · H. Wang (✉) · X. Yu
Department of Pediatric Cardiology, Shengjing Hospital of China Medical University, Shenyang, Liaoning, P. R. China

J. Dong
Department of Cardiology Function, Shengjing Hospital of China Medical University, Shenyang, Liaoning, P. R. China
e-mail: dongj@sj-hospital.org

B. Gao
Department of Neurology Function, Shengjing Hospital of China Medical University, Shenyang, Liaoning, P. R. China

11.1 Case 38: Recurrent KD at Sub-acute Phase

A previously healthy 2-year-old girl presented with an unremarkable past medical and family history.

She presented on Day 7 of illness, with fever for 7 days along with congestive rashes, red lips, and bilateral conjunctival congestion for 6 days. She was treated with cefotaxime sodium for 4 days in a local clinic, but her symptoms were not improved. Echo showed dilated coronary artery. She was admitted in our pediatric cardiology ward. Examination revealed the following findings: afebrile, smooth breath, HR 102 bpm, RR 22 bpm, warm hands and feet (BP 90/60 mmHg). There were congestive rashes all over the body. The laterocervical lymph nodes were swollen. She had nonsuppurative bilateral conjunctivitis, red lips and strawberry tongue, edema in feet, and erythema in hands. Others were normal. Admission blood test revealed WBC 18.6 × 10^9/L, HGB 108 g/L, PLT 294 × 10^9/L, CRP 57.1 mg/L (Table. 11.1). Blood gas ion analysis and myocardial markers were normal. Cervical ultrasonic at the local hospital showed bilateral lymphadenopathy; the bigger one was 2.7 cm × 1.2 cm. Echo showed LCA dilated about 3.0 mm, RCA was normal, tricuspid regurgitation (mild), normal LVEF. Chest DR showed lung texture enhancement. She was treated with (1) oral aspirin 30–50 mg/kg/days, divided in three doses and dipyridamole 3–5 mg/kg/days, divided in three doses; (2) IVIG (2 g/kg/day) over 12 h. On Day 8, blood test revealed liver function was normal, MP-IgM and CP-IgM were negative, MP IgG was 1:160. Virus culture was negative. Oral azithromycin 10 mg/kg/day for 3 days. On Day 11, after IVIG, her temperature was settled over 48 h and the dosage of aspirin was reduced to 3–5 mg/kg/days. Echo showed coronary artery was normal (Fig. 11.1). On Day 13, she was in good condition. Retested results showed WBC 5.1 × 10^9/L, N% 35.4%, HGB 114 g/L, PLT 296 × 10^9/L. CRP 4.35 mg/L. Liver function was normal except ALB 34.0 g/L. She was discharged.

On Day 17, she had fever again, accompanied by cough and runny nose. New rashes with small needle-tip hemorrhagic

H. Wang (ed.), *Paediatric Kawasaki Disease*, https://doi.org/10.1007/978-981-15-0038-1_11

Table 11.1 The comparison of first time and recurrent KD laboratory parameters

	First time KD	Recurrent KD
WBC ($\times 10^9$/L)	18.6	3.28
NE ($\times 10^9$/L)	10.3	0.7
HGB (g/L)	108	106
PLT ($\times 10^9$/L)	294	132
CRP (mg/L)	57.10	4.77

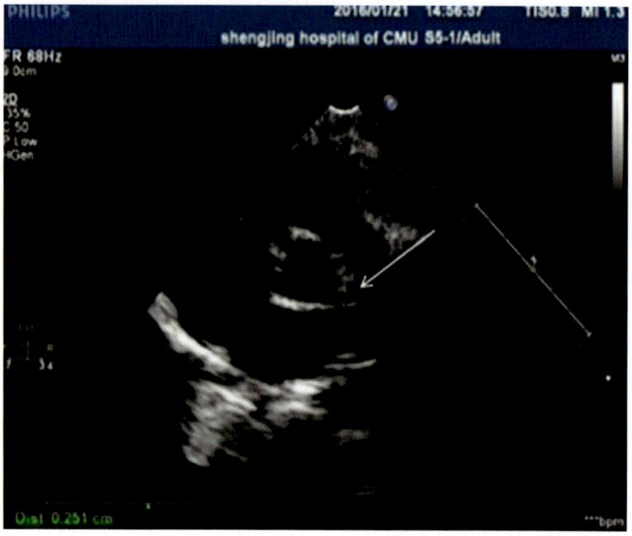

Fig. 11.1 On Day 11, echo showed normal LCA

spots scattered around the body. She had reoccurrence of red lips and strawberry tongue, but no conjunctival congestion. She was admitted again. Blood test revealed WBC 6.23 × 10^9/L, HGB 119 g/L, PLT 186 × 10^9/L. CRP 10.0 mg/L (Table. 11.1). Liver function was normal except AST 48 U/L. DIC was normal. She was given azithromycin infusion and oral esberitox. On Day 18, she still had high-grade fever reaching 39.5 °C. Retested results showed HSV-IgM(−), EBV-IgM(−). Infectious diseases were excluded after consultation with infectious disease specialist. On Day 22, she had persistent fever up to 39.5 °C. Retested blood work revealed WBC 3.28 × 10^9/L, N 10.3 × 10^9/L, HGB 106 g/L, PLT 132 × 10^9/L. CRP 4.77 mg/L. Cervical ultrasonic showed bilateral lymphadenopathy; the bigger one was 3.3 cm × 1.9 cm. Echo showed coronary artery was normal. She had met the criteria for recurrent KD, and she was treated with (1) IVIG 1 g/kg/days for 2 days; (2) aspirin resumed to 30–50 mg/kg/days and dipyridamole, both in three divided doses; (3) bone marrow puncture recommended but turned down by her parents.

On Day 25, her fever improved and rashes disappeared. Retested blood work revealed WBC 4.31 × 10^9/L, HGB 103 g/L, PLT 179 × 10^9/L. Liver function tests showed ALB 30.3 g/L. ALT 32 U/L, AST 49 U/L. NSE 21.07 ng/ml. Ferritin 198.6 ng/ml. LDH 291 U/L. Serum lipoprotein was normal. She was given infusion of albumin. On Day 27, her temperature was normal for 2 days and the dosage of aspirin was reduced to 3–5 mg/kg/days. On Day 32, she was in good condition. Retested blood work results showed: WBC 6.71 × 10^9/L, N% 28.8%, HGB 113 g/L, PLT 301 × 10^9/L. CRP was normal. Liver function was normal except AST 45 U/L. She was discharged.

11.1.1 Clinical Course of the Patient with the First Time Kd

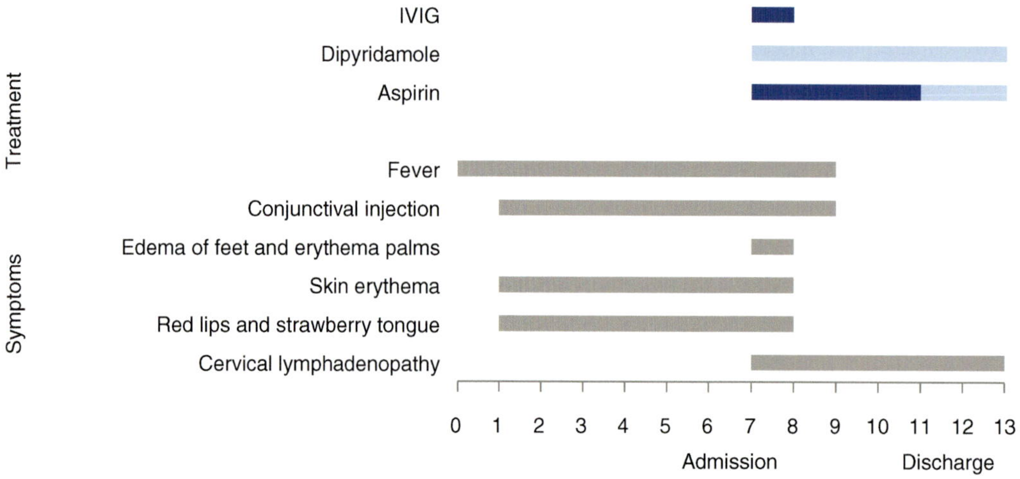

11.1.2 Clinical Course of the Patient with the Second Times KD

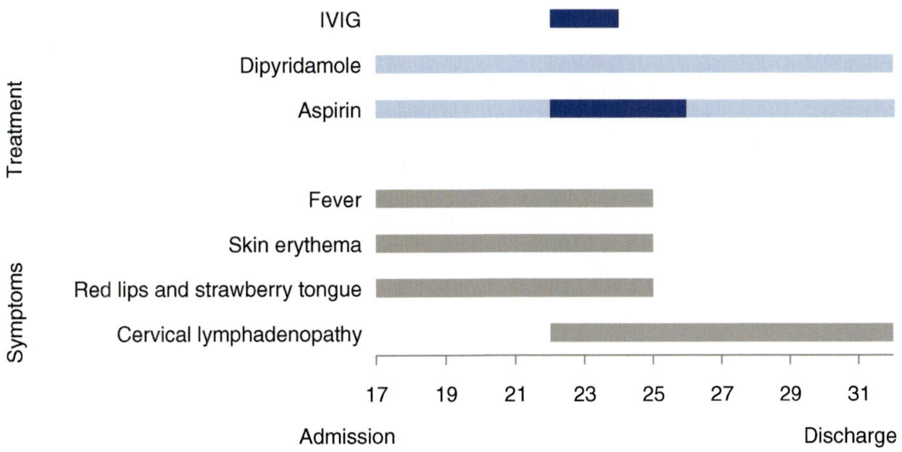

11.1.3 Follow-Up

Since discharged, she took oral aspirin and dipyridamole. Echo was performed 1 week later. On Day 60, she had a normal PLT, ESR; then all medications were stopped.

At 6 months, echo showed normal coronary artery.

11.1.4 Diagnosis

1. KD recurrence.
2. MP infection.
3. Hypoalbuminemia.

11.1.5 Discussion

She had met the criteria of KD: fever lasting for 5 days and antibiotics infusion was not effective, along with (1) conjunctival congestion without exudation; (2) generalized rashes; (3) edema in hands and feet; (4) red lips and strawberry tongue; (5) cervical lymphadenopathy shown in ultrasonography with the biggest one over 1.5 cm; (6) mildly dilated LCA shown in echo.

She also met the criteria of recurrent KD. She had diagnosed KD 17 days ago, all clinical symptoms disappeared and fever settled over 1 week. Then (1) she had recurrent fever for 5 days and infusion of antibiotics was not effective; (2) congestive rashes; (3) red lips and strawberry tongue; iv) cervical lymphadenectasis, the biggest one about 3.3 cm.

11.1.6 Case Specific Clinic Features

1. KD is a syndrome with unknown causes. It typically affects infants and toddlers, and causes systemic vasculitis. Although the incidence rates of KD vary among countries, it happens mostly in Asian children. The US surveys showed that the proportion of recurrent KD among all of the patients was 1.5% and Japan 3.5% [1]. Korea's national epidemiological survey reported a recurrence rate of 2.2% from 2006 to 2008 [2]. The cause of recurrent KD is not clear. It may be related to infections, immune disorders, irregular medication, and genetic susceptibility [3]. The incidence of recurrence is higher for patients less than 3 years of age. At the first onset of recurrent KD, children had longer durations of fever before IVIG treatment, higher levels of ALT and AST, and lower hemoglobin levels compared to those with a single episode of KD [4].
2. MAS is a clinical syndrome, caused by excessive activation and proliferation of well differentiated macrophages [5]. It could occur secondary to a diverse group of diseases including infections, neoplasms and rheumatic disorders, such as systemic onset juvenile idiopathic arthritis, systemic lupus erythematosus and, rarely, KD [6].
3. In this case, the patient was diagnosed with KD for the first time at the age of 2 years. After IVIG treatment, fever settled, and aspirin was reduced after afebrile 48 h. But 9 days later, she had fever again, with cough, expectoration, runny nose, new congestive skin rashes, red lips and strawberry tongue, but had neither conjunctival congestion nor edema in hands and feet. Retested blood work

revealed normal WBC and slightly elevated CRP. Considering a possibility of infection, she was given infusion of azithromycin for 3 days, but her fever did not improve. At this time, the reexamination of CBC suggested reduction in whole blood cells, combined with hypoalbuminemia. The sonography of the cervical lymph nodes indicated that the lymph nodes were larger than before. She was diagnosed with recurrent KD. IVIG was given for another 5 days to treat fever symptom. Then her body temperature returned to normal. Her parents denied bone marrow puncture test. MAS may not be excluded in children who have recurrent fevers with reduced WBC. Test results revealed normal NSE, ferritin, DIC, blood lipid series, ALT, and LDH, which may have resulted from the timely diagnosis of recurrent KD and the treatment with IVIG. The patient had no coronary artery injuries, and needed further long-term follow-up.

Xue-mei Li

11.2 Case 39: Recurrent KD After Cease Medicine

A previously healthy 2-year-old boy presented with an unremarkable past medical and family history.

He presented on Day 5 of illness with a fever lasting for 5 days, along with bilateral conjunctivitis and rashes for 2 days. He was treated with cefuroxime sodium and vidarabine monophosphate for 2 days at a clinic, but the treatment failed to improve his symptoms. He was admitted in pediatric cardiology ward as a KD patient. *Examination* revealed the following findings: afebrile, smooth breath (HR 107 bpm, RR 30 bpm), warm hands and feet (BP 92/58 mmHg), rashes on his back, cervical lymphadenopathy on the left side, bilateral conjunctivitis without purulent secretion, red lips and strawberry tongue, edema in feet, and erythema in palms. Others were normal. *Admission blood* test revealed WBC 6.0 × 10^9/L, HGB 104 g/L, PLT 296 × 10^9/L. CRP 57.5 mg/L. ESR 36 mm/h. ALB 34.2 g/L, ALT 196 U/L, AST 34 U/L. MP-IgM and CP-IgM negative. Cervical ultrasound showed lymphadenopathy on both sides, and the bigger one was 2.0 cm × 1.0 cm. He had met 4 out of 5 of the criteria for KD, and he was treated with (1) IVIG 1g/kg/day, for 2 days; (2) oral aspirin 30–50 mg/kg/days and dipyridamole 3–5 mg/kg/days in three divided doses; (3) infusion of polyene phosphatidyl choline and compound glycyrrhizin.

On Day 8, his fever settled over 48 h and his general condition improved. The dosage of aspirin was reduced to one dose of 3–5 mg/kg/days. Echo showed coronary artery was normal (Fig. 11.2a, b). On Day 11, he was in good condition. Retested blood work found: WBC 5.5 × 10^9/L, HGB 103 g/L, PLT 477 × 10^9/L. CRP 4.55 mg/L. ESR 69 mm/h. Liver function was normal except ALB 34.3 g/L. He was discharged.

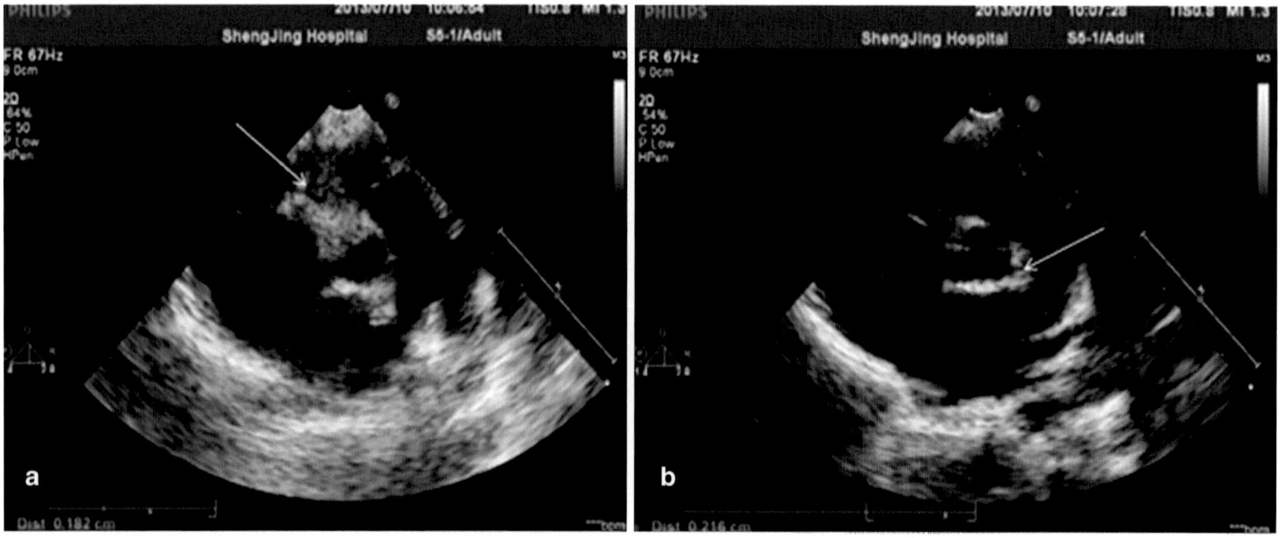

Fig. 11.2 On Day 8, echo showed RCA (**a**) and LCA (**b**) were normal

11.2.1 Clinical Course of the Patient with the First Time KD

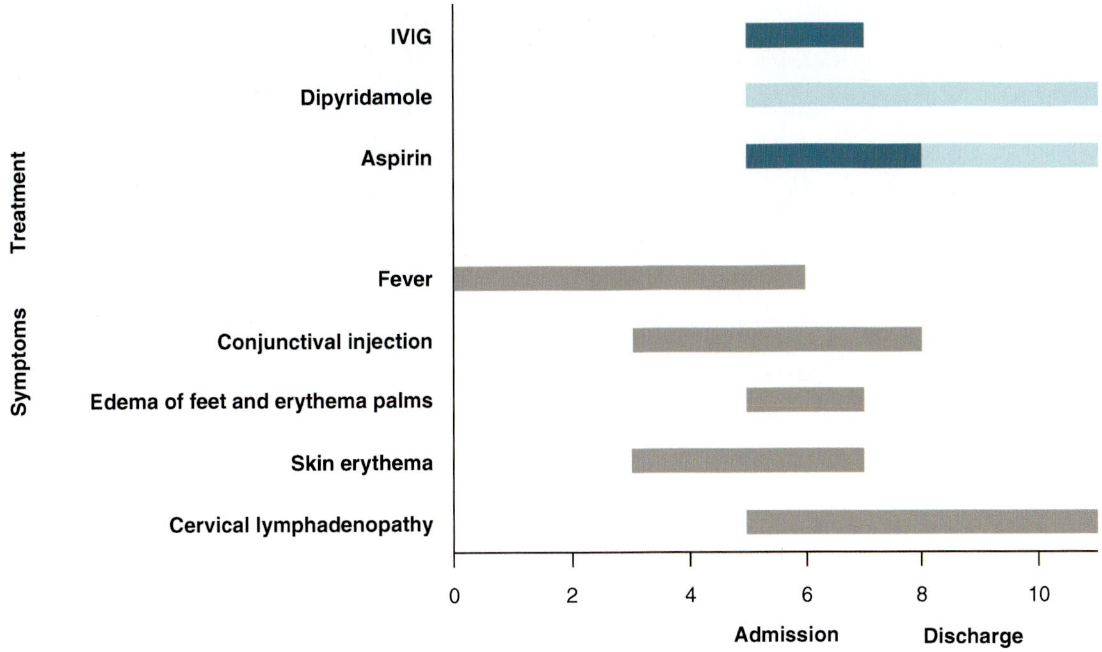

11.2.2 Follow-Up

Since discharged, he took oral aspirin and dipyridamole. Echo was performed 1 week later. Examination at follow-up 2 months revealed that he had normal PLT, ESR, and echo results. Then all medications were stopped.

At 9 months of diagnosis, he presented with a 5 day history of fever, along with bilateral conjunctival congestion and rashes for 1 day. Then he was admitted in our pediatric cardiology ward second time. Examination showed his general condition was good, his vital signs included the following findings: axillary temperature 37.0 °C, PR 100 bpm, RR 25 bpm. He had congestive rashes on the back, cervical lymphadenopathy on the left, nonsuppurative bilateral conjunctivitis, red lips and strawberry tongue, edema in hands and feet. Examination confirmed lungs, heart, abdominal, and neurological system were normal. Admission blood test revealed WBC 21.1 × 10^9/L, HGB114g/L, PLT 355 × 10^9/L. CRP 84 mg/L. Cervical ultrasound showed lymphadenopathy on both sides, the bigger one was 1.6 × 1.2 cm on the left. He was diagnosed with recurrent KD and treated with: (1) IVIG 1 g/kg/day for 2 days; (2) oral aspirin 30–50 mg/kg/days and dipyridamole 3–5 mg/kg/days, in three divided doses; (3) infusion of creatine phosphate sodium 1 g/days. On Day 6, he continued to have fever. Tests were repeated and showed: ESR 53 mm/h; liver function ALB 35.3 g/L, ALT 244 U/L, AST 50 U/L, negative virus antibody titer, and negative MP-IgM and CP-IGM. He was given compound glycyrrhizin infusion.

On Day 8, the dosage of aspirin was reduced to one dose of 3–5 mg/kg/day since he did not have fever for 2 days. Echo showed coronary artery was normal (Fig. 11.3a, b). On Day 11 of illness, he was in good condition. Retested blood work showed WBC 7.1 × 10^9/L, HGB 99 g/L, PLT 489 × 10^9/L, CRP 9.95 mg/L, ESR 73 mm/h, and normal liver function. He was discharged.

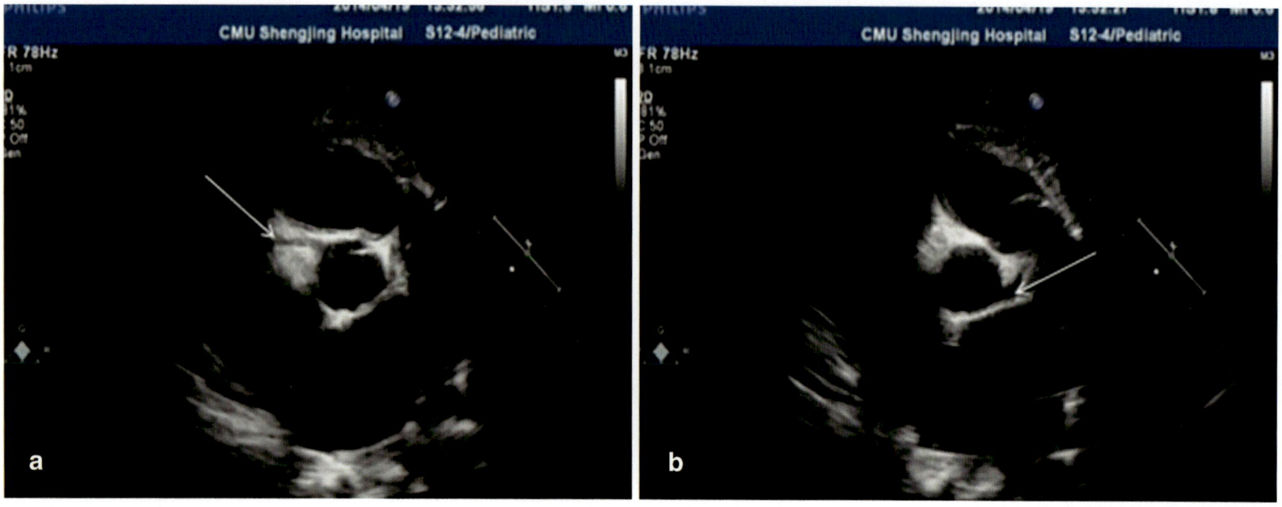

Fig. 11.3 Recurrent KD on Day 8, echo showed RAC (**a**) and LAC (**b**) were normal

11.2.3 Clinical Course of the Patient with the Second Times KD

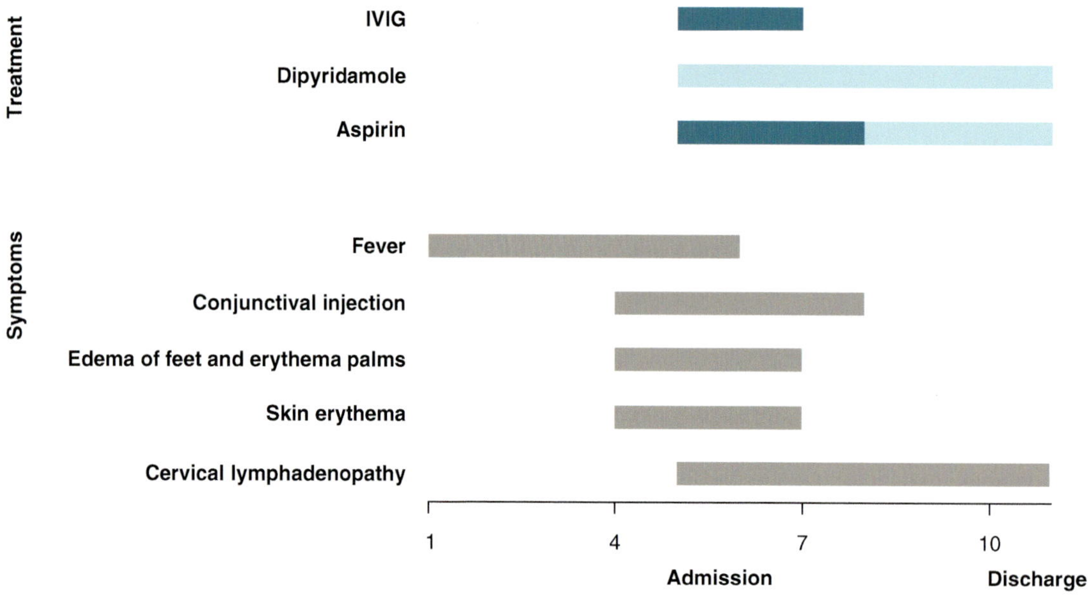

11.2.4 Follow-Up

Since discharged, he took oral aspirin and dipyridamole. Echo was performed at 2, 3, 4, and 8 weeks of illness, and results were normal. At 2 months of illness he had a normal PLT and ESR. All medications were stopped.

11.2.5 Diagnosis

1. Recurrent KD.
2. Liver dysfunction.

11.2.6 Discussion

He had met the criteria for KD; he had fever for 5 days and unresponsive to oral antibiotics, along with (1) cervical lymphadenopathy over 1.5 cm; (2) conjunctival congestion without exudation; (3) generalized congest rashes; (4) edema in feet and erythema in palms, WBC > 15 × 10^9/L. CRP > 30 mg/L. ESR > 40 mm/h.

He had met the criteria of recurrent KD, (1) fever for 5 days and oral antibiotics were not effective; (2) left cervical lymphadenopathy about 1.6 cm × 1.2 cm; (3) conjunctival congestion without exudation; (4) generalized congest rashes; (5) red lips and strawberry tongue; (6) edema in hands and feet. And he was diagnosed with KD 9 months ago.

11.2.7 Case Specific Clinic Features

1. KD was a syndrome with unknown causes. It typically affects infants and toddlers, and causes systemic vasculitis. Although the incidence rates of KD vary among countries, it is much higher in children in Asian countries.
2. The incidence of recurrence was higher for patients less than 3 years old. It was reported that incidence of recurrence within 2 years from the first episode is higher than after 2 years [7]. It is believed that the patients with recurrent KD might develop more serious illness than that of the first onset, and relapse of CAA [8]. Study suggests that a longer duration of fever, lower levels of hemoglobin, and higher AST levels could help to identify children who were at an increased risk of recurrent KD [4]. The mechanism of anemia caused by KD was not very clear. Some people believed that non-bacterial inflammatory reactions inhibit bone marrow hematopoietic function [9].
3. In this case, the child was 2 years old at first KD onset, and KD recurred 9 months later. Results showed mild anemia (RBC 3.7×10^{12}/L, HGB 104 g/L), liver dysfunction (ALT 196 U/L), consistent with KD recurrence risk factors described in the literature. However, there was no prolonged fever in this child, and his fever regressed after IVIG.
4. The results of initial and recurrent assays were compared:

KD	First time KD	Recurrent KD
WBC ($\times 10^9$/L)	6.0	21.1
CRP (mg/L)	57.50	84
ESR (mm/h)	36	53
ALT (U/L)	196	244
AST (U/L)	34	50

It was consistent with that the patients with recurrent KD might associate with the more serious illness than that of the first onset. However, there was no significant difference in the duration of fever, both of which were regressed after IVIG.

5. Although recurrent KD was confirmed, no coronary artery injury was detected. The risk factors for developing coronary artery injury include boy, age < 12 months, hypoalbuminemia, persistent fever for more than 2 weeks, and unresponsive to IVIG. Although this child was a boy, and WBC > 30.0×10^9/L, ESR > 100 mm/h, CRP > 100 mg/L, he did not have any other risk factors for coronary artery injury. Even with recurrent KD, there were no complications of coronary artery injury.

Xue-mei Li

11.3 Case 40: Recurrent KD Before Cease Medicine with CAA

A previous healthy 3-month-old girl presented with unremarkable past medical and family history.

She presented, on Day 9 of illness, with persistent fever, rashes, and conjunctivitis for 9 days. Prior to having fever, she vomited 1 day. Secondary-generation-cephalosporin and liquid infusion were given in a local hospital, and her non-projectile vomiting was relieved. Although consequently high fever (39 °C) and rashes were temporarily relieved for 2 days, lab results revealed worse findings as listed in Table 11.2. Then she was admitted to our pediatric cardiology ward as a patient with unknown fever and rash. *Examination* revealed she had fever (39.3 °C). She was irritable. Red congestive rashes were all over the body, along with bilateral conjunctivitis, red and cracked lips. Others were normal. *Admission blood* tests revealed CMV-IgM (+), EBV-IgM (−). She had met 4/5 criteria for KD, and she was treated with (1) oral aspirin 30–50 mg/kg/day and dipyridamole 3–5 mg/kg/day, both in two or three divided doses; (2) IVIG 1 g/kg/day for 2 days; (3) erythromycin infusion.

On Day 10, her fever settled, and her mental state and rashes were improved. Lymphadenectasis regressed. Skin peeled around left thumb, and there was redness at distal interphalangeal joints. Investigation revealed WBC 13.4×10^9/L, NE 55.3%, HGB 81 g/L, PLT 70×10^9/L. ESR 35 mm/h. NT pro-BNP 14193 pg/ml. ALB 23.8 g/L. CK, CK-MB mass, cTnI, hs-cTnT, ALT, AST, and renal function was normal. CKMB 50 U/L. CRP 119.00 mg/L. ASO 75.0 U/ml. MP-IgG 1:160. CP-IgM positive. HSV-IgM and CMV-IgM were positive. Chest DR showed bilateral blurred pulmonary markings. Cervical ultrasound showed right lymphadenectasis about 1.2 cm × 0.4 cm. On Day 11, she was afebrile, rashes gradually regressed. Blood routine results were listed in Table 11.2. ABEP was normal. She was treated with (1) reduced dose of aspirin at 3–5 mg/kg/day; (2) infusion of ganciclovir 7.5 mg/kg/day; (3) infusion of albumin 1 g/kg/day, for 2 days; (4) oral iron protein succinate 5 ml, bid.

On Day 12, she had mild fever (37.5 °C), with new rashes on her right cheek. On Day 13, her fever was up to 38 °C. Echo revealed LVED 21.8 mm, LVEF 69%, mitral valve mono-wave, LCA dilated 3.4–3.7 mm, RCA dilated about 2.6–3.7 mm. She had met the criteria of IVIG resistance, and was given additional infusion of IVIG 1 g/kg/day for 2 days. On Day 14, she was afebrile, and conjunctivitis was settled.

Table 11.2 The dynamic changes of laboratory parameters

	First time KD							Recurrent KD		
Time of illness	1 day	4 days	8 days	10 days	11 days	15 days	17 days	5 days	9 days	12 days
WBC (×10⁹)	12.6	8.43	18.6	13.4	10.4	14.8		8.3	5.1	5
NE (%)	72.7	79.19	44.2	55.3	18	10.1		66.6	17.9	7.5
HGB (g/L)	120	109	107	81	79	73		118	105	97
PLT (×10⁹)	452	195.5	101	70	113	1097		357	553	596
ESR (mmHg)				35		60	60	75	50	
CRP (mg/L)	11.2	96.5	97.5	119		18.4	15.3	110	19.	6.08
ALT (U/L)				16		58	106	83	19	
AST (U/L)				28		93	171	40	28	
Alb (g/L)				23.8		34.3	37.2	40.8	34.4	
NT-pro BNP (pg/ml)				14193				810.5		

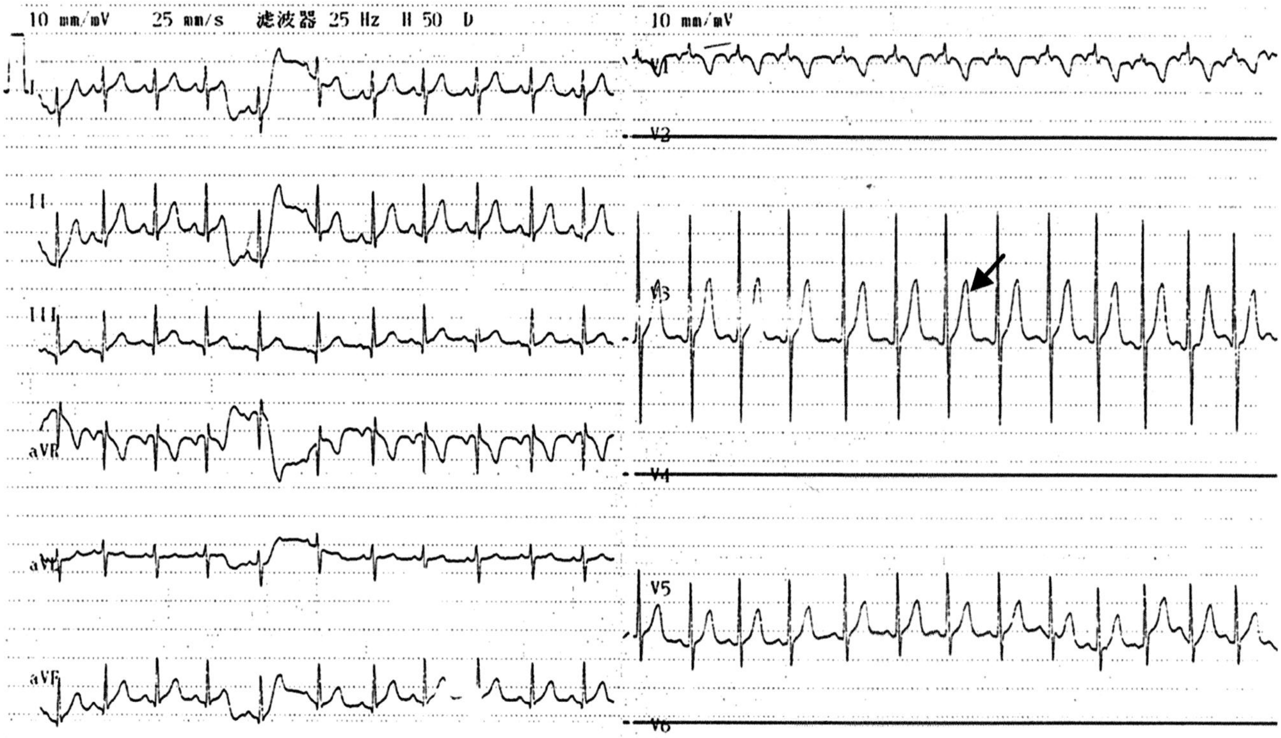

Fig. 11.4 On Day 19 of illness, ECG showed slightly elevated T wave

On Day 15, laboratory test revealed normal NT pro-BNP, ESR 60 mm/h, ASO 129 IU/ml, CRP 18.40 mg/L, ALB 34.3 g/L, ALT 58 U/L, AST 93 U/L, serum K^+5.68 mmol/L. Myocardial enzyme was normal. Blood culture for bacteria was negative. She was given compound glycyrrhizin 20 ml/day and oral furosemidum 1 mg/kg. On Day 18, re-checked echo revealed LVED 25.2 mm, LVEF 67%. Mitral valve E-wave 0.8, A-wave 0.7. LCA 3.0–3.7 mm, LAD 3.1 mm. RCA 3.3–3.4 mm. Serum K^+ 6.68 mmol/L, thus she was remained on furosemide 1 mg/kg infusion.

On Day 19, she was afebrile, and all the symptoms were settled. Examination found desquamation around toenails. Laboratory tests were improved and listed in Table 11.2. ECG showed slightly elevated T wave (Fig. 11.4). She was discharged.

11.3.1 Clinical Course of the Patient at the First Time KD

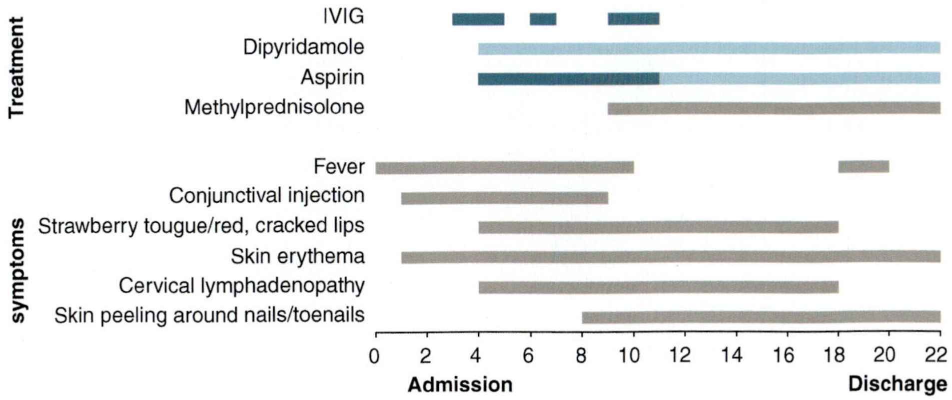

11.3.2 Follow-Up

Three days after discharge, tests found serum K^+ 5.97 mmol/l; thus she was given additional oral furosemide, qd. Ten days after discharge, serum K^+ was 5.07 mmol/l, ALT was normal, and AST was 62 U/L. Repeated echo results were listed in Table 11.3. She took oral aspirin and dipyridamole.

11.3.3 Diagnosis

1. KD, IVIG resistance.
2. Bilateral CAA.
3. Acute bronchitis.
4. Liver dysfunction.
5. Hypoalbuminemia.
6. Moderate anemia.
7. Thrombocytopenia.
8. Mixed virus infection (CMV, HSV).
9. Hyperkalemia.

11.3.4 Case Presentation of Second Course

Seventeen months after the initial onset, the girl presented again with fever (38.5 °C) 2 days, spot-like rashes on her back and bilateral conjunctival congestion. After infusion of erythromycin for 2 days, her fever was not subsided and the rashes spread to chest and arms with partial merge. *Examination* revealed fever (38.5 °C), red congestive rashes distributed on her trunk and arms, partially merged rashes on the back, along with bilateral conjunctivitis, and red dry lips. Others were normal. She was suspected to have KD recurrence, and she was treated with second-generation cephalosporin and erythromycin. She was also given recombinant human interferon aerosol inhaler.

On Day 5 of second illness onset, her body temperature reached 38 °C, rashes increased on the trunk and hip, and she developed strawberry tongue and cervical lymphadenectasis. Investigation findings were listed in Table 11.1. ALT 83 U/L, AST 40 U/L. MP-IgG 1:320. CP-IgM and MP-IgM were positive. Mumps virus-IgM positive. HSV-IgM positive. Chest DR and ECG were normal. Echo revealed diffuse dilation of bilateral coronary artery, LCA 3.5–4.8 mm, LAD 3.0 mm, LCX 2.3 mm. RCA 3.0 mm, LVEF 60% (Figs. 11.5 and 11.6). Cervical ultrasound showed lymphadenopathy about 1.5 x 0.8 cm. She had met 4/5 criteria for KD, and she was treated with (1) IVIG 1 g/kg/day for 2 days; (2) azithromycin infusion; (3) vidarabine monophosphate infusion; (4) oral aspirin 30–50 mg/kg/day, dipyridamole 3–5 mg/kg/day, both in two or three divided doses; (5) oral compound glycyrrhizin to protect liver.

On Day 6, she was afebrile, with mild cough. The rashes, lymphadenopathy, strawberry tongue, and conjunctivitis

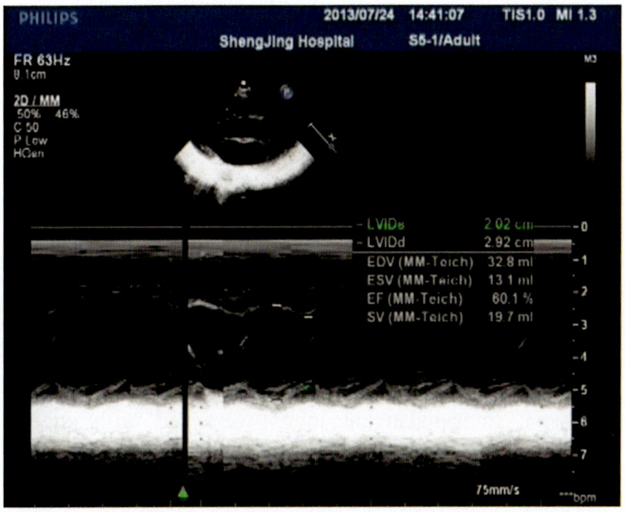

Fig. 11.5 On Day 5 of second illness, echo revealed LVEF 60.1%

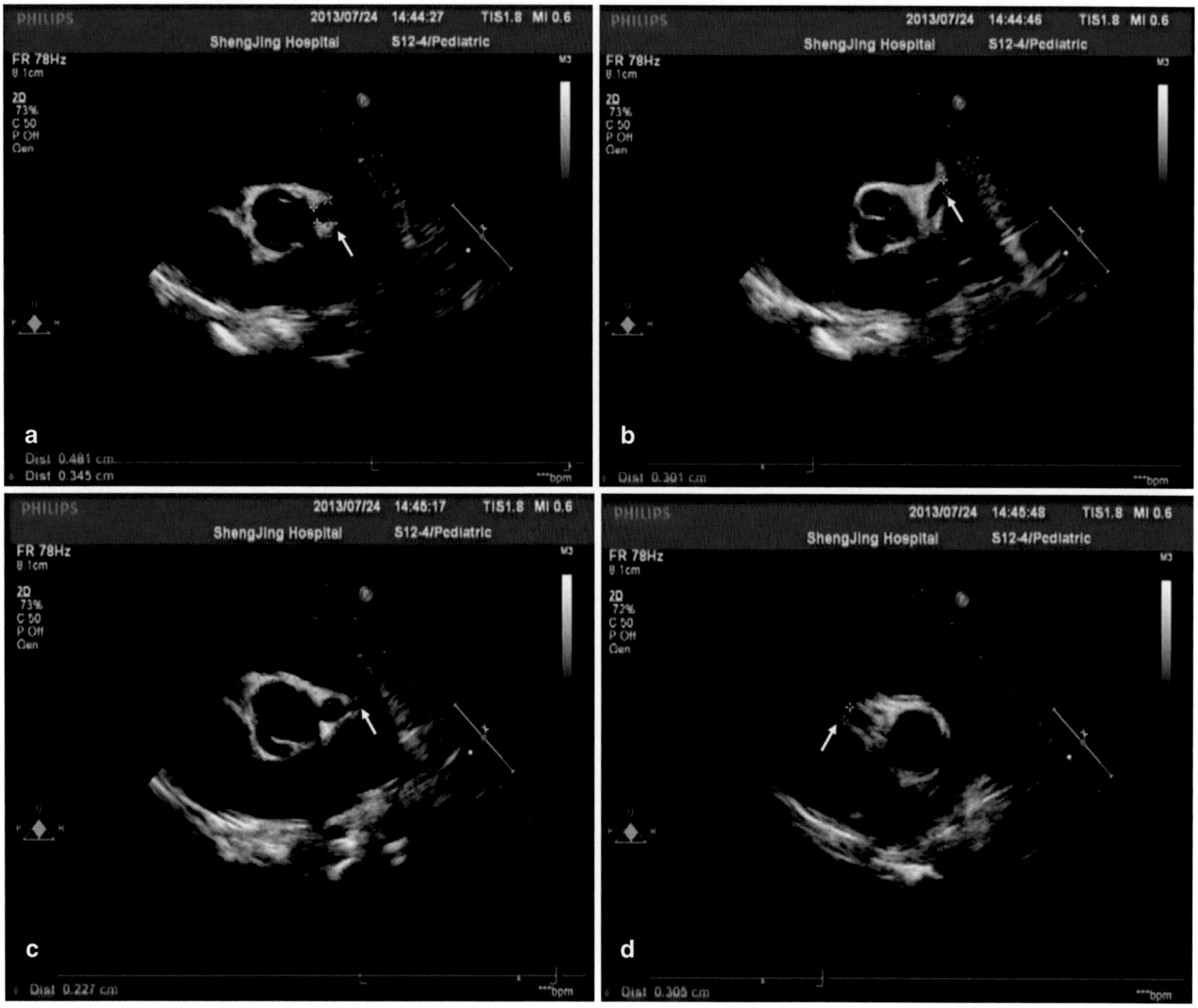

Fig. 11.6 On Day 5 of second illness onset ECHO revealed LCA 3.5–4.8 mm (**a**), LAD 3.0 mm (**b**), LCX 2.3 mm (**c**). RCA 3.0 mm (**d**)

Table 11.3 The dynamic changes of coronary artery

Time of illness	12 days	7 weeks	11 weeks	16 weeks	5.5 months	9 months	14 months	17 months	17 months + 7 days	18 months	27 months	35 months	51 months	58 months
LCA (mm)	3.4–3.7	5.3	5.2	4.26	4.1	3.6	3.5	3.5–4.8	3.2–4.5	3.6	3.8	3.7	3.8	3.0–3.6
LAD (mm)		5.2	5.3		3.7–4.7	3.1–3.7	2.6	3	2.4–2.9	2.4			3.2	
LCX (mm)		3.5				2.1	2.2	2.3	2.4	1.7				
RCA (mm)	2.6–3.7	5.2	4.8	3.48	3.5	3.1–2.6	3	3	2.9–3.1	2.9	2.8	2.7	2.9	2.9

regressed. Interphalangeal joints were red with edema. Parotid gland was normal as shown in ultrasound, so are serum and urine amylase and serum lipase, which indicated the absence of mumps. On Day 9, 48 h after IVIG infusion, all the symptoms were settled. Retested results were listed in Table 11.3. Aspirin was reduced to 3–5 mg/kg/day. On Day 12, investigations revealed WBC 5.0 × 10^9/L, NE 7.5%, HGB 97 g/L, PLT 596 × 10^9/L. CRP 6.08 mg/L. Echo revealed LM 3.2–4.5 mm, LAD 2.4–2.9 mm, LCX 2.4 mm. RCA 2.9–3.1 mm, LVEF 60%. She was discharged.

11.3.5 Clinical Course of the Patient at the Second Times KD

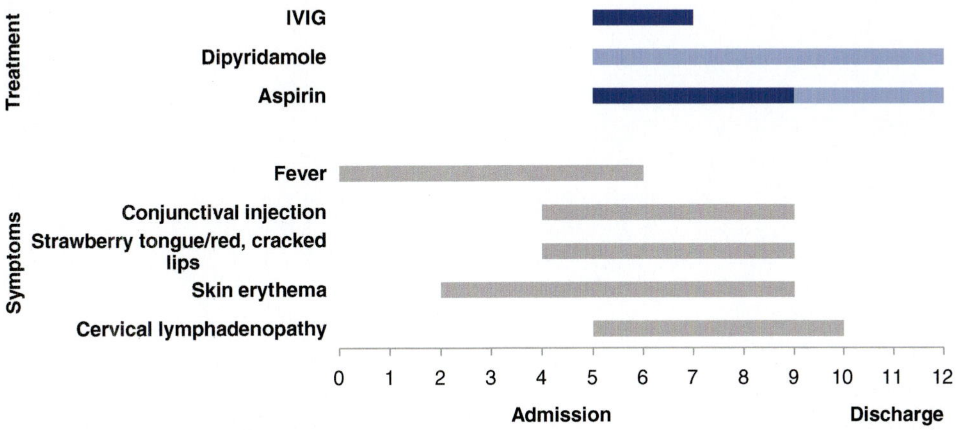

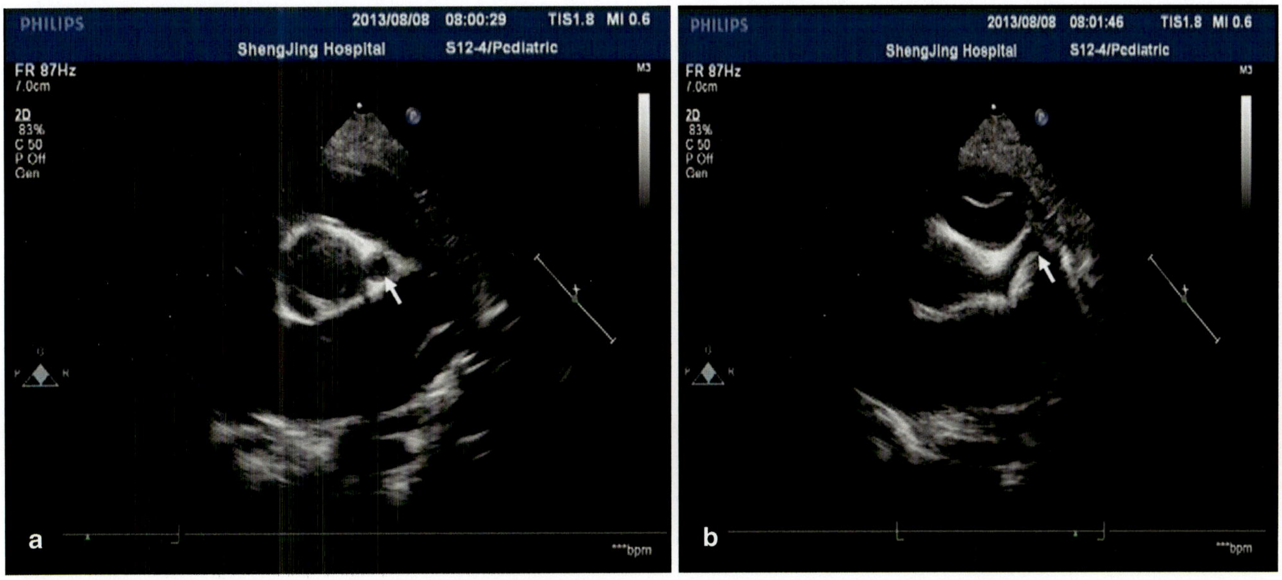

Fig. 11.7 At 18 months of first illness, echo showed LCA 3.6 mm (**a**), LAD 2.4 mm (**b**)

11.3.6 Follow-Up

After discharged, echo was performed at 18, 20, 27, 35, 51, 58, and 64 months, and revealed LCA 3.5 mm, RCA 2.5 mm (Figs. 11.7, 11.8, 11.9, 11.10, 11.11, 11.12 and 11.13). RCA was recovered at 18 months of illness, while LCA remained dilated over 64 months.

11.3.7 Diagnosis

1. KD recurrence.
2. Bilateral coronary artery dilation.
3. Liver dysfunction.
4. HSV infection.
5. MP infection.
6. CP infection.

11.3.8 Discussion

At the initial onset, the girl met all the criteria of KD for persistent fever more than 5 days that was unresponsive to antibiotics and along with (1) bilateral conjunctivitis, without purulent discharge; (2) rashes on her trunk and hands; (3) cervical lymphadenopathy 1.2 cm (3 months old); (4) red and cracked lips; (5) skin membranous peeling around nails; (6) diffuse dilation of coronary artery; additional WBC 18.6 × 10^9/L, NE 44.2%; CRP 96.5 mg/L; NT pro-BNP 14193 pg/ml. At the second time of KD onset, she had persistent fever more than 5 days, antibiotics treatment was ineffective; and she had (1) bilateral conjunctivitis, without purulent discharge; (2) rashes on trunk and hands; (3) cervical lymphadenopathy over 1.5 cm; (4) red and cracked lips; (5) wider coronary artery than shown in the latest echo. ESR 75 mm/h. CRP 110 mg/L.

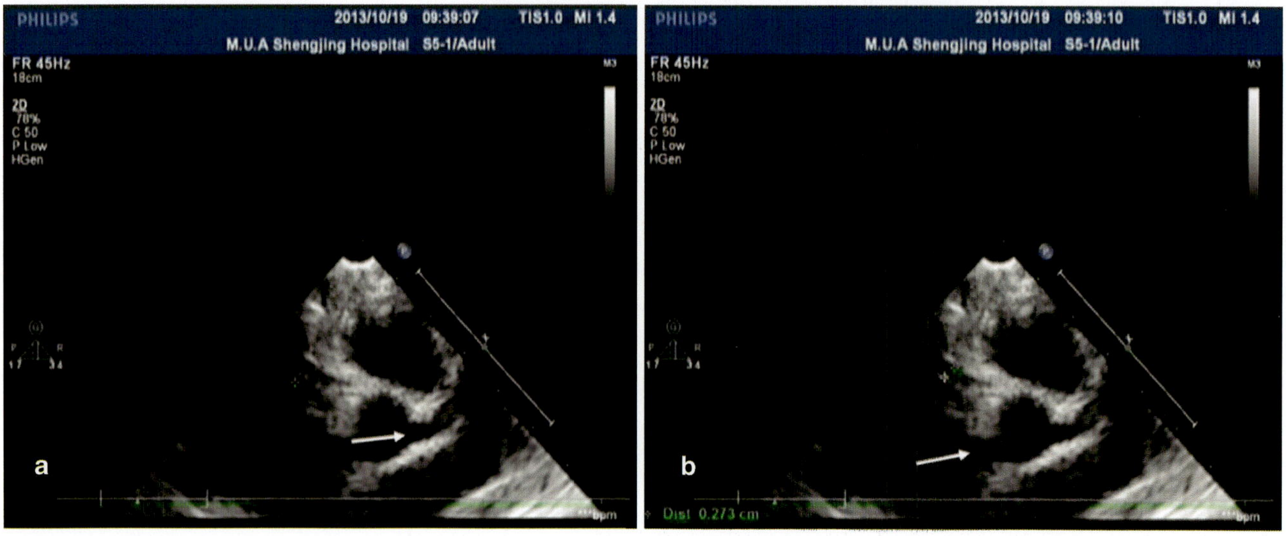

Fig. 11.8 At 20 months of first illness, echo showed LCA 3.7 mm (**a**), RCA 3.0 mm (**b**)

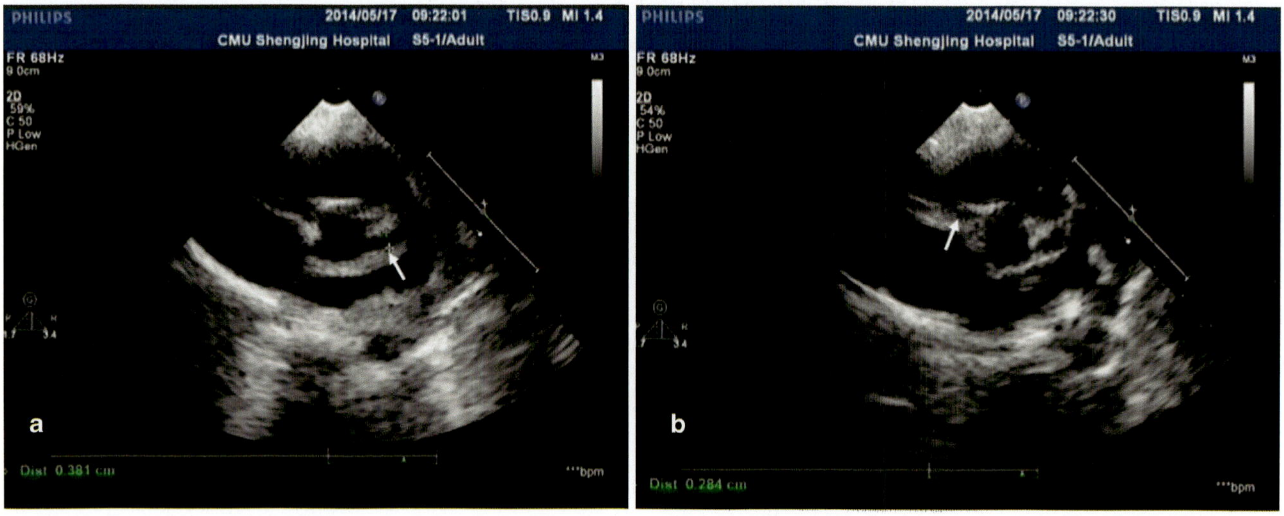

Fig. 11.9 At 27 months of first illness, echo showed LCA 3.8 mm (**a**), RCA 2.8 mm (**b**)

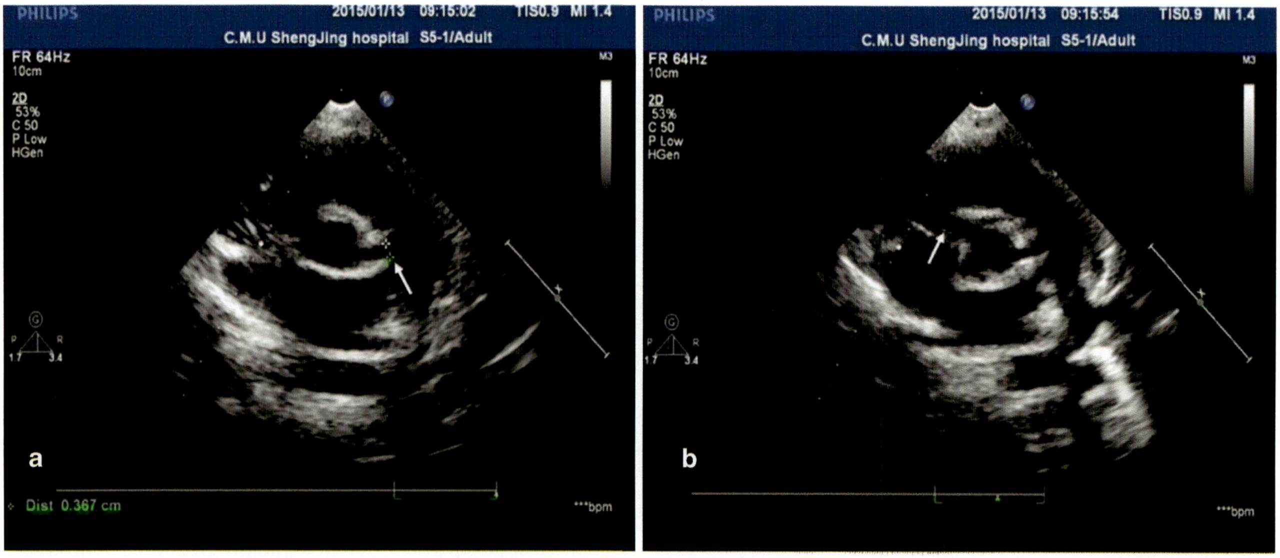

Fig. 11.10 At 35 months of first illness, echo showed LCA3.7 mm (**a**), RCA 2.7 mm (**b**)

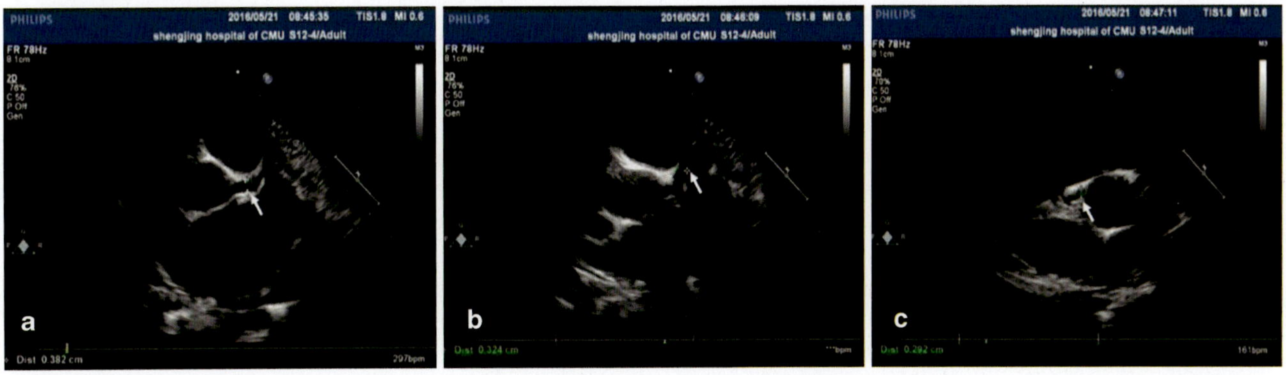

Fig. 11.11 At 51 months of first illness, echo showed LCA 3.8 mm (**a**), LAD 3.2 mm (**b**), RCA 2.9 mm (**c**)

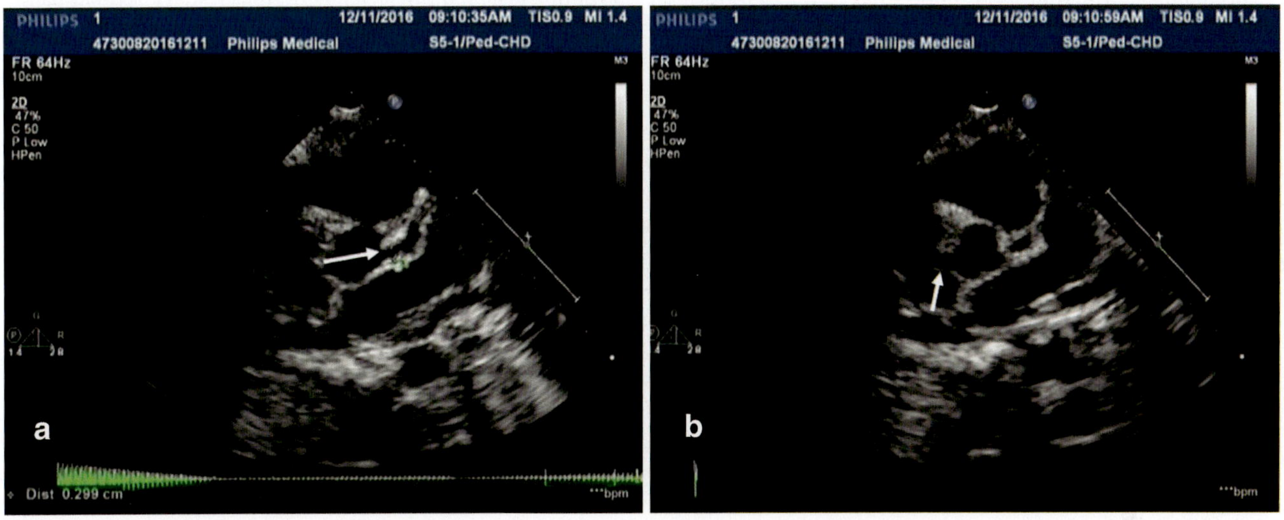

Fig. 11.12 At 58 months of first illness, echo showed LCA 3.0–3.6 mm (**a**), RCA 2.9 mm (**b**)

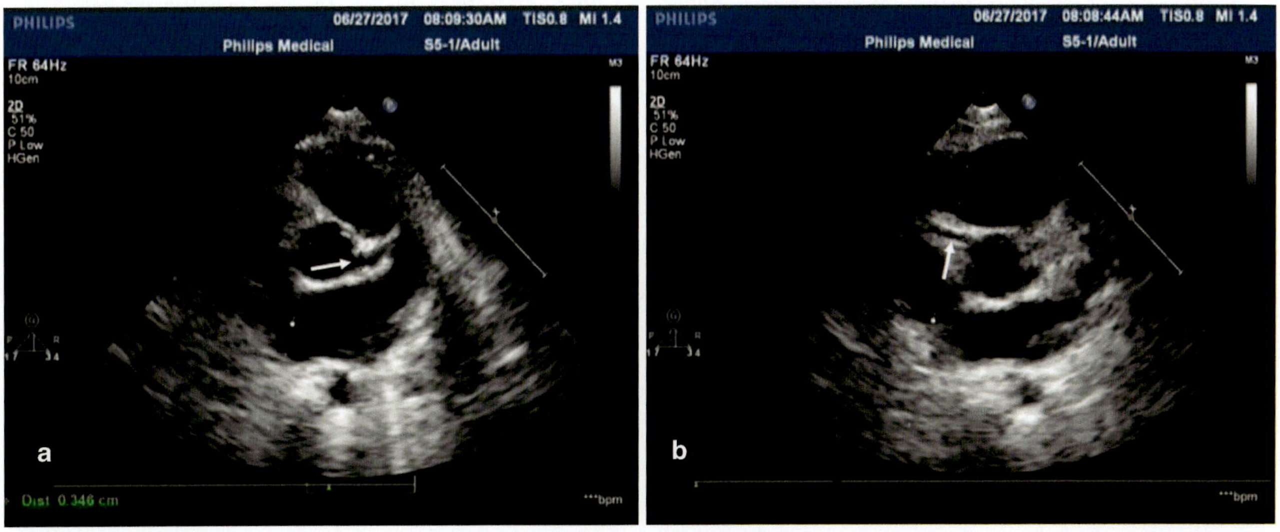

Fig. 11.13 At 64 months of first illness, echo showed LCA 3.5 mm (**a**), RCA 2.5 mm (**b**)

11.3.9 Case Specific Clinical Features

1. The patient was 3 month old when she had the first KD onset. She was admitted to hospital until Day 9 of illness. There have been reported that approximately 35% of infant patients belonged to IKD, which in fact, result in delayed clinical recognition and treatment [10]. KD in children below 6 months seems to have significantly different clinical presentation compared with elder ones. Furthermore, KD in younger patients appears to run a more aggressive clinical course and causes a significant higher risk of developing CAA even with IVIG treatment. Delays in diagnosis, with consequent delays in treatment, could have been responsible for development of complications. In young infants with unexplained fever lasting more than 5 days, a possibility of clinical KD must be considered and appropriate investigations should be ordered. Delays in diagnosis and treatment can have catastrophic consequences.
2. IVIG was applied 9 days after fever onset during the initial KD, 10 days after vomiting symptom. Timely IVIG treatment should be determined by fever instead of the initial symptoms involving gastrointestinal system, respiratory system, nervous system, etc. So the clinician should require detailed medical history, to prevent delaying IVIG treatment beyond Day 10.
3. In this case, recurrent KD occurred 17 months after the initial onset, when aspirin and dipyridamole were taken for the persistent dilation in coronary artery. Recurrence of KD is rare but not impossible. It is generally regarded as a new episode after at least three months from the initial episode. Previous surveys have shown that the incidence of recurrent KD ranges from 1.4% in China to 3% in Japan [11]. Data from a Japanese nationwide survey showed that coronary artery complications are more likely to be observed among children with recurrent disease than among patients with the first episode of recurrent KD. It is reported the incidence of recurrent KD within 2 years from the first episode is higher than after 2 years [7]. This indicates that it is important to follow patients carefully for 2 years after the initial episode. The incidence of recurrent KD was high for children with coronary artery complications in the first episode, and the presence of coronary artery complications in the first episode was a risk factor for recurrence [7]. There was no increased risk of aneurysm with repeated episodes of vasculitis in the second-onset KD compared to that in single episodes. Recent study suggested [12] that circulating levels of AST and hemoglobin can be used as predictive markers for recurrence KD, and they may serve as a therapeutic target for presenting recurrent KD in the future. Risk factors for the sequelae at the second episode of KD are male and the existing sequelae from the initial onset of KD. Older age at recurrent onset and the longer interval between the two episodes are risk factors for developing cardiac sequelae/complication in patients with recurrent KD [13].
4. During the second episode of KD, the patient had positive MP IgM. MP is one of the most reported pathogen in KD. Previous researches have reported that there is no statistic difference between MP induced KD and controls, in terms of duration of fever, levels of HGB, WBC, PLT, ESR, CRP, and albumin, and the incidence of coronary arterial lesions. Abe et al. [14] suggested the process of T cell activation by superantigens may play a role in pathophysiology of KD. By interacting directly with class two major histocompatibility complex molecules, superantigens can stimulate polyclonal T cell activation with subsequent massive cytokines release. Mycoplasma pneumoniae is the major pathogen causing respiratory infections in school-aged children and young adults. The most common manifestations include sore throat, hoarseness, fever, cough, headache, chills, coryza, and myalgia. Chest auscultation may detect rales, scattered or localized rhonchi, and expiratory wheezes. The diagnosis of Mycoplasma pneumoniae is based on clinical manifestations, culture of sputum, cold agglutinins, and antibody titer of Mycoplasma pneumoniae specific IgM. In children, a single positive IgM assay may be considered diagnostic in most cases, as IgM titer typically rises within 7–10 days of infection and appears approximately 2 weeks before IgG [15]. Lung complications in KD may be a consequence of vessel inflammation with increased vascular permeability and perivascular edematous changes.
5. During the initial course, PLT fluctuated from 101×10^9 to 70×10^9 and then 1097×10^9. Thrombocytopenia can be seen as a rare finding in KD and may be present in the acute phase of the disease, usually on days 5–12, then disappear within 3–4 days [10]. Thrombocytopenia in the first week of illness is often considered a marker for poor prognosis in KD and may presage the development of macrophage activation syndrome [16]. Krowchuk et al. suggested that thrombocytopenia is related to the destruction of thrombocytes via immunoglobulins or non-immune mechanisms [17]. Incidence of thrombocytopenia associated with KD has been reported as 1%–2% [18]. Thrombocytopenia can also be seen as a presenting feature in KD instead of thrombocytosis, anemia, leukocytosis, and thrombocytopenia should alert the clinician of severe disease and coronary artery aneurysm development. Frequent follow-up with echocardiographic examinations may be a better approach for these patients.

Xue-mei Li

11.4 Case 41: Recurrent KD (the Third Time)

A 17-month-old boy presented without significant past medical history or family history.

He presented on Day 8 of illness, with persistent high fever (axillary 39.6 °C) for 8 days, along with bilateral conjunctival congestion and rashes for 6 days, chills accompany a rapid rise in body temperature. On Day 3, fever did not regress and developed congest rashes on his trunk along with bilateral conjunctival congestion. He was admitted to local hospital, and was given infusion of erythromycin and the first-generation cephalosporin for 4 days, but the treatment failed to have fever under control. On Day 7 he had significant red lips. Thus, he was transferred to our pediatric cardiology ward. He lost appetite and had watery stool 3 or 4 times per day since fever onset. Physical examination revealed he was in generally good state and had normal vital signs. T 37 °C, PR 105 bpm, RR 22 bpm. Congest rashes were all over body, and he had bilateral conjunctivitis without purulent secretion. Lips were red and cracked, with strawberry tongue and pharyngeal hyperemia. Bilateral lymphadenopathy was about 2 cm. Edematous palms and soles, bilateral interphalangeal joints were red and swollen. Redness was around anus. Admission blood test revealed elevated WBC and CRP, as shown in Table 11.4. He met all criteria for KD and was treated with: (1) oral aspirin 30–50 mg/kg per day, in three divided doses. Dipyridamole 3–5 mg/kg per day, in 3 divided doses. (2) IVIG 2 g/kg over 12 h and 20% mannitol 2.5 ml/kg infusion after IVIG 1 g/kg; (3) second-generation cephalosporin was infused after blood drawn for culture. Chest DR was normal (Fig. 11.14).

On Day 9, fever improved and was 37.8 °C. Laboratory test revealed positive MP-IgM and CP-IgM. On Day 10, ECG showed tachycardia HR 167 bpm (Fig. 11.15). Echo showed normal LCA (Fig. 11.16a), RCA (Fig. 11.16b), and LVEF (Fig. 11.16c). Azithromycin infusion was given. On Day 11, all clinic symptoms improved and was afebrile for 36 h. Aspirin was reduced to 5 mg/kg/day. Afternoon, he had fever spiking to 38.2 °C, along with running nose, cough, and sputum in the throat. Physical examination revealed that both conjunctivitis and edema in hands and feet were settled, skin peeling around fingernails. Auscultation revealed normal lungs. On Day 12, his body temperature was up to 39.3 °C, had congested skin rashes on lower limbs, and conjunctivitis represented. Retested blood routine results were listed in Table 11.4, showing CRP level and NT pro-BNP at 150.0 pg/ml. DIC routine showed D-dimer 606μg/L. ALB 34.8 g/L. ESR 70 mm/h. He met the criteria for IVIG resistance. He was given another dose infusion of IVIG 2 g/kg within 24 h. On Day 13, fever remained around 39.1 °C. He continued to take both methylprednisolone 1.5 mg/kg per day and second-generation cephalosporin. On Day 14, he was afebrile and both conjunctivitis and red lips were settled. But on the following day, he still had fever at 38.4 °C but without additional symptoms. Examination revealed skin peeling off around fingernails; others were normal. Infusion of methylprednisolone was increased to 2 mg/kg per day, in two divided doses. Chest CT scan showed no abnormal findings (Fig. 11.17). Azithromycin infusion was given for another 3 days. Third-generation cephalosporin was applied to replace the previous antibiotics. On Day 16, fever was up to 39.4 °C. Retested blood work results were listed in Table 11.4, showing negative HSV-IgM, EBV-IgM, and EBV DNA. On Day 17, his temperature was still 39 °C. The dosage of methylprednisolone was increased to 4 mg/kg per day, in two divided doses. On Day 19, fever regressed to38.8 °C. Aspirin was resumed to 30–50 mg/kg/day, in three divided dose. On

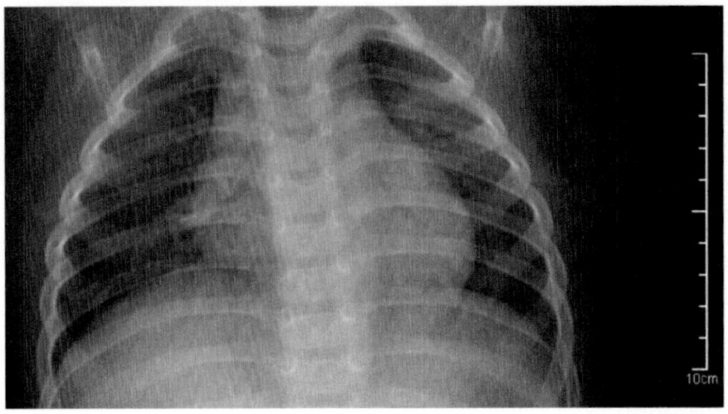

Fig. 11.14 On Day 8 of illness, chest DR was normal

Table 11.4 The dynamic changes of lab parameters

	First-KD			Second-KD		Third-KD	
Day of illness	12 days	18 days	24 days	8 days	13 months	3 days	7 days
WBC (×10⁹)	12.48	19.34	11.91	10.19	8.69	21.07	
NE (%)	63.2	68.8	25.4	40.1	25	75.7	
HBG (g/L)	93	86	90	91	112	111	106
PLT (×10⁹)	440	503	390	615	370	332	303
CRP (mg/L)	29.5	19.6	1.79	19.7	1.48	77.6	86.4
ESR (mm/h)	70			59			60
ALB (g/L)	34.8						32.6
NT pro-BNP (pg/ml)	150						564.1

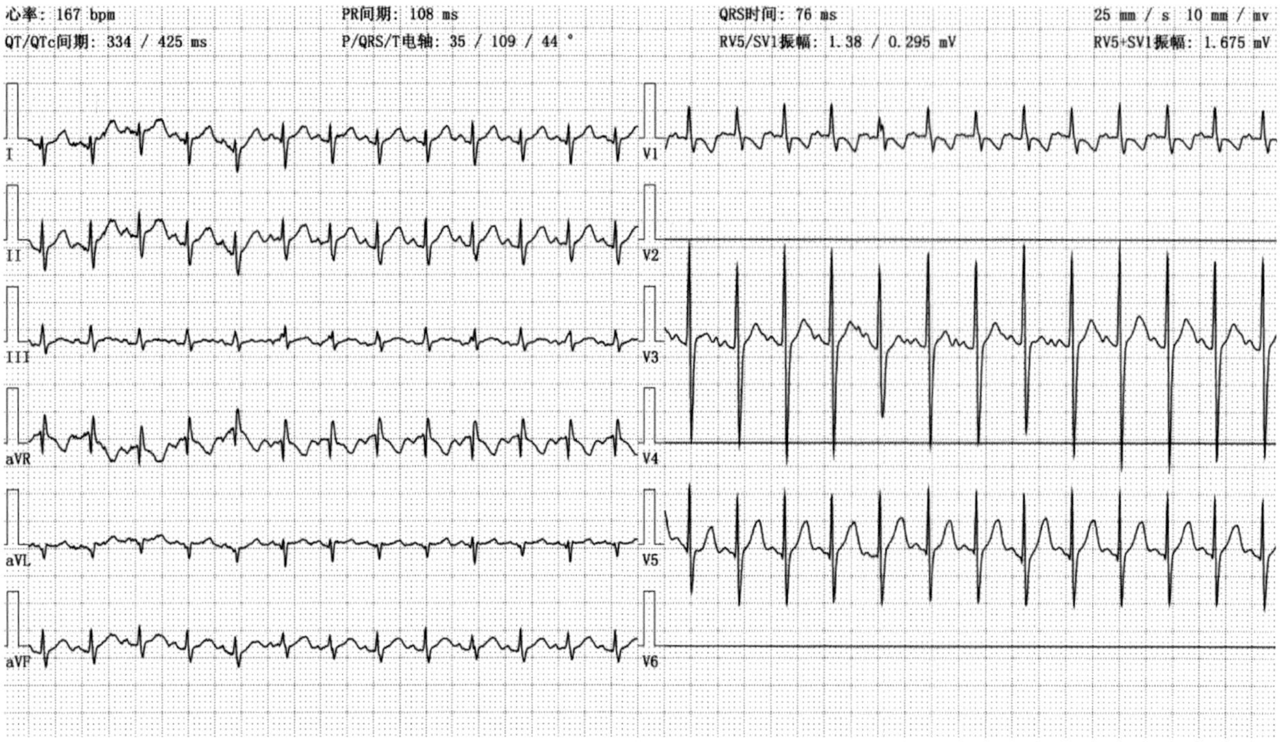

Fig. 11.15 On Day 10 of the first illness, ECG showed tachycardia, HR was 167 bpm

the following days, he was afebrile. Repeated blood test showed HGB down to 92 g/L, CRP dropped to 19.6 mg/L. Antibiotics treatment was switched to first-generation cephalosporin. Oral ferralia and vitamin C were given to him. Methylprednisolone was reduced to 2 mg/kg, in two divided doses. Echo showed normal results (Fig. 11.18a–d). On Day 21, fever settled for 48 h, aspirin was reduced to one dose 3–5 mg/kg/day. On Day 23, he was afebrile over 6 days. Methylprednisolone was reduced to one dose of 1 mg/kg per day (infusion) and 2 days later reduced to one dose of 5 mg (oral). On Day 26, his temperature was 37.2°C, and one hour later his body temperature was back to normal. On Day 27, oral methylprednisolone was reduced to one dose of 4 mg in the morning. Aspirin was reduced to one dose of 5 mg/kg per day. Retested blood work revealed HBG 90 g/L. Normal CRP and DIC. He was discharged.

On Day 32 (Day 7 of second fever onset), he was admitted again with interval fever for 1 week, along with bilateral conjunctivitis for 1 day. Since last discharged, he continued to take oral methylprednisolone 4 mg/day and aspirin 5 mg/kg/day as scheduled. However, his body temperature rose from 37 °C up to 38 °C on Day 33, and he developed rashes on the trunk and bilateral conjunctivitis. Physical examination found bilateral conjunctivitis, red lips, and rashes all over the body. Others were normal. Laboratory examination results were shown in Table 11.4. On the following days, he had fever at 38 °C. He was diagnosed with recurrent KD, and was treated with IVIG 2 g/kg (on Day 8 of the second illness), increased aspirin dosage at 30–50 mg/kg/day. On Day 10 of the second illness, his fever, conjunctivitis, and red lips were settled, rashes regressed too. ECG was normal (Fig. 11.19). On Day 12 of second KD, methylprednisolone was reduced to 2 mg/day. On Day 38 of the first illness (Day 13 of the second illness), echo showed LCA 3.5 mm (Fig. 11.20a), LAD 2.4 mm, RCA 1.9–2.4 mm (Fig. 11.20b), LVED 32 mm, LVEF 79% (Fig. 11.20c). Cervical ultrasonic showed bilateral lymphadenectasis, the bigger one was 1.3 × 0.8 cm on left, the right one was 1.2 × 0.8 cm. Aspirin was reduced to 5 mg/kg/day. On Day 16 of second illness, he was afebrile for 6 days. Then he was discharged.

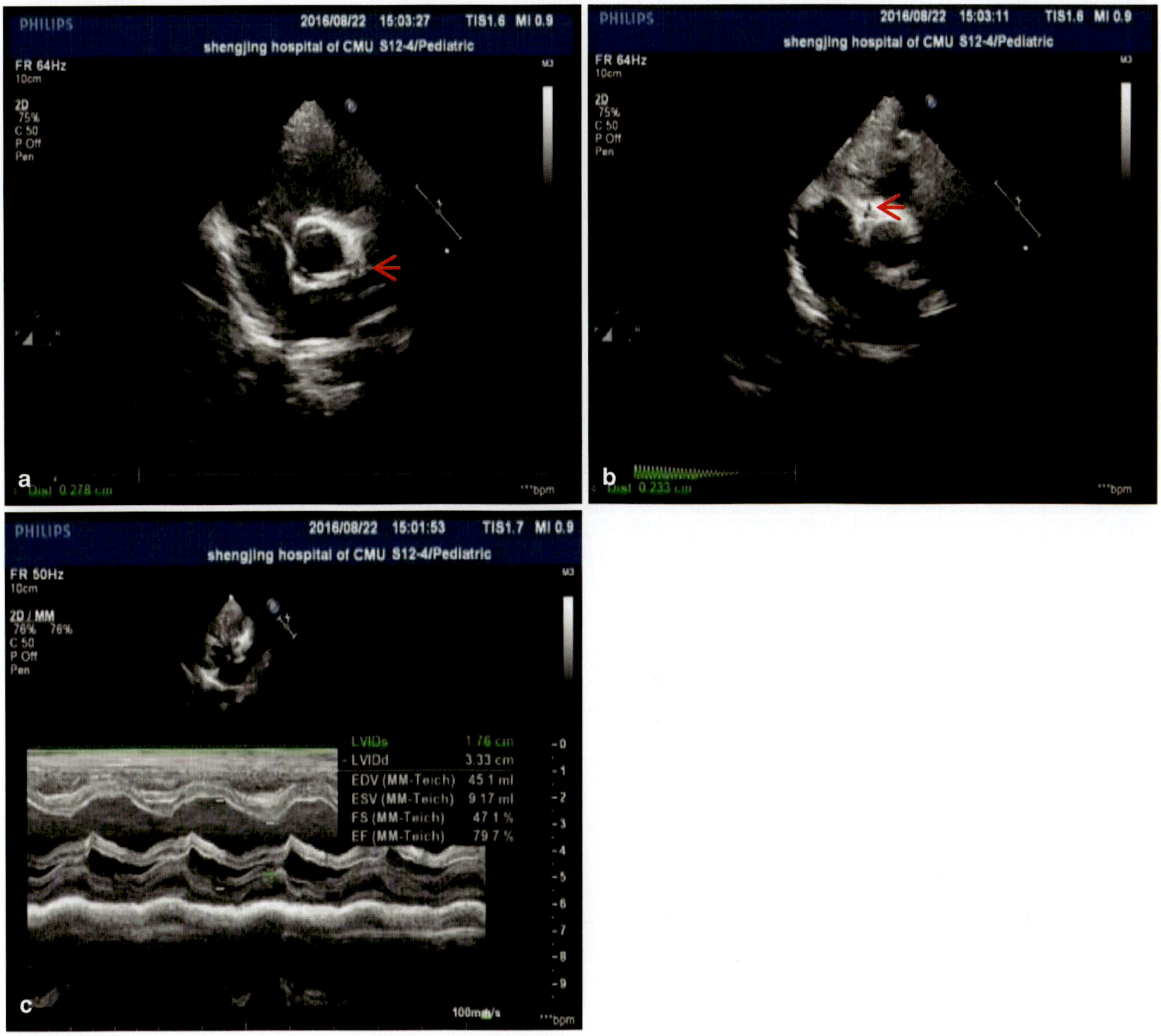

Fig. 11.16 On Day 10 of the first illness, echo showed normal LCA (**a**), RCA (**b**), and LVEF (**c**)

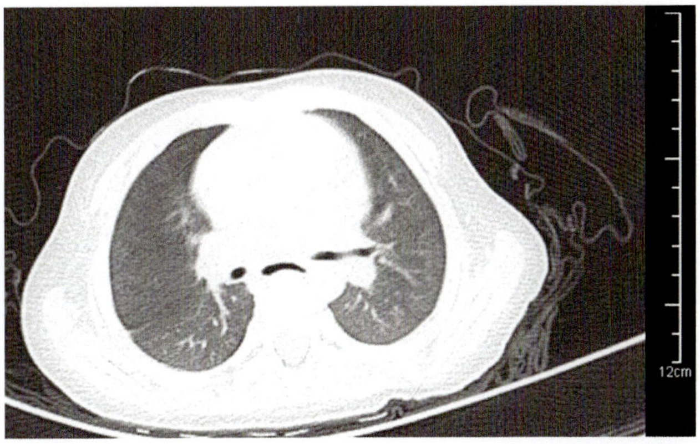

Fig. 11.17 On Day 15 of the first illness, chest CT showed almost normal

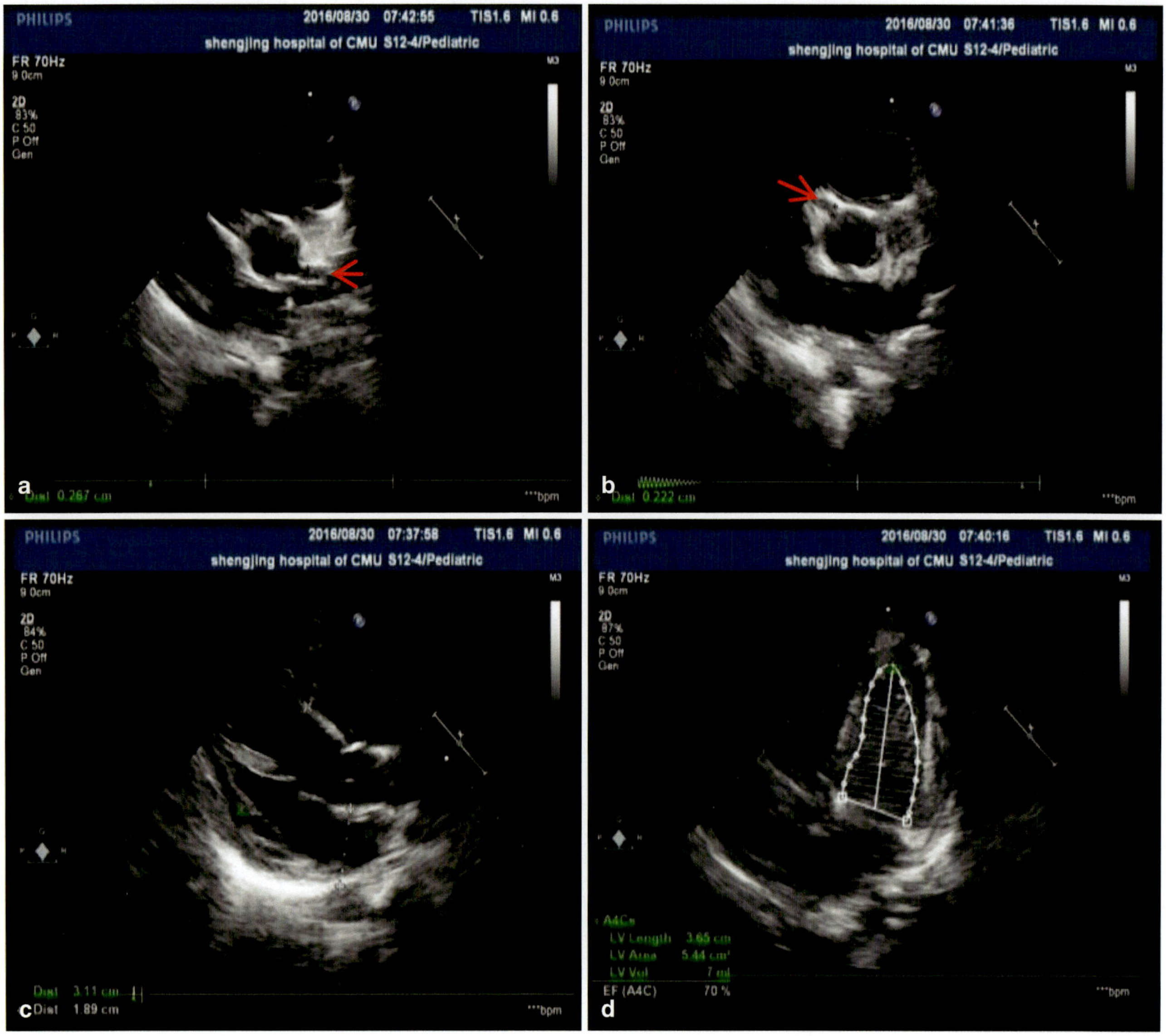

Fig. 11.18 On Day 19 of the first illness, echo showed normal LCA (**a**), RCA (**b**), LVED (**c**), and LVEF (**d**)

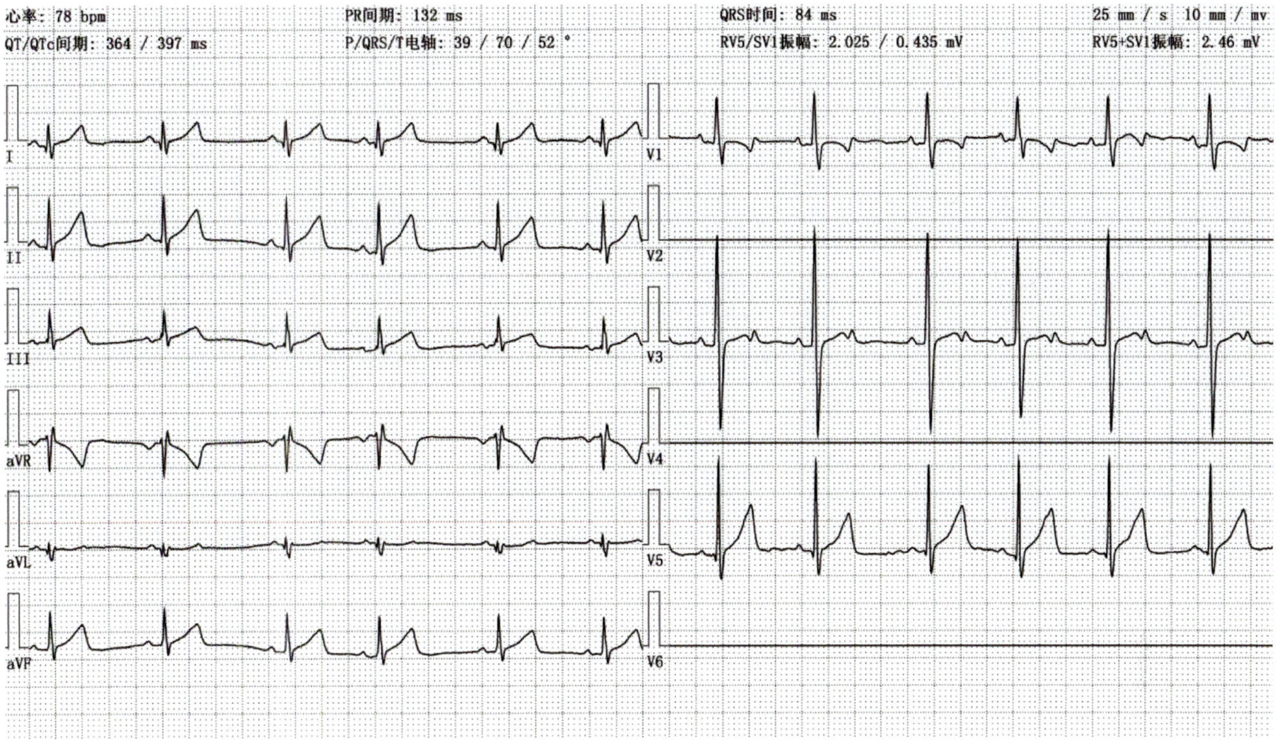

Fig. 11.19 On Day 32 of the first illness, ECG was normal

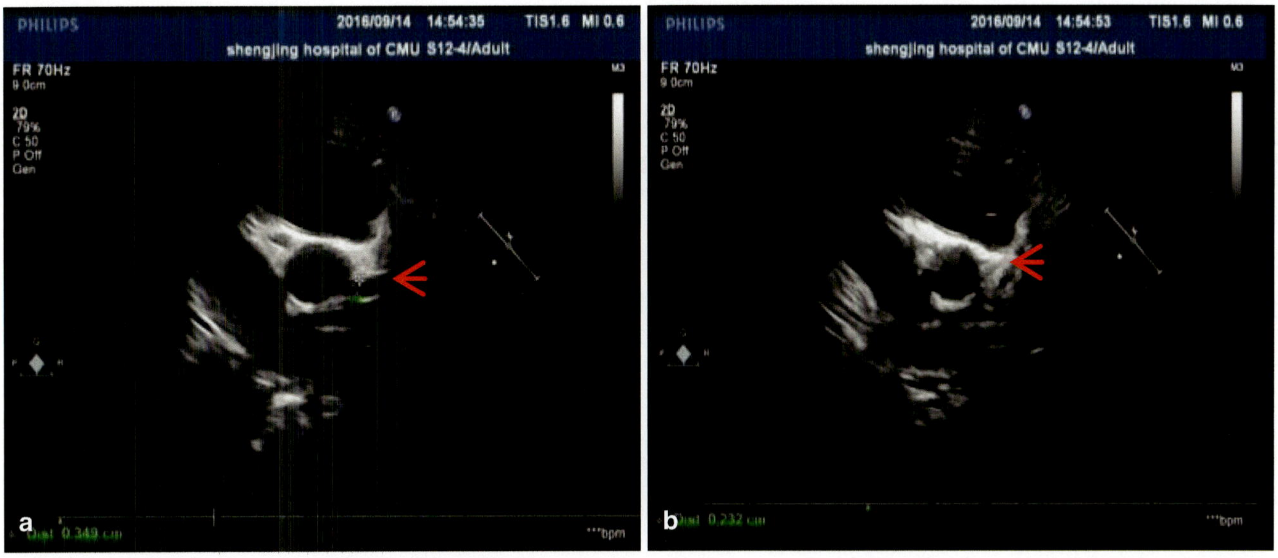

Fig. 11.20 On Day 38 of the first illness, echo showed LCA dilated about 3.5 mm (**a**), normal LAD (**b**), RCA (**c**) and LVEF (**d**)

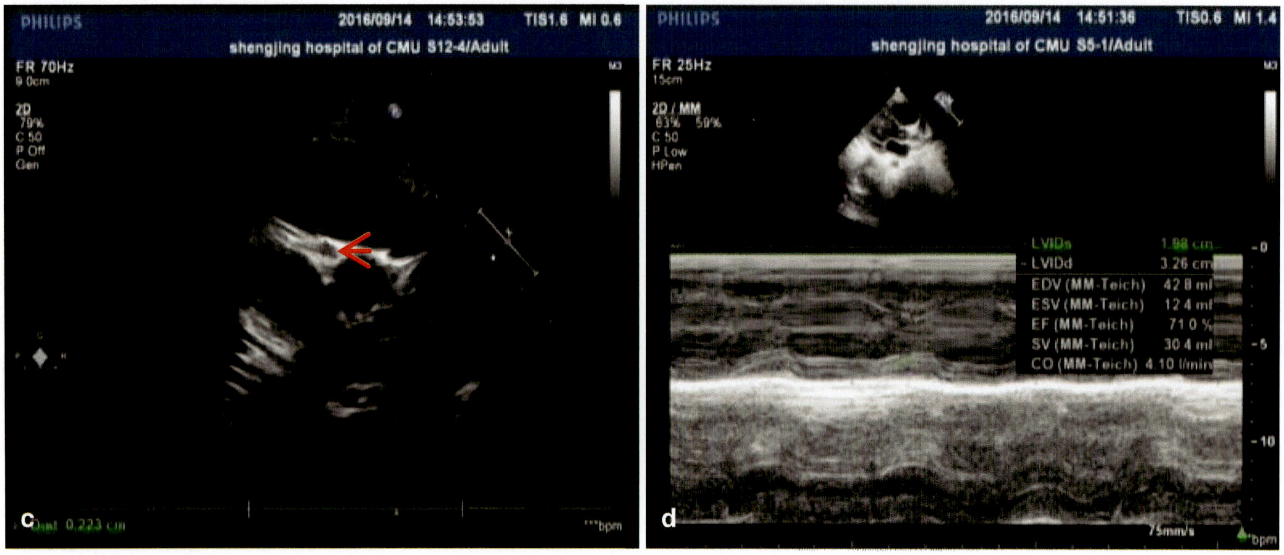

Fig. 11.20 (Continued)

11.4.1 The First Time KD Clinical Course of the Patient

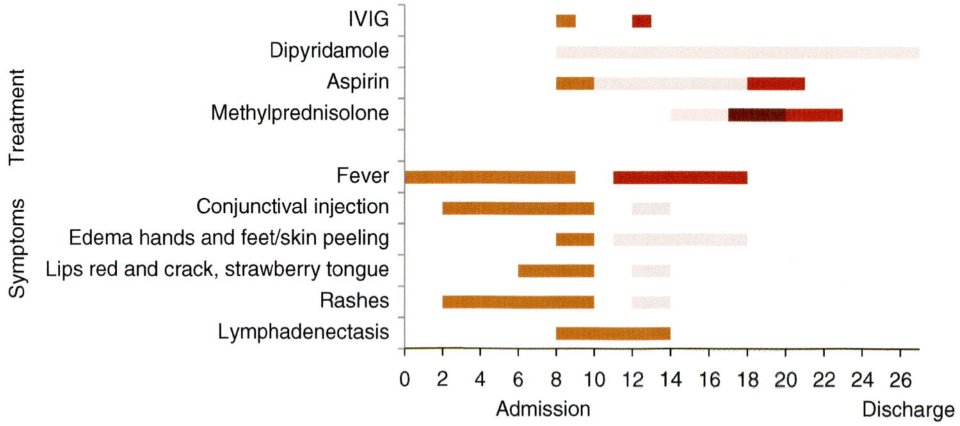

11.4.2 The Second Time KD Clinical Course of the Patient

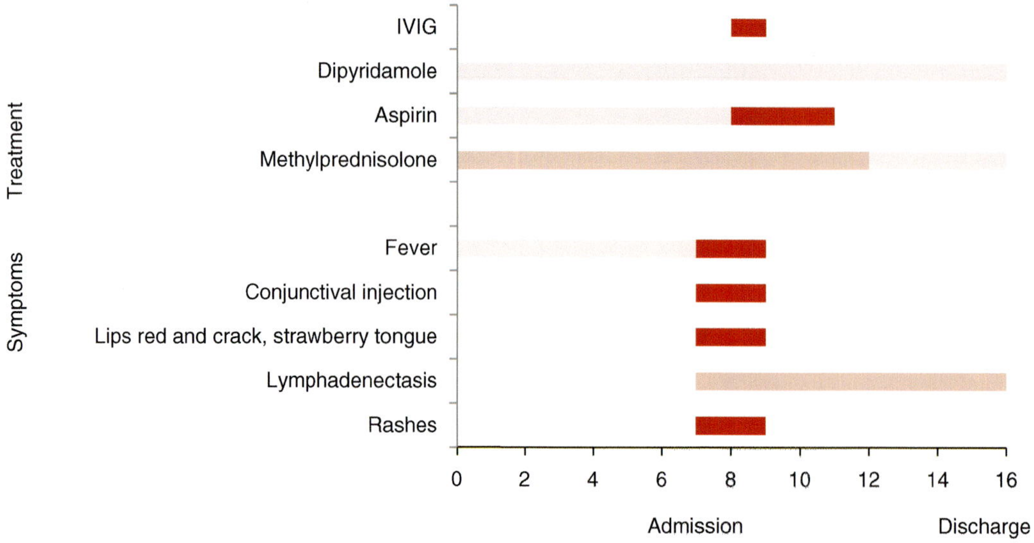

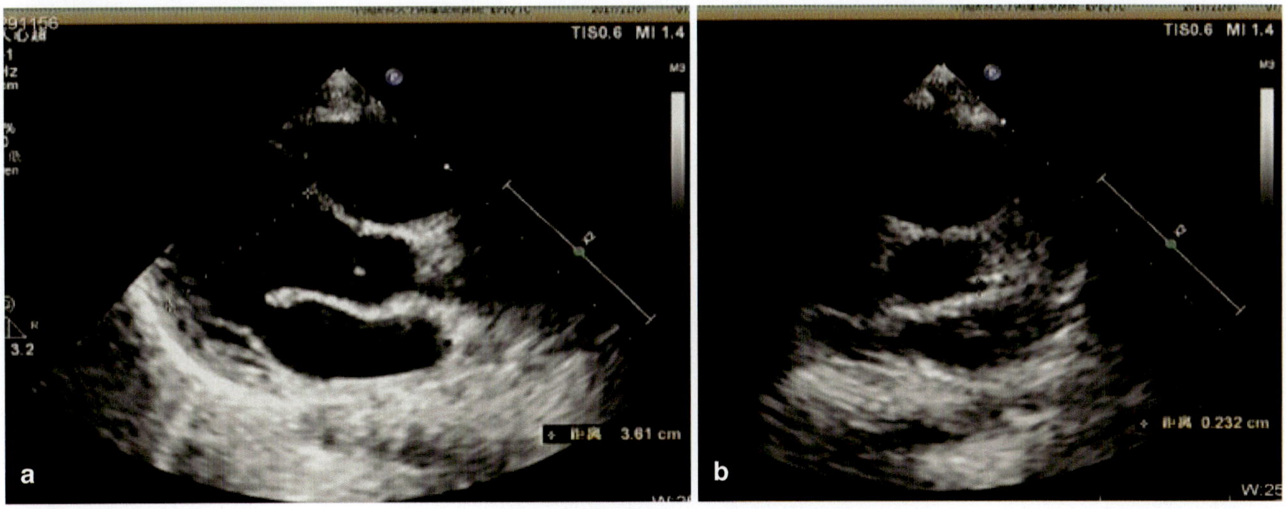

Fig. 11.21 At 13 months of the first illness, echo showed LVED enlarged about 36.1 mm (**a**), LCA was normal (**b**)

11.4.3 Follow-Up

Echo was performed at 2 months of second KD. LCA returned to normal. At 5 months of the second KD, repeated echo was normal. Aspirin and dipyridamole were discontinued. Echo was rechecked at 13 months of second KD. LVED was enlarged to 36 mm (Fig. 11.21a), LVEF (70%) and coronary arteries (Fig. 11.21b) were normal. Physical examination was normal. Investigation revealed blood routine, CRP, ESR, ASO, immunoglobulin, CK, cTnI, NT pro-BNP, hs-cTnT, liver function, DIC, blood gas analysis, K^+, and Na^+ 138 mmol/L were normal. ECG was normal (Fig. 11.22). Chest DR and AECG were normal. His parents turned down coronary artery CTA and he was only given oral FDP and levocarnitine. Echo was performed at 18 months of the second KD, LVED (32 mm) was almost normal. All medications were stopped.

Twenty months after second KD, he presented on Day 5 of illness with persistent fever for 5 days (spiking at 39.2 °C). He was given infusion of third-generation cephalosporin and adenosine monophosphate for 2 days at our emergency room, but fever was not regressed. He developed red lips, edema in hands and feet, and rashes on the trunk on Day 4. This was the third time for him being admitted in our ward for KD. Since the onset, he lost appetite and vomited once. Physical examination showed well general state. Rashes were all over the body, and he had red and cracked lips, strawberry tongue. He had bilateral lymphadenopathy which was about 2 cm. Both palms and toes were congested. Finger joints were red with edema. Others were normal. Blood test on Day 3 of the third illness showed WBC, NE, and CRP elevated significantly. Cervical ultrasound showed left lymphadenopathy about 2.0 cm × 1.5 cm. ECG showed tachycardia (Fig. 11.23). He had met the 4 out of 5 criteria for KD (the third time KD). Blood culture result was negative. He was treated with IVIG 1 g/kg/day for 2 days. Aspirin 30 mg/kg/day, dipyridamole 3–5 mg/kg/day were initiated, in three divided doses. On Day 7 of the third KD, he had fever up to 39.0 °C, lost appetite, and was sleepy. Examination showed the rashes and swollen finger joints regressed. Laboratory evaluation revealed blood and gas analysis were normal, urine protein ±0.2 g/L. Mildly positive acetone. ESR 60 mm/h. DIC routine revealed PT13.2s, APTT 31s, D-dimer 571μg/L. NT-pro BNP 564.1 pg/ml. CK, CKMB, CKMB-M, cTnI, MYO, immunoglobulin, ASO, 25-OH-vitamin D, IgE, ACA, and sodium were normal. ALB 32.6 g/L, ALT was normal. Tb-Ab was negative. EB NA-IgG (+) (>600), EB VCA-IgG (+) (>750), EB EA-IgG (−). EBV-IgM and PINF-IgM were positive. PPD was normal. He had met the criteria for IVIG resistance. The plan was to administrate another 2 g IVIG within 24 h, but the parents refused to accept the plan, only gave consent on GC [30 mg intravenous infusion of methylprednisolone (16 kg)]. On Day 8, he was afebrile. IVIG another 2 g/kg was given within 24 hours for his parents were concerned that he might develop CAA again. On Day 10, his fever subsided over 48 h, and his appetite was improved. Aspirin was reduced to one dose of 50 mg and methylprednisolone to 20 mg/day. Examination found skin peeling around fingernails. Others were normal. Repeated echo showed normal LCA (Fig. 11.24a), LVEF (Fig. 11.24b), and LVED (Fig. 11.24c). On Day 11, his general condition got worse with agitation. Examination showed left palmar chin reflex was positive. EEG or ordered, but his mother refused to give consent. On the following days, he was still agitated, and left palmar chin reflex was positive. Meningeal irritation was negative. His mother allowed EEG test, which showed more 4–7 Hz slow wave on bilateral occipital (Fig. 11.25). He was treated with continuous GCs and mavericks protein infusion.

On Day 13 of the third time KD, his mental station improved. Head CT was normal, methylprednisolone was reduced to 8 mg morning oral. On Day 16, repeated EEG showed almost normal (Fig. 11.26). He was discharged.

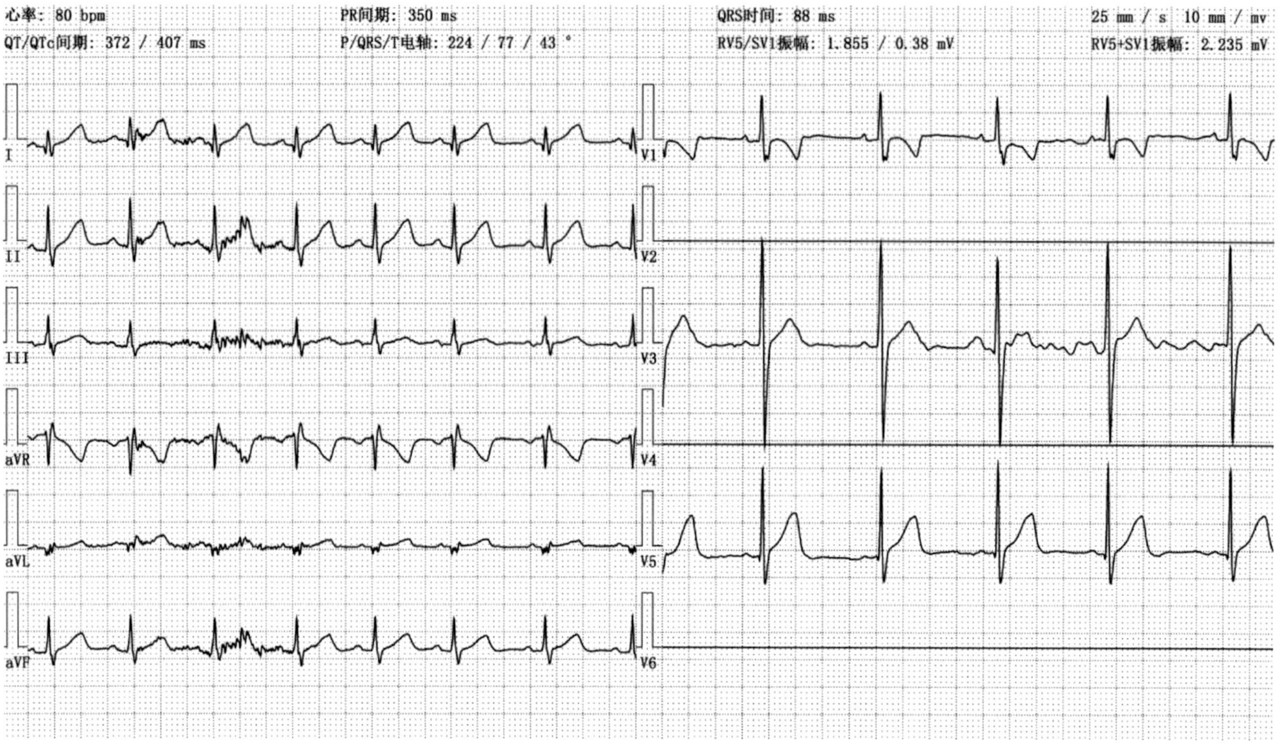

Fig. 11.22 At 20 months of the first illness, ECG was normal

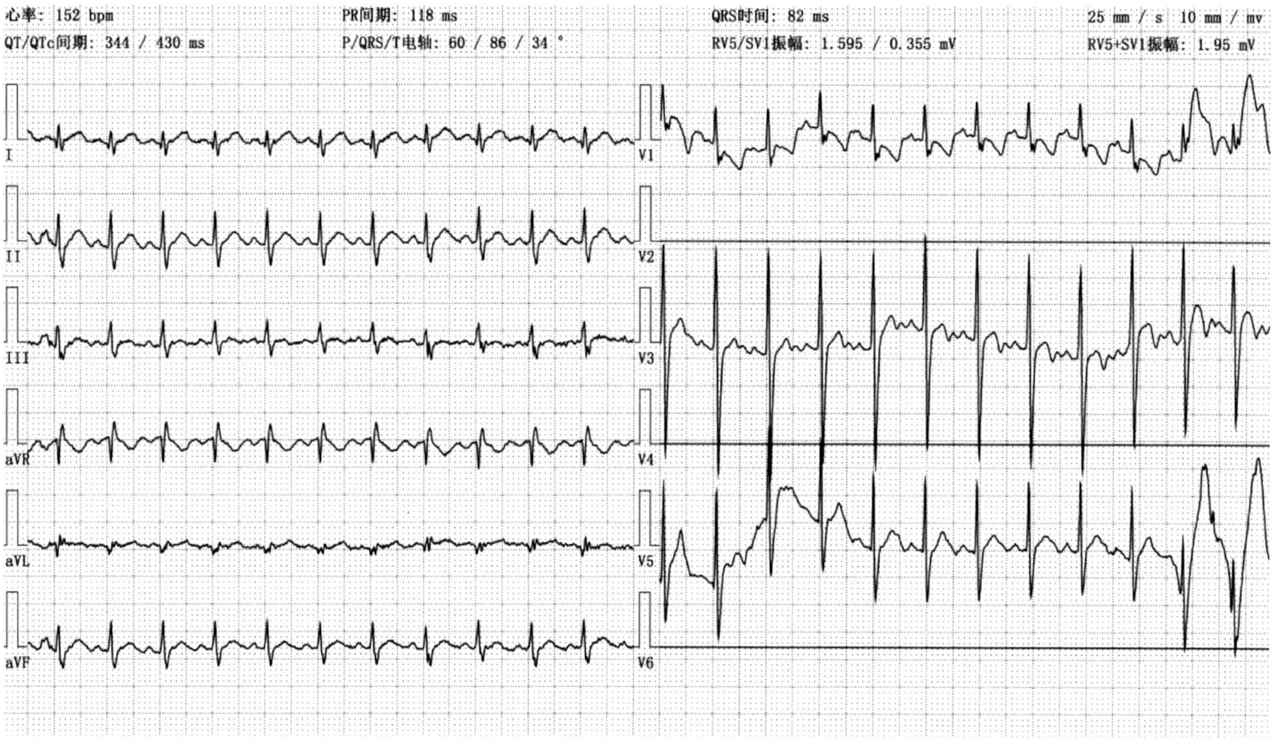

Fig. 11.23 On Day 5 of the third illness, ECG was tachycardia, HR 152 bpm

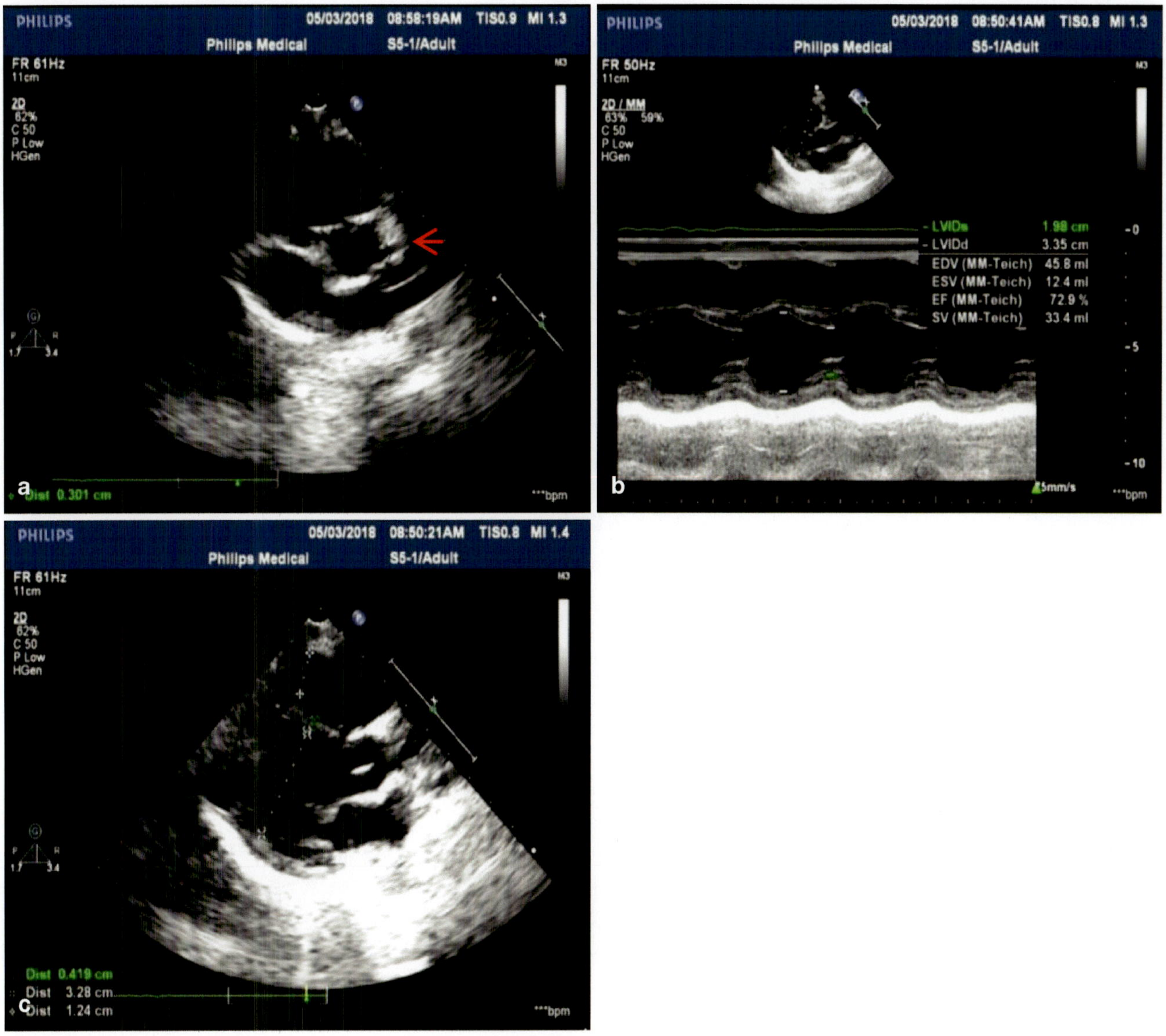

Fig. 11.24 On Day 10 of the third illness, echo showed normal LCA (**a**), LVEF (**b**), and LVED (**c**)

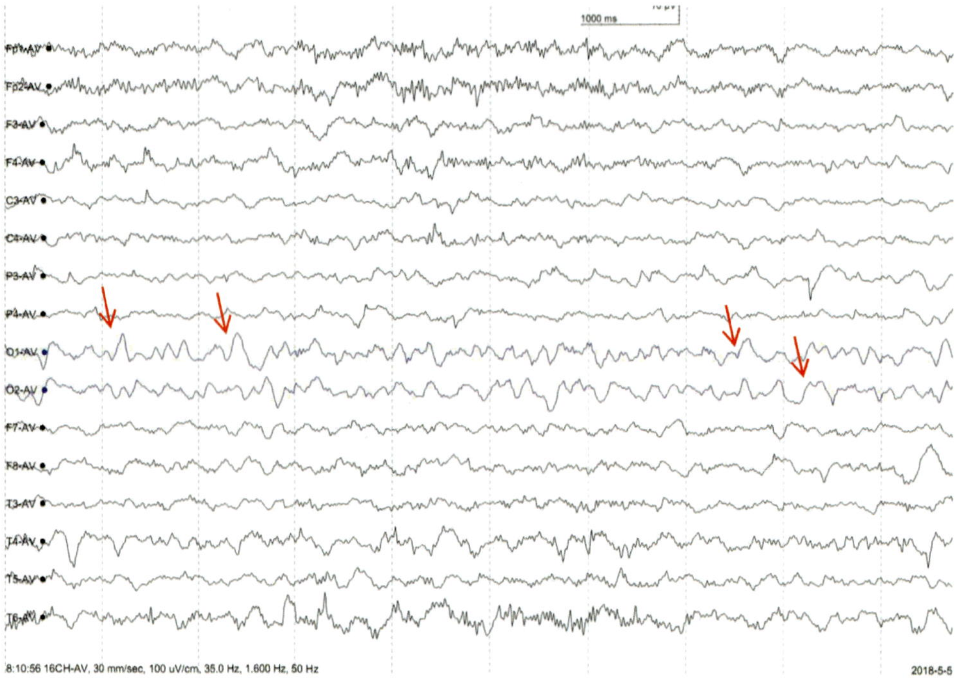

Fig. 11.25 On Day 11 of the third illness, EEG showed more 6–7 Hz slow waves

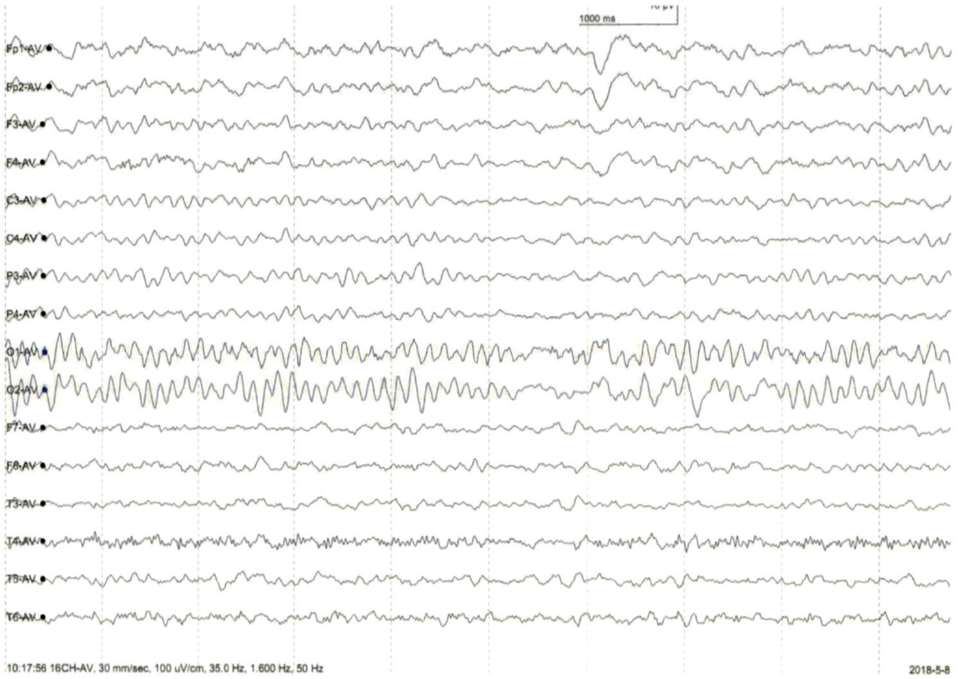

Fig. 11.26 On Day 16 of the third illness, EEG showed almost normal

11.4.4 The Third Time KD Clinical Course of the Patient

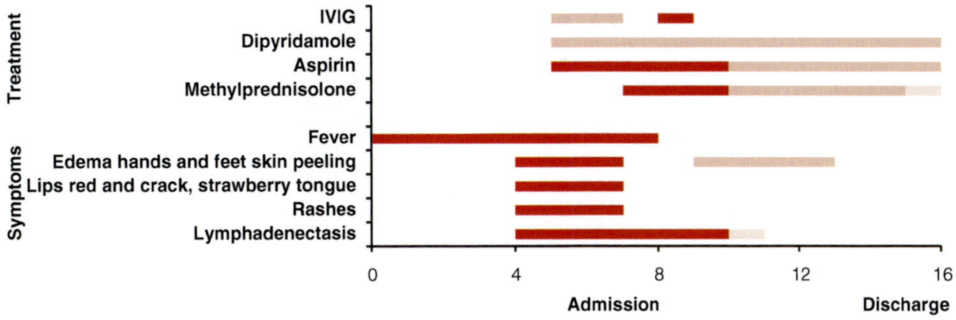

11.4.5 Follow-Up

Since discharged, methylprednisolone was gradually weaned within a week. He continued to take oral brain protein hydrolysate tablets, aspirin and dipyridamole. On Day 22, repeated echo showed LCA was at critical value (3.0 mm) (Fig. 11.27a). One week later it regressed to normal (Fig. 11.27b), while LVED and LVEF were always normal. EEG was normal, too. He stopping taking brain protein hydrolysate tablets. Echo performed 2 months after the third KD showed normal results. He stopped taking all medications.

11.4.6 Diagnosis

1. Recurrent KD (the third time).
2. IVIG resistance.
3. Sterile urethritis.
4. Moderate anemia.
5. MPI.
6. CPI.

11.4.7 Discussion

When admitted the first time, he met all criteria for KD. He had persistent high-grade fever over 5 days, along with (1) rashes all over the body; (2) bilateral conjunctivitis; (3) cervical lymphadenectasis; (4) red and cracked lips, strawberry tongue and pharyngeal hyperemia; (5) red and edema finger joints and later skin peeling around fingernails. At his second time admission, he had prolonged fever over 5 days (during oral methylprednisolone and aspirin) along with all the same symptoms as shown at the first time except edema

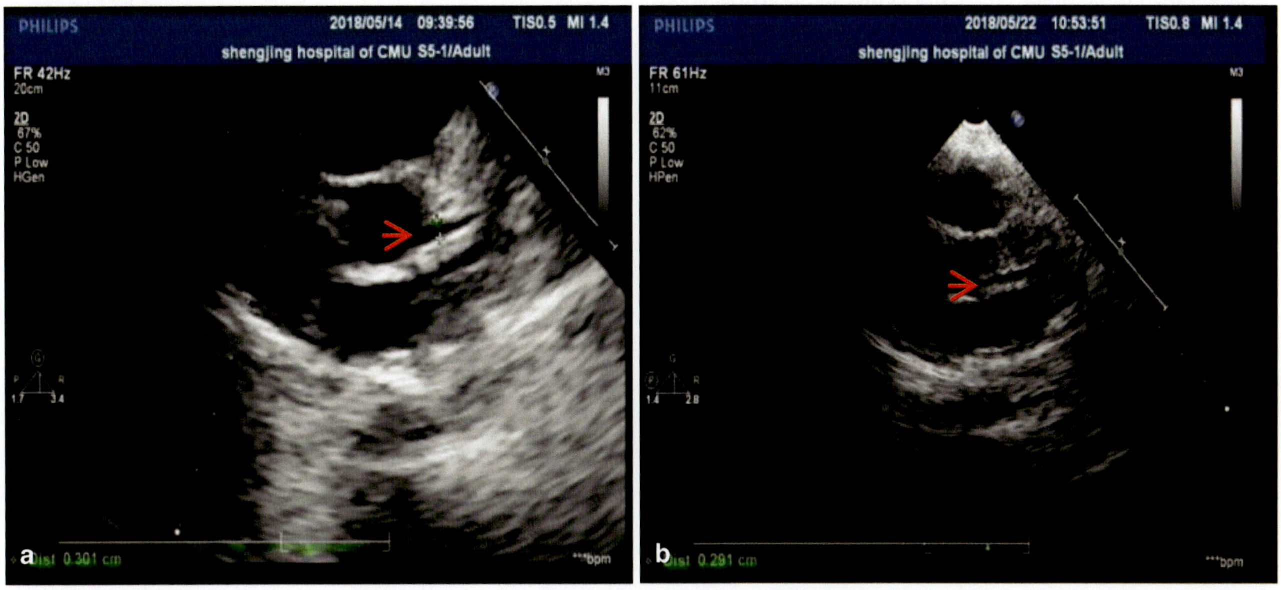

Fig. 11.27 Echo showed LCA 3.0 mm (**a**) at 3 weeks, and 2.9 mm (**b**) at 4 weeks of the third illness

hands and feet. Thus he met the 4 out of 5 criteria for KD. When admitted at the third time, he had fever over 5 days along with all the same symptoms presented before except for conjunctiva congestion. His blood routine revealed WBC over 15 × 10^9, NE% over 75%. CRP was significantly elevated whereas blood culture was negative. He had KD three times.

11.4.8 Case Specific Clinical Features

1. Both initial and the third time with KD, he was IVIG standardly and 48 h later, fever not regressed and spiking over 38.5 °C, with more than one KD symptom. Thus he was definitely diagnosed IVIG no-response [19]. For the second incidence of coronary artery dilatation, it may be related to the literature report that re-KD is prone to coronary artery dilatation [20]. It suggests that more aggressive treatment strategies in conjunction with IVIG may be indicated for the second episode of KD [21]. Thus, though he was afebrile after infused 2 mg methylprednisolone in the third time KD, we persuaded his parents to IVIG another 2 g/kg and his prognosis was nice which confirmed our therapy was appropriate.
2. One literature reported after initial IVIG there was nearly a third KD patients who had recurrent fever. In two-thirds of these patients, the fever had subsided spontaneously without retreatment [22]. Thus recurrence in the USA was 1.7%. Among the US Asian/Pacific Islanders KD recurrence was 3.5%, which is same as with Japan (3.5%) [21]. As to incidence of three times of KD, we have no idea, nor the long-term prognosis of such patients because the third time KD was rare [22]. Totally there were 2 cases with three times KD in our center in 30 years. Their prognoses were well.
3. With the publicity of KD and the recognition of its symptoms, parents of children with KD, even if they are not doctors, often can diagnose by themselves when KD reappears due to its special clinical manifestations, and can come to see the doctor within 5 days after the onset of KD. Therefore, once the symptoms of KD are recognized, usually there will be no misdiagnosis [23].

Hong Wang

References

1. Nakamura Y, Yashiro M, Uehara R, et al. Epidemiologic features Kawasaki disease in Japan: results of the 2007-2008 nationwide survey. J Epidemiol. 2010;20(4):302–7.
2. Park YW, Han JW, Hong YM, et al. Epidemiological features of Kawasaki disease in Korea, 2006–2008. Pediatr Int. 2011;53(1):36–9.
3. Uehara R, Yashiro M, Nakamura Y, et al. Clinical features of patients with Kawasaki disease whose parents had the same disease. Arch Pediatr Adolesc Med. 2004;158(12):1166–9.
4. Yang HM, Du ZD, Fu PP. Clinical features of recurrent Kawasaki disease and its risk factors. Eur J Pediatr. 2013;172(12):1641–7.
5. Janka GE. Familial and acquired hemophagocytic lymphohistiocytosis. Eur J Pediatr. 2007;166(2):95–109.
6. Suresh N, Sankar J. Macrophage activation syndrome: a rare complication of incomplete Kawasaki disease. Ann Trop Peadiatr. 2010;30(1):61–4.
7. Hirata S, Nakamura Y, Yanagawa H. Incidence rate of recurrent Kawasaki disease and related risk factors: from the results of nationwide surveys of Kawasaki disease in Japan. Acta Padiatr.2001; 90(1):40–4.
8. Nakada T. Clinical features of patients with recurrent Kawasaki disease. Nippon Rinsho. 2008;66(2):296–300.
9. Eladawy M, Dominguez SR, Anderson MS, et al. Abnormal liver panel in acute Kawasaki disease. Pediatr Infect Dis J. 2011; 30(2):141–4.
10. Newburger JW, Takahashi M, Gerber MA, et al. Diagnosis, treatment, and long-term management of Kawasaki disease: a statement for health professionals from the committee on rheumatic fever, endocarditis, and Kawasaki disease, council on cardiovascular disease in the young, American Heart Association. Pediatrics. 2004;114(6):1708–33.
11. Zhang Y, Du Z, Zhao D, et al. The epidemiologic study on Kawasaki disease in Beijing from 2000 through 2004. Pediatr Infect Dis J. 2007;26(5):449–51.
12. Yang H, Du Z, Fu P. Clinical features of recurrent Kawasaki disease and its risk factors. Eur J Pediatr. 2013;172(12):1641–7.
13. Nakamura Y, Oki I, Tanihara S, et al. Cardiac sequelae in recurrent cases of Kawasaki disease: a comparison between the initial episode of the disease and a recurrence in the same patients. Pediatrics. 1998;102(6):E66.
14. Abe J, Kotzin BL, Meissner C, et al. Characterization of T cell repertoire changes in acute Kawasaki disease. J Exp Med. 1993;177(3):791–6.
15. Ferwerda A, Moll HA, de Groot R. Respiratory tract infections by Mycoplasma pneumoniae in children: a review of diagnostic and therapeutic measures. Eur J Pediatr. 2001;160(8):483–91.
16. Beken B, Unal S, Cetin M, et al. The relationship between hematological findings and coronary artery aneurysm in Kawasaki disease. Turk J Haematol. 2014;l3(2):199–200.
17. Krowchuk DP, Kumar ML, Vielhaber MM, et al. Kawasaki disease presenting with thrombocytopenia. Am J Dis Child. 1990;144(1):19–20.
18. Nofech-Mozes Y, Garty BZ. Thrombocytopenia in Kawasaki disease: a risk factor for the development of coronary artery aneurysms. Pediatr Hematol Oncol. 2003;20(8):597–601.
19. Tavli V, Yilmazer MM, Güven B, et al. Evaluation of unresponsiveness to standard high-dose gamma globulin therapy in Kawasaki disease. Turk Kardiyol Dern Ars. 2010; 38(1):20–4.
20. Yoshida M, Oana S, Masuda H, et al. Recurrence of fever after initial intravenous immunoglobulin treatment in children with Kawasaki disease. Clin Pediatr (Phila). 2018;57(2):189–92.
21. Maddox RA, Holman RC, Uehara R, et al. Recurrent Kawasaki disease: USA and Japan. Pediatr Int. 2015;57(6):1116–20.
22. Verma P, Agarwal N, Maheshwari M. Recurrent Kawasaki disease. Indian Pediatr. 2015;52(2):152–4.
23. Tissandier C, Lang M, Lusson JR, et al. Pediatrics. 2014;134(6):e1695–9.

Misdiagnosed KD

12

Hong Wang, Yali Zhang, Yang Hou, and Xiaona Yu

Abstract

Among all the complications associated with KD, the most dangerous one is the damage of coronary arteries, which can have a long-term impact on life even becomes life threatening [Suda et al. Circulation 123(17):1836–1842, 2011]. According to the literature, a quarter of untreated patients developed coronary artery aneurysms (CAA) [McCrindle et al. Circulation 135(17):e927–e999, 2017]. As to the retrospective diagnosis, usually CAA was discovered, and then patient recalled had a prolonged fever, rashes, changes of conjunctiva, oral and lips, and lymphadenectasis about 6 months ago. Thus diagnosis of KD was established. If the CAA was found by chance, then patients will have good prognosis in the future. Even if the thrombus is found in CAA some time, as long as it is found in time and the patient has grown up, it can be removed by interventional thrombectomy or by coronary artery bypass grafting. But, if CAA is found after heart failure, the prognosis will be troublesome, because it is likely that a blood clot has formed in CAA and affects the blood supply to the heart. This condition progresses gradually. When patients under 5 years old, who have thin blood vessels, develop thrombosis at unknown point and also heart failure, it is generally impossible for physicians to perform thrombectomy for this group of patients. Furthermore, it may aggravate the occurrence of myocardial ischemia. Because of the chronic thrombosis, it is difficult for oral warfarin to work using as anticoagulant treatment.

In this chapter, we presented four cases. CAA in case 42 and case 43 were found by chance; now patients in these two cases are just like normal kids. While CAA in case 44 and case 45 were found after heart failure, one lost his life forever, and the other one have a DCM.

H. Wang (✉)
Department of Pediatric Cardiology, Shengjing Hospital of China Medical University, Shenyang, Liaoning, P. R. China

Y. Zhang
Department of PICU, The First Affiliated Hospital of Zhengzhou University, Zhengzhou, Henan, P. R. China

Y. Hou
Department of Radiology, Shengjing Hospital of China Medical University, Shenyang, Liaoning, P. R. China

X. Yu
Department of Ultrasound, Shengjing Hospital of China Medical University, Shenyang, Liaoning, P. R. China
e-mail: yuxn@sj-hospital.org

12.1 Case 42: Misdiagnosed KD with Coronary Artery Dilatation and Chronic Myocardial Damage

A 19-month-old boy was presented with an unremarkable personal, allergy, and family history.

He presented on Day 3 of illness with a history of cough for 3 days along with fever for 1 day and increased cTnI for 6 h. On the second day, he developed fever (up to 40.5 °C) with sputum. On admission day, he continued to have fever and elevated cTnI. He was treated with penicillin, adenine arabinoside monophosphate once. From the onset, his mental status was poor, but he had good diet and sleep. Examination revealed he was irritable, breathe smoothly, T38°C, HR 94 bpm, RR 22 bpm, Weight 9.5 kg. Physical examination found no positive signs except pharyngeal congestion. Before admission blood test revealed CBC: WBC 8.3×10^9/L, NE 55.40%, HGB 118 g/L, PLT 189×10^9/L. CRP 6.74 mg/L. cTnI 0.059 μg/L. Admission investigation revealed normal MYO, CK-MB mass, NT-pro BNP. CTnI 0.048 μg/L, hs-cTnT 0.020 ng/ml. DIC parameters and ECG were normal. For he had myocardial damages, he was given infusion of creatine phosphate sodium, levocarnitine, and azithromycin after blood drawn for culture. On Day 4, he had remittent fever up to 38.8 °C. His cough was the same as prior to admission. Auscultation of the lungs revealed rales on both sides. Blood gas analysis showed that ESR, ASO,

H. Wang (ed.), *Paediatric Kawasaki Disease*, https://doi.org/10.1007/978-981-15-0038-1_12

total IgE were normal. MP IgG, MP IgM, viral and tuberculosis antibody were negative. CK 185 U/L, CK-MB 50 U/L. Serum iron was 4.0 (NR 9–32 μmol/L). AST and ALT were normal. Lymphocyte subsets: CD_3^+ normal, CD_3^+ CD_8^+ 10.6%decreased (13–41). CD_3^+ CD_4^+ normal, CD_4/CD_8, Th/Ts 3.65and CD19 + 28.1% elevations, D16+ CD56+ normal.

On Day 5, he was afebrile more than 24 h, and still had paroxysmal cough without wheezing, especially in the morning. Physical examination found rales were improved. Blood culture showed G^+ coccus growth on both bottles, while CBC and CRP were normal. He was given infusion of first-generation cephalosporin after blood re-drawn for culture. On Day 7, he was afebrile for 3 days, his cough reduced, and pharyngeal herpes disappeared. Repeated cTnI was normal, hs-cTnT 0.036 ng/ml. The result from original (admission) blood culture test indicated the positive growth of staphylococcus epidermidis. MP IgG was still negative. Echo showed LCA dilated about 3.5 mm (Fig. 12.1a), LAD 3.5–3.7 mm (Fig. 12.1b). RCA was normal. After discussion with his mother, we learned he had fever for more than 10 days 9 months ago, with rashes and red lips. At that time, WBC increased, mainly in lymphocytes, PLT increased. Combined with his past medical history, the diagnosis of recovered stage of KD was possible, and he was treated with (1) oral aspirin and dipyridamole, in 3–5 mg/kg/day; (2) IVIG 2 g/kg; (3) mannitol and furosemidum added half way of IVIG infusion, slow infusion for more than 12 h.

On Day 9, he had a fever 38 °C after catching cold, without any uncomfortable feelings. He was given oral ibuprofen. On Day 11, his fever settled, and repeated test revealed WBC 8.2 × 10^9/L, NE 11.4%, HGB108g/L, PLT 387 × 10^9/L. hs-cTnT 0.029 ng/ml. The repeated blood culture test for bacteria was negative and he was discharged.

12.1.1 Diagnosis

1. KD, recovery stage.
2. LCA dilatation.
3. Bacteremia (Staphylococcus epidermidis).
4. Myocardial injury.
5. Herpes angina.

12.1.2 Follow-Up

After discharged, he was followed up as scheduled at our clinic. 2D echo was performed at 9, 10, 21, 24, and 35 months of illness. LCA was remained dilated (Figs. 12.2a, b, 12.3a, b and 12.4) without thrombus in it. LAD and RCA remained normal. ECG was normal (Fig. 12.5).

12.1.3 Discussion

The diagnosis of KD was established for he had fever more than 5 days 9 months before admission, along with (1) rashes on the back during fever; (2) red lips; (3) coronary artery dilated shown in echo. At that time, blood tests showed increased WBC and PLT. It has been reported in literature

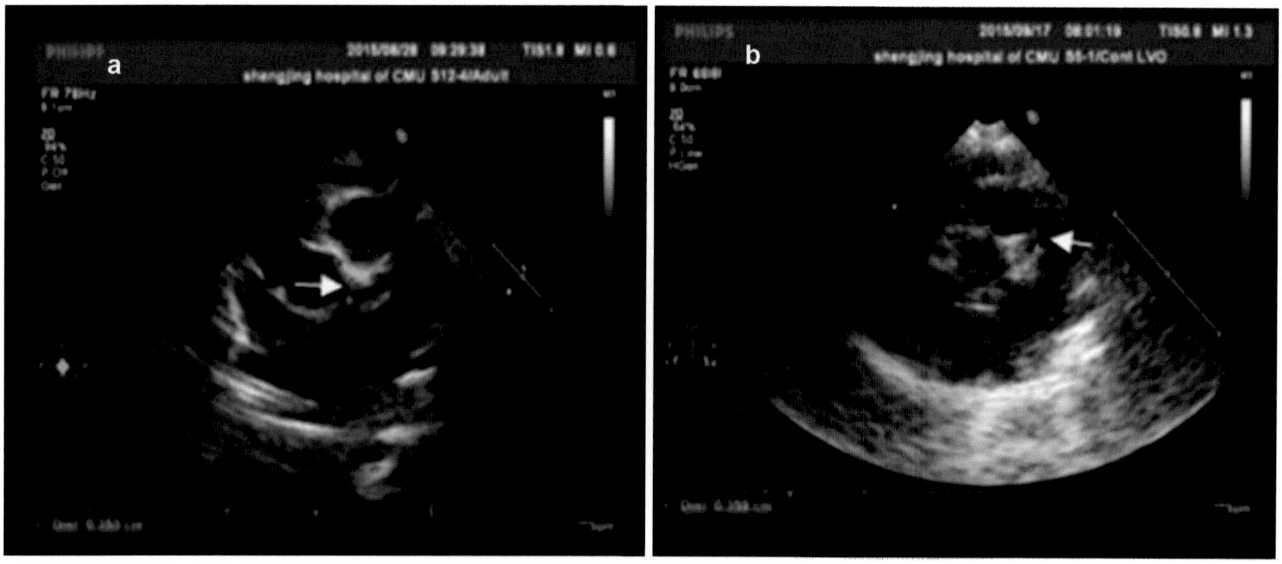

Fig. 12.1 About 9 months of illness, echocardiography showed LCA dilated to 3.5 mm (**a**), LAD dilated about 3.5–3.7 mm (**b**)

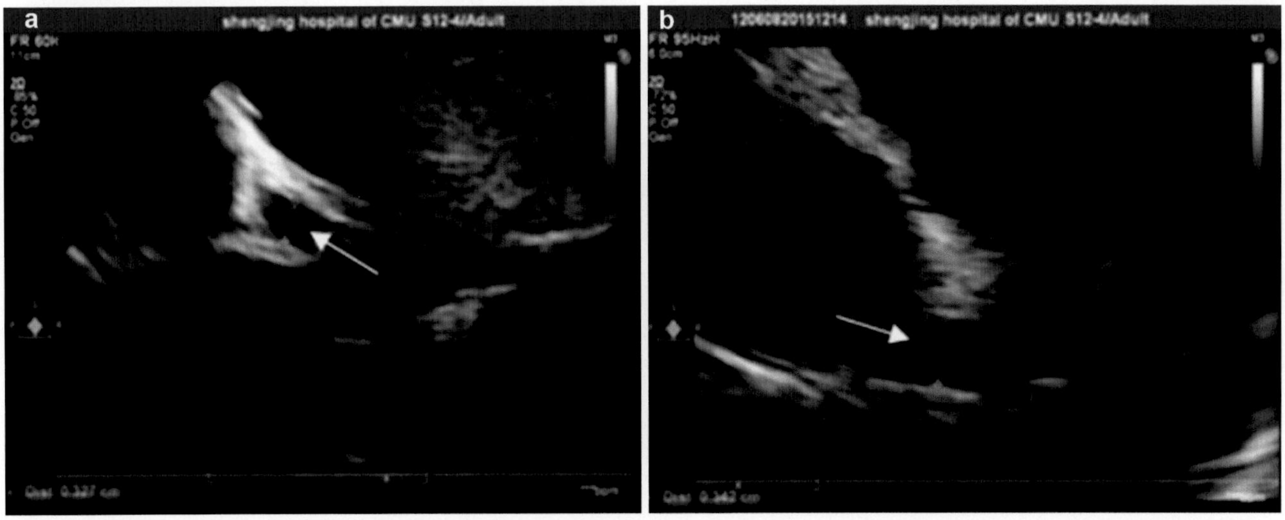

Fig. 12.2 Echocardiography showed LCA dilated to 3.3 mm (**a**) at 10 months, 3.4 mm (**b**) at 12 months of illness

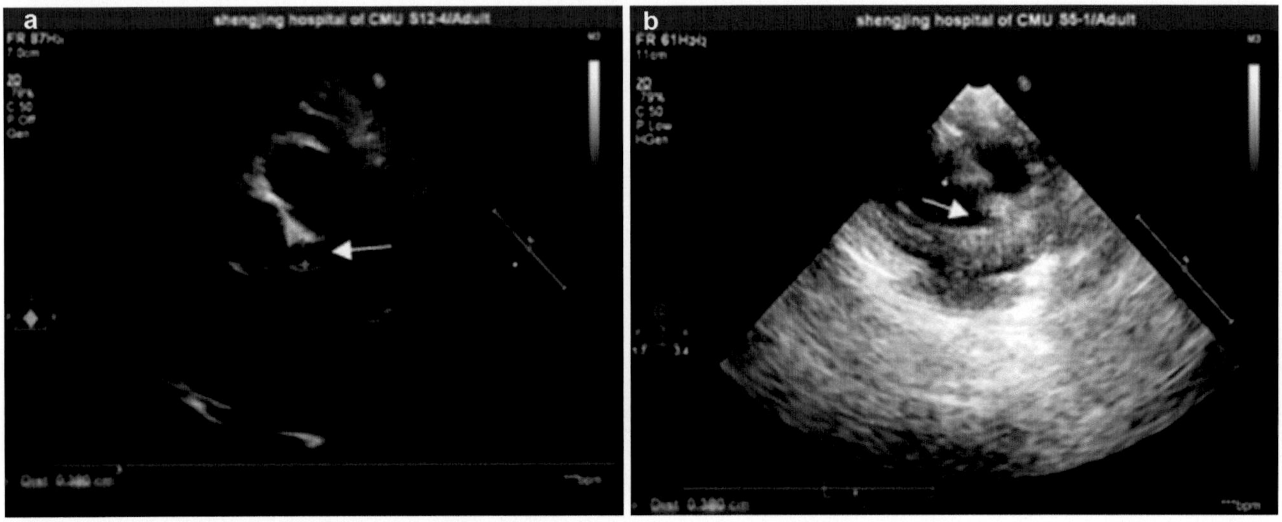

Fig. 12.3 Echocardiography showed LCA dilated to 3.8 mm at 21 months (**a**), and the same at 2 years (**b**)

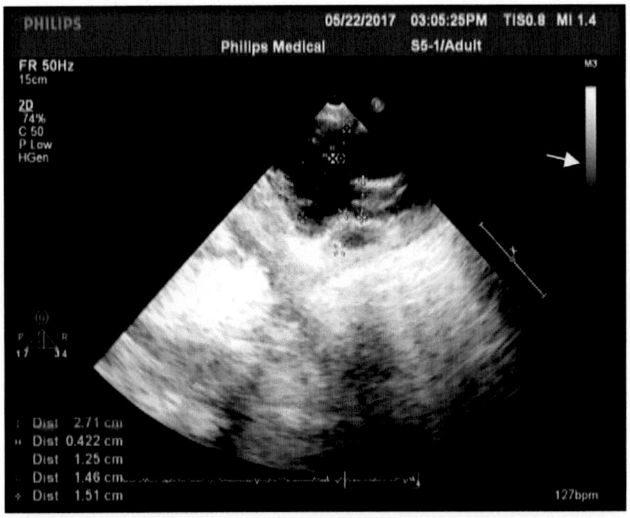

Fig. 12.4 Echocardiography showed LCA dilated to 3.3 mm at 35 months

that about 10–25% of untreated KD patients have coronary artery injuries [1]. If elevated troponin detected, routine ECG and echo should be performed.

12.1.4 Case Specific Clinical Features

1. In the acute phase of KD, myocardial injury and even acute myocarditis can occur (see case 1). But there are rare cases showing persistent troponin elevation after coronary artery injury, coronary thrombosis, and ischemic cardiomyopathy. Troponin continues elevated in some patients (see case 62). This patient had an upper respiratory tract infection. It was unknown whether troponin elevation was a result of current infection or of previous coronary artery injury. In the following 15 months, the patient did not present with infection during follow-ups at

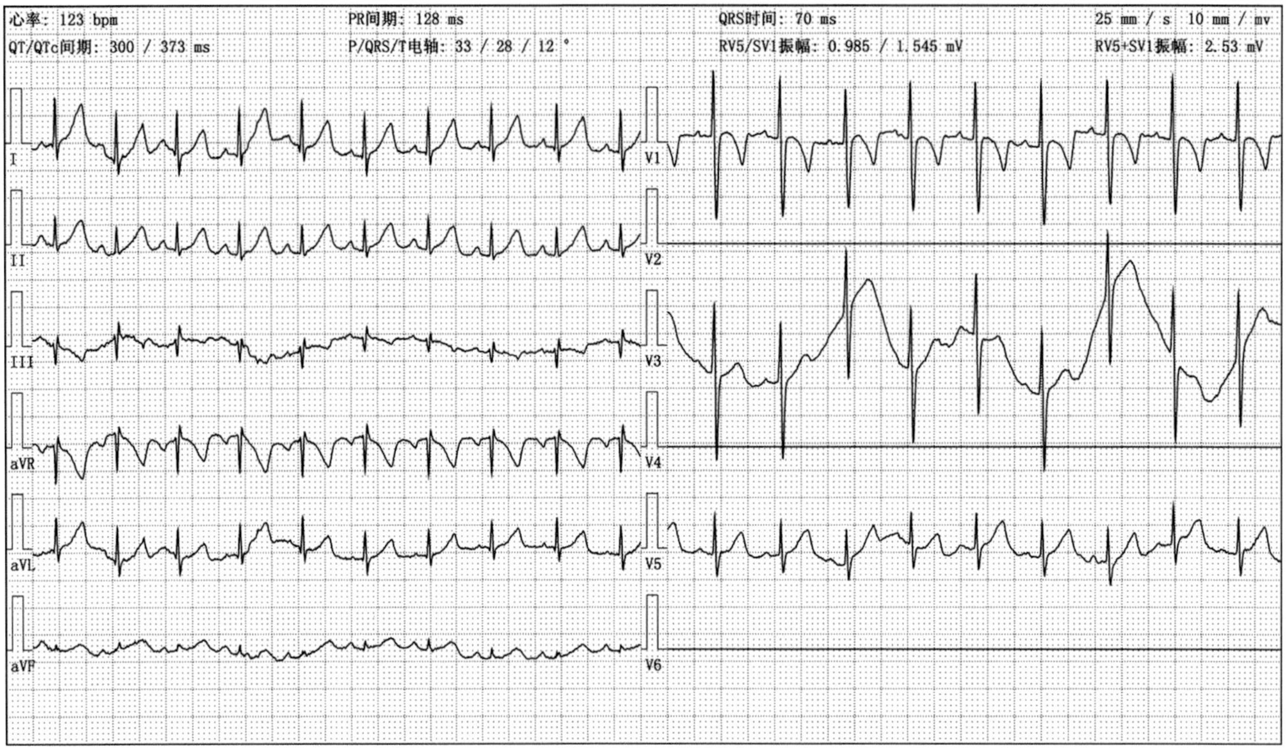

Fig. 12.5 ECG was normal at 35 months

the outpatient clinic. CK/CK-MB = 245/41 was increased. The possibility that this elevated cTnI was a result of coronary artery injury could not be excluded.

2. For this boy was in the recovering phase of KD even with coronary artery dilatation. Theoretically, IVIG application was not necessary. The patient had elevated cTnI (hs-cTnT) at the time of admission. Based on literature reports that KD can result in myocardial damage for a long time [2], thus IVIG 2 g/kg infusion was given to him. It may have no effect on protection of coronary arteries, but at least it may be beneficial in protecting myocardium. After 4 months treatment, his cTnI was reduced to normal.
3. In the 90s of the last century, few Chinese patients could afford IVIG. Therefore only aspirin was used as treatment in most cases, which might underlie the high incidence of coronary artery lesions [3]. At present in China, there are no detailed data analyzed from multiple centers on the incidence of CAA in KD patients. Data collected from our center have shown that there are rare ST-T changes in ECG when LVEF is reduced in KD patients who only have coronary arteries dilations with neither coronary thrombosis nor cardiac enlargement. We conclude that ECG is not sensitive enough to detect myocardial damages in these cases.
4. Literatures reported that the occurrence of KD is related to IgA and the inhibition of CD_8^+ [4, 5]. After 9 months of onset, he still had IgA reduction and normal CD_3^+. $CD_3^+CD_8^+$ 10.6% indicated CD_8^+ was reduced and $CD_3^+CD_4^+$ were normal. Elevation of CD_4/CD_8 and Th/Ts also indicate that CD_8^+ is in inhibitory state.

Ya-li Zhang

12.2 Case 43: Misdiagnosed KD with Giant CAA

A 6-year-old girl presented with a significant past medical history. When she was 2 or 3 years old, she had fever for 7–10 days, along with red eyes, dry and red lips, desquamation of fingernails. Coronary artery was not examined at that time.

She presented on Day 8 of illness with a history of cough and fever for 4 days and coronary artery dilation for 7 days. Eight days ago, she had fever up to 38.6 °C, twice a day, with paroxysmal cough, sigh, and fatigue. She was treated with antiviral, antitussive medications for 4 days. Her fever and cough regressed. Seven days ago, she came to our clinic. Echo showed LCA dilation. She was admitted to our pediatric cardiology ward. Since the onset, her mental state, diet, and sleep were normal, as well as her activities. Examination revealed afebrile (T 36.9 °C), and breathing smoothly (PR 98 bpm, RR 20 bpm, BP 106/62 mmHg). Her weight was 20 kg. Cervical lymphadenectasis was detected, along with congested pharynx and tonsil. Liver was enlarged 2 cm below right costal margin, medium hard. Others were normal. One week before admission, investigation revealed WBC 2.5 × 10^9/L, NE 1.34 × 10^9/L, HGB 116 g/L, PLT 123 × 10^9/L. MP IgG, MP IgM and CP IgM antibodies were negative. CK-MB 28 U/L, cTnI, CK-MB mass, myoglobin, and CRP were normal. Chest CT did not show abnormal findings. Six days ago, echo showed LAD dilated about 3.6–5.4 mm (Fig. 12.6a), while RCA (Fig. 12.6b), LVED (Fig. 12.6c), and LVEF (Fig. 12.6d) were normal. Five days before admission, WBC 3.4 × 10^9/L, NE 1.42 × 10^9/L, HGB 117 g/L, PLT 134 × 10^9/L. After admission, WBC 4.6 × 10^9/L, NE 1.74 × 10^9/L, HGB 126 g/L, PLT 206 × 10^9/L. She had met 4/5 criteria for KD (sequela period), with left CAA. She had upper respiratory tract infection at admission. She was treated with aspirin 3–5 mg/kg/day, in one dose, and dipyridamole 3–5 mg/kg/day, in three divided doses.

On the second day of admission, she was afebrile but had good condition in general.

On Day 4 of admission, coronary artery CTA confirmed that there were no calcified plaques in all segments of LAD and RCA. LCA opening was 2.1 mm. LAD proximal aneurysm dilation was about 7 mm, with 16.8 mm in length (Fig. 12.7a). LCX was 2.9 mm. RCA was 1.4 mm (Fig. 12.7b). She was discharged.

12.2.1 Follow-Up

After discharged, she continued to take oral aspirin and dipyridamole and was informed to avoid strenuous activities. One week after discharged, echo showed LVED was 36 mm, LVEF 65%, dilated LAD remained unchanged (3.6–5.4 mm) (Fig. 12.8). RCA was 2.3 mm. She has not followed up with us since then.

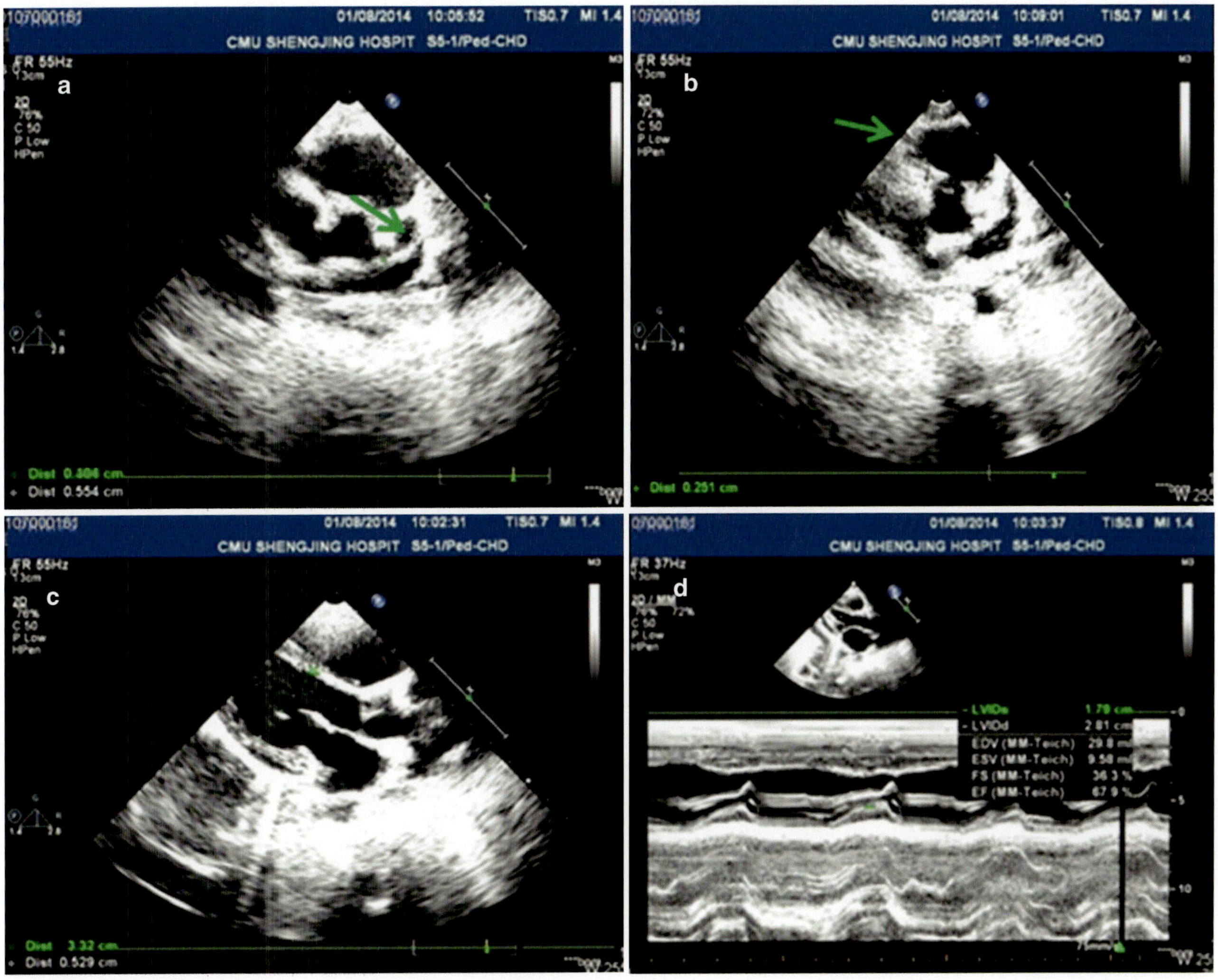

Fig. 12.6 Six days before admission, echocardiography showed LAD dilated to 5.4 mm (**a**), while RCA (**b**), LVED (**c**), and LVEF (**d**) were normal

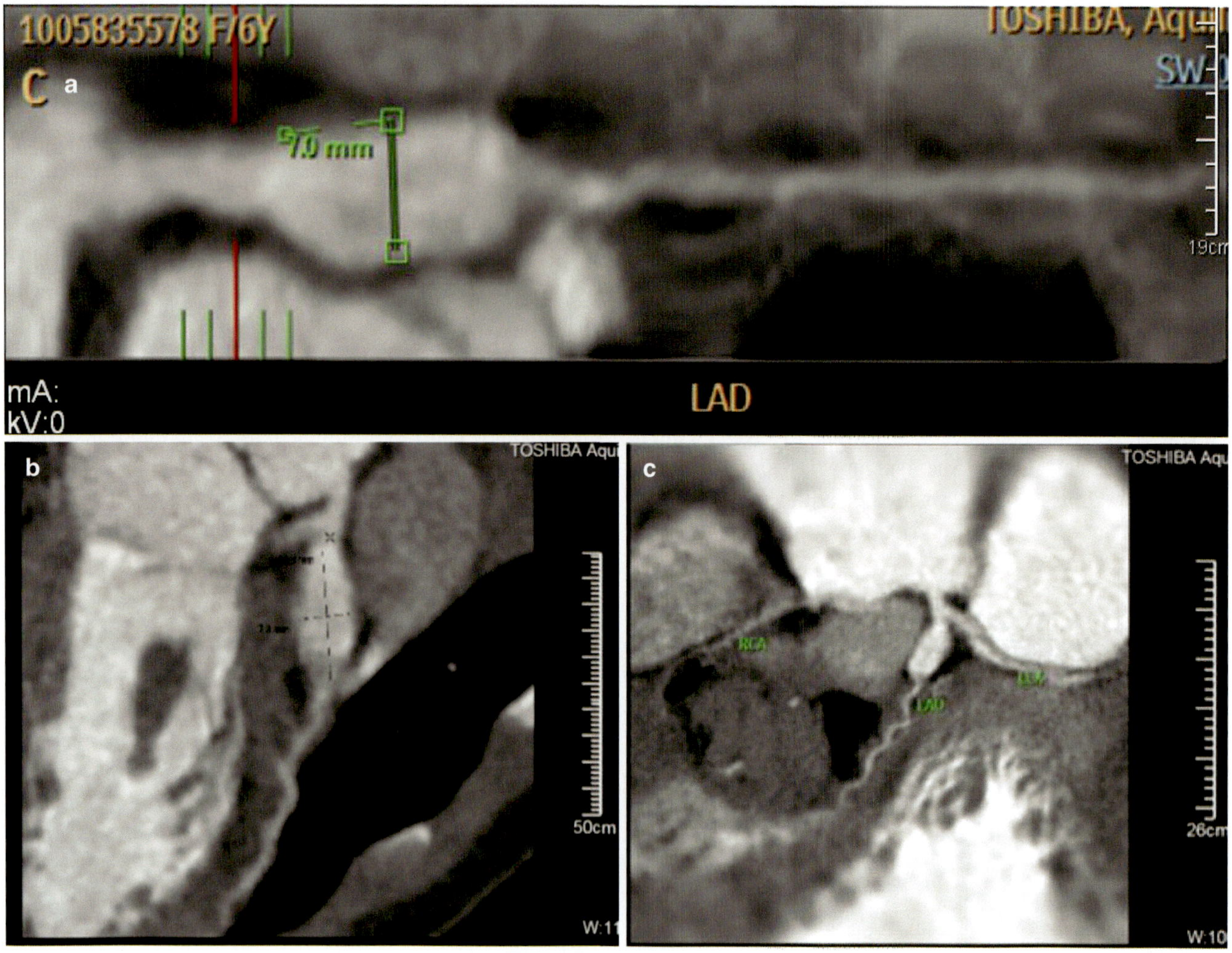

Fig. 12.7 On Day 4 of admission (about 3.5 years of the illness), coronary artery CTA showed LCA starting segment diameter 2.1 mm, LAD proximal tumor expansion, diameter 7 mm (**a**), length 16.8 mm (**b**), while RCA and LCX were normal (**c**)

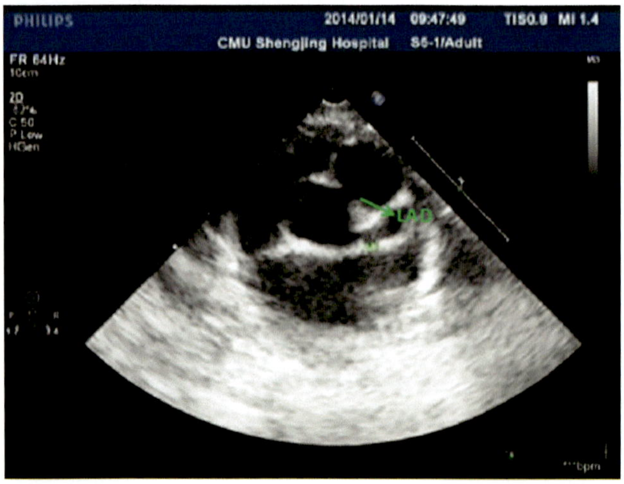

Fig. 12.8 On Day 7 after admission, echocardiography showed no significant change in diameter of the dilated LAD (5.4 mm)

12.2.2 Diagnosis

1. KD (sequela period).
2. Left CAA.
3. Acute upper respiratory tract infection.

12.2.3 Discussion

She had met the criteria of KD for she had persistent fever for more than 5 days 3 or 4 years ago, along with (1) red lips; (2) conjunctiva hyperemia in both eyes; (3) desquamation around fingernails; (4) echo and CTA confirmed left CAA.

12.2.4 Case Specific Clinical Features

1. KD is a febrile disease with unknown causes. The main pathological change is systemic small vasculitis, coronary artery dilatation in about 1/5 of untreated patients, and likely thrombosis formed by myocardial infarction within 2 years [6]. After 2 years of medication, most can be recovered. But about 5% of patients, even with IVIG treatment, still have CAA after 15 years [7].
2. Since the Japanese doctor Kawasaki Fusuke's report in 1967, more pediatricians have recognized KD. But here are still misdiagnosed cases. Fortunately, for this girl, a coronary aneurysm was discovered without ischemic cardiomyopathy developed, and anticoagulant was applied timely. If there is neither coronary thrombosis formed nor ischemic cardiomyopathy developed, patients can undergo coronary artery bypass surgery when they grow up. The long-term prognosis is optimistic. But for cases with coronary aneurysm developed for 3–4 year, it is less likely for heart to return normal.
3. In our center, for patients whose KD diagnosis was delayed, those with CAA on the right have better prognosis than those with CAA on the left (see case 15). Furthermore, prognosis in patients with delayed diagnosis is better than in patients with misdiagnosis. Even patients miss the best window to receive IVIG, they can take oral aspirin to prevent coronary thrombosis. If patients have developed giant CAA, they need to take oral warfarin to prevent the thrombus formed in CAA (see case 42). But eventually, the majority of these patients have small amount of thrombus adhering to the inner wall of CAA, and gradually develop into irreversible calcification in CAA wall (case 4 and case 7). If misdiagnosed patients were admitted due to other symptoms, they would have better prognosis than those admitted due to heart failure symptoms (see case 43). Thus, as long as heart failure does not occur, prognosis in KD patients is generally good.

Ya-li Zhang

12.3 Case 44 Misdiagnosed KD with Giant CAA, LCA Thrombus, and Chronic Heart Failure

A 3-year-old boy presented with a past medical history of prolonged fever over 10 days, along with red eyes, cervical lymphadenopathy, dry and red lips about 6 months ago, without rashes and desquamation around fingernails or toenails. He had unremarkable allergy and no family history.

He presented with an interrupt cough for nearly 20 days, fever for 2 days, along with stomachache for 6 days. On the second day of admission, he was diagnosed with pneumonia and was given infusion of second-generation cephalosporin for 1 week in a local hospital. His cough regressed. On Day 12, chest DR showed heart enlargement. On Day 14, he developed paroxysmal stomachache around navel. On Day 18, his cough got serious. Chest CT scan showed poor local inflation in bilateral inferior lobes, interstitial edema, right pleural effusion, pericardium effusion. Echo showed RCA aneurysm dilation, LCA dilation, heart enlargement, weak left ventricular wall motion, mitral and tricuspid regurgitation (moderate), pericardial effusion (mild). LVEF was decreased. He was admitted in our pediatric cardiology ward as a patient with CAA and heart failure. He had paroxysmal cough along with fatigue, sweaty, lack of appetite since the onset. *Examination* revealed he was afebrile, irritable, tachypnea (RR 40 bpm). Auscultation in lungs was normal. He had enhanced heart apex beats, weak heart sounds, and tachycardia (HR 138 bpm), with mild murmur at apex of the heart. Liver was enlarged 5 cm below right costal margin, moderate hard. Others were normal. *Investigation revealed* enlarged heart in chest DR (Fig. 12.9) on Day 12 CBC results were shown in Table 12.1. On Day 18, CK 254 U/L, CK-MB 33 U/L, total 25-OH vitamin D was 23.79 ng/ml; CRP, ASO, RF, serum ions, and urine were normal. On Day 20, chest CT showed local dilatation of the lower lobe and possible interstitial edema (Fig. 12.10a), right pleural effusion, pericardial effusion (Fig. 12.10b). Echo showed LVED 46 mm, LVEF 45% (Fig. 12.11a), RCA dilated about 8.4 mm, LAD dilated about 5.3 mm (Fig. 12.11b), left ventricular wall moved weakly, mitral and tricuspid regurgitation (moderate) (Fig. 12.11c), pericardial effusion (mild) (Fig. 12.11d).

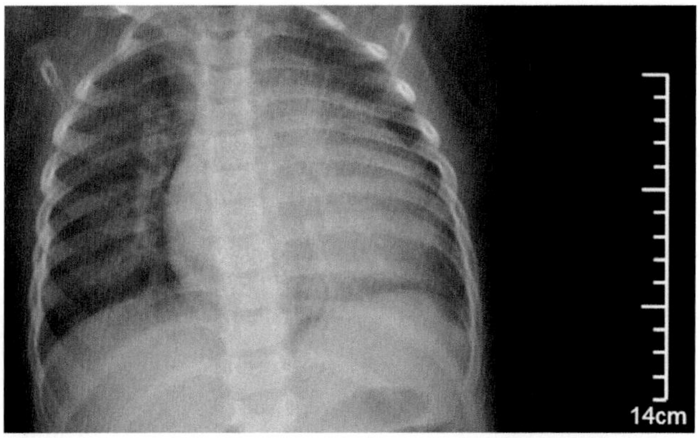

Fig. 12.9 On Day 12 of admission, chest DR showed left side of the heart was significant enlarged

Table 12.1 Dynamic changes of lab parameters

Time	1 day	5 days	12 days	2 months	13 month	36 months	38 months	40 months
WBC (×10^9/L)	10.6	9.3		7.5	6.68	8.59	6.2	8.4
NE (%)	38.6	37.2		30.2	32.5	41.2	38.3	71.5
HGB (G/L)	128	118		125	126	131	125	132
PLT (×10^9/L)	204	223		214	220	246	210	183
NT pro-BNP (pg/ml)	9952	3361	2929	1698	318	319.8	275	253
Hs-cTnT (ng/ml)	0.045	0.031	0.016	0.01	0.009	0.006	0.007	0.005

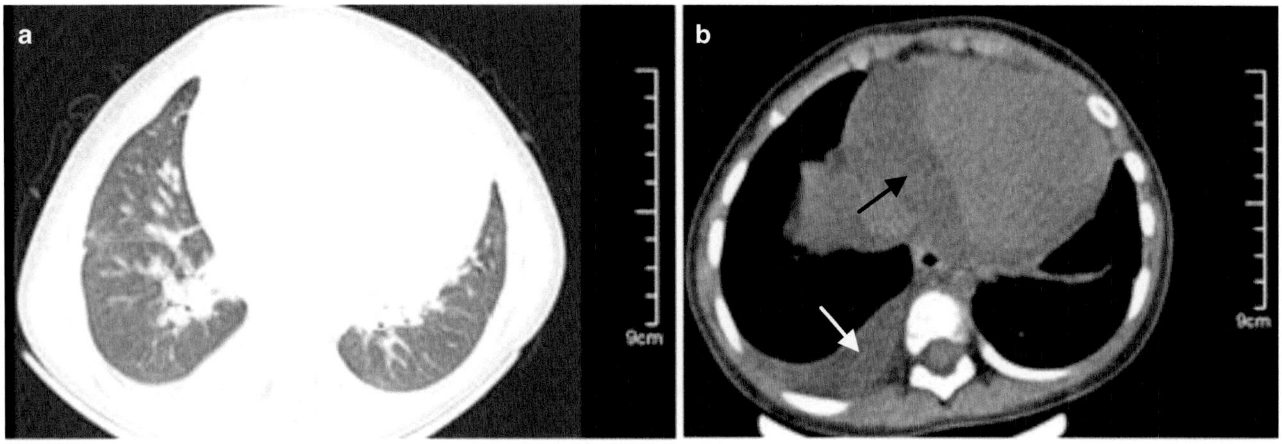

Fig. 12.10 On Day 18 of admission, chest CT showed local dysplasia of the lower lobe of both lungs and possible interstitial edema (**a**), right pleural effusion (**b**-white arrow), and pericardial effusion (**b**-black arrow)

Overall systolic function of left ventricle was reduced. *Admission blood* test was summarized in Table 12.1. CK-MB mass, cTnI, blood gas ion analysis, CRP, D-dimer, and INR were normal. PT was 16.3s. ECG showed low-flat and inverted T wave and the enlarged left atrium (Fig. 12.12). He had acute episode of chronic heart failure. He was monitored for ECG, BP, blood oxygen, and was advised bed rest. He was treated with cedilanid 0.03 mg/kg, fast saturated in 24 h, IV furosemidum 1 mg/kg/day, oral spironolactone in 1 mg/kg/day, qd, 4 days of every week, oral captopril 1 mg/kg in two divided doses. Considering his previous medical history, he was diagnosed with KD at recovered stage, and he was given oral aspirin and dipyridamole 3–5 mg/kg/day.

On Day 21, his urine volume increased, and dyspnea regressed. Under ECG monitoring, HR was reduced to 110 bpm. Percutaneous oxygen saturation was maintained above 95%. Examination found heart sounds were more powerful than before. Investigation revealed normal liver function and myocardial enzymes, negative MP-IgM and CP-IgM, MP-IgG 1:40. He was given oral digoxin 0.01 mg/kg/day after cedilanid fast saturated. On day 22, he urinated a lot and could lay on the back. All monitoring procedures were stopped.

On Day 23, physical examination found his heart sound was powerful. 2/6 systolic murmur could be heard around the apical area. The liver was regressed to 2.5 cm below the right costal margin. Blood test revealed lymphocyte subsets analysis was normal. ACA was negative. On Day 24, everything went well, and physical examination found no hepatomegaly. Repeated echo showed LVEF 39%, LCA and its branches were filled with a substantial weak echo reflex (Fig. 12.13a), LCA expanded about 6.4 mm (Fig. 12.13b). LAD slightly widened about 4.4 mm, RAD 8.4 mm (Fig. 12.13c). Left ventricle showed spherical dilatation, and its wall movement was generally weak and inharmonious, with moderate mitral regurgitation, tricuspid valve mild reflux, pericardial effusion 3–10 mm. There was no obvious abnormality in liver ultrasound. For LCA thrombosis, he was treated with oral warfarin at dose of 0.1 mg/kg/day.

On day 25, he had abdominal pain along with vomiting three times, and abdominal pain was relieved after vomiting. ECG showed low-flat T wave. He received infusion of saline solution with supplemental potassium. He was on a watch for possible digoxin toxicity. On day 26, his abdominal pain regressed. Investigation revealed: NT-pro BNP 3361 pg/ml, hs-cTnT 0.031 ng/ml. Liver function and levels

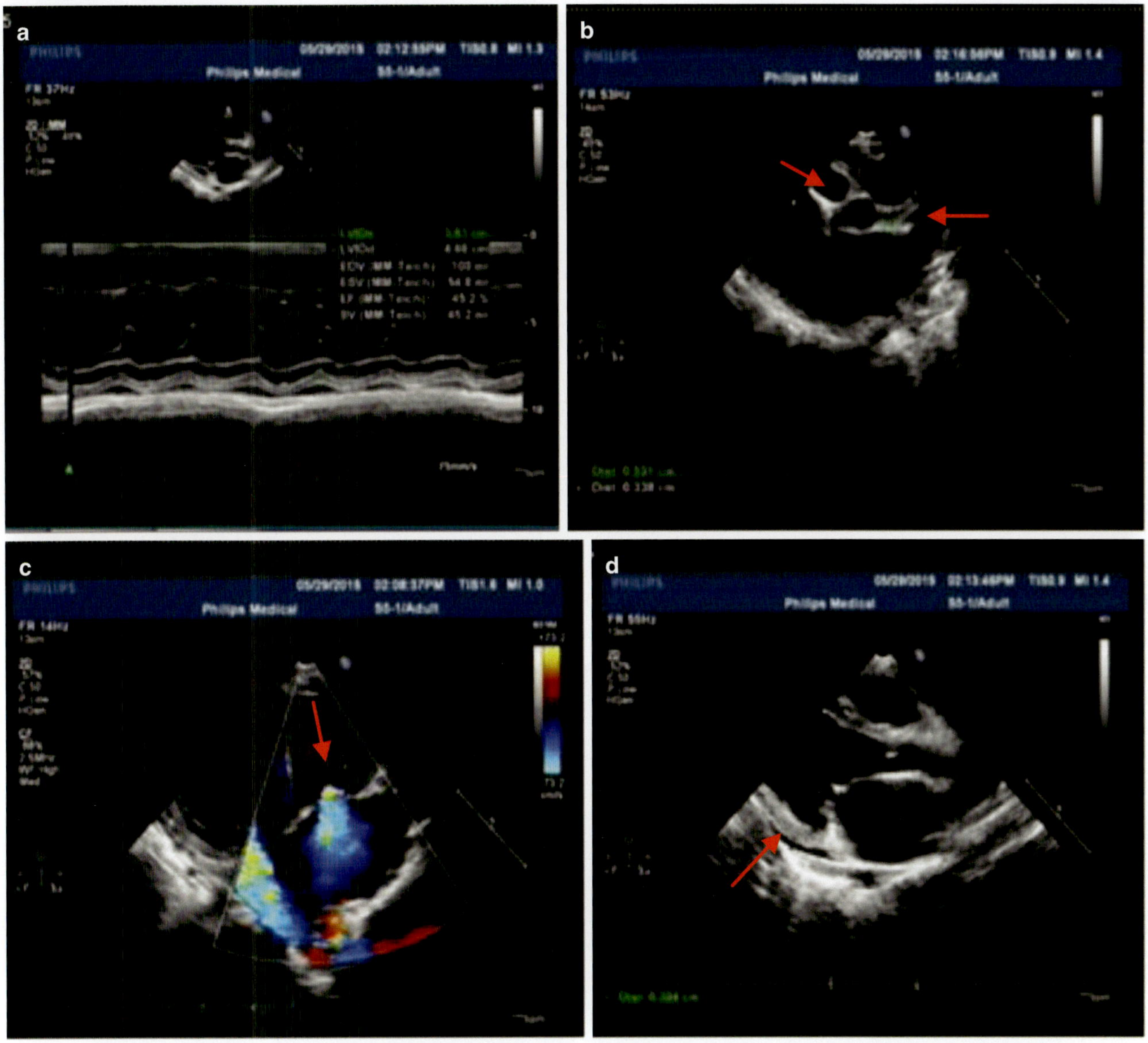

Fig. 12.11 On Day 18 of admission, M-mode echocardiography showed LVED 46 mm, LVEF 45% (**a**). RCA aneurysm dilated about 8.4 mm, LCA about 3.3–5.3 mm (**b**), mitral regurgitation (moderate) (**c**), 3 mm pericardial effusion behind the posterior wall of LV (**d**)

of potassium, sodium, and chlorine were normal. INR was 1.3. On day 27, ECG showed low-flat T wave. On Day 28, blood test revealed INR 1.4. ECG showed HR was 84 bpm, ST segment downshifted by 0.05 mv, and T wave was low-flat. On day 31, blood test revealed normal potassium level, NT-pro BNP 2929 pg/ml, hs-cTnT 0.016 ng/ml, and INR2.0. Repeated echo showed LVED 52 mm, LVEF 37%, LCA 4.9 mm, LAD 4.4 mm. LCA and LAD were filled with a substantially weak echo signal, RCA 12.6 mm, others were the same except that pericardial effusion was reduced to 3–8 mm. ECG parameters were significantly improved (Fig. 12.14). Oral dipyridamole was stopped, and he was discharged.

12.3.1 Follow-Up

He was followed up at clinic every month since discharged. DIC and coronary artery dynamic changes were listed in Tables 12.1 and 12.2. Echo was performed at 2 (Fig. 12.15a, b), 5 (Fig. 12.16a–c), 10 (Fig. 12.17), and 13 months (Fig. 12.18a, b). During this section, his echo showed there was thrombus in his LCA and LAD till 6 months of illness. He took oral traditional Chinese medication along with warfarin and aspirin. At 9–10 months of illness, the thrombus disappeared and his LVEF was increased over 45%. He could move anywhere without any uncomfortable feeling and he had no hepatomegaly. Coronary artery CTA (Fig. 12.19a–c) confirmed that

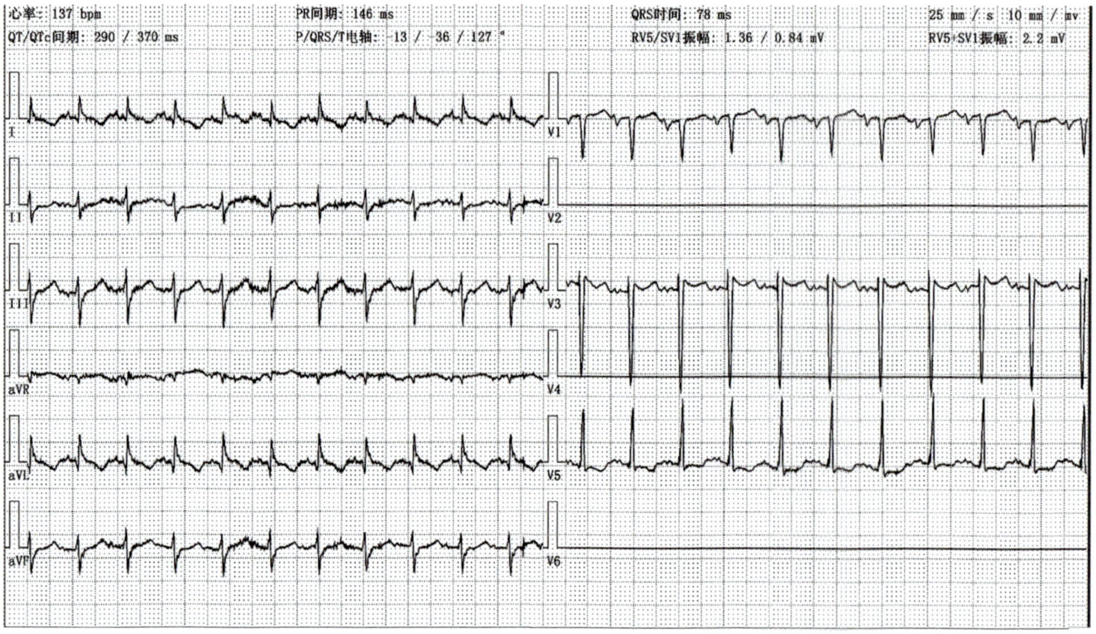

Fig. 12.12 On Day 20 of admission, ECG showed T wave low-flat and invert. LA enlarged was not excluded

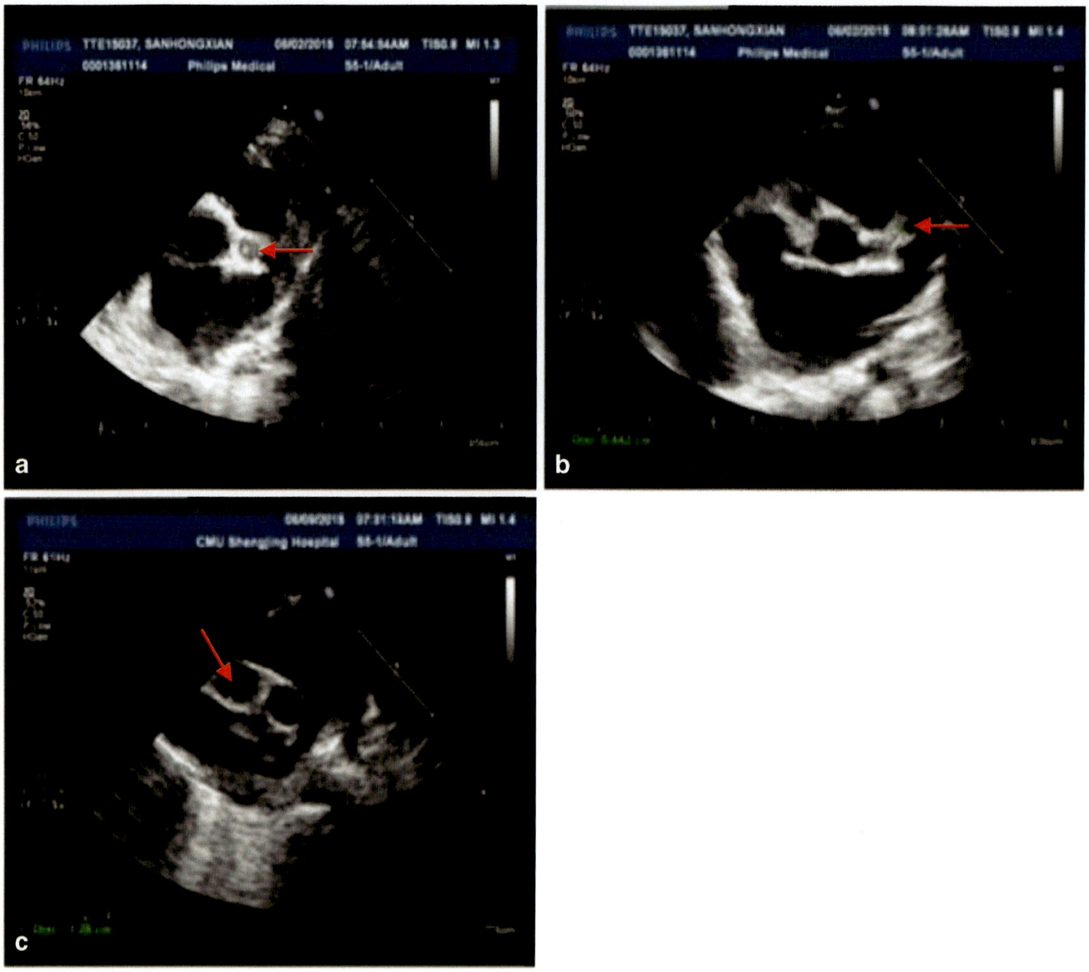

Fig. 12.13 On Day 24 of admission, echocardiography showed the hypoechogenicity in the dilated LAD (**a**, **b**), RCA aneurysm dilated up to 12.6 mm (**c**)

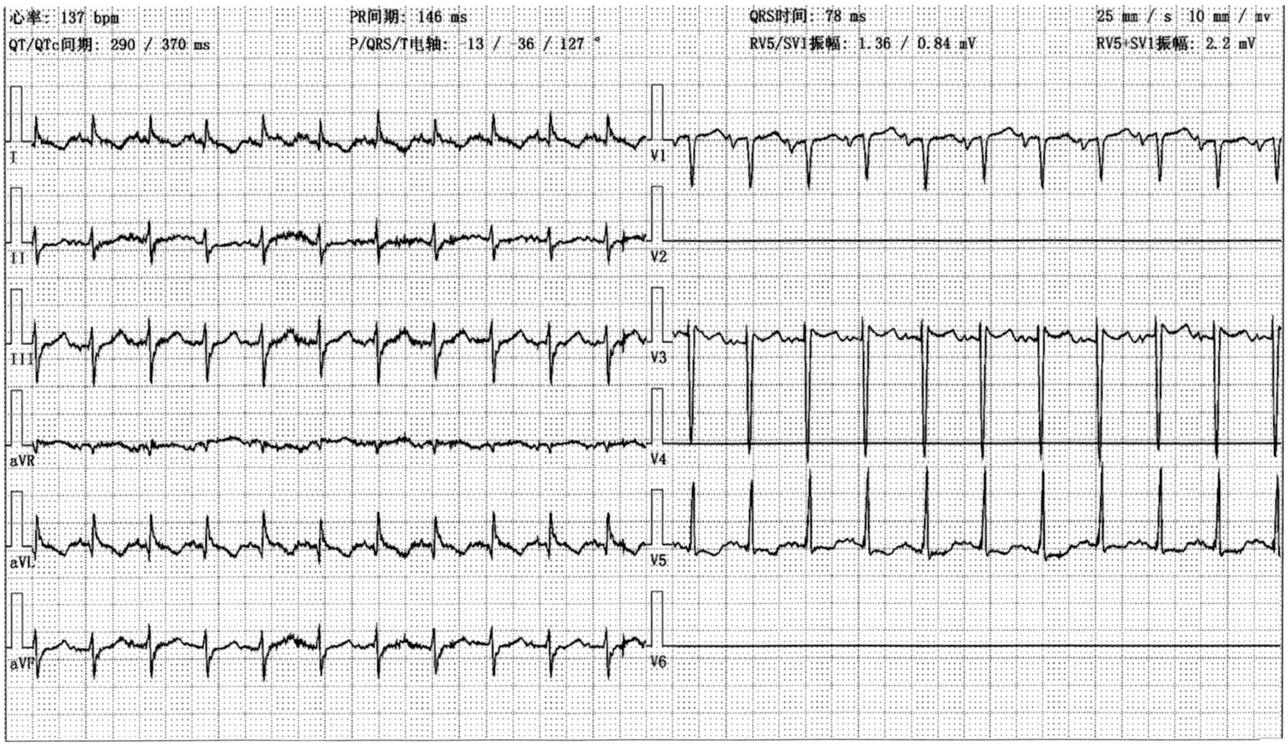

Fig. 12.14 On Day 31 of admission, ECG showed T wave was regressed on inferior wall

Table 12.2 The dynamic changes of coronary artery

Time of Diagnosis	1 day	5 days	12 days	2 months	5 months	10 months	13 months	22 months	34 months	40 months
Warfarin (mg/kg/day)	0.1	0.1	0.1	0.1	0.1	0.1	0.1	0.09	0.08	0.08
INR	1.1	1.3	2	1.2	1.9	1.5	1.3	1.8	1.8	2.5
LVED (mm)	46	52	52	52	53	49	48.5	50	47.5	45.4
LVEF (%)	45	39	33	44	38	42	44	35	48	47.5
LM (mm)		6.4	4.9	4.3	4.3	4.1	4.8–5.0	3.4	3.1	5.3–3.7
LAD (mm)	5.3	4.4	4.4	4.1	4.1	4.4	3.7	5.8	4.5	5.4
RCA (mm)	8.4	8.4	12.6	11.8	15	14	13.1	13.8	14.2	14.2
Thrombus		LCA + LAD	LCA + LAD	LCA + LAD	LCA + LAD	No	No	No	RCA 5.8 × 2.4	RCA 5.0 × 4.6
LCA blood		No	No	No	No	Yes	Yes	Yes	Yes	Yes
Calcification									RAC	

there was blood flow in LAC and LAD. At 17 months of illness, echo showed LCA was dilated about 2.6–6.2 mm (Fig. 12.20). But At 26 months, ECG still showed ST segment shifts ≥0.05 mv, negative and positive bipolar T wave, anomalous q-waves on leads I and AVL.

By now, he was diagnosed with giant RCAA over 3.5 years. DIC was monitored every month and warfarin dosage was adjusted timely to keep his INR from 2.0 to 3.0. Unfortunately, at 29 months of diagnosis, and echo showed LCA dilation, there was a thin blood flow in LCA, but the distal LCA was blurred (Fig. 12.21a, b). At 30 months of illness, coronary artery CTA was performed. LCA was dilated, with block-shape expansions in local segments, and the distal segment was blurry (Fig. 12.22a). LCX was almost normal (Fig. 12.22b). RCA showed aneurysm dilatation about 17 mm × 12 mm. Calcification was detected on the wall, and inner echo was not uniformed (Fig. 12.22c). The distal segment was clear. There was aneurysm-like dilatation shown in RCA (Fig. 12.22d-fasade). At 32 months of illness, echo showed RCA expansion with giant aneurysm was about 14.2 mm. There were a few in situ clots formed: the biggest one was 5.8 mm × 2.4 mm, without activity. (Fig. 12.23).

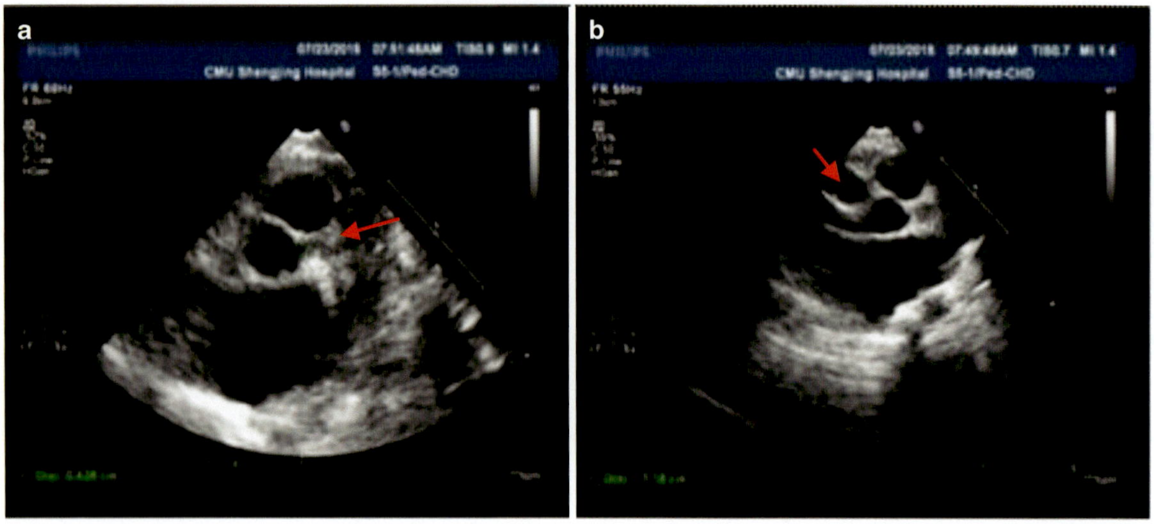

Fig. 12.15 At 2 months of illness, echocardiography showed the hypoechogenicity in the dilated LAD (**a**), RCA aneurysm dilated up to 11.8 mm (**b**)

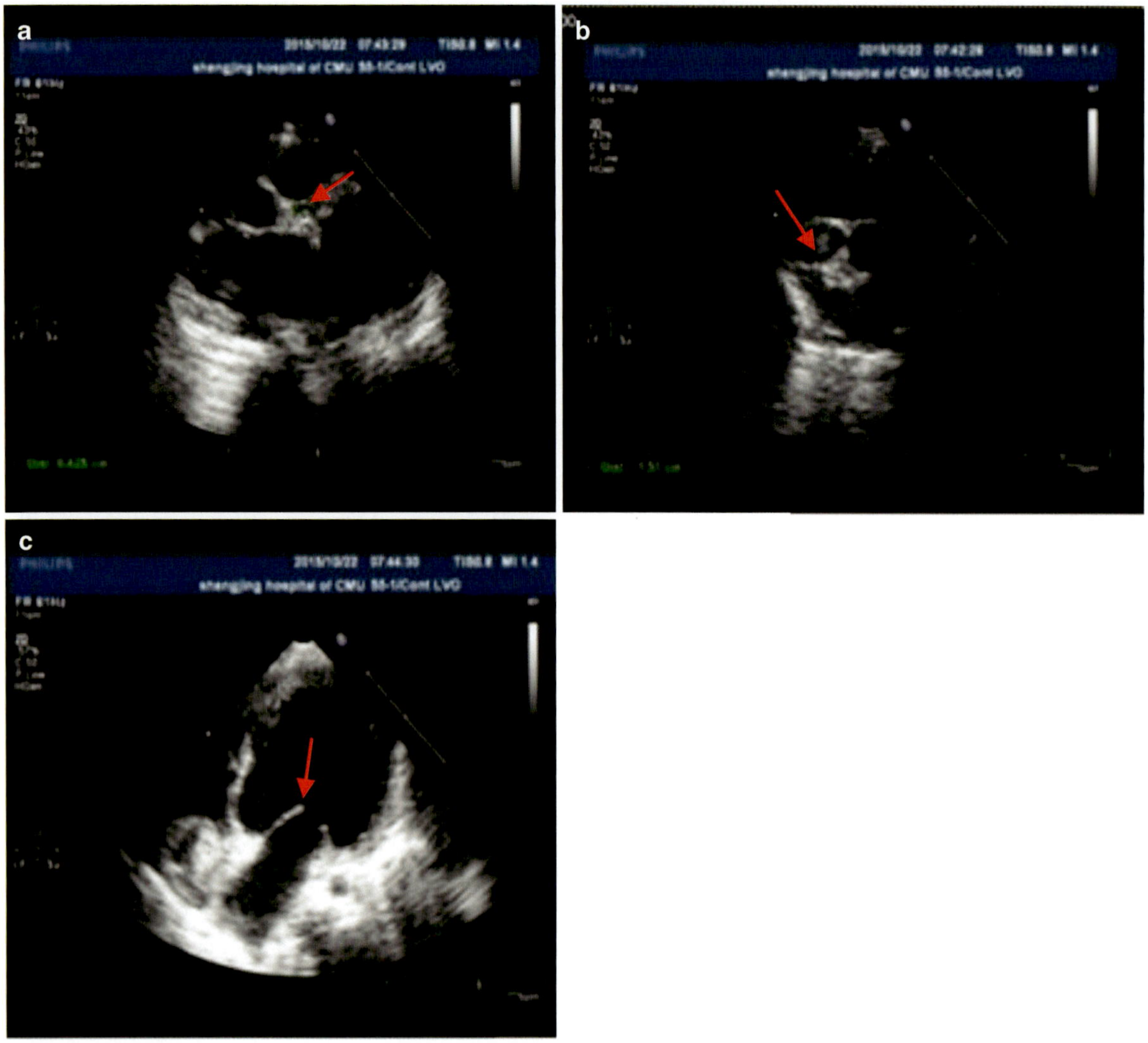

Fig. 12.16 At 5 months of admission, echo showed LCA was significantly dilated and filled with a substantial hypoechoic (**a**), RCA aneurysm dilated to 15 mm (**b**), hyperechoic mitral valve (**c**)

At 34 months, repeated echo showed some strong echo reflex. The biggest one was increased to 5.8 mm × 2.4 mm in RCA, without activity. There were no other changes. At 40 months of illness, ECG showed lower ST segment ≥0.05 mv (Fig. 12.24). Echo showed LVED 46.5 mm, LVEF 40% (Fig. 12.25a). Left ventricular wall moved weakly and inharmoniously. LCA was dilated about 6.6 mm (Fig. 12.25b), and there was a 5.3 mm × 3.7 mm soft echo reflex in it (Fig. 12.25c). LCX was dilated. The aneurysm dilatation in RCA was about 14.2 mm (Fig. 12.25d). There were many strong wall-attached echo reflexes in it. The biggest one was 5.9 mm × 4.6 mm, without activity (Fig. 12.25e). The dynamic changes of INR were shown in Fig. 12.26.

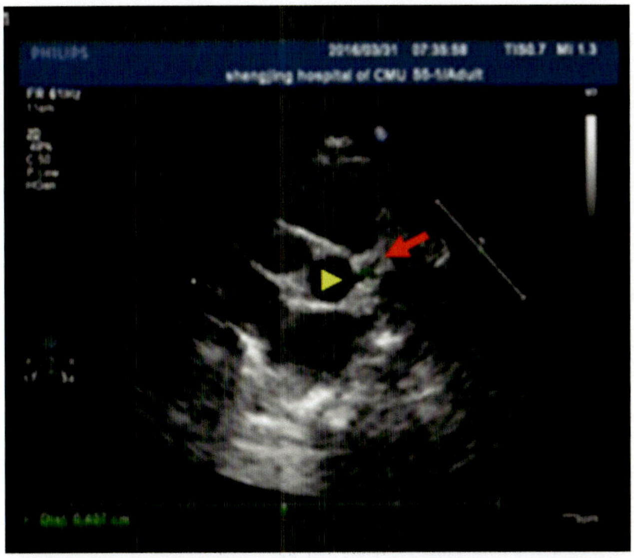

Fig. 12.17 At 10 months of admission, echocardiography showed both LCA (yellow arrow) and LAD (red arrow) dilated to 4.1 mm, without hypoechogenicity inside

12.3.2 Diagnosis

1. KD, recovered stage.
2. Giant CAA.
3. LCA thrombosis.
4. Ischemic cardiomyopathy.
5. Chronic heart failure (NYHA Class IV).
6. Right pleural effusion.
7. Pericardial effusion (mild).
8. Mitral regurgitation (moderate).

12.3.3 Discussion

He had met the criteria of KD. He had fever for 10 days half year ago, along with (1) red lips, (2) bilateral conjunctival congestion; (3) cervical lymphadenopathy; (4) bilateral CAA.

Differential diagnosis of dilated cardiomyopathy should be considered.

12.3.4 Case Specific Clinical Features

1. KD is an autoimmune disease, mainly affecting middle and small arteries. Diagnosis is mainly based on clinical symptoms [8]. KD can result in some heart-related diseases. Thus, it has become a major cause underlying acquired heart diseases in children in developed countries.

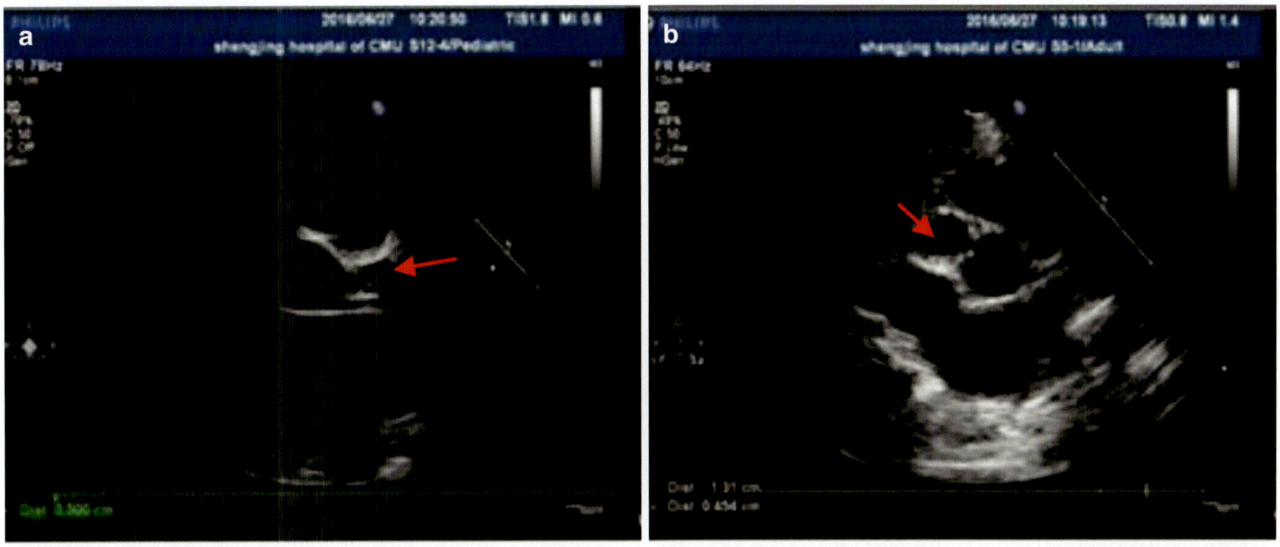

Fig. 12.18 At 13 months of admission, echocardiography showed LCA was dilated to 4.8–5.0 mm (**a**), RCA aneurysm dilated to 4.8–13.1 mm (**b**), no additional echogenicity in both LCA and RCA

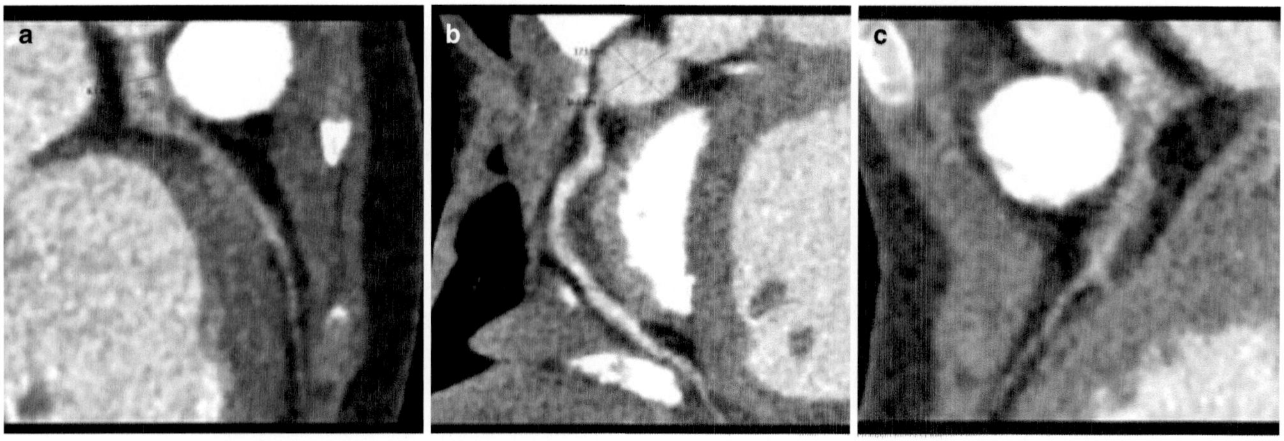

Fig. 12.19 At 13 months of illness, coronary artery CTA showed LCA dilated to 6.1 mm (**a**), RCA aneurysm dilated to 17.1 mm × 16.6 mm (**b**), LCA proximal was enlarged and far end normal (**c**)

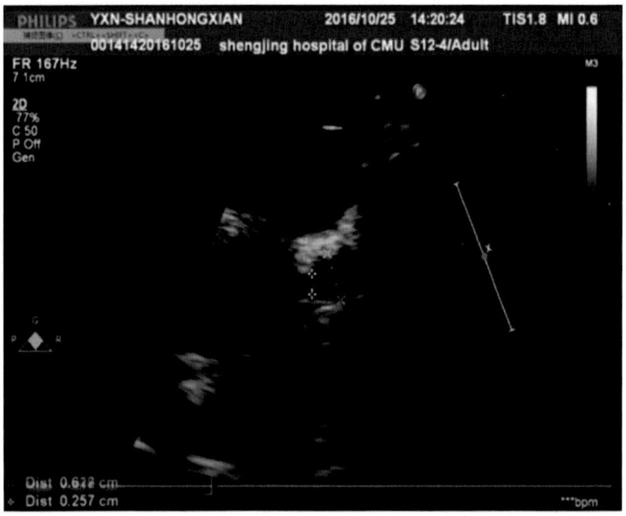

Fig. 12.20 At 17 months of illness, echo showed LCA was dilated to 2.6–6.2 mm

When the patient presented to hospital, he had developed chronic heart failure. Coronary arteries were dilated. After talking with his parents, we learned that he had fever for 10 days half year ago, along with red lips, cervical lymphadenopathy, and bilateral conjunctival congestion. Local clinic suspected that he had viral infection and drug allergies. For KD is a self-limited disease, symptoms can disappear even without proper treatment. Therefore, we highly suspected that he had KD at that time.

2. In KD patients without formal treatments, there is 20% chance to develop coronary artery injuries, and the risk to develop myocardial infarction with coronary thrombosis is the highest in the first 2 years [6]. One percent of them can suddenly die due to heart failure and thrombosis [9]. Despite treatment, there are still several risk factors that can lead to coronary artery injuries in patients, and they are male, age, elevated WBC, and fever that does not respond to IVIG or prolonged treatment. It has been reported in the literature that serum albumin <30 g/L may indicate coronary artery injuries [10].
3. Coronary artery injury will enhance thrombosis risk, thus anticoagulant therapy is necessary [11]. It is very important to predict the occurrence of coronary artery injuries, and treat patients timely at the early stage of disease. It has been reported in literature that when NT-pro BNP is 950 pg/ml, the sensitivity of cardiovascular injury is 88.1% while the specificity is 89.0% [12]. Another study finds that elevated serum 25-(OH) D3 can be used to predict coronary artery injury. When serum 25-(OH) D3 concentration is higher than 65 μg/L, the sensitivity is 78% and specificity is 73% [13].
4. To date, no randomized clinical trials have evaluated the safety and efficacy of antithrombotic regimens for prophylaxis of coronary thrombosis in KD [14]. Small dosage of aspirin combined with warfarin is recommended as treatment plan, for the nose bleeding is common in children, thus, it is difficult to maintain INR at 2.0–3.0 [14].
5. The patient has been taking warfarin and aspirin regularly for 6 months, and the thrombosis in LCA remained unchanged. When combined with of traditional Chinese medication for 3 months, the thrombus disappeared. The coronary CTA also showed there was flow in it without thrombus. The giant aneurysm occurred in RCA not in LCA. This maybe the reason that his prognosis is better, though KD was not confirmed at the acute stage which might delay the correct diagnosis (see case 43). The thrombus in LCA would result in left ventricular ischemia, which may lead to incoordinated motion in left ventricular wall. By now, the first and advanced choice for therapy is to absorb thrombus by applying ultrasound to coronary artery. This procedure has been performed in adults [15], and patients must fit in acute cases. It was not a common practice in mainland China 3 years ago. The

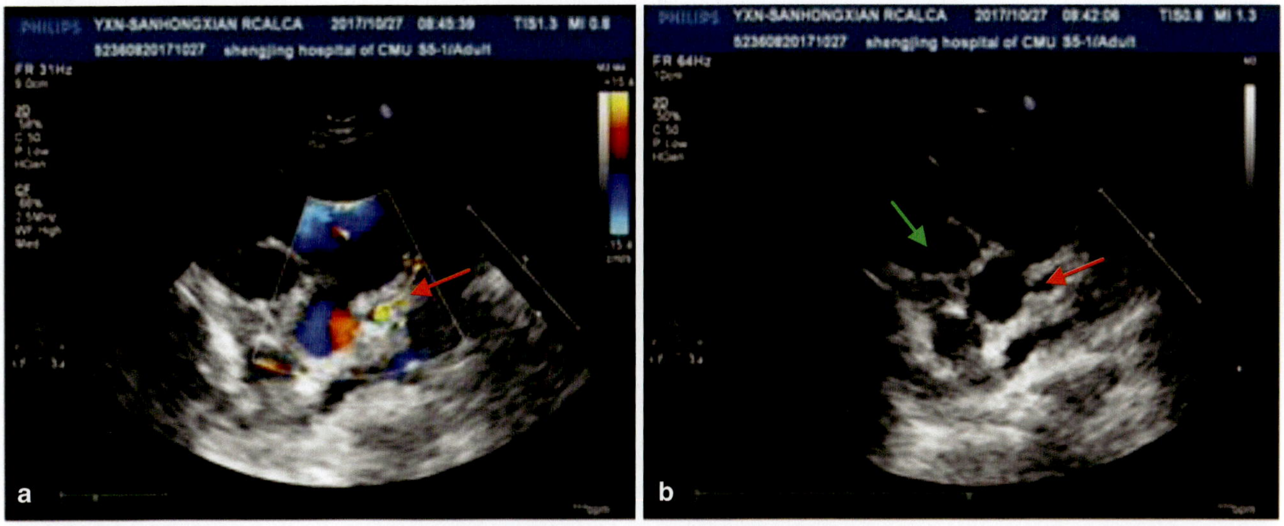

Fig. 12.21 At 29 months of admission, echocardiography showed the blood flow in LCA (**a**). LCA was 3.1 mm at beginning, it dilated to 4.5 mm after 3.4 mm away from beginning and branches off the LAD (**b**-red arrow). RCA was 4.0 mm at beginning, it dilated up to 14.2 mm after 2 mm away from beginning with substantial hyperechogenicity inside, the maximum one was 4.2 mm × 2.8 mm (**b**-green arrow), no significant activity

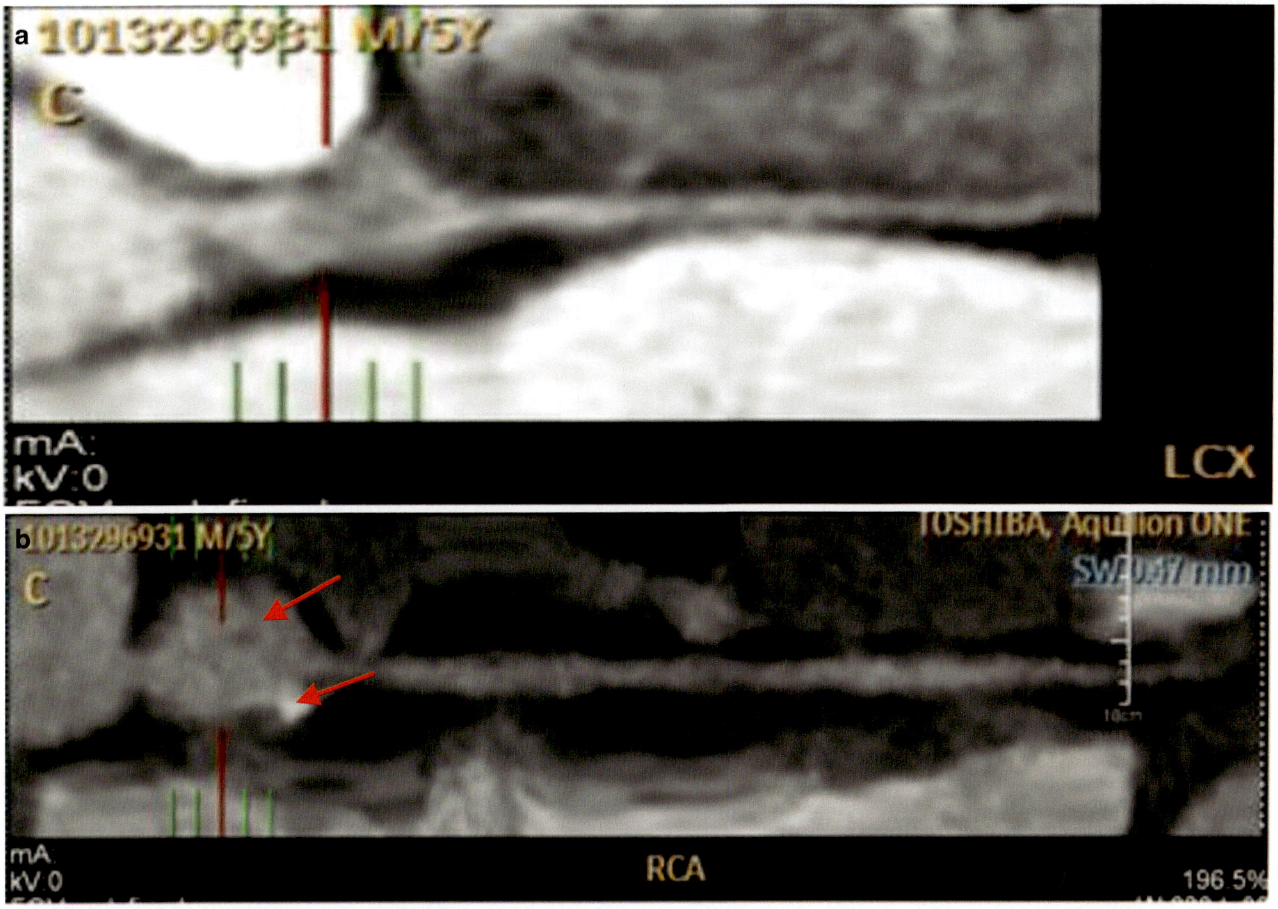

Fig. 12.22 At 30 months of admission, coronary artery CTA showed that LCA was dilated, local block-like expansion, and was unclear at far-end (**c**). LCX was almost normal (**a**). RCA was dilated to form an aneurysm, about 17 mm x 12 mm. it had calcification on the wall (**b**-lower arrow) and had uneven penetration (**b**-upper arrow) in it. It was clear at the far-end. RCA was dilated as an aneurysm (**d**-outlook)

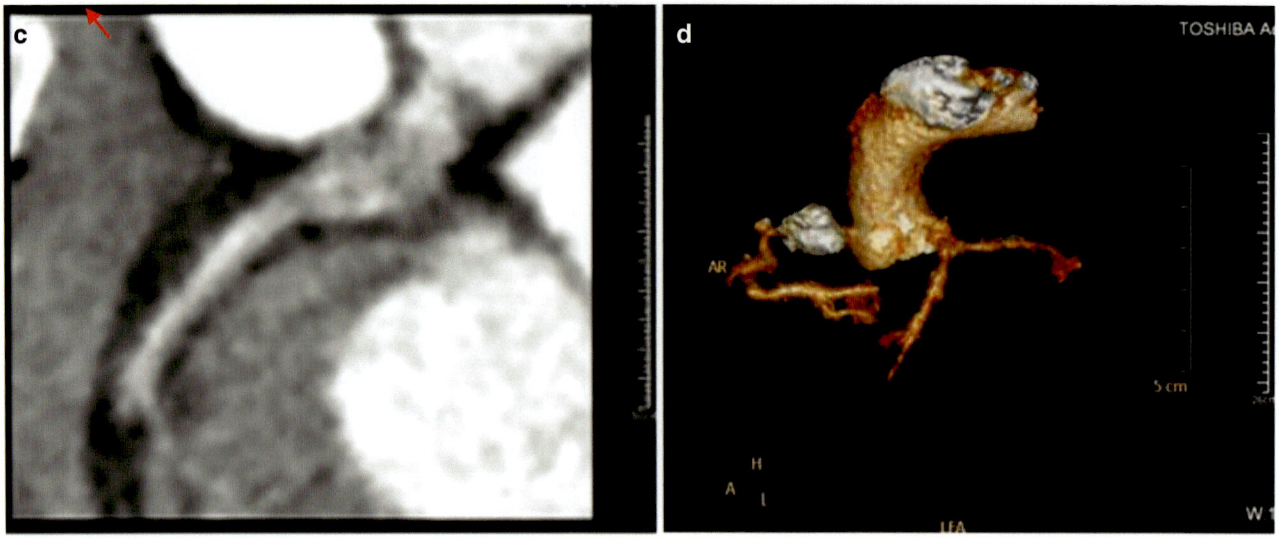

Fig. 12.22 (continued)

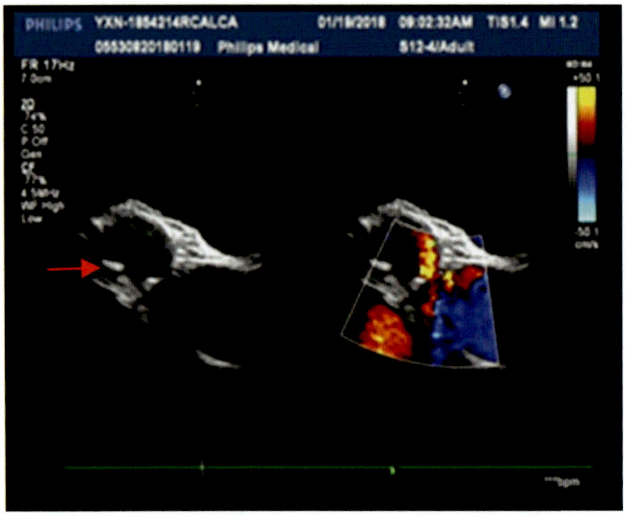

Fig. 12.23 At 32 months of admission, echocardiography showed the gigantic aneurysm of RCA, maxmium diameter 14.2 mm. Arrow shows one of the biggest hyperechogenicity inside of it, size 5.8 mm × 2.4 mm

second therapy choice is to apply heparin infusion. He was too young to tolerant daily blood sample drawn and consequences of possible risk of intracranial hemorrhage. At acute stage of disease (less than 48 h of onset), ECG usually shows ST segment elevation. But his ST segment was low–flat at admission, suggesting an ischemia. Echocardiography confirmed a low density clot. Taken together, there had been significant improvements in heart failure symptoms based on ECG results. We highly suspected he already developed thrombus before admission [16]. The third therapy choice is to apply oral warfarin. For his nose bleeding and skin hemorrhage, warfarin dosage was adjusted from 0.1–0.06–0.15 mg/kg.

6. MI signs in young children and infants are either silent or associated with nonspecific symptoms. Suddenly decline in ventricular function (like this case) or change in electrocardiographic findings should be highly considered as a link to coronary artery thrombosis. After active treatment, the left coronary artery thrombosis disappeared 9–10 months after admission. ECG was also significantly improved. He had no symptoms in his usual activities. Left ventricular enlargement, incoordination of wall motion, and declined ejection-function failed to recover due to long-term ischemia. His long-term prognosis was not optimistic.

Hong Wang

12.4 Case 45: Misdiagnosed KD with Giant CAA, LCA Occlusion, and Chronic Heart Failure

A 3-year-old male was presented with an unremarkable personal, allergy, and family history.

He presented on Day 20 of illness, with a history of stomachache for 20 days, along with fever and cough for more than 10 days, and body edema for 10 days. He came in with a 20-day history of abdominal pain described as intermittent lower abdominal pain, with fever up to 39 °C, along with pharyngalgia. He was given infusion of first-generation cephalosporin for 1 day and erythromycin for 3 days at a local clinic, and then fever regressed. On Day 5, he had fever again and developed paroxysmal coughing with wheezing which was more serious in the morning and at night. He was treated with first-generation cephalosporin again for 7 days,

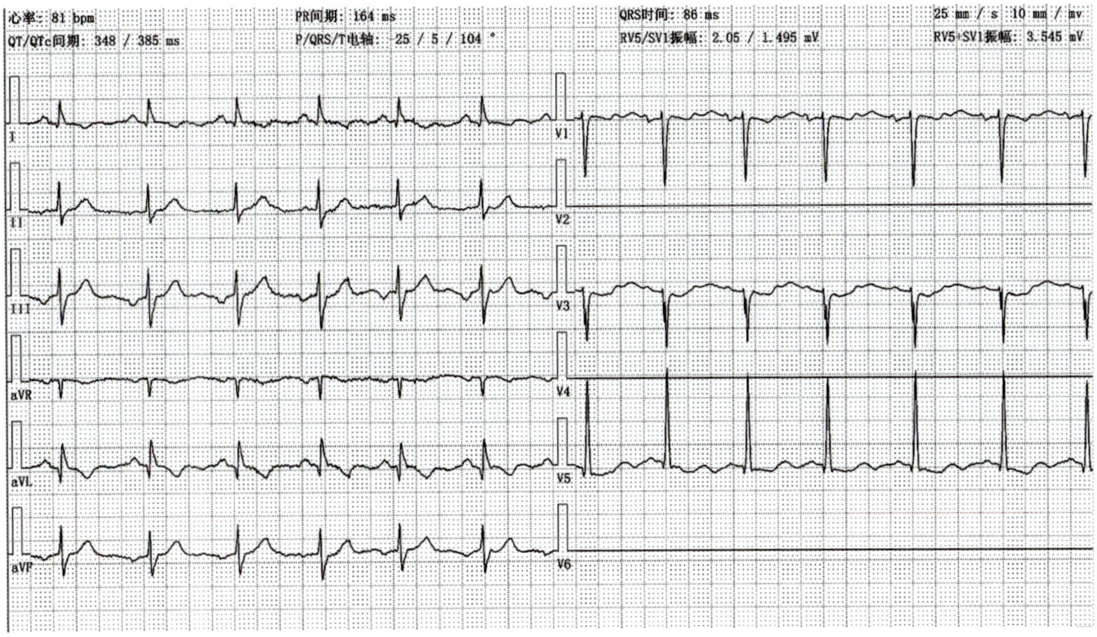

Fig. 12.24 At 40 months of illness, ECG showed ST segment was depressed ≥0.05 mv

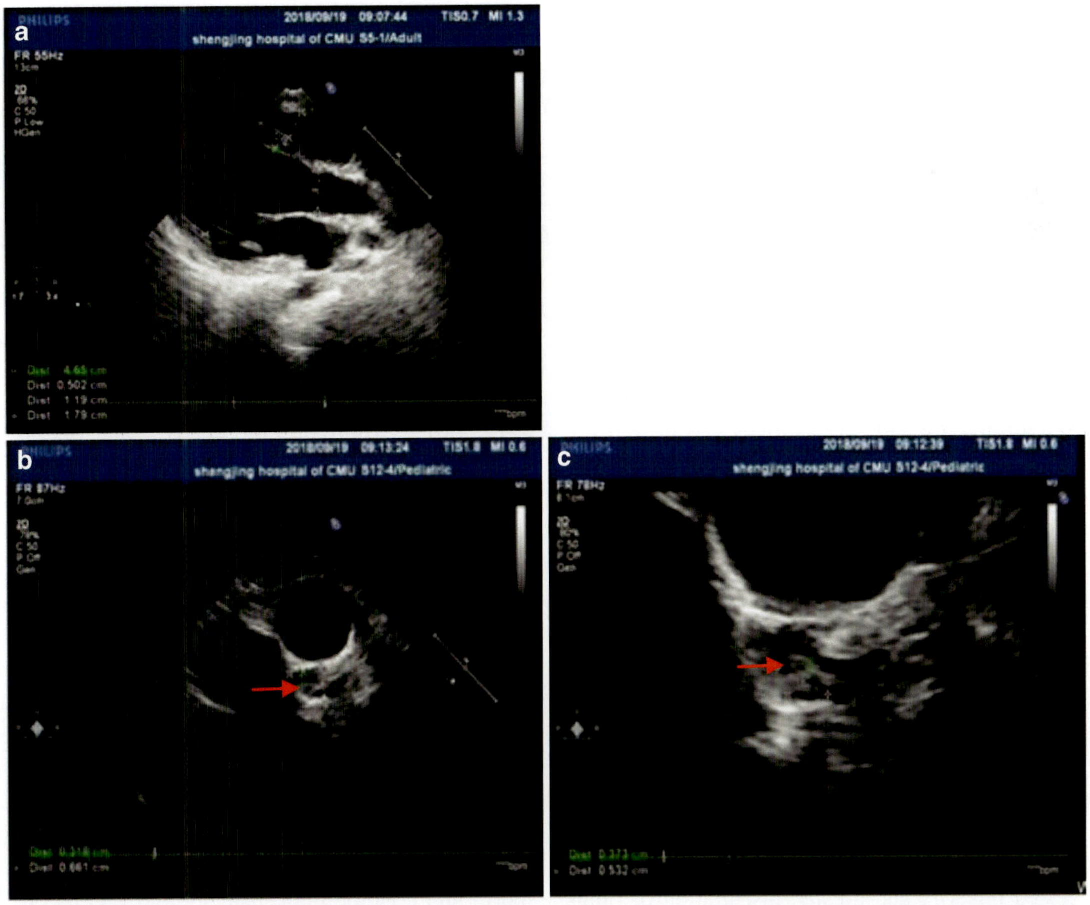

Fig. 12.25 At 40 months of admission, M-mode echocardiography showed LVEDD 46.5 mm(**a**), LVEF 40% . The dilated LCA with thrombus, size 5.3 × 3.7 mm (**b**). The gigantic aneurysm of RCA, maximum diameter 14.2 mm. Arrow showed one of the biggest hyperechogenicity inside of it, size 5.8 mm × 2.4 mm (**c**)

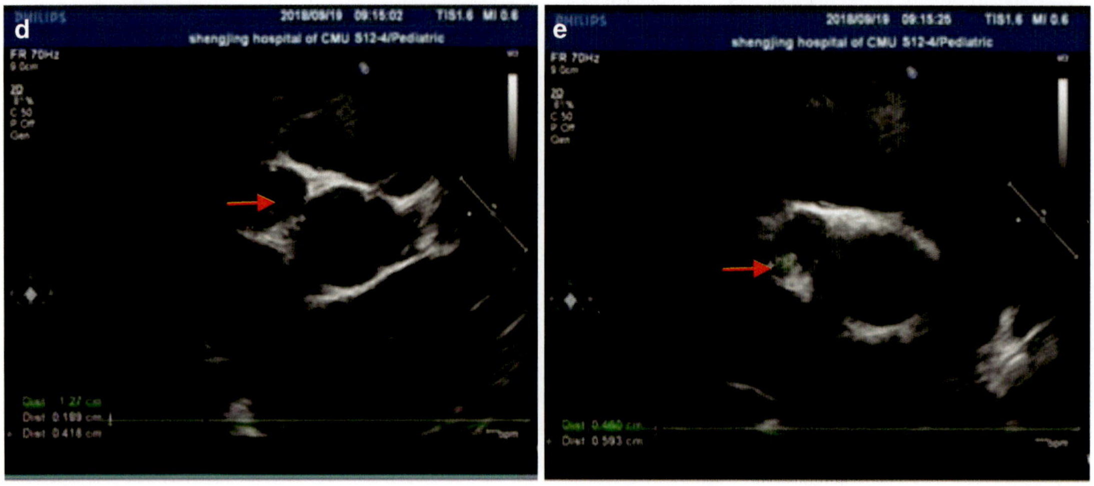

Fig. 12.25 (continued)

Fig. 12.26 The dynamic changes of INR

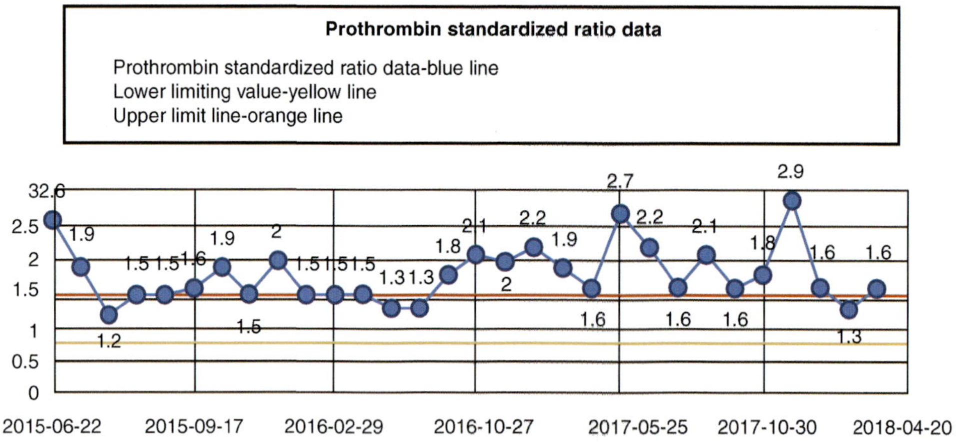

the fever subsided. But he developed facial and body edema, and oliguria. Vitamin C was given one time and azithromycin infusion was given for 1 day. His facial edema, cough, and wheezing all deteriorated, and dyspnea was developed. After he received diuretics for 2 days and took traditional Chinese medication for 7 days, his edema improved. Sputum could be coughed up easily. But he still had cough with wheezing at night. The patient was fatigue, pale, sweaty when moving. He was hospitalized at a local hospital. The chest DR showed cardiomegaly. Echo showed significantly enlarged left ventricle, weak wall movement, and mild pericardial effusion. He was transferred to our pediatric cardiology ward as a patient with dilated cardiomyopathy. Since the onset of illness, he had to sleep on his right side and gradually had oliguria. Examination revealed his mental state was bad, pale, dyspnea. Axillary temperature 36 °C, HR 96 bpm, RR 35 bpm. His weight was 15 kg. Physical examination found congested pharynx and tonsil. Auscultation of lungs revealed some phlegm sound. Precordial area was uplifted and heart sound was weak. Abdominal area was soft with slight tenderness in umbilical region. Liver enlarged 3 cm below the margin of right costal, spleen enlarged 2 cm below left costal margin, moderate hard. Edema was in bilateral lower limbs. Peripheral oxygen saturation was 96%. Others were normal. Admission blood test revealed a normal complete blood count, slightly elevated NT-pro BNP 2557 pg/ml, venous blood gas analysis PH7.33, PO_2 49.4 mmHg, PCO_2 39.6 mmHg, BE −5.3 mmol/L, arterial oxygen saturation was 82.6%, serum potassium was 3.8 mmol/L. ECG showed decremented R_{V1}, R_{V3}, and R_{V5}, abnormal LV Q wave and inverted T wave on LV side wall. For he had a serious chronic heart failure, he was monitored for ECG, BP, blood oxygen and advised to rest in bed. He was treated with (1) cedilanid at a total dose of 0.03 mg/kg, divided in three (one half, a quarter, followed by a quarter) to fast saturate in 24 h; (2) oral furosemidum 1 mg/kg/day every day, spironolactone 1 mg/ kg/day for 4 days per week, captopril 1 mg/kg in three divided doses; (3) infusion of second-generation cephalosporin and creatine phosphate sodium 1 g/day; (4) infusion speed limited to 3 ml/kg/h.

On Day 21, his fever settled and mental state was improved. Investigation revealed serum ALB 33.7 g/L, while urine routine, CRP, ASO, ALT, AST, CK, CKMB, and CK-MB mass were normal. cTnI 0.29μg/L (Table 12.3). MP-IgG 1:320. Abdominal ultrasound was normal. Chest CT showed inflammatory lesions in bilateral lung multi-lobe (Fig. 12.27a). He was treated with (1) infusion of azithromycin 10 mg/kg/day for 3 days; (2) digoxin 0.005 mg/kg/day after cedilanid quickly saturated; (3) digoxin adjusted to 0.01 mg/kg/day, after 3 days of azithromycin.

On day 24, his urine volume increased, and he could lie on the back. Physical examination found no changes. His mother confirmed that he had fever for more than 10 days about 6 months ago, with rashes, red conjunctiva, red lips, red hands and feet, dark urine, without hard swollen hands and feet or skin peeling around fingernails. Echo showed that the RVED was 13.5 mm, the interventricular septum thickness was 4.5 mm, the LVED was 49 mm (Fig. 12.27b), and the thickness of the left posterior wall was 4.9 mm. Mitral valve E = 1.0, A = 0.5, LVEF 30%. In LCA, there were a dilatation about 3–4 mm at the opening, and an aneurysm at the middle section dilated about 18 mm in diameter (Fig. 12.28a) with a 3–4 mm mixed echo in it (Fig. 12.28b). Its far end was tapered to normal. LAD was normal. The middle and lower myocardium of left ventricle was unevenly thin about 1–2 mm. The left ventricular apex showed diffuse aneurysm dilatation (Fig. 12.29), and the regional myocardial centripetal motion was generally weakened and almost disappeared. Left ventricular pump function was reduced, and no additional echo was observed in left ventricular cavity. Mitral valve was incompatible, and there was a mild-moderate regurgitation. There was 3–5 mm pericardial effusion. Combined with his previous medical history,

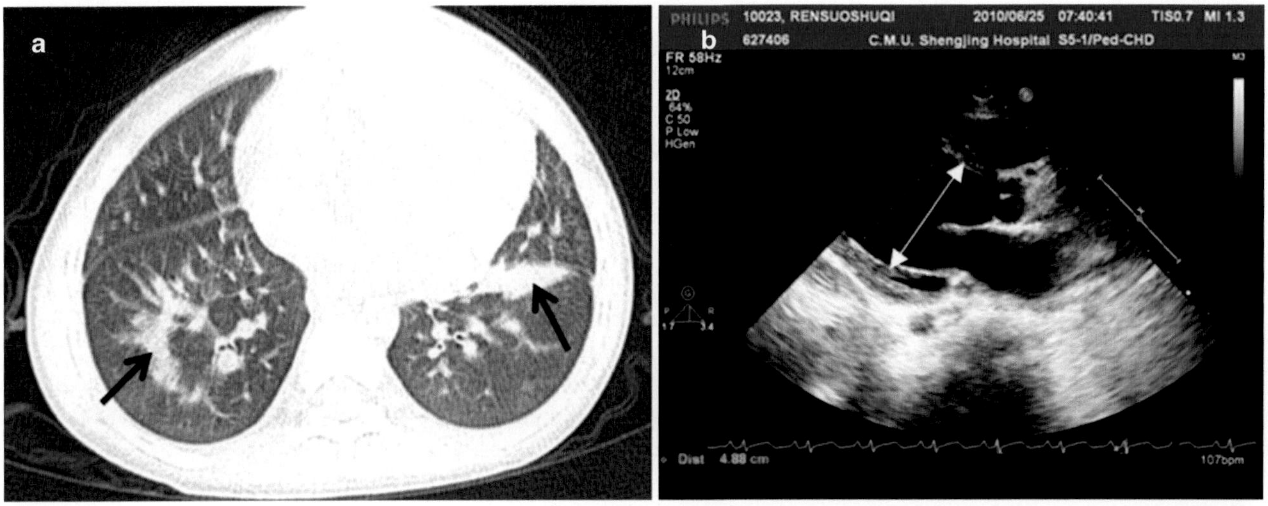

Fig. 12.27 On the second day of admission, chest CT showed bilateral lung multi-lobe inflammatory lesions (**a**). Echocardiography showed LVED dilated to 49mm (**b**)

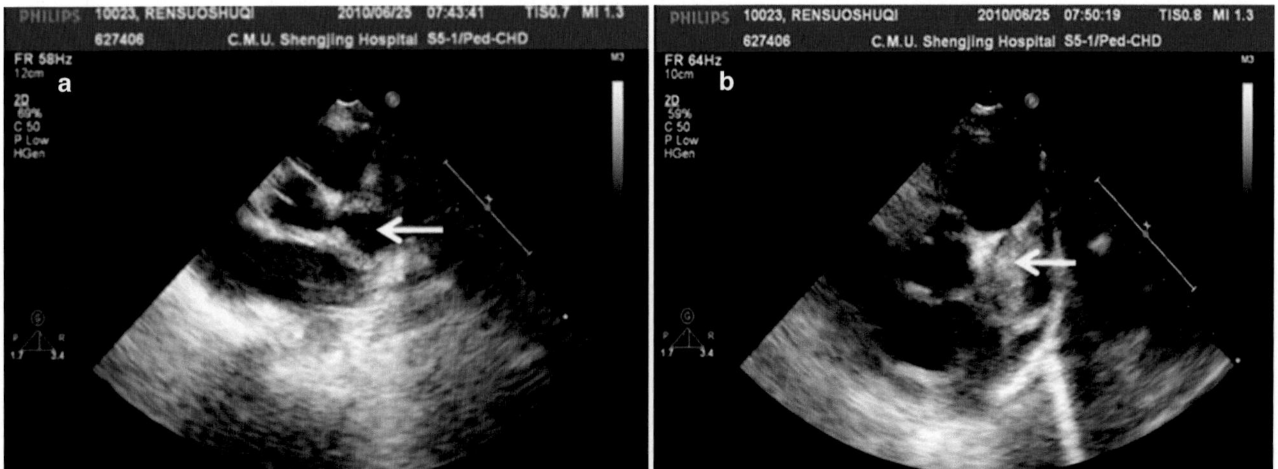

Fig. 12.28 On Day 4 of the first time admission, echocardiography showed the LCA dilated up to 18 mm after 3–4 mm from beginning (**a**), with a 3–4 mm mixed echogenicity inside (**b**)

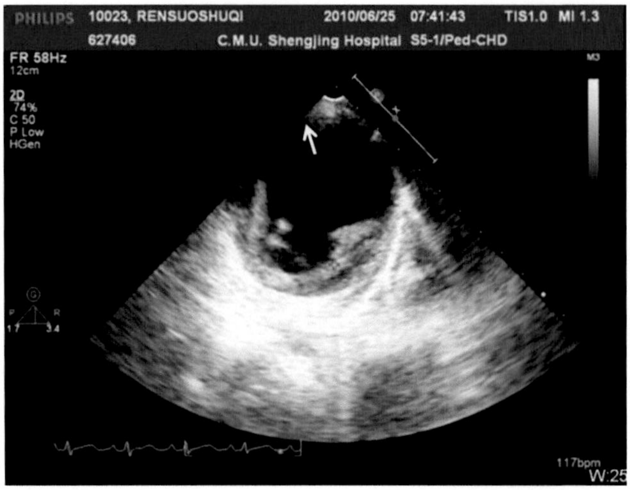

Fig. 12.29 On Day 4 of the first time admission, echocardiography showed diffuse dilation of left ventricular apex (white arrow)

he was diagnosed with KD at recovered stage, and was given oral aspirin and dipyridamole, in 3–5 mg/kg/day. He was critically ill and had a poor prognosis. We advised him to take oral warfarin thrombolytic therapy and informed his parents of his critical condition. They decided to pursue further treatment at Beijing children hospital. Then he was discharged.

12.4.1 Follow-Up

After discharge, he was followed up for five times. He was admitted in our pediatric cardiology ward for cough, fever, or other infection four times. He was treated with oral warfarin in Beijing children hospital, but his parents were resistant to this medication. They either reduced the dose or stopped the medication. He stayed on other medications, and he receives regular DIC monitoring in local clinic. INR was always less than 1.5.

At 4 months of first admission, he was admitted in our pediatric cardiology ward with paroxysmal cough and short breath for 2 days. Chest CT showed inflammation at right upper lobe, a little pleural effusion at right side (Fig. 12.30a). Echo showed LVED 65 mm (Fig. 12.30b), left ventricular posterior wall thickness was 5 mm. The diameter of the pulmonary artery was 18 mm. LVEF was 31%. The anterior wall of the left ventricle, the interventricular septum, and the apical myocardium became thin. The thinner part was about 2.6 mm (Fig. 12.31a). It was extended outwards and the movement disappeared. The movement of the remaining walls was weakened. The left ventricle was significantly enlarged in spherical shape, and so was left atrial. There were no ventricular aneurysm and mural thrombosis. There was mild-moderate regurgitation at mitral valve and tricuspid valve. Pulmonary artery systolic pressure was 40 mmHg, left ventricular diastolic function decreased (restricted type) (Fig. 12.31b). LCA aneurysm dilated about 8.6–20.5 mm (Fig. 12.32a) and RCA 2.1–3.5 mm (Fig. 12.32b). ECG showed that sinus rhythm, V_3-V_6 lead ST elevation, declined R wave, abnormal Q wave, T wave inversion; I, avL with abnormal q wave, T wave inversed. After 10 days treatment, his symptom subsided, but repeated chest CT and echo showed no significant improvement.

At 6 months of first admission, he presented with paleness and weakness, and extreme fatigue after strenuous activities. He was admitted to our pediatric cardiology ward. Coronary artery CTA was performed and revealed giant left CAA (Fig. 12.33a), the proximal segment of LAD was occluded? (Fig. 12.33b), RCA's proximal was bulging (Fig. 12.34a). Lymphocyte was 14%. EBV-IgM was negative. EB IgG (EA, NA, and VCA) was positive. He was given infusion of ganciclovir 7.5 mg/kg/day for 1 week. Echo showed that left ventricular end diastolic diameter was 63 mm, EF 24% (Fig. 12.34b). LCA was about 6.3 mm at opening, and, 1 cm below, there was aneurysm dilated about 25 × 24 mm (Fig. 12.35a), with a visible 1–2 mm weak echo clot in it (Fig. 12.35b). RCA was about 3–3.4 mm. The posterior inferior endocardium was slightly thickened, approximately 2–3 mm, with enhanced echogenicity. Echocardiography showed the hyperechoic thick mitral valve (Fig. 12.36), and mild reflux at closure. Reflux was detected, trace to small amount, at tricuspid valve. He took warfarin again at a dose of 0.1 mg/kg/day.

At 13 months of diagnosis, he presented with cough for 3 days and fever for 1 day and was forth admitted in our pediatric cardiology ward.

At 7 months of first admission, he presented with a history of cough for 3 days, and could not cough up sputum easily, without wheezing. Echo showed significantly spherically dilated left ventricle, LVED 62 mm, mitral regurgitation, and diffuse dilatation of left ventricular apex (Fig. 12.37a). LCAA about 22 mm × 19 mm (Fig. 12.37b). RCA was slightly widened. The endocardium was 3 mm, LVEF 28%. There were no improvements in others.

At 1 year of first admission, he presented with cough and along with fever for 1 day. Echo showed that left ventricular end diastolic diameter was 68 mm, EF was 27%. The inner diameter of the LCA was about 4.4 mm. 1 cm away from this, LCAA was about 18 mm × 22 mm. Left wall of the coronary artery had a massive weak echo. The diameter of RCA trunk was approximately 3–3.4 mm. Echocardiography showed the thick endocardium 2–3 mm at the posterior wall (Fig. 12.38). The mitral valve was diffusely thickened, with echo enhancement and mild reflux at closure. The chest CT showed the left side of heart was significantly enlarged (Fig. 12.39a). A high-density patch-like shadow was detected at the upper ligule segment of the left lung (Fig. 12.39b). The density of the lower lobe of the left lung was reduced

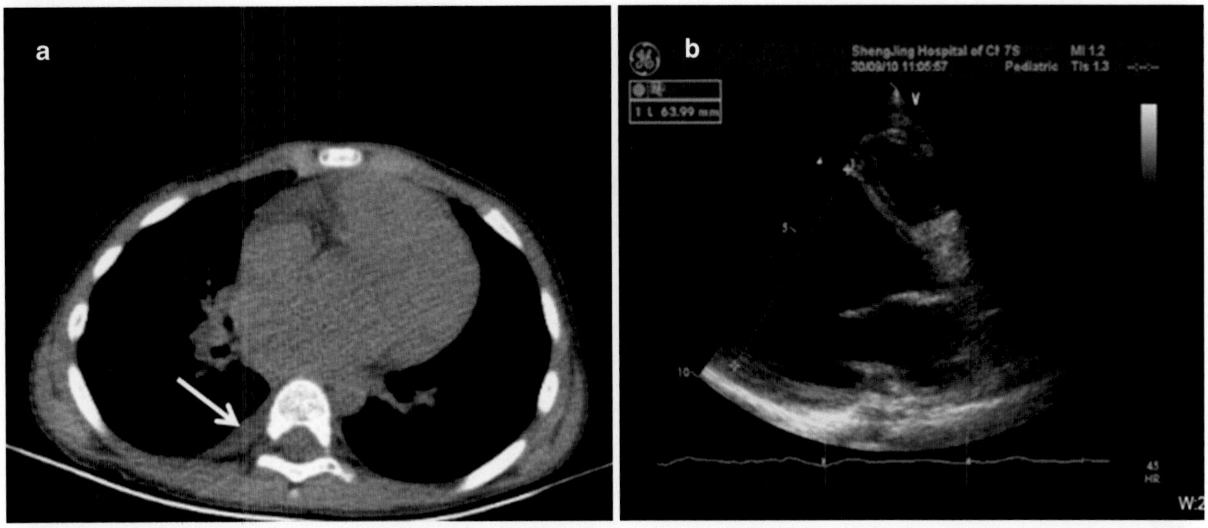

Fig. 12.30 At 4 months of the first time admission, Chest CT showed inflammation at right upper lobe, a little pleural effusion at right side (**a**). Echocardiography showed the significantly enlarged LV, LVED 65 mm (**b**)

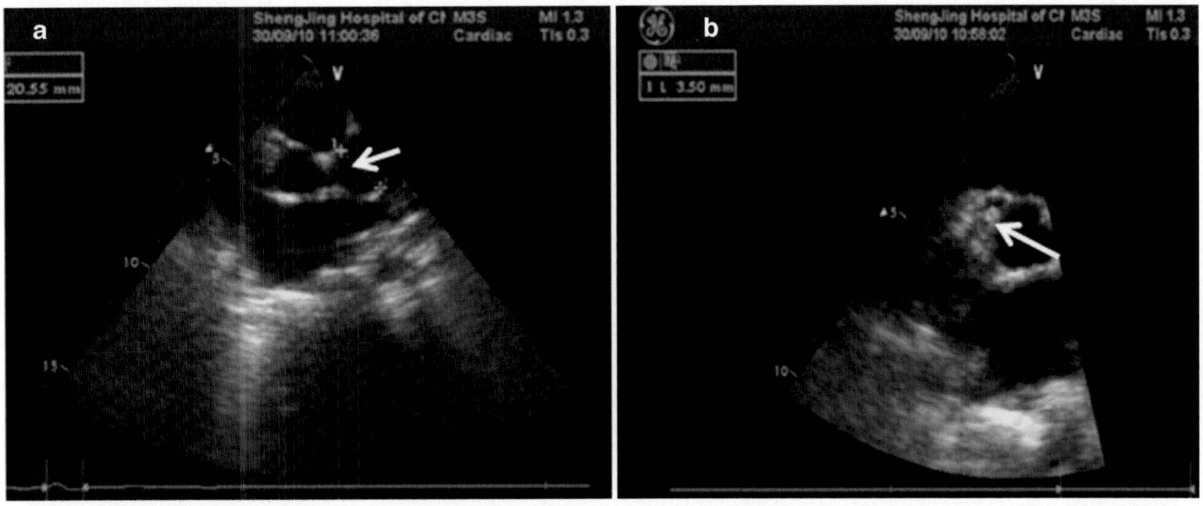

Fig. 12.31 At 4 months of the first time admission, echocardiography showed LM dilated up to 20.5 mm (**a**), RCA dilated to 3.5 mm (**b**)

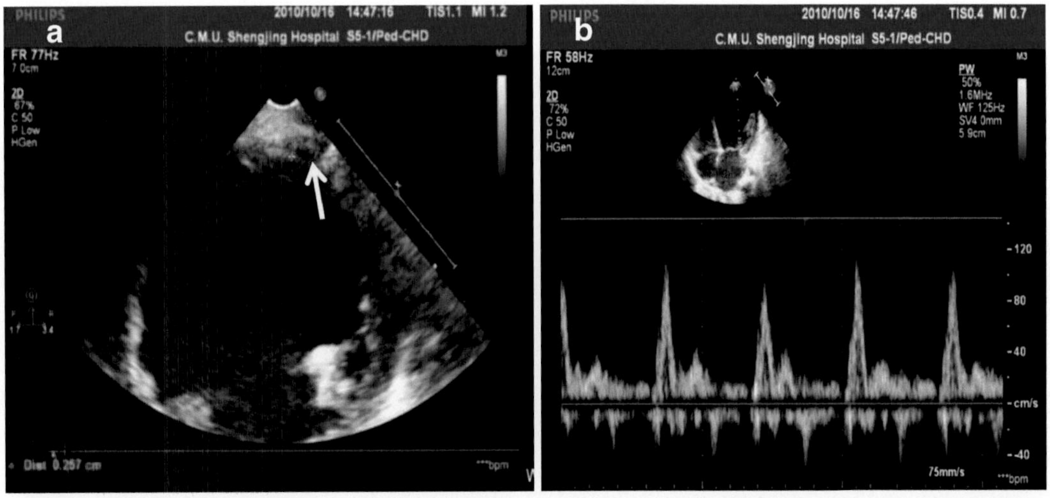

Fig. 12.32 At 4 months of the first time admission, echocardiography showed the dilated left ventricular apex with the thinnest point 2.6 mm (**a**), left ventricular diastolic function decreased (restricted type) (**b**)

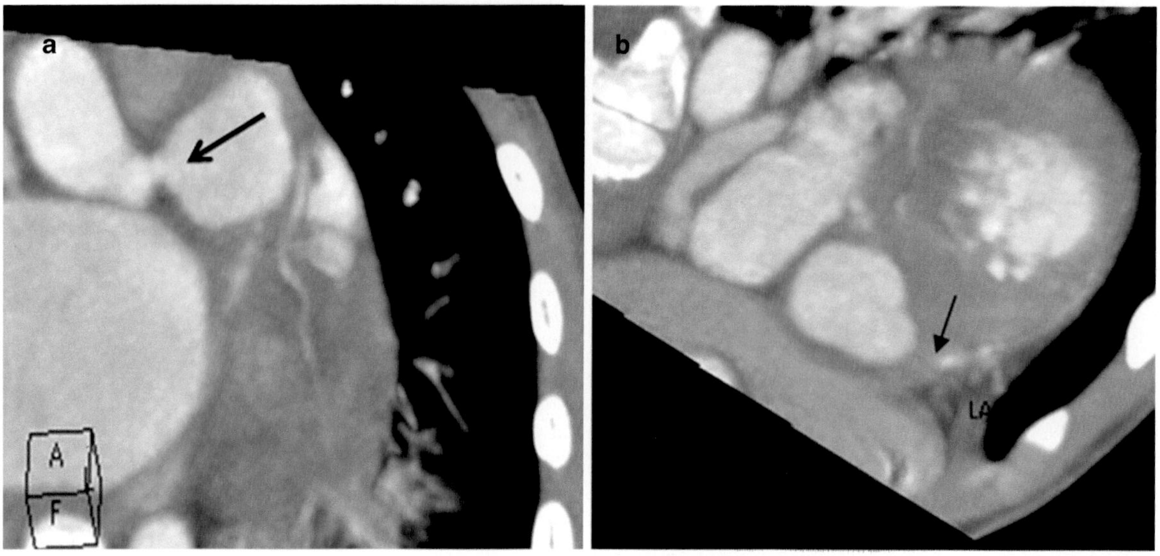

Fig. 12.33 At the 6 months of the first time admission, coronary artery CTA showed LCA giant CAA about 18 mm × 22 mm (**a**), proximal occlusion of the LAD (**b**)

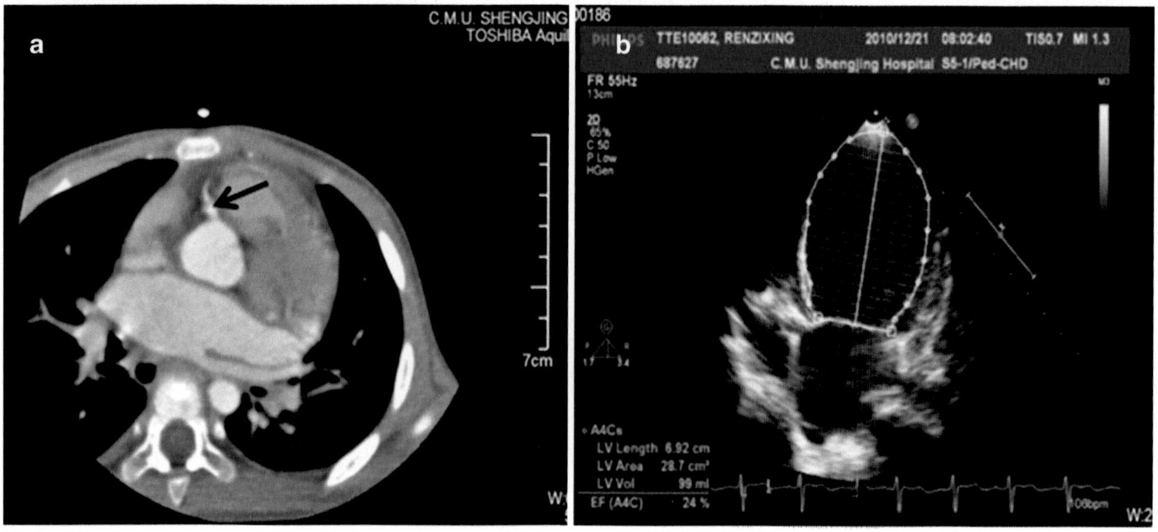

Fig. 12.34 At 6 months of the first time admission, coronary artery CTA showed RCA proximal expansion (**a**). Echocardiography showed the left ventricular ejection function was significantly reduced (LVEF 24%) (**b**)

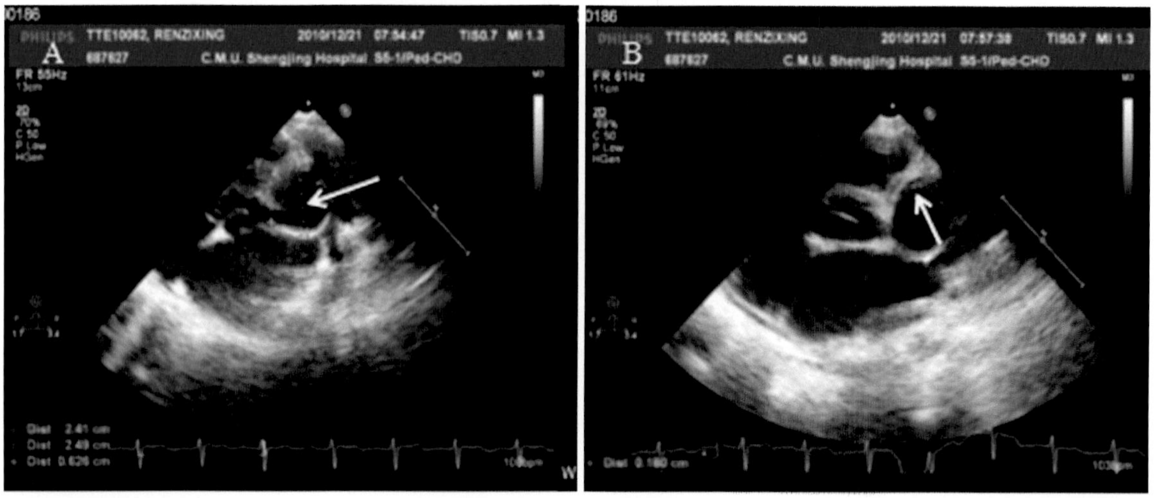

Fig. 12.35 At 6 months of the first time admission, echocardiography showed the giant left CAA (24 mm × 25 mm) (**a**), with 1–2 mm hypoechogenicity inside (**b**)

compared to 6 months ago. He was treated with aspirin (75 mg/day, PO), warfarin (1.5 mg/day, QD, PO), and regular reviews of DIC. We advised him to consult with heart transplant specialists in Beijing or Shanghai.

About 2 years of first admission, he followed-up with us at our clinic. Echo showed there were no changes for left giant CAA and cardiac dilatation. About 3.5 years of first admission, he suddenly died while playing at home (Tables 12.3, 12.4 and 12.5).

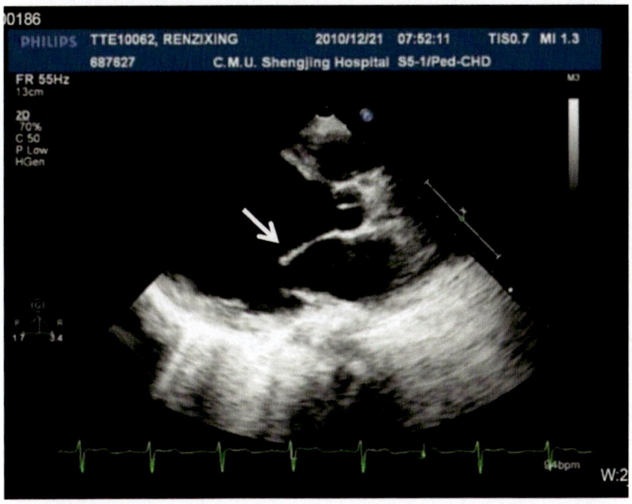

Fig. 12.36 At 6 months of the first time admission, echocardiography showed the hyperechoic thick mitral valve

12.4.2 Diagnosis

1. KD, recovery phase.
2. Giant left CAA.
3. Coronary thrombosis.
4. Dilated cardiomyopathy.
5. Left ventricular aneurysm.
6. Pericardial effusion.
7. Mitral regurgitation (severe).
8. Pulmonary hypertension (moderate).
9. Chronic heart failure (NY class IV).
10. Acute bronchopneumonia.
11. MP infection.
12. Right pleural effusion.
13. Mild anemia.
14. Infectious mononucleosis.

12.4.3 Discussion

He had met the criteria of KD for he had persistent fever for more than 5 days about 6 months ago, along with (1) rashes; (2) conjunctiva hyperemia without purulent discharges in both eyes; (3) red lips; (4) left giant CAA. Differential diagnosis of myocarditis and primary cardiomyopathy should be considered.

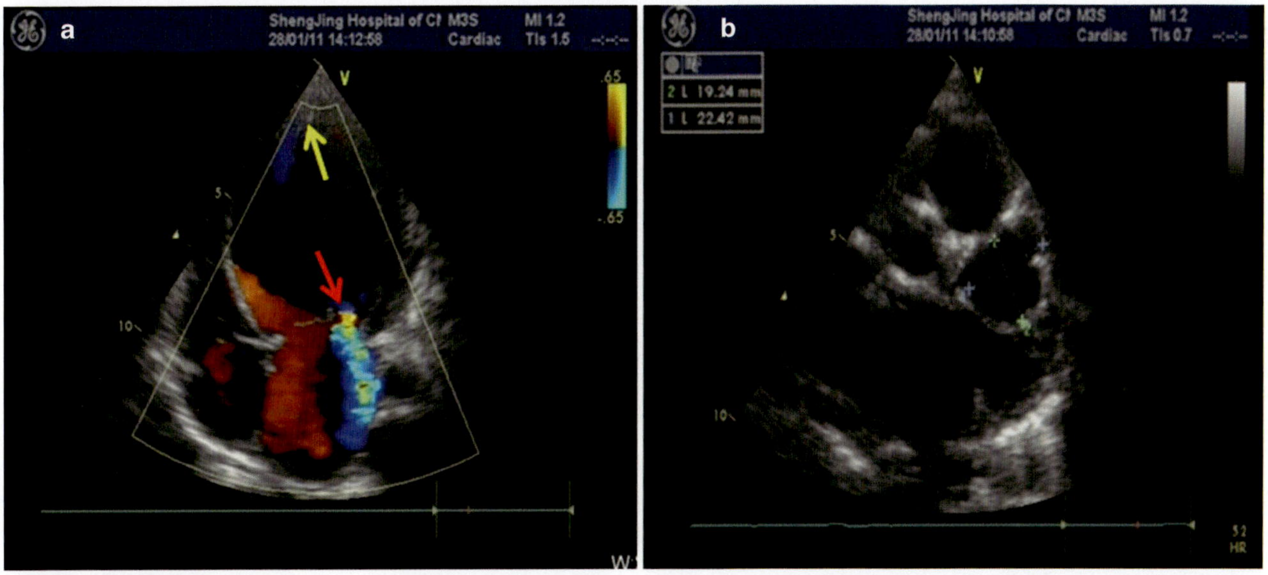

Fig. 12.37 At the 7 months of the first time admission echocardiography showed mitral regurgitation (red arrow), and diffuse dilatation of left ventricular apex (yellow arrow) (**a**), giant left CAA (19 mm × 24 mm) (**b**)

12.4.4 Case Specific Clinical Features

1. KD is the most common cause for childhood acquired cardiovascular diseases in developed countries. In the USA, the incidence of KD among children under 5 years old is 20:ten million [17]. The most common prognosis is coronary artery lesion, especially coronary artery aneurysm (CAA) [18]. The incidence is about 78% within 2 years of illness onset. If a patient is misdiagnosed, for its character of self-limitation, he/she may have no symptoms if there is no coronary lesion (blocking) even with mild CAA. CAA is only occasionally found in coronary angiography [1] or echo like case 44 and 45. Once coronary artery blocking occurred, especially on the LCA, the heart failure symptom usually appeared at 6 months after onset of illness, such as case 42 and this case.

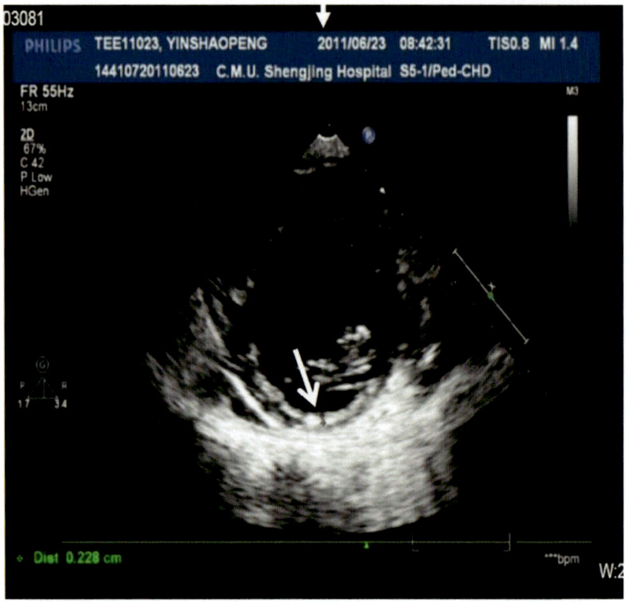

Fig. 12.38 At 1 year of the first time admission, echocardiography showed the thick endocardium 2–3 mm at the posterior wall

2. Each time he was admitted to hospital, he always had coughs. In addition to the first time admission showed heart failure, there was no fever for two times, most no edema and oliguria. Lung CT showed almost the same changes every time examined. We speculated the following possibilities made he cough all the time: in addition to infection, pulmonary edema, abnormal heart enlargement causing lung compression leading to defects in lobe inflation, and oral captopril. As his left ventricular systolic function was deteriorating, he needed to stay on medications for cardiac, diuresis, and blood vessel dilations.
3. KD is also named as mucocutaneous lymph node syndrome. It is an inflammatory disease with unknown origin. The mainly affected system in this disease is the coronary artery where CAA, and coronary artery stenosis and obstruction can be developed, leading to myocardial ischemia, infarction, and even sudden cardiac death [18]. The incidence of coronary artery lesions is 20% in untreated children [1], and is 3%–5% in treated ones [19]. Even with CAA, there is still half recovered [20].
4. In moderate or large CAA, the incidence of thrombotic occlusion is up to 16% shortly after onset, 78% occurred within 2 years of onset of illness, and some die of sudden

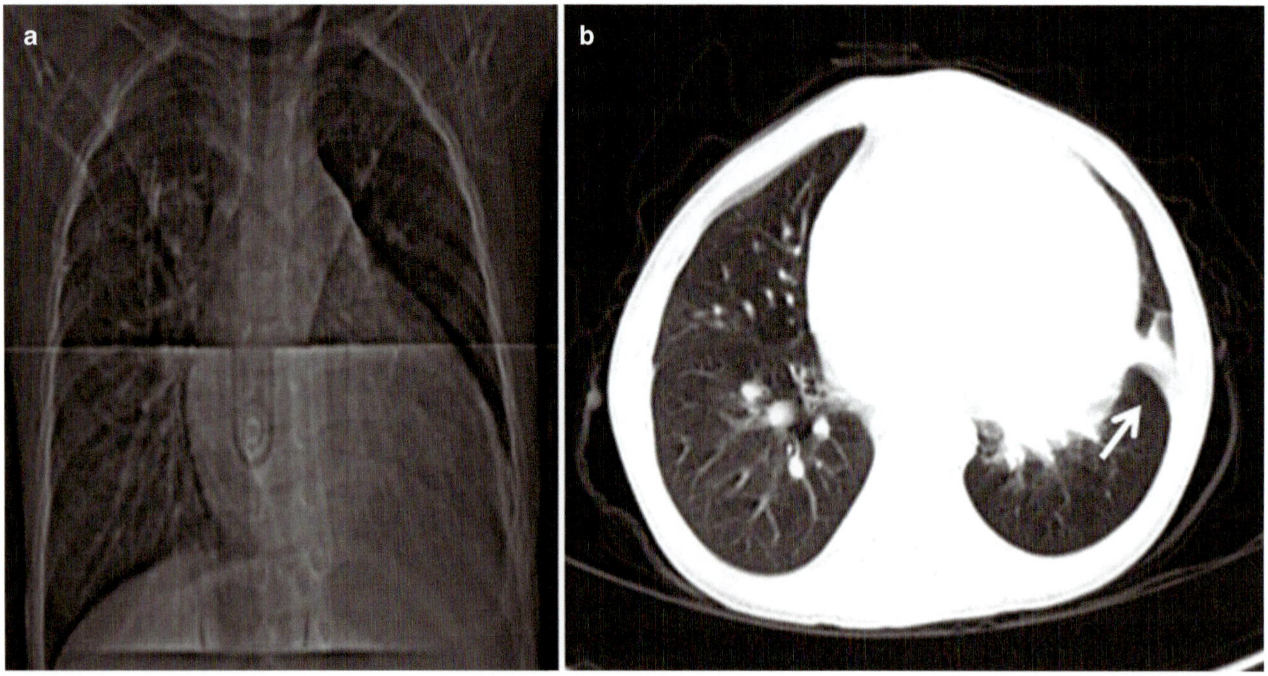

Fig. 12.39 At 1 year of the first time admission, chest DR showed the heart was enlarged significantly, the ratio of heart to chest was 0.67 (**a**). Chest CT showed new high density plaque on left upper lobe of tongue segment (**b**)

Table 12.3 The dynamic changes of clinical symptoms

Time of diagnosis	4 days	4 months	6 months	7 months	12 months
Edema					
Facial	Yes	–	–	–	–
Limbs	Yes	Yes	Yes	Yes	Yes
Liver (cm)					
Below right costal margin	3	2	3	0.5	–
Below xiphoid	3	3	3	3	–
Spleen (cm)	2	1	0.5	0.5	–
HR (bpm)	96	126	106	106	120
cTnI (ng/ml)	0.29		0.18	0.07	
NT pro-BNP(pg/ml)	2557	1289			

Table 12.4 The dynamic changes of echo

Time of diagnosis	4 days	4 months	6 months	7 months	12 months
LVED (mm)	49	65	63	62	68
LVEF (mm)	30	31	24	28	27
PA (mmHg)		40–54			
E	1	1.2			
A	0.5	0.5			
MI	Mild	Severe	Mild		
TI	–	Trace	Mild		
Endocardium (mm)	–	–	2–3	3	2–2.5

Table 12.5 The dynamic changes of coronary artery

Time of diagnosis	4 days	4 months	6 months	7 months	12 months
INR	1.1	1.3	1	1.3	1.2
Aspirin (mg/kg)	3–5	3–5	3–5	3–5	3–5
Warfarin (mg/kg)	Refused	0.1	Stop	0.1	Refused
Dipyridamole(mg/kg)	3–5	3–5	3–5	3–5	3–5
LAC(mm)	4–18	8.6–20.5	6.3–25	5–22	4–22
RCA(mm)		2.1–3.5	3–3.4	3.4	3–3.4

death. But 2/3 of patients who have no symptoms are found to have CAA in coronary angiography [21]. Once giant CAA is discovered, it is recommended to give patients anticoagulant therapy as soon as possible [19].

5. Grading system is established according to the severity of coronary artery diseases. Grade III is single small or medium CAA; grade IV is ≥1 giant CAA, or multiple CAA, without stenosis; grade V lists stenosis or occlusion shown in coronary angiography. Grade IV or V requires oral warfarin treatment for anticoagulation [21]. There are individual differences when taking warfarin, especially in infants and young children. INR is very unstable and is required to repeat testing to follow up. To patients who only take oral warfarin, it is safe to maintain INR in the range of 2.0–3.0. But KD patients should take warfarin together with aspirin (with dipyridamole usually in cases of giant CAA), therefore INR is maintained between 1.5 and 2.5 which is a safe range. When taking warfarin, it is necessary to monitor whether there is diarrhea or abnormal bleeding. Patients should avoid contacts with sharp or hard objects and competitive sports. Vitamin K treatment should be given immediately if there is a serious bleeding. Regular anticoagulation therapy can effectively reduce coronary artery thrombosis.
6. Coronary artery bypass grafting is an effective treatment for severe coronary artery disease with myocardial ischemia. It can significantly improve KD patients' quality of life, reduce the incidence of sudden death and other cardiovascular events. Post-operative vascular patency rate is 94.4%, and is higher in children under 12 years of age [22]. This child has developed ischemic cardiomyopathy, but he was too young to undergo a bypass grafting. Even if he was old enough, bypass grafting does not reverse the necrotic myocardium. As a result, he needs heart transplantation. Unfortunately, transplantation can be rarely completed due to lack of donors.
7. Endocardial elastic fibrosis is a special condition in this case. A literature reports [23], it may also be one of the reasons why heart function does not recover, and may be also related to giant CAA on the left side. Thrombosis and occlusion result in insufficient blood flow to the left ventricle. With proper treatment in later stage, LVEF was increased to 50%. But heart failure cannot be improved if left ventricle undergoes uncoordinated contraction and relaxation. Ventricular arrhythmia is the leading cause in sudden death of KD patients.

Hong Wang

References

1. Senzaki H. Long-term outcome of Kawasaki disease. Circulation. 2008;118(25):2763–72.
2. Haneda N, Mori C. Histopathologic and coronary angiographic assessment of effectiveness of aspirin or aspirin-and-gammaglobulin in Kawasaki disease. Acta Paediatr Jpn. 1993;35(4):294–7.
3. Wang H, Yu XY, Piao YA, et al. The significance of intravenous IVIG in the treatment of Kawasaki disease. J China Med Univ. 2000;29(2):156–7.
4. Rowley AH, Shulman ST, Spike BT, et al. Oligoclonal IgA response in the vascular wall in acute Kawasaki disease. J Immunol. 2001;166(2):1334–43.
5. Brown TJ, Crawford SE, Cornwall ML, et al. CD8 T lymphocytes and macrophages infiltrate coronary artery aneurysms in acute Kawasaki disease. J Infect Dis. 2001;184(7):940–3.
6. Newburger JW, Takahashi M, Burns JC. Kawasaki disease. J Am Coll Cardiol. 2016;67(14):1738–49.
7. Holve TJ, Patel A, Chau Q, et al. Long-term cardiovascular outcomes in survivors of Kawasaki disease. Pediatrics. 2014;133(2):e305–11.
8. Ayusawa M, Sonobe T, Uemura S, et al. Revision of diagnostic guidelines for Kawasaki disease (the 5th revised edition). Pediatr Int. 2005;47(2):232–4.
9. Kuo HC, Yang KD, Chang WC, et al. Kawasaki disease: an update on diagnosis and treatment. Pediatr Neonatol. 2012;53(1):4–11.
10. Honkanen VE, McCrindle BW, Laxer RM, et al. Clinical relevance of the risk factors for coronary artery inflammation in Kawasaki disease. J Pediatr Cardiol. 2003;24(2):122–6.
11. Eleftheriou D, Levin M, Shingadia D, et al. Management of Kawasaki disease. Arch Dis Child. 2014;99(1):74–83.
12. Lu HL, Liu YP, Hu XF. The significance of N-terminal pro-brain natriuretic peptide precursor in early prediction of coronary artery lesions in Kawasaki disease. Chin J Pediatr. 2015;53(4):300–3.
13. Chen YL, Wang JL, Li WQ. Prediction of the risk of coronary arterial lesions in Kawasaki disease by serum 25-hydroxyvitamin D_3. Eur J Pediatr. 2014;173(11):1467–71.
14. Sugahara Y, Ishii M, Muta H, et al. Warfarin therapy for giant aneurysm prevents myocardial infarction in Kawasaki disease. Pediatr Cardiol. 2008;29:398–401.
15. Fry J, Naqvi A, Bahia A, et al. Aspiration thrombectomy and intracoronary tirofiban via GuideLiner catheter for a thrombosed aneurysmal vessel. Futur Cardiol. 2017;13(2):131–5.
16. Potter EL, Meredith IT, Psaltis PJ, et al. ST-elevation myocardial infarction in a young adult secondary to giant coronary aneurysm thrombosis: an important sequela of Kawasaki disease and a management challenge. BMJ Case Rep. 2016;2016:bcr2015213622. https://doi.org/10.1136/bcr-2015-213622.
17. Holman RC, Belay ED, Christensen KY, et al. Hospitalizations for Kawasaki syndrome among children in the United States, 1997–2007. Pediatr Infect Dis J. 2010;29(6):483–8.
18. Tsuda E, Hamaoka K, Suzuki H, et al. A survey of the 3-decade outcome for patients with giant aneurysms caused by Kawasaki disease. Am Heart J. 2014;167(2):249–58.
19. Durongpisitkul K, Gururaj VJ, Park JM, et al. The prevention of coronary artery aneurysm in Kawasaki disease: a meta-analysis on the efficacy of aspirin and immunoglobulin treatment. Pediatrics. 1995;96(6):1057–61.
20. Kato H, Sugimura T, Akagi T, et al. Long-term consequences of Kawasaki disease. A 10 to 21-year follow-up study of 594 patients. Circulation. 1996;94(6):1379–85.
21. Liu F, Zhao L, Wu L, et al. Treatment and management evaluation of Kawasaki disease coronary artery disease based on severity clinical grade. Chin J Pediatr. 2015;53(9):690–5.
22. JCS Joint Working Group. Guidelines for diagnosis and management of cardiovascular sequelae in Kawasaki disease (JCS 2008) -digest version. Circ J. 2010;74(9):1989–2020.
23. Orenstein JM. Kawasaki disease has so much to teach us! Ultrastruct Pathol. 2014;38(2):83–5.

Atypical KD

13

Hong Wang, Jing Dong, Bai Gao, and Ce Wang

Abstract

Kawasaki disease (KD), first reported by Dr. Tomisaku Kawasaki in Japan in 1967, is an acute febrile illness in children with systemic non-specific vasculitis as the main disease. KD infringes on coronary arteries, and KD has replaced rheumatic fever as the most common cause of acquired heart disease in children [Agarwal and Agarwal, Expert Rev Clin Immunol. 13(3): 247–58, 2017; Guo et al., Chin Med J. 123(12):1533, 2010]. If patients have less than three clinical symptoms, they will be diagnosed with atypical Kawasaki disease (AKD). AKD usually occurs in infants less than 6 months old [Minich et al., Pediatrics 120:e1434–40, 2007]. The cause of KD is not completely clear, and the diagnosis is made mainly depending on a group of clinical manifestations. For lacking specific clinical manifestations and characteristic laboratory tests, the diagnosis is often delayed due to lack of conjunctival congestion or changes in oral mucosa. Delayed diagnosis affect effective treatment. Therefore CAA is more likely to occur [Imagawa et al., Eur J Pediatr. 163(4–5):263–4, 2004].

Because the clinical features in AKD children are less than those in KD children, the symptoms from systems outside the cardiovascular system are often the main manifestations, including symptoms from nervous system, respiratory system, hematopoietic system, digestive system, and urinary system symptoms (the main or primary symptoms). Therefore, diagnosis is easily missed [Imagawa et al., Eur J Pediatr. 163(4–5):263–4, 2004]. Once bilateral conjunctival congestion occurs, KD is usually considered even without sufficient symptoms in patients. When infants have prolonged fever and acute heart failure, with other diseases excluded, they should be considered to have IKD, especially if they receive glucocorticoid therapy at onset of illness. At subacute stage, peeling skin around fingernails or nail groove should be concerned.

H. Wang (✉) · C. Wang
Department of Pediatric Cardiology, Shengjing Hospital of China Medical University, Shenyang, Liaoning, P. R. China

J. Dong
Department of Cardiology Function, Shengjing Hospital of China Medical University, Shenyang, Liaoning, P. R. China
e-mail: dongj@sj-hospital.org

B. Gao
Department of Neurology Function, Shengjing Hospital of China Medical University, Shenyang, Liaoning, P. R. China

13.1 Case 46: AKD with Gallop Rhythm

A previous healthy 1-year-old boy had no significant past medical and family history.

He presented on Day 8 of illness, with an intermittent fever 8 days, along with cough. On Day 2, he was given infusion of first-generation cephalosporin for 3 days at a local hospital and fever was not regressed. On Day 4 of illness, he received infusion of dexamethasone 3 mg. Fever was only under control for nearly 2 days, and he took oral second-generation cephalosporin at home. On Day 6 of illness, he had fever again, up to 40.1 °C. He was sleepy and had loose stools two times. Examination revealed mild fever 37.8 °C, smooth breath (HR 132 bpm, RR 28 bpm). Pharynges were congested without conjunctiva congestion. Cardiac auscultation found gallop rhythm. Others were normal. Admission blood test revealed WBC 17.16 × 10^9/L, NE 53.8%, HGB 106 g/L, PLT 403 × 10^9/L. CRP 16.6 mg/L, ESR 80 mm. MP-IgM mild positive, MP-IgG was negative. HSV (I + II)-IgM and EBV IgM were negative. NT pro-BNP 994.1 pg/ml. It was certain that he had mycoplasma pneumoniae infection, but it was not certain whether he had acute cardiac insufficiency. After blood sample drawn for culture, he was treated with (1) infusion of creatine phosphate sodium,

H. Wang (ed.), *Paediatric Kawasaki Disease*, https://doi.org/10.1007/978-981-15-0038-1_13

L-carnitine; (2) infusion of azithromycin 10 mg/kg/day for 3 days; (3) all infusion velocity controlled under 3 ml/kg/h.

On Day 9, he had fever repeatedly, and had strikingly red lips. Investigation revealed WBC 8.05 × 10^9/L, NE 67.0%, HGB 100 g/L, PLT 381 × 10^9/L. CRP 34.20 mg/L. CKMB-M, hs-cTnT, and cTnI were normal. Cervical ultrasound found cervical lymphadenectasis, about 2.1 cm × 0.7 cm on the left and 2.2 cm × 0.9 cm on the right. ECG revealed tachycardia, HR 141 bpm, I°AVB (Fig. 13.1). EEG was normal (Fig. 13.2). For he was suspected to have KD and had persistent fever for 9 days, he was treated with (1) IVIG 2 g/kg over 12 h, 20% mannitol 2.5 ml/kg and furosemidum 1 g/kg also infused after IVIG 1 g/kg; (2) oral aspirin 30–50 mg/kg/day and dipyridamole 3–5 mg/kg/day in two divided doses. His condition rapidly evolved favorably to IVIG treatment. His fever and red lips were settled subsequently on Day 10 of illness. Cardiac gallop rhythm disappeared. On Day 12, echo showed normal results except ASD 3.2 mm. He was afebrile over 48 h, and aspirin was reduced to one dose 3–5 mg/kg/day.

On Day 13, he coughed but without sputum. Retested blood revealed WBC 5.43 × 10^9/L, NE 15.7%, HGB 108 g/L, PLT 321 × 10^9/L. Normal CRP and NT-pro BNP. ALT 74 U/L, AST 99 U/L. ESR 69 mm/h. ECG showed sinus rhythm, I°AVB (Fig. 13.3). Chest CT scan showed uniform in bilateral lungs (Fig. 13.4). Blood culture was negative. He was discharged.

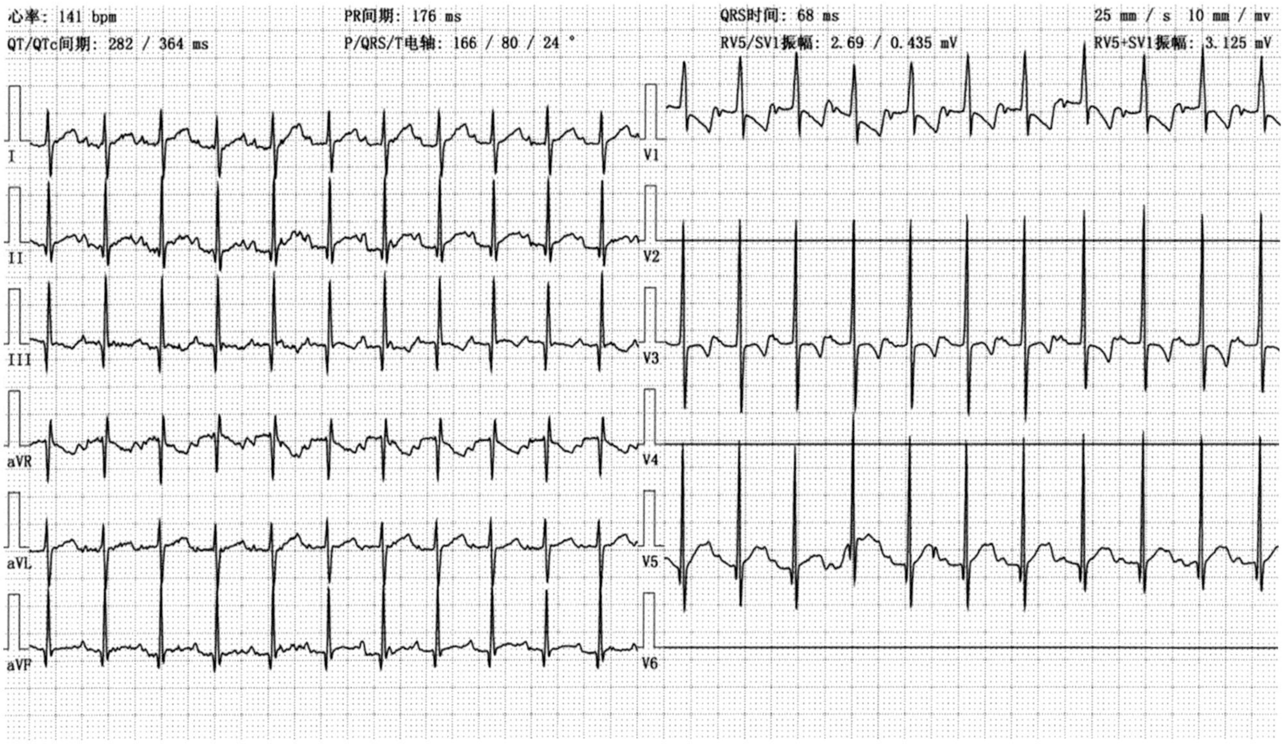

Fig. 13.1 On Day 9 of illness, ECG showed sinus tachycardia, HR 141 bpm, I°AVB (PR interval 176 ms)

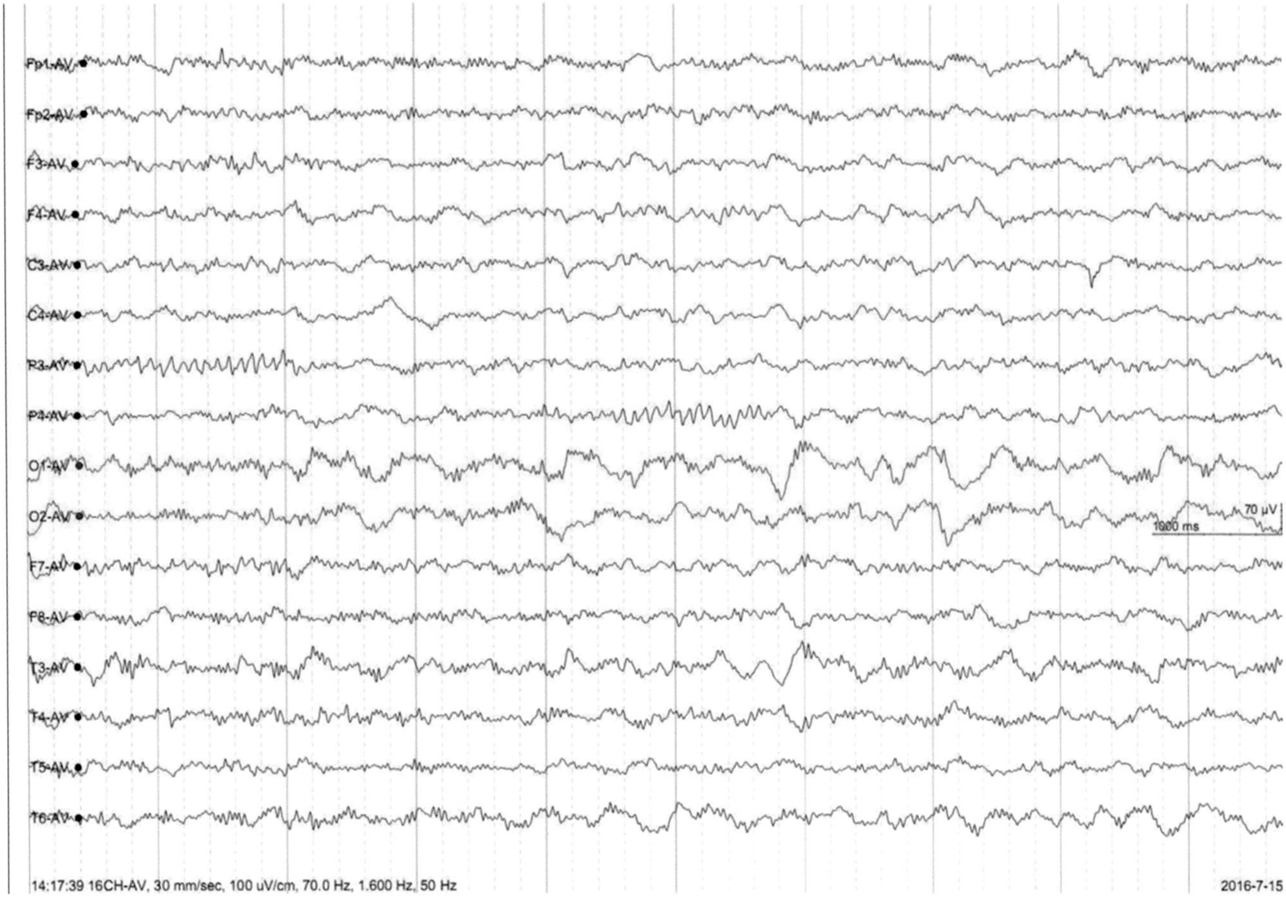

Fig. 13.2 On Day 13 of illness, EEG was normal

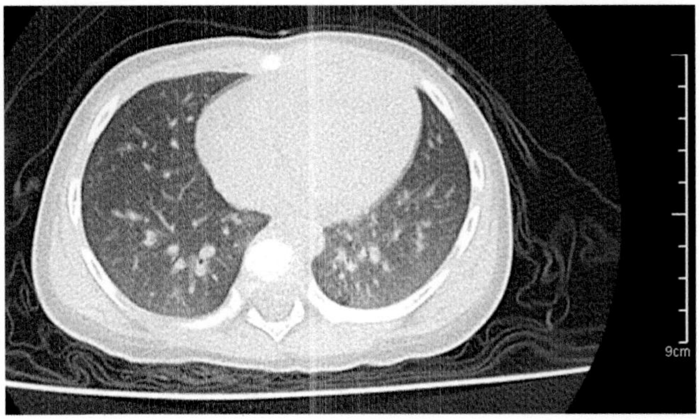

Fig. 13.3 On Day 13 of illness, chest CT scan showed penetration was not uniform in bilateral lungs

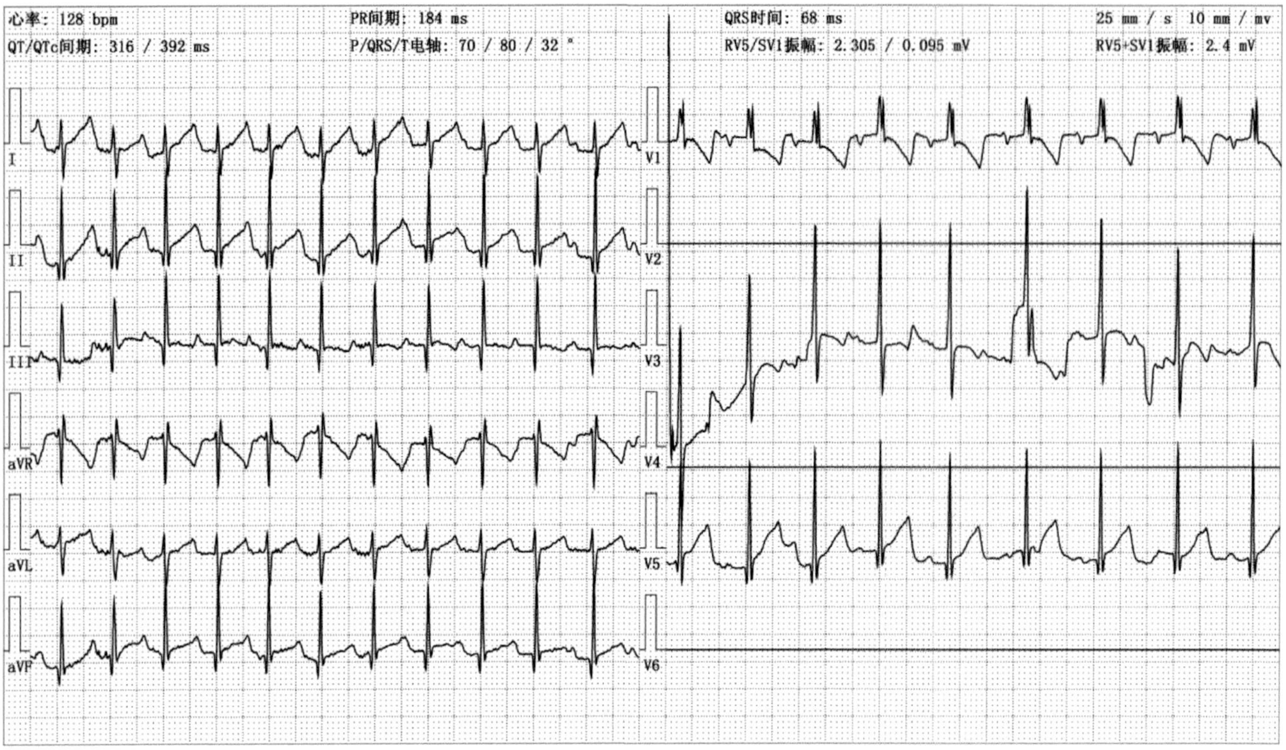

Fig. 13.4 On Day 13 of illness, ECG showed sinus rhythm, HR 128 bpm, I°AVB(PR interval 184 ms)

13.1.1 Clinical Course of the Patient

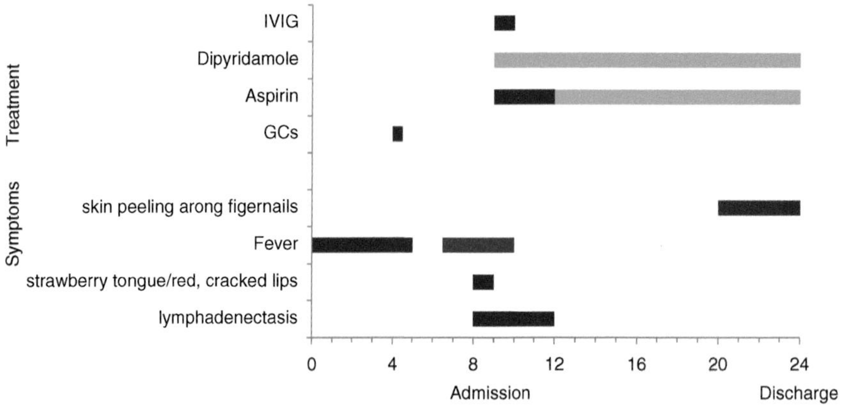

13.1.2 Follow-Up

Since discharged, he took oral aspirin, dipyridamole, and compound glycyrrhizin, once daily, azithromycin 85 mg, once daily, for 3 days.

On Day 20, peeling skin occurred around fingernails. At this point, his atypical KD diagnosis was established. On Day 25, both liver function and ESR settled. On Day 39, PLT was normal. Echo performed at both one and 2 months revealed normal results. ECG was not repeated. At 2 months, medications were stopped.

13.1.3 Diagnosis

1. AKD
2. Liver dysfunction
3. I°AVB
4. Pneumonia

13.1.4 Discussion

With peeling skin around fingernails, he had met the 3/5 criteria for AKD. He had prolonged fever over 5 days, along with (1) strikingly red lips; (2) cervical lymphadenectasis; (3) peeling skin around fingernails after he was discharged.

There is no direct correlation between galloping and KD. Galloping is a sign of heart failure. Because it occurs in infants, there are no myocarditis, no cardiomyopathy, or congenital heart disease, it is not easy to explain this galloping rhythm. However, he had fever for a long period of time which was unresponsive to antibiotics, with obviously dry and red lips and enlarged lymph nodes in the neck. Blood test showed elevated WBC, mainly neutrophils, and significantly increased erythrocyte precipitation. He had a history of glucocorticoid injection at the fourth day of the onset. So we had a reason to speculate that he had IKD. Some of the children with IKD may develop heart failure combined with galloping rhythm. Thus, we can explain all his clinical symptoms. Fortunately, the subsequent skin peeling around the nails supported our conclusion.

Differential diagnosis of acute heart failure should be considered.

13.1.5 Case Specific Clinical Feature

1. Patient had persistent fever for 9 days, intermittent fever after given injection of dexamethasone. Thus, his clinical symptoms were not obviously significant, especially he had no rashes, conjunctiva, or edema in hands and feet. When he was admitted, auscultation revealed gallop rhythm, and blood test supported typical KD: CRP >30 mg/L, ESR > 40 mm/h, combined with increased NT pro-BNP, the latter one indicated either heart or brain damage. This patient's mental state was stable, and EEG found normal signals. Thus, mild branch pneumonia could not be used to explain gallop rhythm. According to the guideline for KD management, he was only given infusion of γ-Globulin and followed up with us. However, when informed that he received infusion of dexamethasone on Day 4 of illness, we highly suspected he had AKD. In patients treated with glucocorticoid alone at early stage of KD, chance to develop coronary artery lesion is significantly higher than in patients treated with glucocorticoid and IVIG together [1]. He had remitted fever for 9 days. After discussing with his parent, they accepted IVIG treatment with oral aspirin and dipyridamole. Before discharge, he was suspected to have AKD. The diagnosis was finalized once skin peeling occurred around his fingernails.

Hong Wang

13.2 Case 47: AKD with CAA

A healthy 3-year-old boy presented with unremarkable past medical or family history.

He presented on Day 8 of illness, with intermittent fever for 8 days along with bilateral conjunctival congestion for 2 days without purulent. He had infusion of ceftriaxone sodium for 6 days, erythromycin for 1 day at a local hospital, but fever no progress. On Day 6, he developed red and cracked lips and bilateral conjunctival congestion. He was intramuscular injection once dexamethasone. His fever settled down for one day. On Day 8 he had fever again and admitted in our hospital. Examination found the followings: T 38.6 °C, HR104 bpm, bilateral conjunctival congestion, red and cracked lips, without strawberry tongue. Others were normal. Tested blood work revealed WBC 4.13 × 10^9/L, NE 62.28%, HGB 103 g/L, PLT 366 × 10^9/L, NT-pro BNP 348.6 pg/ml, and normal CRP. He was diagnosed with unknown fever, suspected to have atypical KD. He was given intravenous azithromycin.

On Day 9, he was irritable along with fever and bilateral conjunctival congestion. Retested blood work revealed ESR 46 mm/h, ALB 29.6 g/L, and positive CP-IgM, MP-IgM, and PINF-IgA, weakly positive tuberculosis antibody, and MP-IgG1:80. Cervical ultrasound showed lymphadenopathy about 1.2 cm × 0.8 cm on the left, and 1.3 cm × 0.8 cm on the right. EEG showed the middle volatility of the bilateral occipital leads was mainly 4–6 Hz θ wave, and the inclusion was slightly more δ wave (the background rhythm was slow, mainly θ and δ waves) (Fig. 13.5). Echo showed LCA about 3 mm (Fig. 13.6), RCA about 2.6 mm. Lumbar puncture test showed CSF flow rate 54 drops/min. CSF was a little pink (puncture bleeding) and non-condensing. Pandy's test was negative. Total cell number was 1120 × 10^6/L, WBC 10 × 10^6/L, RBC 1110 × 10^6/L. Chlorine 119.3 mmol/L, glucose 3.21 mmol/L, protein 0.41 g/L. CSF pathogens were negative. He had met the criteria for atypical KD, with aseptic meningitis. He was treated with (1) IVIG 2 g/kg; (2) albumin 10 g/day, for 2 days; (3) infusion of calf serum deproteinized 0.4 g once a day; (4) mannitol and furosemide, qd; (5) aspirin 200 mg/time, three times a day oral; dipyridamole 25 mg/time, three times a day oral route.

On Day 10, he developed peeling skin around fingernails of right hand. Lung CT scan showed his lungs had clear texture but pericardial effusion. He received infusion of (1) cefuroxime sodium; (2) methylprednisolone at 1 mg/kg once a day. On Day 12, he was afebrile over 48 h. Retested blood work revealed WBC 3.8 × 10^9/L, NE 19.6%, HGB 102 g/L, PLT 353 × 10^9/L, NT-pro BNP 1106 pg/ml, ALB normal. Head MR showed low-signal shadow at the edge of cerebellar hemisphere edge; sinus artifacts was not excluded. He had sinusitis. He was treated with (1) traditional Chinese

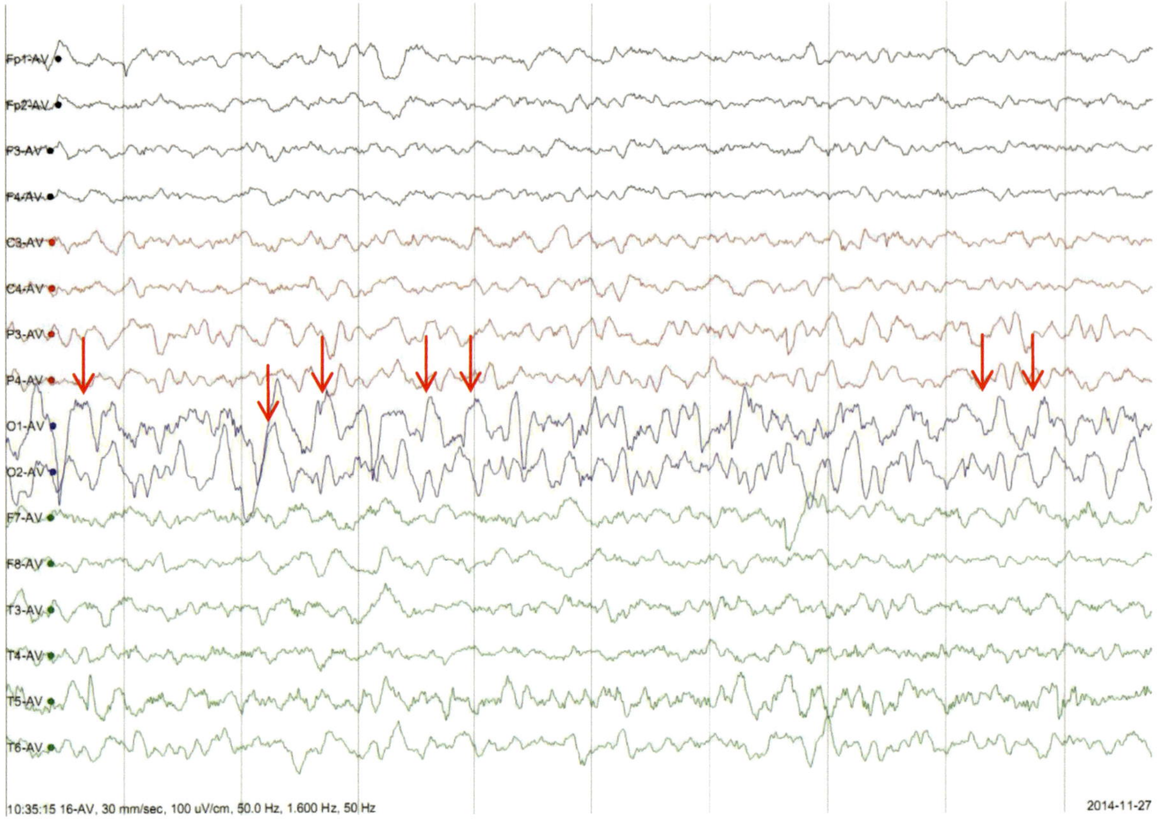

Fig. 13.5 On Day 9 of illness, EEG showed the middle volatility of the bilateral occipital leads was mainly 4–6 Hz θ wave

Fig. 13.6 On Day 9 of illness, echo showed LCA about 3 mm

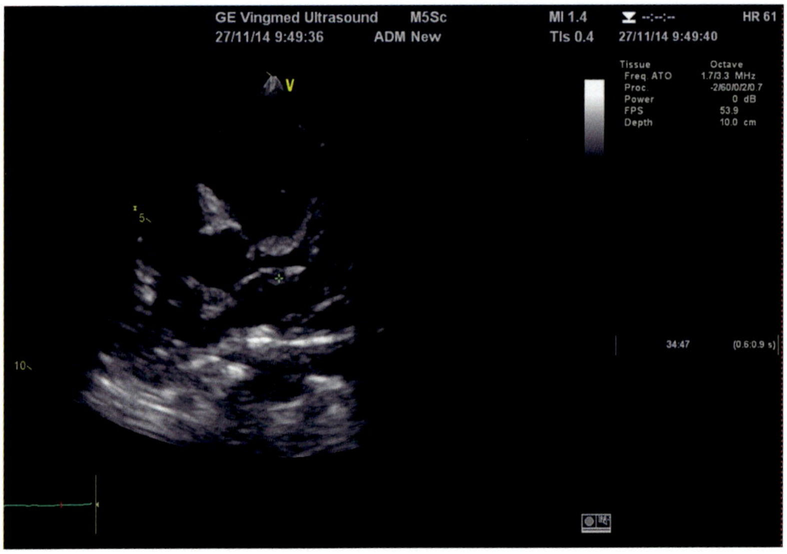

medication orally for increasing granulocytes; (2) aspirin reduced to one dose of 3–5 mg/kg. On Day 14, he developed cough. Retested blood work showed positive MP-IgM. He was give infusion of (1) azithromycin for 3 days; (2) methylprednisolone reduced to 0.5 mg/kg once a day for 3 days. Two days later, repeated echo showed LCA dilated to 2.6–3.9 mm (Fig. 13.7a), LAD dilated to 6.1 mm (Fig. 13.7b), while RCA 2.5 mm was normal. On Day18, repeated EEG was normal (Fig. 13.8). Retested blood work showed WBC 9.1 × 10^9/L, NE 42.2%, HGB 105 g/L, PLT 232 × 10^9/L, ESR 54 mm/h, and normal NT-pro BNP. He was discharged.

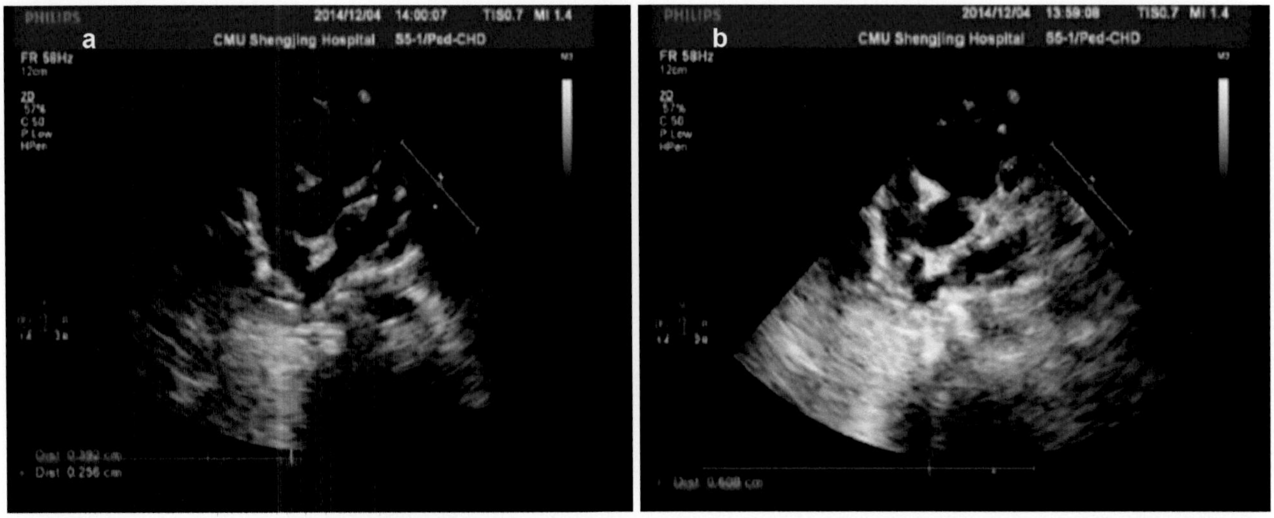

Fig. 13.7 On Day 16 of illness, LCA dilated to 2.6–3.9 mm (**a**), anterior descending coronary dilated to 6.1 mm (**b**)

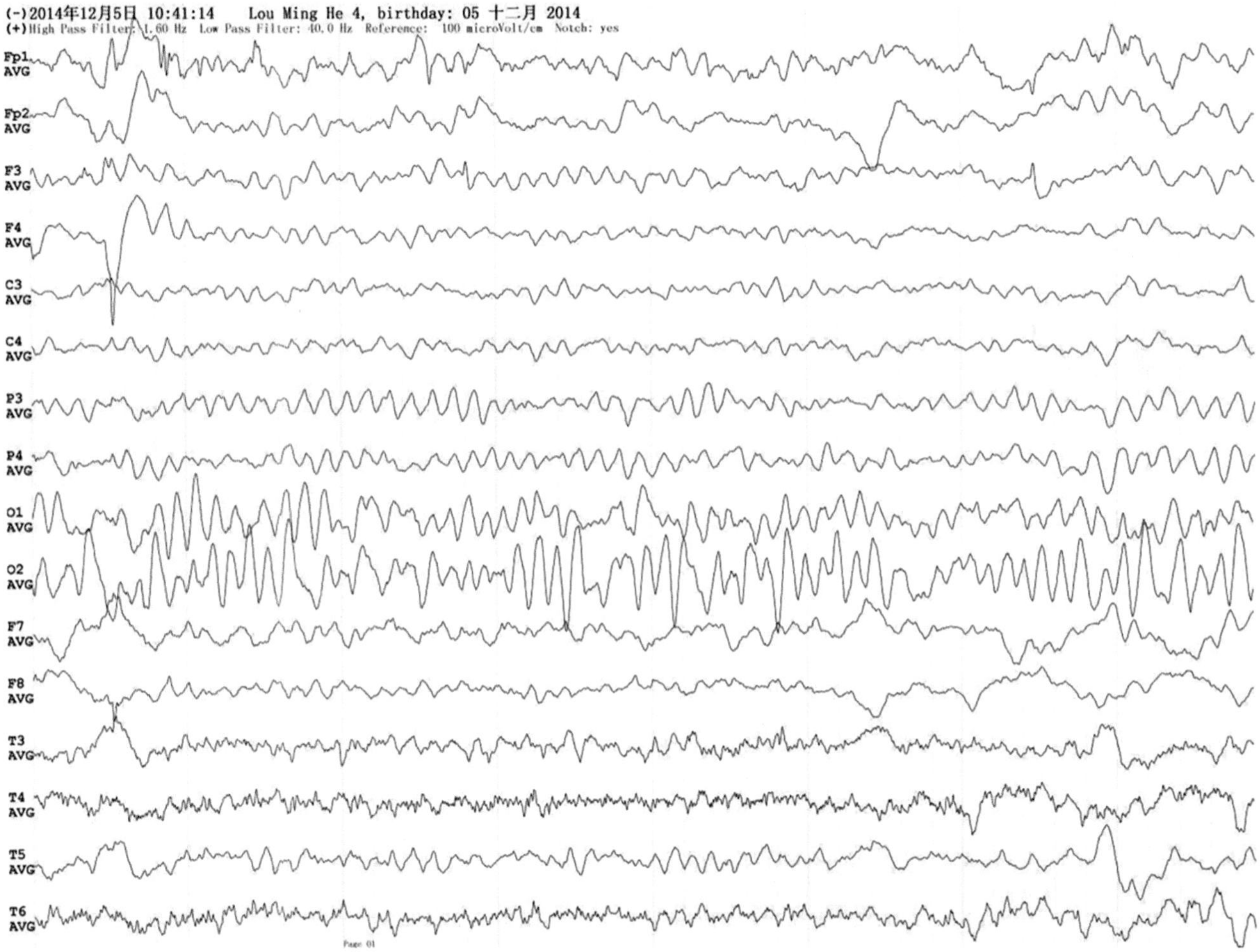

Fig. 13.8 On the Day 18 of illness, EEG was normal

13.2.1 Clinical Course of the Patient

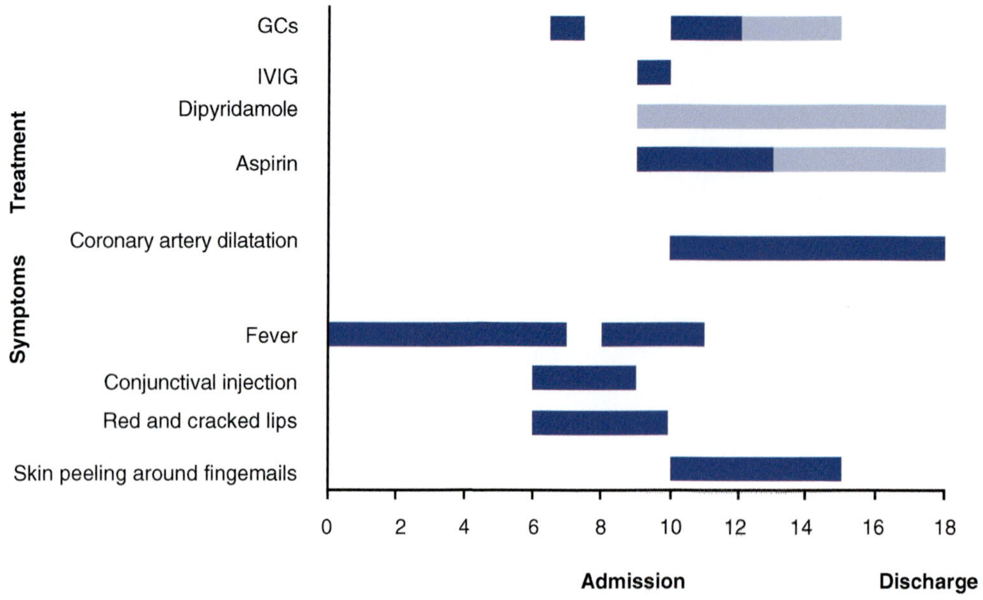

13.2.2 Follow-Up

On Day 25 of illness, blood work revealed both ESR and DIC were normal. At 1 year of illness, echo showed LAD about 3.5 mm (Fig. 13.9). He continued to take aspirin. After that, he did not followed up with us.

13.2.3 Diagnosis

1. KD
2. Left CAA
3. Aseptic meningitis
4. Hypoproteinemia
5. Pericardial effusion (mild)
6. Parainfluenza virus infection
7. MP infection.

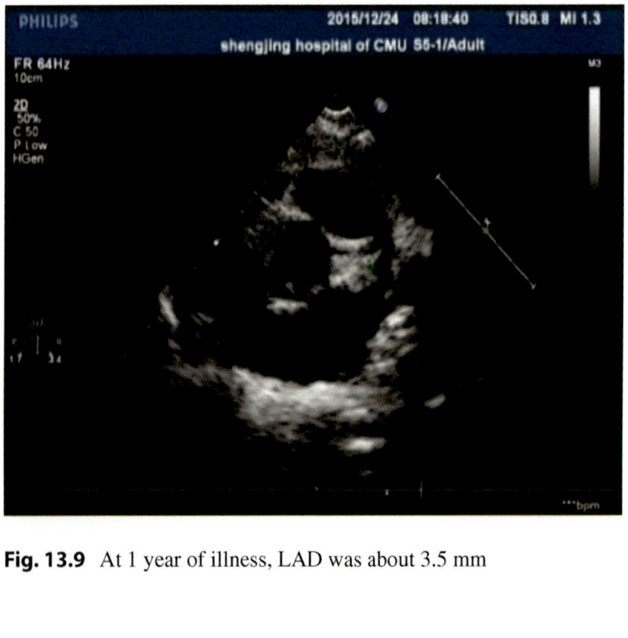

Fig. 13.9 At 1 year of illness, LAD was about 3.5 mm

13.2.4 Discussion

When he was admitted to the hospital, there were insufficient evidences to support the diagnosis of atypical KD. He had fever for 8 days, and antibiotic treatment was ineffective. He also had (1) transient bilateral conjunctival congestion; (2) erythema and cracked lips. The cervical lymph nodes were < 1.5 cm and the CRP was normal, which disagreed with KD. Of course, we could assume that the lymphadenopathy was big enough at beginning, but regressed to less than 1.5 cm on Day 8 of illness.

Differential diagnosis of ocular membrane thermal was considered. Supporting evidences include fever, conjunctival hyperemia. WBC and CRP were normal. However, negative test in adenovirus, especially along with no purulent secretions in both eyes, the most important symptom to distinguish it from KD, did not support ocular membrane thermal.

Echo performed earlier indicated that the diameter of coronary artery was normal in the high range. However, there was a significant decrease in albumin, which may be one of the causes of CAA in the later stage. Hypoproteinemia may aggravate coronary artery injury. Although this boy had MP infection, chest CT did not find severe pneumonia or pleural effusion, and physical examination did not find edema changes on both legs. It is difficult to explain hypoalbuminemia, thus, we highly suspected he was a typical KD.

The patient was admitted on the Day 8 of illness, and antibiotics treatment was ineffective. On the following day, the diameter of coronary artery was at a critical value. KD was highly suspected in this case. However, parents were concerned with possible complications associated with procedures, i.e. IVIG, and insisted on diagnosis confirmation first followed by treatment. They turned down IVIG treatment. Persuaded by professionals repeatedly, his parents agreed on IVIG treatment. As stated in guideline, it is better to give IVIG at Day 5-Day 10 of illness. Based on our experience, infants would be crying and be irritated, and older babies would have headache symptom, if infusion of IVIG 2 mg/kg lasts less than 10 h. Blood colloid osmotic pressure raised rapidly, which may result in headaches due to increased circulating blood volume. He received infusion of mannitol (20%) and furosemide after 1 g/kg IVIG. He had no discomforts.

On the Day 11 of the illness, periungual desquamation occurred which supported the AKD diagnosis. Repeated echo showed CAA, which confirmed KD diagnosis. This also supports that early diagnosis and timely IVIG therapy are very important. MP antibody gradually turned positive, while tuberculosis antibodies were weakly positive. PPD was negative, and lung CT showed no signs of tuberculosis changes. After 6 months of follow-up, tuberculosis antibodies were negative without anti-tuberculosis treatment. It was possible a false positives that could be a result of cross immunoreaction.

13.2.5 Case Specific Clinic Features

1. The number of CSF cells was normal. The patient should be diagnosed with aseptic meningitis, because of lethargy, high pressure in CSF, and abnormal slow wave of EEG. At the beginning of admission, both WBC and CRP were normal, which does not meet the criteria for classic KD. There was specific bilateral conjunctival congestion with no purulent secretion. Adenovirus titer was negative. NT pro-BNP was increased. Together they support KD. It has been reported that the combination treatment using IVIG and glucocorticoids is beneficial for KD patients with severe myocarditis and meningitis [2]. Diagnosis tends to be delayed in atypical cases, which can cause severe coronary artery damage. Therefore it was important to explain his conditions and prognosis to his parents as soon as possible, so he could get treatment on time.
2. KD is characterized with systemic vessel inflammation, and complications in nervous system are often overlooked. Histopathological examination in KD nervous system finds edema, necrosis, glial cell hyperplasia, lymphocyte invasion, etc. [3]. Children with KD have diverse neurological involvement. Aseptic meningitis is the most common complication in KD, followed by seizures, whereas temporary hemiplegia, facial paralysis, ataxia, hearing impairment, visual abnormalities, behavioral abnormalities [4–7] are rare. For children with poor mental state, sleepness, abnormal EEG; lumbar puncture test with aseptic meningitis changes, doctors could give mannitol to lower intracranial pressure along with therapy for maintaining nutrition in brain and nerves. EEG would be normal in 2 weeks or occasionally last for 4 months (case 18). Most children with KD symptoms would improve after treatment, and would not have sequelae found.

Ce Wang

13.3 Case 48: AKD Diagnosed after Finding CAA

A 2-month-old girl presented without remarkable past medical history or family history.

She presented on Day 14 of illness, with intermittent fever for 2 weeks. She had fever up to 39 °C, without shivering and convulsion, fever twice a day. She took ibuprofen and roxithromycin for 10 days. Intramuscular injections of unknown antipyretic medication were given twice on Day 2 and 4 of illness, her body temperature maintained 38.0 °C–39.0 °C. Then she was admitted to a local hospital. Due to significantly elevated WBC and CRP, she was suspected to have sepsis, and was given infusion of third-generation cephalosporin plus vitamin C for 7 days and IVIG 2.5 g for 3 days. She was afebrile for 4 days. On Day 13, her fever reoccurred, and her body temperature was 38.5 °C. She was transferred to our pediatric cardiology ward. Since the onset, she had good appetite and sleep. Physical examination could not find any abnormal signs. Her temperature was 37.0 °C, HR 130 bpm, RR 32 bpm, weight 5 kg. Her general condition was stable. Bregma was flat and normal strain. Tested blood work on Day 8 revealed WBC 17.21 × 10^9/L, NE 5.6 × 10^9/L, RBC 3.04 × 10^{12}/L, HGB 87 g/L, PLT 917 × 10^9/L, CRP 274.7 mg/L. She was suspected to have sepsis and thrombocythemia, and was treated with (1) infusion of zinacef after blood sample drawn for culture; (2) aspirin and dipyridamole 3–5 mg/kg/day oral; (3) intramuscular injection of vitamin K_1 for 3 days.

On Day 16, she was afebrile without any discomforts. On Day 17, her body temperature was 37.6 °C but recovered automatically 1 h later, along with diarrhea 4–6 times a day. Retested blood work revealed WBC 7 × 10^9/L, NE1.92 × 10^9/L, RBC 3.1 × 10^{12}/L, HGB 90 g/L, PLT

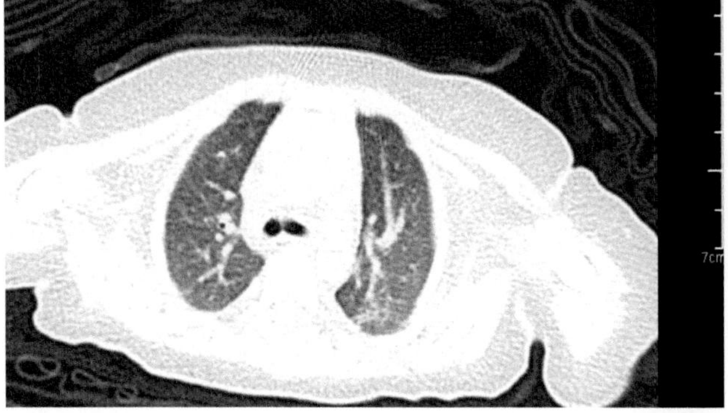

Fig. 13.10 On Day 16 of illness, chest CT scan showed mild bronchopneumonia on the left lower lobe

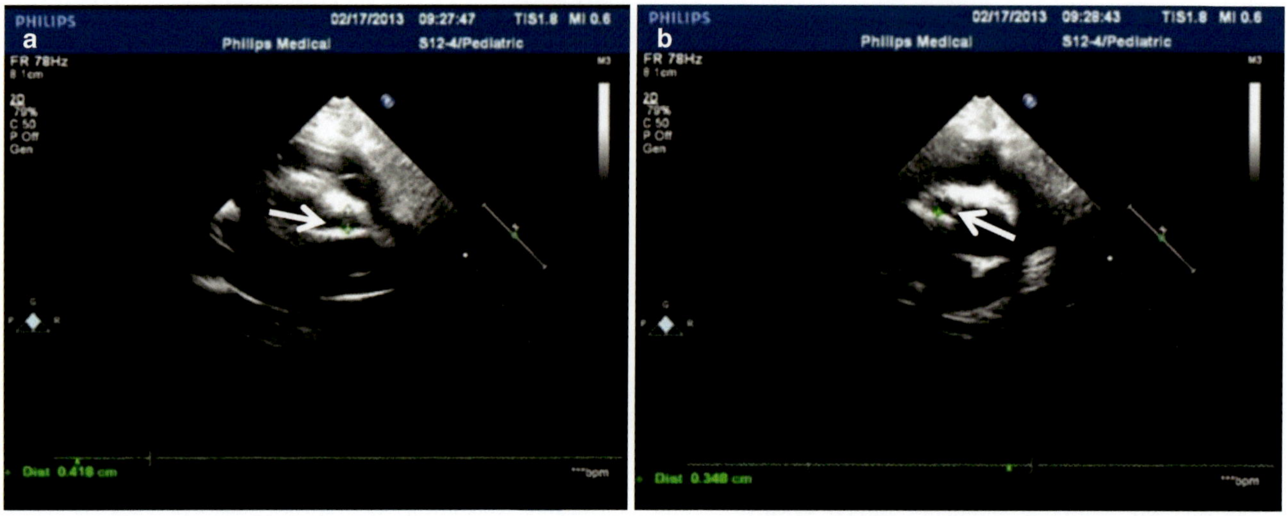

Fig. 13.11 On Day 20 of illness, echo showed LCA dilatation about 4.2 mm (**a**), RCA dilatation about 3.5 mm (**b**)

644×10^9/L, CRP 8.07 mg/L, ESR 38 mm, ALT 52 U/L, AST 73 U/L, AKP 432 U/L. CKMB 100 U/L, and hs-cTnT 0.023 ng/ml. CK and NT pro-BNP were normal. CMV-IgM was positive. Chest CT scan showed mild inflammation at left lower lobe (Fig. 13.10). After talking with her parents we learned that she had transient rashes on her hands when visiting at a local outpatient clinic. AKD was highly suspected, thus echo and BAVEP were ordered and she was given infusion of compound glycyrrhizin. On Day 18, she was afebrile for 36 h, diarrhea was reduced to three times per day. She developed some rashes on her face, varying along with body temperature, without itch. Echo showed dilated coronary arteries, LCA 4.4 mm (Fig. 13.11a), RCA 3.4 mm and the length of 5 mm (Fig. 13.11b), ASD 2 mm. Thus, AKD was diagnosed. She was diagnosed with sepsis at a local hospital, and she had been given IVIG 7.5g. It was on Day 18 of illness and afebrile over 36 h, CRP was almost normal when we confirmed AKD. We did not treat her with IVIG, instead we only gave her aspirin and dipyridamole.

On Day 19, retested EBV-IgM showed it was increased from 21.3 AU/ml to 33.3 AU/ml. BAVEP was normal. She was given infusion of ganciclovir 7.5 mg/kg/day for 5 days. On Day 21, her body temperature was 37.2 °C, no discomfort. On Day 22, body temperature up to 38.4 °C, accompanied with pharyngeal congestion. She took bufferin. On Day 23, her fever settled. Retested blood work revealed hs-cTnT 0.027 ng/ml, ALT 48 U/L, AST 50 U/L, CRP 15.90 mg/L, and ESR 47 mm/h. On Day 24, her temperature was 37.7 °C at midnight and dropped to normal after she drank water. She was discharged.

13.3.1 Clinical Course of the Patient

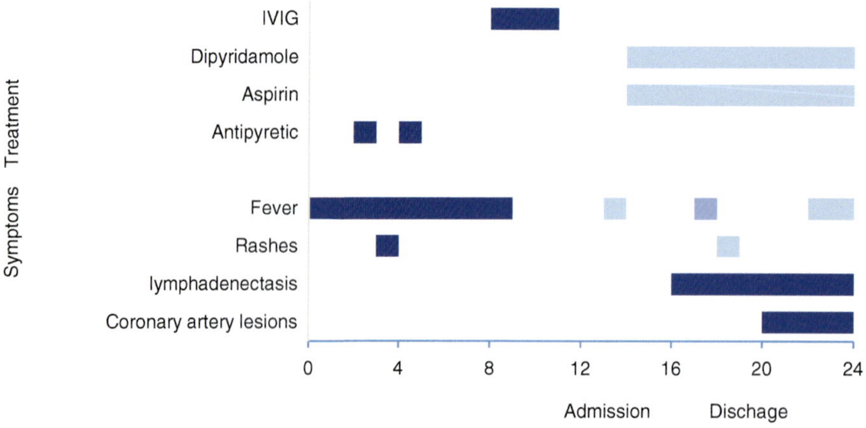

13.3.2 Follow-Up

Echo was performed at 3 (Fig. 13.12a, b), 7, and 21 months (Fig. 13.13). RCA (2.2 mm) returned to normal at 7 months of illness, and LCA (3.5–3.7 mm) did not recover. Her parents stopped all medication at 10 months of illness. At 21 months of illness, repeated echo showed LCA 3.3–3.7 mm (Fig. 13.14), RCA was normal. Then she has never followed up with us.

13.3.3 Diagnosis

1. AKD
2. Left CAA
3. Myocardium damage
4. Liver dysfunction
5. Viral infection (CMV + EBV)
6. Acute bronchopneumonia
7. Diarrhea
8. Mild anemia

13.3.4 Discussion

She had met the 3/5 criteria of IKD for she had continuous fever over 5 days and did not respond to broad spectrum antibiotics, and (1) lymphadenectasis (2 months old, after 18 days, her cervical lymphadenopathy 1.2 cm); (2) rashes; (3) both LCA and RCA were dilated, RCA had CAA.

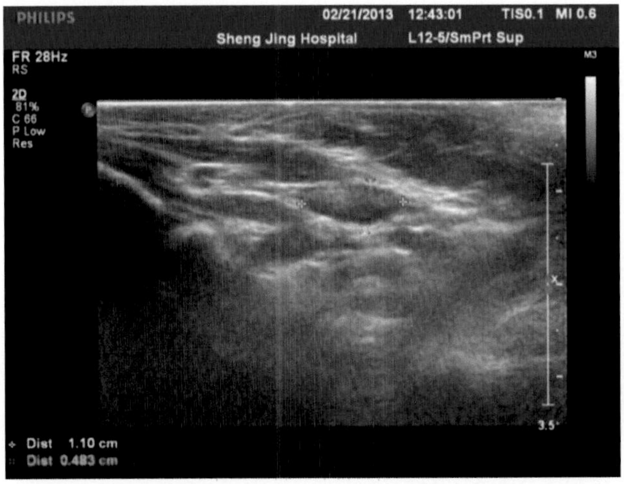

Fig. 13.12 On Day 20 of illness, cervical ultrasound showed cervical lymphadenectasis about 1.2 cm × 0.5 cm on the left

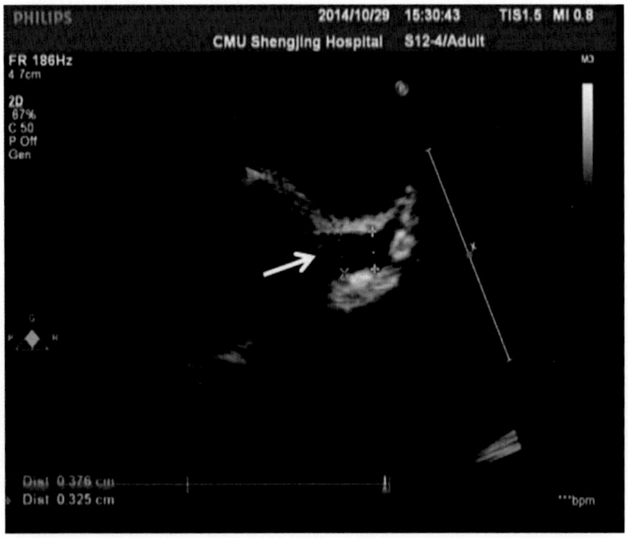

Fig. 13.14 At 21 months of illness, echo showed LCA dilatation about 3.3–3.7 mm

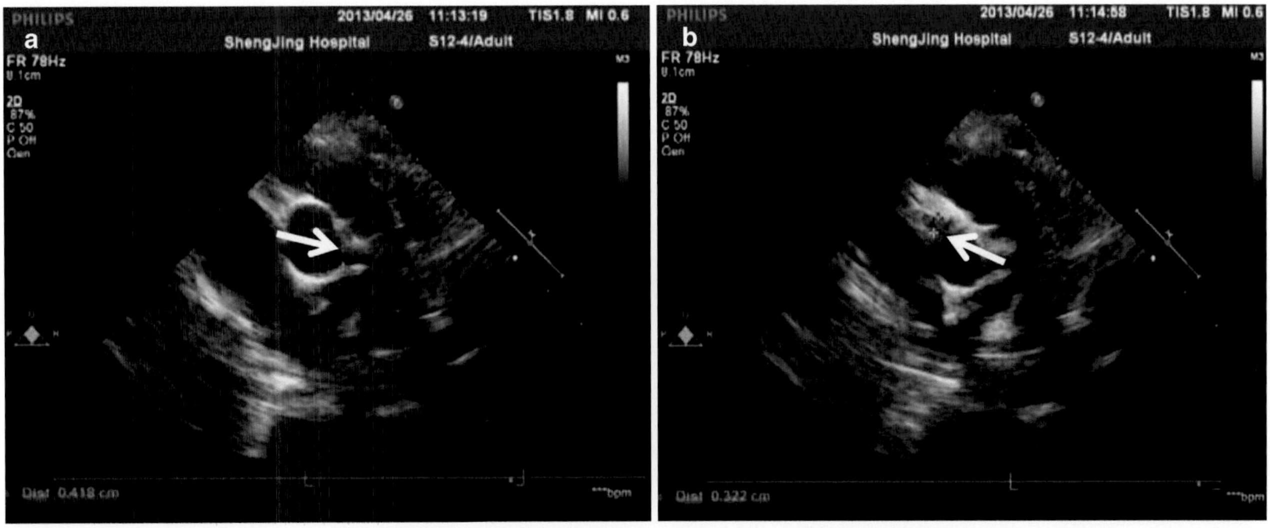

Fig. 13.13 At 3 months of illness, echo showed LCA opening dilatation about 4.2 mm (**a**), RCA 3.2 mm (**b**)

Differential diagnosis of infectious mononucleosis should be considered.

13.3.5 Case Specific Clinical Features

1. Her clinical symptoms were very atypical. We hypothesized that, at the early stage of her fever, the intramuscular injection of antipyretic medication she received was glucocorticoid. Thus, symptoms of KD were masked. Fortunately, she was given IVIG treatment for having sepsis before it was too late in a local hospital, which was the main reason of thrombocytosis when she was admitted in our ward, and she was in the subclinical stage of KD, platelets usually elevated. Because she was very young, had a persistent fever, had a poor response to antibiotic treatment, and her CRP was significantly increased, we suspected that she had KD. Echo test revealed coronary artery dilation, and then AKD was diagnosed. Though the doses of IVIG did not reach 2 g/kg, it was 18 days of illness, and fever retreated for more than 36 h. The inflammatory index was close to normal, so we did not continue to make up for it.
2. When applying glucocorticoid (GC) to KD patients, the chance and the medication compatibility were important. Studies have shown that an initial treatment using combination of GC and IVIG can reduce the incidence of CAL and of unresponsiveness to initial treatment, and shorten fever duration. Also the combined treatment increases neither recurrence of KD nor incidence of adverse events [8, 9]. A moderate-quality evidence shows that use of steroids in the acute phase of KD can improve coronary artery abnormalities, reduce hospitalization time, and decrease duration of clinical symptoms [10, 11]. But single glucocorticoid is not recommended, indeed. Some doctors said single glucocorticoid treatment in KD was independent risk factor of coronary artery dilatation or CAA [12]. Most clinicians concern about that glucocorticoid usage at the early stage may mask typical symptoms in KD including conjunctival congestion, rashes, strikingly red lips, edema in hands and feet. She received two intramuscular injections of unidentified antipyretic reagents at the early stage of fever. They were very possible GCs.
3. KD patient with coronary artery dilatation needs to take aspirin for a long period of time. Most coronary artery dilatation can be recovered within 2 years if patients continue to take aspirin. CAA remained stationary even after 2 years of onset similar with this case. However, some patients do develop thrombosis and coronary calcification in CAA 2 years later, even though they continue to take warfarin, aspirin, and dipyridamole (see case 7).

Hong Wang

References

1. Newburger JW, Takahashi M, Gerber MA, et al. Diagnosis, treatment, and long-term management of Kawasaki disease: a statement for health professionals from the Committee on Rheumatic Fever, Endocarditis, and Kawasaki Disease, Council on Cardiovascular Disease in the Young, American Heart Association. Pediatrics. 2004;114(6):1708–33.
2. Suga K, Inoue M, Ono A, et al. Early combined treatment with steroid and immunoglobulin is effective for serious Kawasaki disease complicated by myocarditis and encephalopathy. J Med Investig. 2016;63(1–2):140–3.
3. Amano S, Hazama F. Neutral involvement in Kawasaki disease. Acta Pathol Jpn. 1980;30(3):365–73.
4. Alves NR, Magalhães CM, Almeida Rde F, et al. Prospective study of Kawasaki disease complications: review of 115 cases. Rev Assoc Med Bras. 2011;57(3):299–300.
5. Poon LK, Lun KS, Ng YM. Facial nerve palsy and Kawasaki disease. Hong Kong Med J. 2000;6(2):224–6.
6. Knott PD, Orloff LA, Harris JP, et al. Kawasaki disease multicenter hearing loss study group. Sensorineural hearing loss and Kawasaki disease: a prospective study. Am J Otolaryngol. 2001;22(5):343–8.
7. Alves NR, Magalhães CM, Almeida Rde F, et al. Prospective study of Kawasaki disease complications: review of 115 cases. Rev Assoc Med Bras (1992). 2011;57(3):295–300.
8. Li J, Wang BL, Feng RB, et al. Efficacy of glucocorticoids combined with immunoglobulin in initial treatment of Kawasaki disease: a Meta analysis. Zhong guo Dang Dai Er Ke Za Zhi. 2016;18(6):527–33.
9. Miura M. Role of glucocorticoids in Kawasaki disease. Int J Rheum Dis. 2018;21(1):70–5.
10. Zhao DM, Yin QL, Ji XH, et al. Glucocorticoid combined with ulinastatin in treatment of Kawasaki disease in children: a non-randomized controlled clinical trial. Zhong guo Dang Dai Er Ke Za Zhi. 2015;17(8):780–5.
11. Wardle AJ, Connolly GM, Seager MJ, et al. Corticosteroids for the treatment of Kawasaki disease in children. Cochrane Database Syst Rev. 2017;1:CD011188.
12. Du ZD, Gao LL. Corticosteroid therapy might be associated with the development of coronary aneurysm in children with Kawasaki disease. Chin Med J. 2016;129(8):922–8.

Controversial KD

14

Hong Wang, Xuan Liu, Jing Dong, Yang Hou, Xiaona Yu, Xiaozhe Cui, and Yunming Xu

Abstract

In the diagnosis of KD, fever is essential and lasts more than 5 days, and is a prerequisite for the ineffectiveness of broad-spectrum antibiotics. But in clinical practice, we have treated a wide variety of patients with no fever, but other characteristics of KD are typical. We have treated one case with no specific symptoms and signs of KD, only with non-specific symptoms such as nausea, vomiting, abdominal distension, but developed CAA and other artery lesions (case 49). We have also treated some cases with recurrent fevers that eventually develop severe damage to the coronary arteries, aorta, and other body arteries, with massive thrombosis inside that leading to death at a young age (case 50 and case 51). According to the AHA guideline (McCrindle et al., Circulation 135(17):e927–e999, 2017), they all didn't meet the diagnostic criteria for KD, which we call the controversial KD.

If coronary and somatic artery damage occurs in infants less than 6 months old, it needs to be differentiated from polyarteritis. It has been reported that multiple arteritis is difficult to be diagnosed in live infants, and it is basically confirmed by postmortem autopsy (Zhu, Practical paidonosology [M]. 6th ed. Beijing: People's Medicine Publishing House, 1996). KD can affect body arteries, but coronary arteries damage is a prerequisite (Newburger et al., Circulation 110(17):2747–2771, 2004; Dionne et al., Pediatr Int 59(3):265–270, 2016). KD can involve the heart valve and cause regurgitation (Printz et al., J Am Coll Cardiol 57(1):86–92, 2011), but the disappearance of the entire valve has not been reported. KD combined with thrombosis almost all occurred in CAA, and rarely reported thrombosis in body arteries.

This chapter presented three cases different from classic KD, two patients died.

14.1 Case 49: Afebrile with CAA

A 3-month girl presented without significant past medical history and family history.

She presented on Day 15 of illness, with a history of vomiting after breeding and ventosity for about two weeks. On Day 5, liquid glycerinum was given via anal injection at home, but did not regress ventosity. On Day 8, she came to our outpatient clinic, and blood work revealed both elevated WBC and CRP. DR on abdomen showed ileus. She had infusion of third-generation cephalosporin for 3 days in local outpatient clinic, and vomiting and ventosity improved, but she still had significant malaise and no appetite. Retested CBC did not show any improvements. She was admitted in our pediatric cardiology ward. Since the onset of illness, she was sleepy and easily frightened; she had no fever, cough or diarrhea. Examination revealed the follows: she was in a bad state but her vital signs were almost normal (T 37.0°C, HR 120bpm, RR30bpm, WT 6kg), along with gloomy complexion and poor response, sunken bregma about 2cm×2cm, fast pupils reflection to light, ventosity abdomen without hepatosplenomegaly, normal bowel sounds. Others were normal. Tested blood work 7 days before admission revealed WBC 17.6×10^9/L, NE 54.5%, HGB 82g/L, and PLT 800×10^9/L. Normal CK and CK-MB. Abdominal ultrasound showed more intestinal gas reflection, without effusion or

H. Wang (✉) · X. Cui · Y. Xu
Department of Pediatric Cardiology, Shengjing Hospital of China Medical University, Shenyang, P.R. China

X. Liu
Department of Hematology Laboratory, Shengjing Hospital of China Medical University, Shenyang, P.R. China

J. Dong
Department of Cardiology Function, Shengjing Hospital of China Medical University, Shenyang, P.R. China

Y. Hou
Department of Radiology, Shengjing Hospital of China Medical University, Shenyang, P.R. China

X. Yu
Department of Ultrasound, Shengjing Hospital of China Medical University, Shenyang, P.R. China

H. Wang (ed.), *Paediatric Kawasaki Disease*, https://doi.org/10.1007/978-981-15-0038-1_14

enclosed mass. Blood work in the morning before admission was listed as following (Table 14.1): WBC 18.2×10^9/L, NE 48.0%, HGB 77g/L, PLT 799×10^9/L, and CRP 62.6mg/L. ALT, AST, CK, and CK-MB were normal. For she was suspected to have sepsis, she was treated with infusion of third-generation cephalosporin after admission.

On Day of 16, she had no fever. Retested blood work revealed WBC 21.4×10^9/L, NE 43.8%, HGB 82g/L, PLT 750×10^9/L, NT-pro BNP 693.1(<300) pg/ml, hs-cTnT 0.158 (<0.014) ng/ml, cTnI 0.137 (<0.04) μg/L, IgG 4.48g/L, IgA 0.234g/L, IgM 1.00g/L, ASO <25.0IU/ml, CRP 39.50mg/L, and serum iron 4.3μmol/L. MP-IgM, CP-IgM, CMV-IgM, HSV(I+II)-IgM and EBV-IgM were negative. Abdominal ultrasound showed normal pylorus, liver, and spleen. Chest CT scan showed the permeability was uneven in both lungs (Fig. 14.1a). Lumbar puncture showed the pressure of CSF was 147 drops/min. Results from CSF routine and biochemistry test were normal. Culture of CSF was negative for pathogens. For the patient also had accompanied with myocardium damage, acute bronchopneumonia, moderate anemia, and intracranial hypertension, and aseptic meningitis, she was treated with (1) infusion of mannitol (20%) and furosemidum; (2) third-generation cephalosporin; (3) deproteinized calf blood extract to natrium cerebral cells; (4) creatine phosphate sodium; (5) muscular injection of vitamin K_1 for three days. On Day 18, she had ventosity and refused breeding again without vomiting. Examination found that her abdomen was slightly expanded. Others were normal. Abdominal stand DR showed there was no free gas shadow under diaphragm, more intestinal gas in abdominal cavity, intestinal dilatation, and clear air fluid level (Fig. 14.1b). Lateral position DR revealed that there is no intestinal gas before sacrum (Fig. 14.2a), and there was no stone or calcification detected. Imaging showed possible intestinal obstruction. Neonatal surgeon recommended recheck next day. Head MR, echo and EEG were ordered. On Day 19, retested blood work revealed WBC 21.1×10^9/L, NE 65.3%, HGB 80g/L, PLT 650×10^9/L, CRP 53.60mg/L, NT-pro BNP 2138pg/ml, cTnI 0.688ug/L, and hs-cTnT 0.320ng/ml. Abdominal DR showed there was intestinal gas before

Table 14.1 The dynamic changes of lab parameters

Time of illness	8 days	15 days	16 days	19 days	**24 days**	**33 days**
WBC ($\times10^9$/ml)	17.6	18.2	21.4	21.1	13.6	9.6
NE (%)	54.5	48.0	43.8	65.3	36.7	33.6
HGB (g/L)	82	77	82	80	64	109
PLT ($\times10^9$/ml)	800	799	750	650	584	412
CRP (mg/L)		62.6	39.5	53.6	18.1	5.6
ESR (mm/h)						
cTnI (μg/L)			0.137	0.688		0.03
Hs-cTnT (ng/ml)			0.158	0.320		0.021
NT pro-BNP (ng/ml)			693.1	2138		1057

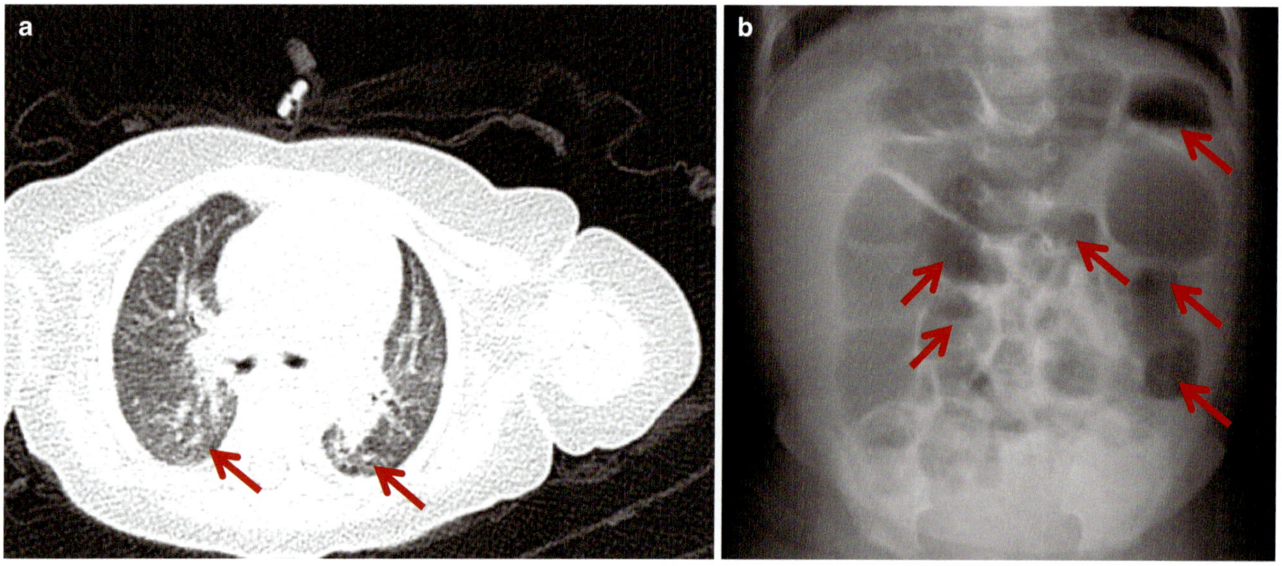

Fig. 14.1 On Day 16 of illness, chest CT showed acute branchopneumonia on bilateral lung (a). On Day 18 of illness, her abdominal stand DR showed liquid-gas level (b)

sacrum (Fig. 14.2b), others were not improved. ECG was normal (Fig. 14.3). Neonatal surgeon stated there was no surgical indication and recommended continuing treatment with medications. On Day 20, she still had ventosity and developed vomiting and watery stool. Pediatric gastroenterologist suggested test food allergens (intolerance), barium enema, abdominal CT, and to take simethicone. Echo showed both LVED (22mm) and LVEF (68%) were normal. Movement of left ventricular wall was normal. There was mild trace reflux at mitral, tricuspid valve. Coronary arteries were clear and

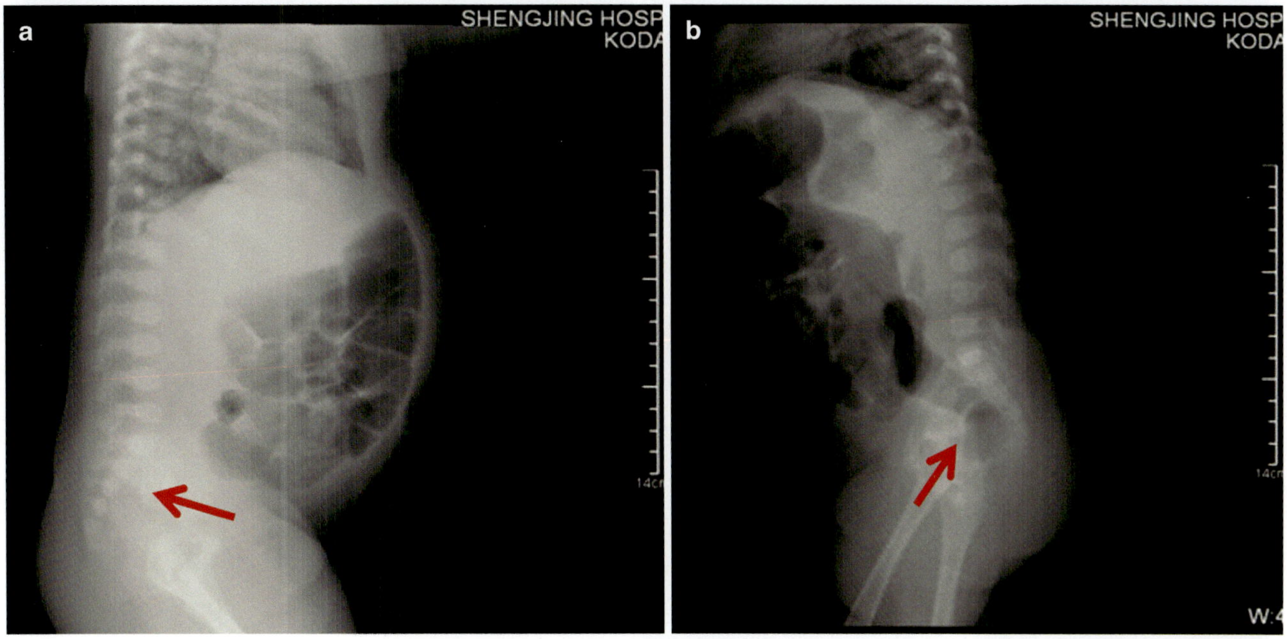

Fig. 14.2 Lateral view of abdomen DR showed intestinal gas can't be seen before sacrum on Day 18 (**a**) and it appeared on Day 19 (**b**) of illness

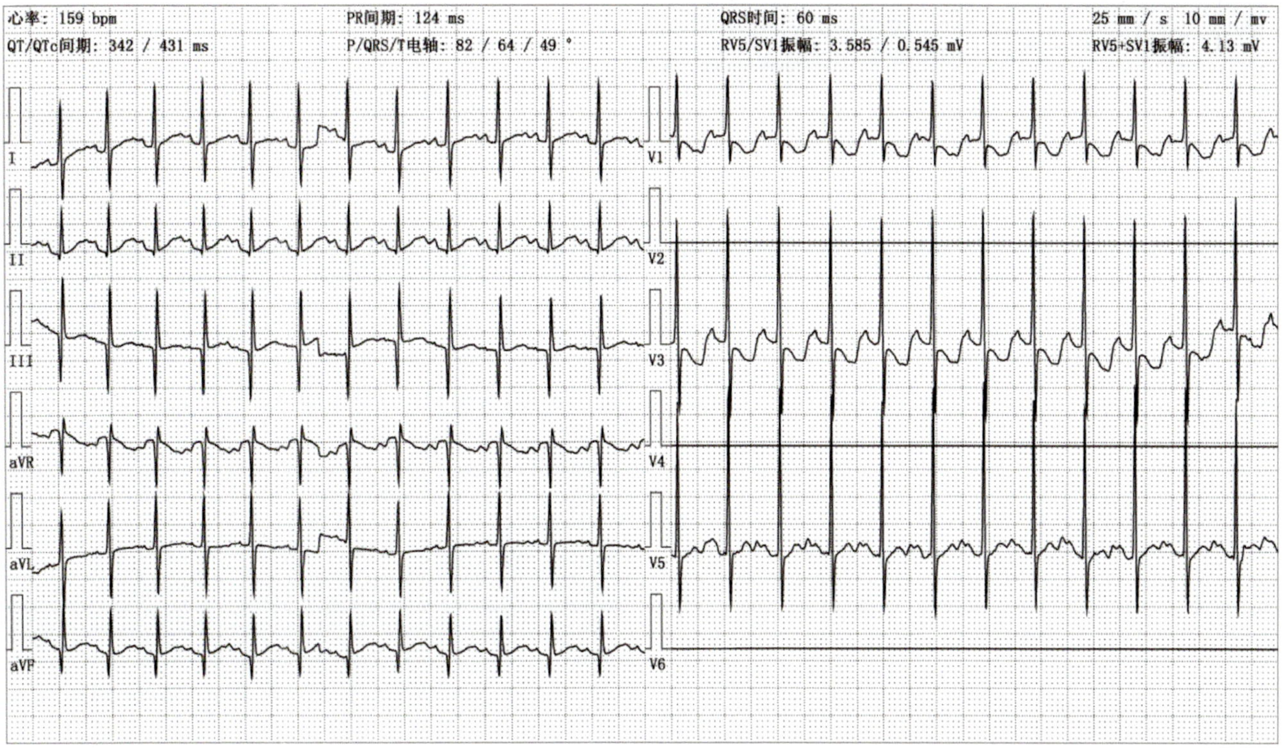

Fig. 14.3 On Day 19 of illness, her ECG was sinus tachycardia

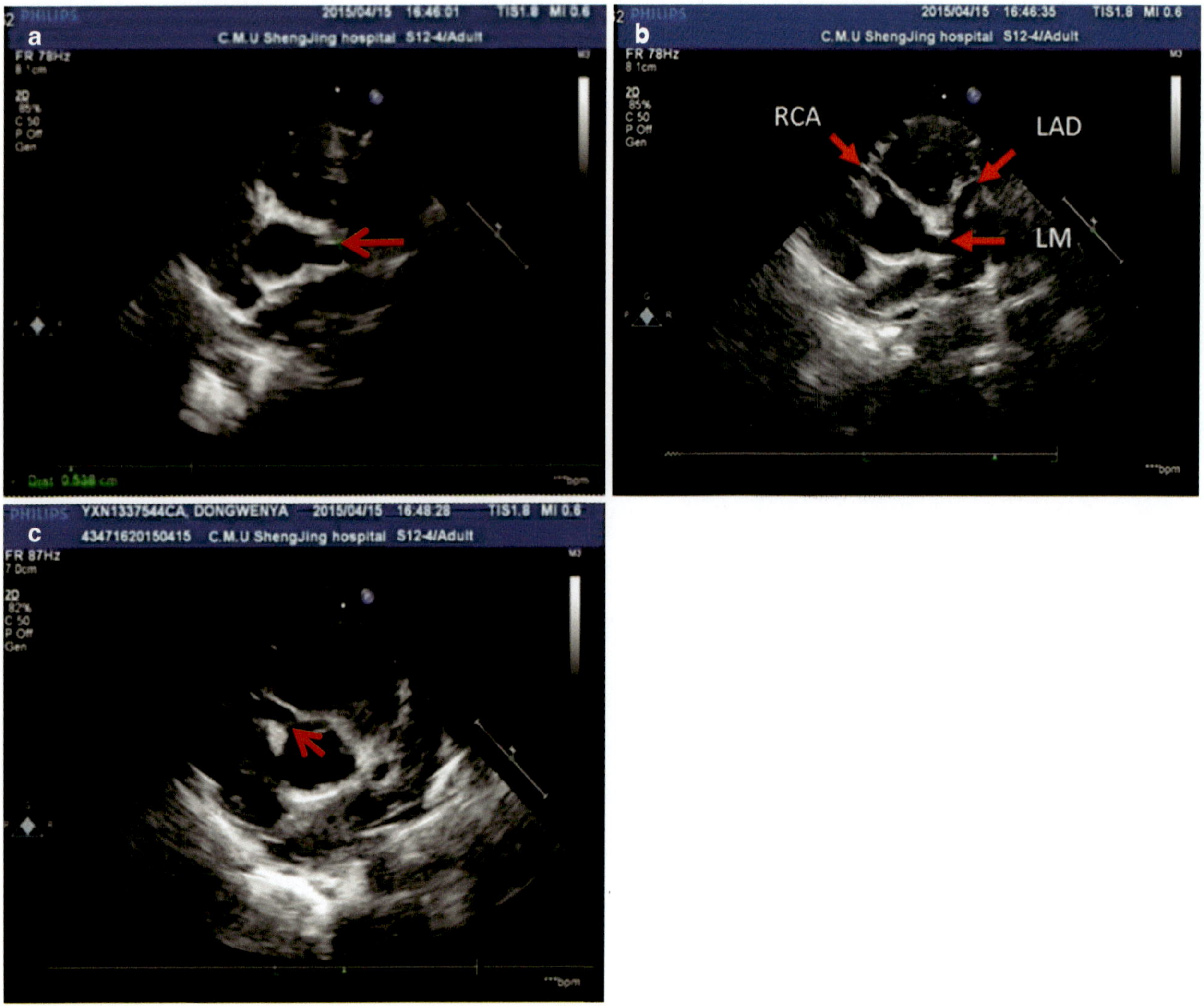

Fig. 14.4 On Day 20 of illness, echocardiography showed LCA dilated to 5.2 mm (**a**), LAD dilated to 3.5 mm (**b**). RCA dilated to 4.1 mm (**c**)

dilated: LCA 5.2 mm (Fig. 14.4a) like salami, LAD 3.3–4.3 mm (Fig. 14.4b), and RCA 4.1 mm (Fig. 14.4c). There was no thrombus in it. Detected ASD 2 mm. There was no pericardial effusion. For incomplete KD could not be excluded, she was treated with (1) aspirin and dipyridamole 3–5 mg/kg/d, dipyridamole 3–5mg/kg/day; (2) single dose of IVIG 2g/kg, over 12 hours, (3) Mannitol and furosemidum infusion after IVIG 1g/kg infusion.

On Day 21, she had fever up to 38.1°C. It regressed after she took bufferin. Examination revealed no positive sign. Coronary artery CTA was ordered to perform. On Day 22, she was afebrile, and her mental state and appetite were improved. Retested blood work revealed NT-pro BNP 1744pg/ml, hs-cTnT 0.207ng/ml, D-dimer 911ug/L, blood gas analysis, K^+, Na^+, and Cl^- were normal. On Day 23, she had cough. Auscultation assessment on lungs were normal. On Day 24, she still had cough without sputum. Retested blood work revealed WBC 13.6×10^9/L, NE 3.7×10^9/L, RBC

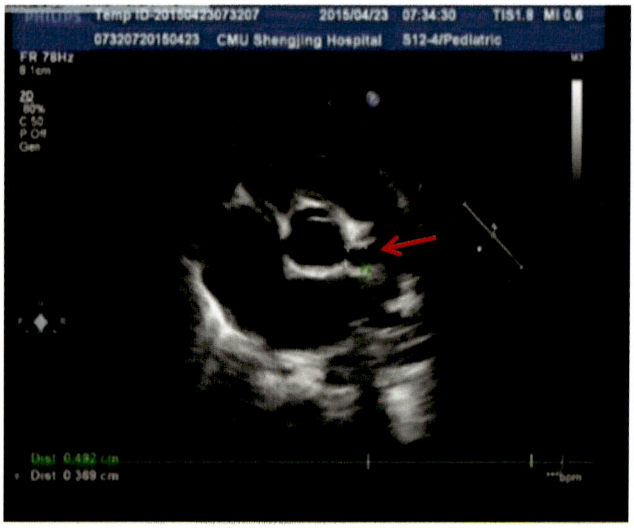

Fig. 14.5 On Day 28 of illness, echocardiography showed LCA dilated to 3.7–5.0 mm

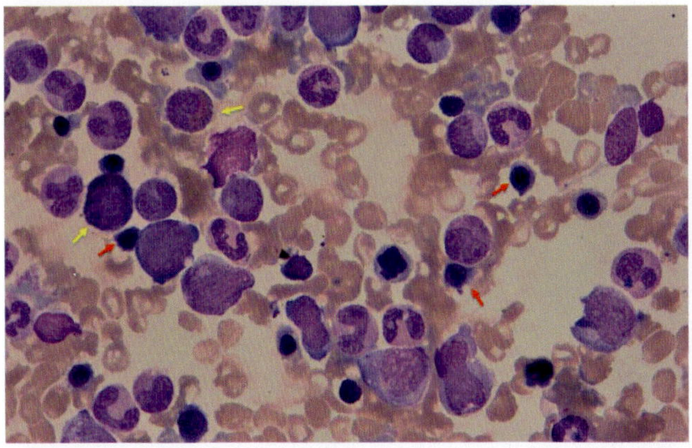

Fig. 14.6 Bone marrow smear: Wright-Giemsa×1000. On Day 30 of illness, bone marrow showed cellular marrow with low myeloid-to-erythrocyte ratio. Infantile erythrocyte (red arrow) body was small, cytoplasm was little. Nucleoplasm was relatively solid shrinkage, showing iron deficiency, (yellow arrow) was eosinophils

2.6×10^{12}/L, HGB 64g/L, PLT 584×10^{9}/L, CRP 18.10mg/L, MP-IgG 1:80, mildly positive Anti-SS-A, and positive anti-Ro-52. She had developed severe anemia, and was given infusion of erythrocyte twice and erythromycin. Coronary artery CTA was not completed for sedation issue. On Day 26, after given infusion of erythrocytes, her mental state was visibly improved, but rashes were developed on the back and legs. On Day 27, coronary artery CTA was failed again for trocar was too thin to perform CTA. Consultation with Pediatric rheumatic immunologist concluded the followings: (1) she was only 3 months old, with mildly positive anti-SS-A, positive anti-Ro-52 and unrecovered CRP. Her disease was so complicated that it was necessary to do further blood tests. (2) All limb blood pressure, bone marrow test and total abdominal CT should be performed. On Day 28, she was afebrile and coughed with sputum. BP: left arm 78/40mmHg, right arm 80/45mmHg, left leg 95/45 mmHg and right leg 100/60mmHg. Retested blood work showed CRP 4.59 mg/L, IgE 28.03 IU/ml, positive ACA, and normal C_3, C_4, RF and ANA. Coomb's test revealed that all anti IgG+C_3d, anti C_3d and anti IgG were negative. Repeated echo showed coronary arteries dilated, LCA 3.7–4.9 mm (Fig. 14.5), LAD 3.4 mm, RCA 3.9 mm, ASD 2.5 mm, and normal LVEF. Bone marrow test was failed for insufficient marrow, and the procedure was repeated.

On Day 30, she still had cough. Auscultation assessment on both lungs found rales. Bone marrow test showed hyperplasia obviously active, the ratio of grain and red decreased. No LE cell was found (Fig. 14.6). She had developed acute bronchopneumonia, and continued to receive infusion of erythromycin, inhaling pulmicort and combivent. On Day 32–33 days, she had mild fever 37.5–37.7°C, her cough improved. Examination findings were the same. Retest blood work revealed WBC 9.6×10^{9}/L, NE 33.6%, RBC 3.9×10^{12}/L, HGB 109g/L, PLT 412×10^{9}/L, NT-pro BNP 1057pg/ml, hs-cTnT 0.021ng/ml, and normal cTnI and CRP. Head MR showed bilateral temporal brain gap widened (Fig. 14.7a), and MRA was normal. Abdominal artery ultrasound showed the internal iliac artery was thicker about 0.6 mm (Fig. 14.7b). Ultrasound on renal arteries showed normal results. On Day 34, she had rashes all over the body. Consultation with a der-

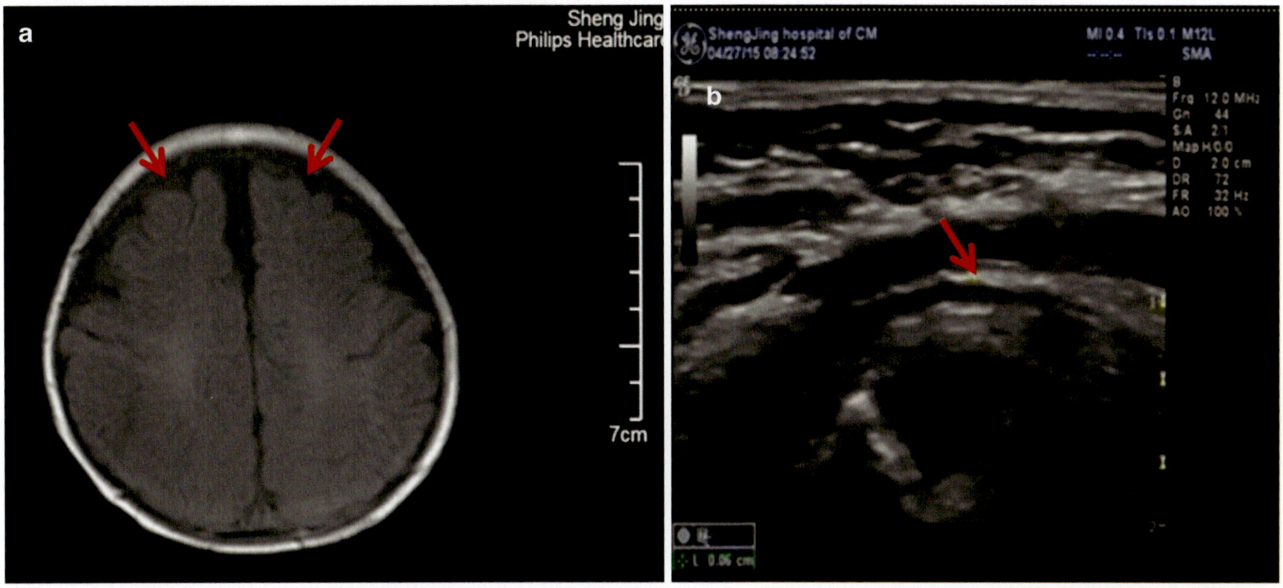

Fig. 14.7 On Day 33 of illness, her head MR showed bilateral temporal brain gap widened (**a**), Ultrasonic of abdominal arteries showed the internal iliac artery was thicker about 0.6mm (**b**)

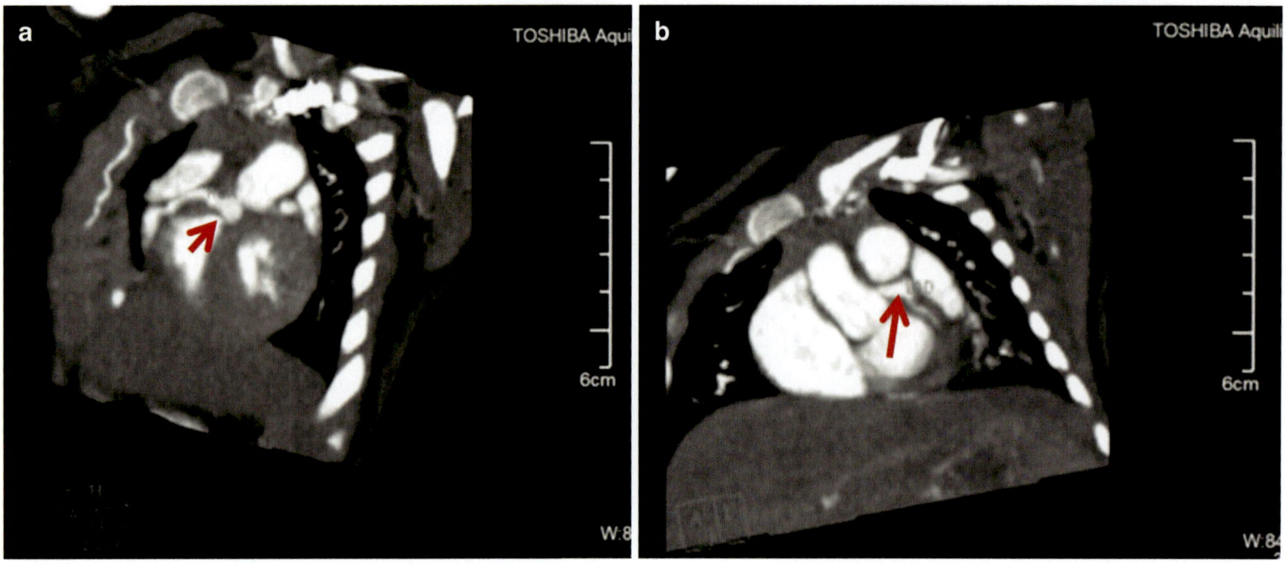

Fig. 14.8 On Day 34 of illness, coronary artery CTA:RCA inner diameter was 3.7mm (**a**), the diameter of LM was 3mm (**b**)

matologist concluded urticarial diagnosis, and she was given chlortrimeton orally. Coronary artery CTA showed aorta inner diameter was 12.5 mm, pulmonary artery inner diameter was11.5 mm. The wall of both aorta and pulmonary artery were normal. The walls of coronary artery branches were thickened at different layers. The diameter of RCA was 3.7 mm (Fig. 14.8a), and the diameter of LM was 3 mm (Fig. 14.8b). The walls of bilateral ventricles, the inner diameter of bilateral auricle and ventricular were normal. On Day 35, her disease was so complicate that we were not sure whether she should be given oral glucocorticoid for a long period of time. Her parents decided to seek treatment for her at Beijing Children Hospital.

14.1.1 Follow-Up

After discharge, she took aspirin and dipyridamole. One week later, her parents informed us they had gone to Beijing Children Hospital, where she was diagnosed with atypical KD and did not need to take glucocorticoid. Since then she had never followed up with us.

14.1.2 Diagnosis

1. Atypical KD? Infantile polyarteritis?
2. Aseptic meningitis
3. Myocardium damage
4. Severe anemia
5. Acute branchopneumonia.

14.1.3 Discussion

She hadn't met the criteria for AKD because she only had coronary artery dilatation shaped like sausage, and she did not have any symptoms of KD, and did not even have fever. But blood work showed WBC >15.0×10^9, NE >75%, CRP >30mg/L, ESR >40mm. We highly suspect she had AKD [1].

14.1.4 Case Specific Clinical Features

1. She had never had fever since she was born, and did not have any symptoms of KD. But she had aseptic meningitis, coronary artery dilation. Afebrile KD was uncommon. In our center, there have been two cases of KD without fever been diagnosed. Those had all other KD symptoms. For this girl differential diagnosis of infantile polyarteritis should be considered. She had mildly positive anti-SS-A titer, positive anti-Ro-52, and positive ACA. Coronary artery was dilated, different layer thickness, and iliac artery thickening, with all these considered, infant polyarteritis could not be completely ruled out.
2. For this patient, results from laboratory tests were similar to those in KD. We performed the echocardiography and found coronary artery dilated. Thus AKD was highly suspected. Cases of KD patients with CAA and iliac artery thickening are reported in literature [1]. We had never seen iliac artery thickening before, though we had treated over 500 KD patients every year for nearly 30 years. It is very possible that misdiagnosis could happen here, for we did

not perform ultrasound to assess iliac artery. By now, without guideline for treating infantile polyarteritis, we don't know its long-term prognosis. Most patients may die [2] and, in that case, diagnosis is only established based on autopsy. If this girl was treated as a polyarteritis patient, she would be given glucocorticoid over 10 years. During this no vaccination, therefore, the opportunity to catch infectious diseases will be significantly increased and that even endanger her life. Furthermore, it could affect her height. So we were very cautious and recommended her have consultation with clinicians who had more experiences.

3. Elevated NT-pro BNP may help the AKD diagnosis NT-pro BNP [3]. In KD infants with cardiovascular complications, increased NT-pro BNP can be used as clinic theory reference for estimating therapeutic effects [4]. This girl was suspected to have AKD just because she had elevated NT-pro BNP combined with elevated WBC/NE and CRP, even though she did not have fever. Otherwise, we only diagnosed sepsis and may missed other diagnosis. According to her symptoms and results from blood work, she was at acute phase of KD or had polyarteritis when she came to our hospital.
4. It has been reported that CAA in some KD patients can be recovered in 2 years, if the right diagnosis is made followed by timely IVIG treatment, and patients continue to take aspirin. But with dilatation in a shape like sausage, her long-term prognosis was alarming. KD can along with body aneurismal, but was rare only with body aneurismal and without CAA [5].

Hong Wang

14.2 Case 50: Recurrent Fever with Coronary Artery, Aortic, and Iliac Artery Dilatation

A 3-year-old girl presented with a history of recurrent fever for 21 months. She was vaccinated as scheduled without allergic history or connective tissue disease history in her family.

She presented at about 21 months of illness. She had continuous fever for one month at beginning. Blood test at a local hospital revealed liver dysfunction. Slight tricuspid regurgitation was detected in echo examination and others were normal. She was admitted in our pediatric gastroenterology ward. After receiving treatment for protecting hepatocyte for 8 days, her fever settled, and liver function recovered. She was discharged as a hepatitis patient associated with infection. Twenty days later her fever recurrent and was sent to Beijing Children Hospital, where she was found to have an enlarged heart and was suggested to receive "chemotherapy" treatment. Her parents refused to give consents and she went home. Since then she had intermitted fever for 2 months. She was never followed up with any clinicians. Since the onset, she had been always weak and fatigue. Ten days before admission, she was irritable and lost appetite, with cough and difficulties in breathing. She had edema and oliguria for 3 days. She did not have sputum or vomit, and her stool was normal. Echo performed at the local clinic revealed coronary dilatation at initial segment, and severe aortic and mitral regurgitation. She was admitted in our pediatric cardiology ward. Examination revealed the follows: she was irritable, facial edema, dyspnea and tachycardia. Her body temperature was 37°C, PR 150bpm, RR 40bpm, BP 98/59mmHg, weight 13kg, SaO_2 was over 95%. Auscultation assessment found dull heart sound and fast HR (150bpm), without murmurs. The second heart sound at pulmonary artery was normal. Abdomen was soft. Liver edge was 7cm below the right costal margin, 5cm below the xiphoid, and hard texture. Her spleen wasn't enlarged. Blood vessel murmurs could be heard 2cm on left side of navel. She had legs edema and positive in dentation test. On Day 7, echo showed enlarged left ventricle, ascending aorta was widened. Bilateral coronary was dilated at initial segment. She had severe aortic regurgitation, severe mitral regurgitation, mild tricuspid regurgitation, and pulmonary arterial hypertension. Tested blood work at admission revealed WBC 14.57×10^9/L, NE 44.5%, HGB105g/L, PLT 318×10^9/L, CRP 11.90mg/L, cTnI 0.182ug/L, hs-cTnT 0.052ng/ml, and NT pro-BNP>35000pg/ml. CKMB-M was normal. ECG showed sinus tachycardia, HR 147bpm, low-flat T wave (Fig. 14.9). Chest CT scan showed inflammation in both lungs (Fig. 14.10). Multiple arteritis and KD weren't excluded, and diagnosis of chronic heart failure (NYHA class VI), myocardium damage, and pneumonia were made. She was treated with (1) infusion of furosemidum; (2) cedilanid rapid saturation; (3) zinacef; (4) creatine phosphate sodium and L-carnitine; (5) spironolactone and captopril oral; (6) monitoring ECG, BP, and SO_2; (7) velocity of all liquid infusion under control at less than 3ml/h/kg.

On Day 11, she was afebrile. PR 134bpm, RR 30bpm, urine volume increased and facial edema improved. Echo showed IVS was 5mm, LVED 48mm, LVW 5mm, and LVEF 56%. Coronary arteries were clear and dilated, LCA 8.8mm (Fig. 14.11a), LAD 7.4mm (Fig. 14.11b), RCA 8.5mm (Fig. 14.11c). Aortic root was dilated about 35mm (Fig. 14.11d). Aortic valves showed three leaves, and the construction of left coronary valve was nearly extinct (Fig. 14.12) leaving behind a significant gap and severe colorful regurgitation at diastolic section. The bloodstream of ascending aorta was eccentric. For her aortic valve disease was associated with severe regurgitation, secondary dilated cardiomyopathy diagnosis was made. She was treated with (1) the dose of furosemidum changed to once a day and spirolactone changed to once a day for 4 days a week; (2) infusion of azithromycin; (3) Tb-T-spot and PPD test; (4) chest CT, aorta CTA, limbs, renal artery ultrasound and ECG. Cardiac surgery specialist suggested aortic valve was

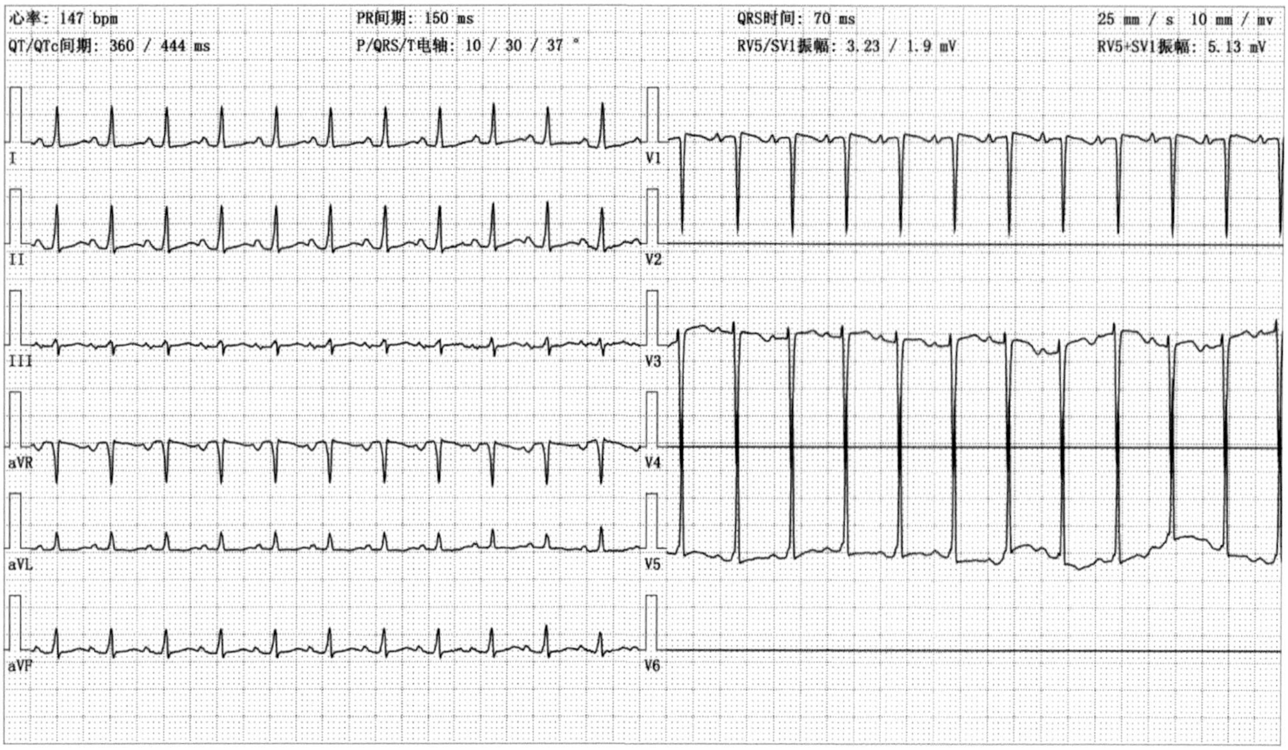

Fig. 14.9 On Day 10 of illness, ECG showed tachycardia, HR was 147bpm, low-flat T waves.

secondary to immunity disease, and the long-term progress was poor. Also she was too young to have the valve replaced with manmade valve.

On Day 12, she was sweaty, and edema in her right eye lid and right leg aggravated when she woke up. HR130bpm. Retest EBV-IgG positive (EA>150, NA>600, VCA>750). Thoracic aorta and abdominal aorta enhanced CT showed the abdominal aortic branches were significantly dilated with uneven size (Fig. 14.13a), arterial tortuosity at the aortic arch and the thoracic aorta, and thickening in vessel wall, which all support arteritis. Three-dimensional reconstruction showed abdominal aortic wall was multi and irregular thickening, with visible multiple collateral vessels. Abdominal aortic

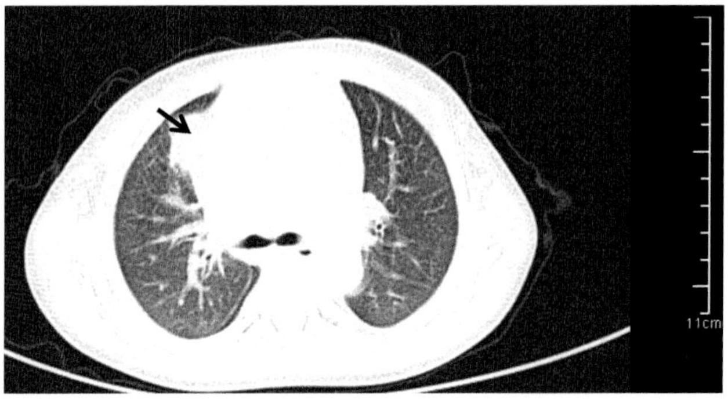

Fig. 14.10 On Day 10 of illness, chest CT scan showed pneumonia on the right lung

enhancement CT scan and three-dimensional reconstruction showed the anterior abdominal aortic bifurcation and significant expansion of bilateral iliac artery (Fig. 14.13b). The diameter of the right iliac artery was 25mm, and left one was 20mm. There was calcification on left iliac artery wall. There was a filling defect in the initial part of the left iliac artery and its far end was not shown clearly (Fig. 14.14). The proximal part of the right iliac artery was bulbous, and the diameter was 11mm. The distal was truncated (Fig. 14.15), the circle shadow was slightly low in density, and diameter was 13mm, with slightly higher density at edges. Lymphadenectasis was found behind peritoneum and in mesentery. For she was with giant abdominal aorta, iliac artery dilation and abdominal aortic thrombus, she was treated with oral warfarin 0.1mg/kg/d and aspirin 3–5mg/kg/d, dipyridamole 3–5mg/kg/d. For she had EBV infection, she had infusion of genciclovir 7.5mg/kg/d for 5 days. We were debating on whether she should be given oral glucocorticoid to treat multi section artery dilatation because it may increase the risk of thrombus. On Day 13, her body temperature was 38.5°C, with worse coughing. Urine volume increased and edema in right eye lid and right foot regressed. Urine routine test revealed WBC 16/HP. She was treated with oral azithromycin. On Day 14, she had fever once and her general state improved. She coughed with sputum, and was given infusion of mucosolvan.

On Day 16, she was afebrile for 2 days, but still had cough. Her urine volume increased to 700–800ml per day,

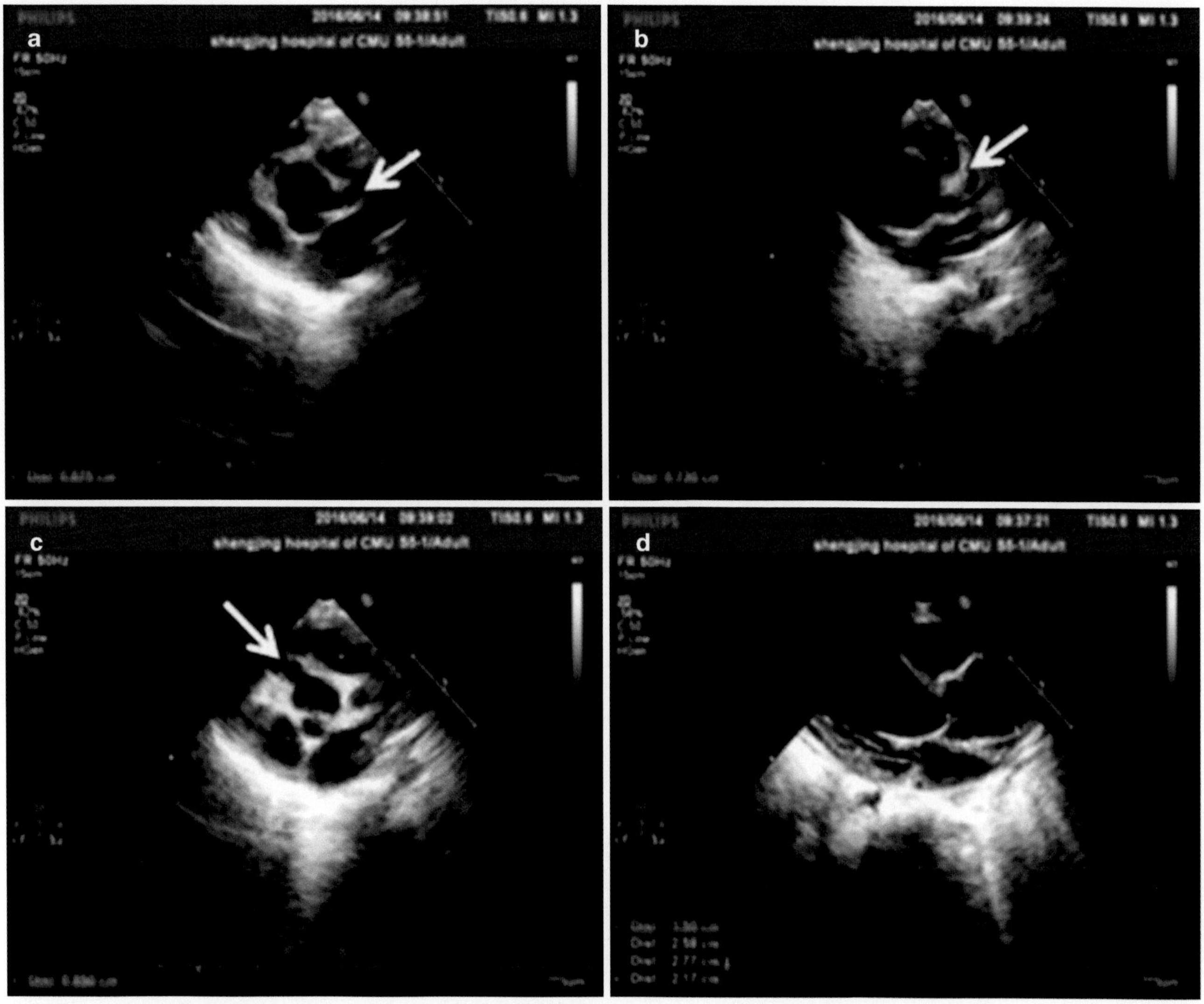

Fig. 14.11 On Day 11 of illness, echocardiography showed coronary arterys dilated, LCA 9.8 mm (**a**), LAD 7.4 mm (**b**), and RAD 8.5 mm (**c**). Aortic root dilated to 35 mm (**d**)

edema in face and feet were regressed. Auscultation assessment on murmurs and hepatomegaly stay unchanged. On Day 17, retested blood work revealed NT-pro BNP 11353pg/ml, PT 33.4s, INR 3.1, and APTT 45s, and blood gas analysis, cTnI, and hs-cTnT were normal. Urine routine test was normal. Warfarin dose was changed to 0.08mg/kg/d. On Day 18, she was still afebrile with mild cough. Retested DIC revealed PT 30.3s, INR 2.8. She was discharged.

14.2.1 Follow-Up

After discharged, she took aspirin, dipyridamole and warfarin and was referred to Beijing children hospital. During waiting in outpatient clinic, she developed nausea, vomiting, oliguria, and edema in face and legs. Her parents stopped giving her all medication and took her back to hometown. Two days later, she developed difficulties in breathing and was sent to a local hospital. 4 hours later, her condition was too severe to rescue, and she died of heart failure.

14.2.2 Diagnosis

1. Polyarteritis? Atypical KD?
2. Abdominal aortic thrombus (the beginning of the left iliac artery);
3. Aortic valve disease with severe regurgitation
4. Secondary dilated cardiomyopathy
5. Chronic heart failure, NYHA class IV
6. EBV infection
7. Acute branch pneumonia

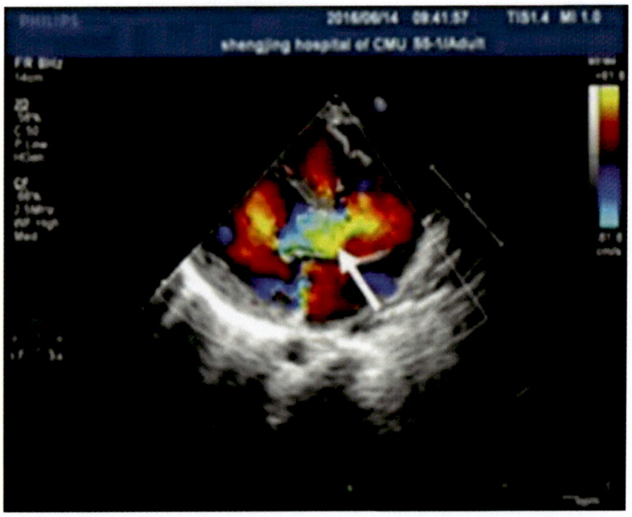

Fig. 14.12 On Day 11 of illness, echo showed severe aortic valve regurgitation at diastolic (white arrow)

14.2.3 Discussion

She didn't meet the criteria of KD, though she had repeated fever for a long time, and not responsive to broad-spectrum antibiotics. She had coronary artery cystic expansion. But the severe damage in her aortic valve can't be explained. Her parents couldn't recall whether she had rashes and other KD symptoms such as changes in lips, edema in hands and feet or bilateral conjunctival congestion at illness onset.

14.2.4 Case Specific Clinical Features

1. Congenital aortic valve dysplasia could be excluded, for there were no aortic valve changes shown in her echo 20 months ago.
2. Differential diagnosis of chronic activated EBV infection (CAEBVI) should be considered. She had repeated fever over 20 months, and every time her fever lasted over half month, along with liver dysfunction and hepatomegaly. Investigation revealed she had EBV infection recently. But we couldn't explain why there were aortic dilatation and severe damage in aortic valve. CAEBVI usually causes hepatosplenomegaly. The patient spleen wasn't enlarged. Immune-reaction induced by EBV maybe result in KD [6].
3. It has been described in literature that KD patients can have complications with. But it is very rare to see limb artery dilatation alone without coronary artery dilatation [4].KD also complicating with valve damage and resulted in heart failure [7]. But hole valve disappeared never be reported [8,

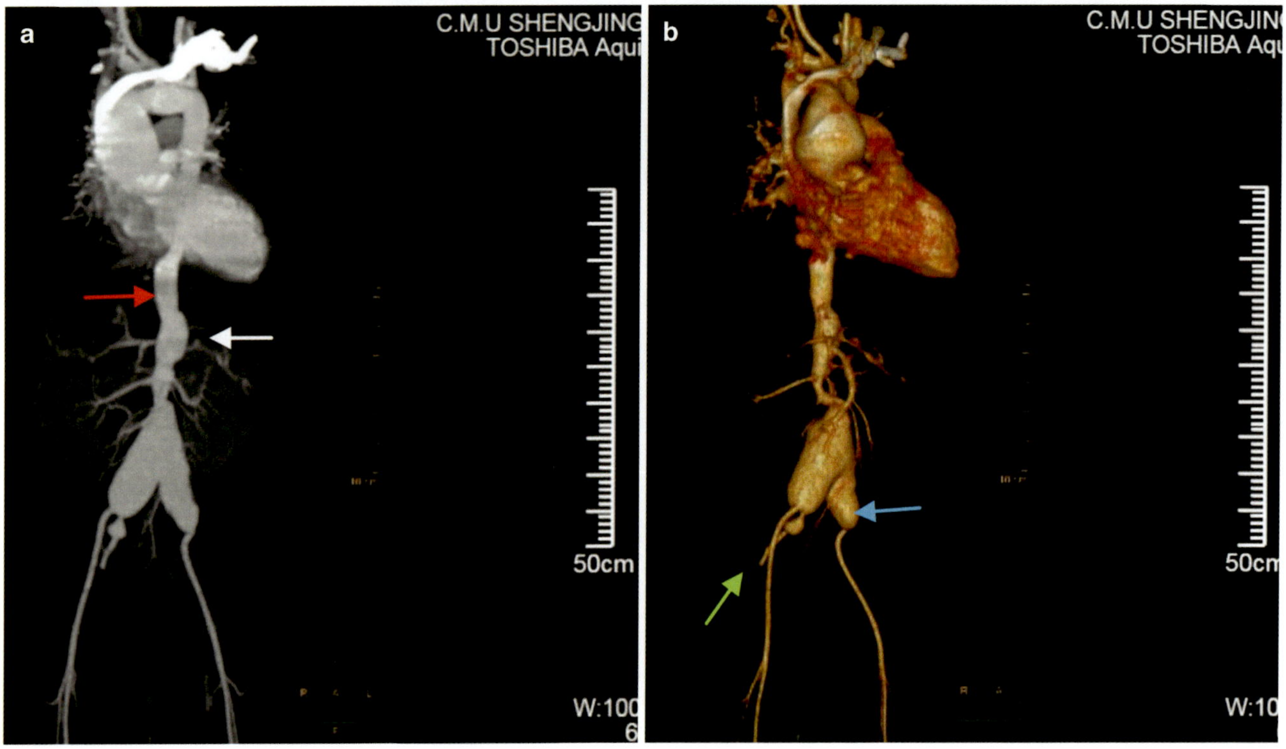

Fig. 14.13 On Day 12 of illness, aortic enhancement CT plus 3D reconstruction: The ascending aorta begins with a cystic dilatation (**a**) (red arrow), the aortic arch and the thoracic aorta are circuitous, the abdominal aortic branches were significantly dilated with uneven size (**a**) (white arrow), the lumen was uneven, and multiple collateral vessels were revealed. The right iliac artery was about 25 mm ( ) (white arrow), the left one about 20 mm (**b**) (blue arrow), iliac artery occlusion from the proximal segment

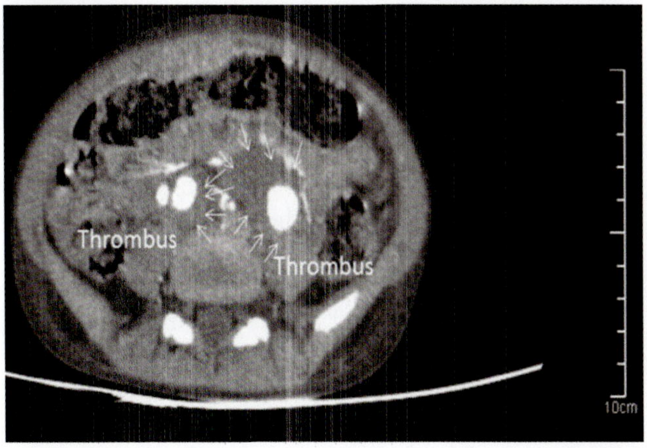

Fig. 14.14 On Day 12 of illness, abdominal aortic enhancement CT scan and 3D reconstruction cross section showed abdominal aortic thrombus (white arrows)

9]. Nodosa polyarteritis can complicate coronary artery dilatation [10]. Thus, the final diagnosis was inclusive, and we had lost her. Based on experience we accumulated in clinic, once chronic heart failure is developed, patients like her had poor prognosis. Despite a lack of final diagnosis, her prognosis was poor, since she had heart failure, especially with jaundice appearing on her sclera.

Hong Wang

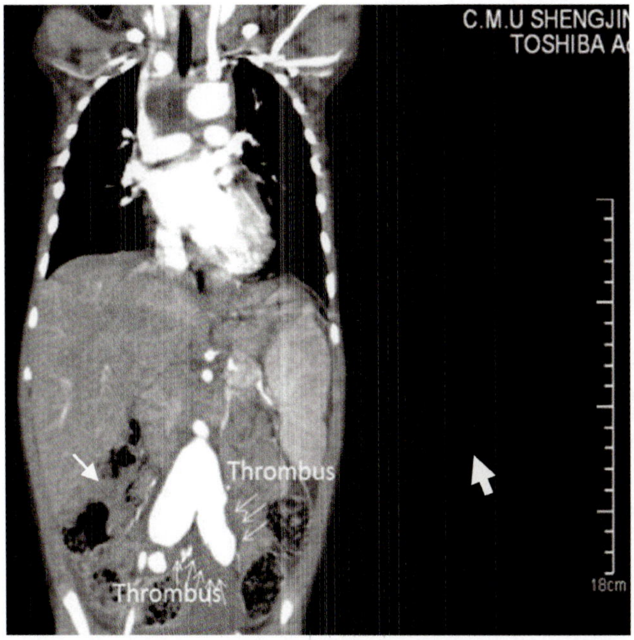

Fig. 14.15 On Day 12 of illness, thoracic aorta and abdominal aortic enhancement coronal showed filling defect (thrombus) in the initial part of the left iliac artery (white arrow), the left internal iliac artery was occluded in the proximal segment. The proximal apex of the right iliac artery was locally bulbous, diameter about 11 mm

14.3 Case 51: Giant CSA with Abdominal Aortic Thrombus and Aortic Valve Disease

A five-year-old girl presented with post medical history of pneumonia, EBV infection, and liver dysfunction seven months ago, and. Myocarditis was suspected six months ago at the local hospital. In addition, she had a chronic allergy to cephalosporin, shrimp, chicken, mutton, sunflower seeds, and egg yolks.

She presented with facial swelling for 6 months, bilateral eyelids edema for two months, and coronary artery dilation for two days. Six months ago, she began to develop fever with no obvious cause along with facial edema that had persisted to this day even though the fever had disappeared. Later she developed blisters on her mouth and lips with yellow snot. She had no cough, vomit or diarrhea. After taking traditional Chinese medicine, the blisters disappeared and snot decreased, but the facial edema was not relieved, and she developed bilateral eyelids edema two months ago, had no changes in vision, bilateral conjunctiva or urine. Meanwhile, there were rashes on her face and trunk, along with pruritus. After treatment with traditional Chinese medicine for 3 days, rashes decreased for some days then resurfaced again, and the venous blood vessels above the lower jaw and at the level of the nipple showed clearly with bluish purple color. She was brought to our clinic two days ago. Echo was performed and revealed coronary artery dilation.

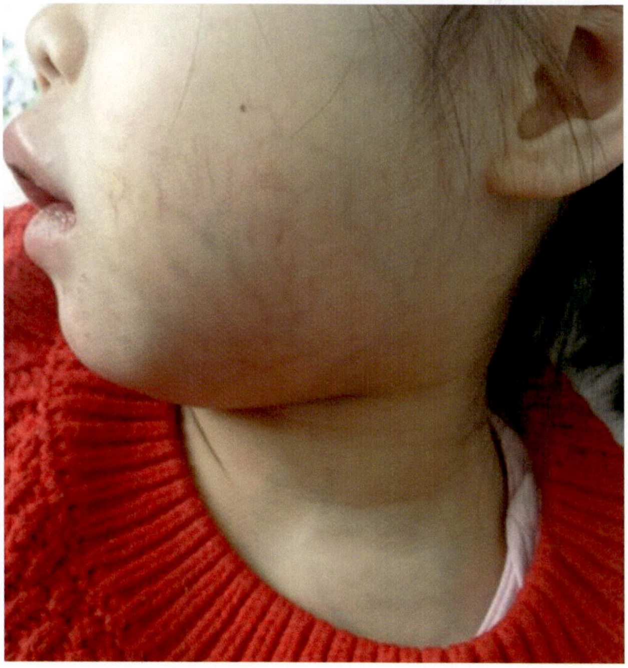

Fig. 14.16 On Day admission, physical examination found veins were prominent over face, neck and superior chest

She was admitted in our pediatric cardiology ward. Examination revealed the follows: her mental stage was stable, her body temperature was 36.6°C, PR 99bpm, RR 24bpm, weight 17.5 kg, BP 90/56mmHg at left arm, 84/53mmHg at right arm, 87/50mmHg at left leg, 78/51mmHg at right leg. She had facial edema and varicose veins all over the mandibular, neck and chest (Fig. 14.16). She also had pharyngeal hyperemia and cervical lymphadenopathy about 1.5cm. Auscultation assessment on heart revealed murmurs on the costal of right 2 and left 3–4, with normal second pulmonary artery sound. Liver was about 5cm below the right costal margin, 4cm below the xiphoid, medium hard. Spleen was about 3cm below the left costal margin, medium hard. There was no nodule along the artery of extremities. Others were normal. Blood work from two days before admission revealed WBC 5.75×10^9/L, NE 47.7%, HGB 123g/L, PLT 158×10^9/L, ALT 69U/L, AST 84U/L, CK 390U/l, CKMB-M 8.9ug/l, NT-pro BNP 308.1pg/ml, cTnT 0.019ng/m. Renal function parameters including CKMB and cTnI were normal. Urine routine showed RBC 3.62 (0.1–2.2/HP), WBC 8.96 (0.1–4.5/HP). EBV-IgG (NA/VCA/EA) were positive. EBV-DNA 1.23×10^4, EBV-IgM and HSV(I+II)-IgM were negative. ECG showed sinus rhythm, HR was 112bpm, PR interval prolonged (168ms) (Fig. 14.17). Chest CT scan showed there were no obvious abnormalities in two lungs. Aortic arch was slightly thick (Fig. 14.18) (Fig. 14.8b). Cervical ultrasound showed bilateral cervical lymphadenectasis. The bigger one was 1.8cm×0.8cm on the left, 1.7cm×0.7cm on the right. Abdominal ultrasound showed both liver and spleen were slightly enlarged. Liver was 1.8cm below the right costal margin, and spleen was 1.2cm below the left costal margin. ECHO showed the aortic sinus aneurysm dilation about 33.4mm (Fig. 14.19a), RCA was about 3.4mm (Fig. 14.19b), LCA about 5.7mm (Fig. 14.20a, b). At the level of atrium, there was a shunt from left to right. TV was mildly regurgitated. She had met the diagnosis of (1) aortic sinus aneurysm dilation, with possible congenital malformation; (2) bilateral coronary artery dilation, and possible KD recovery phase; (3) ASD; (4) chronic active EB virus infection wasn't except. Thus, she was treated with: (1) aspirin and dipyridamole 3–5mg/kg/d, in 3 divided doses; (2) infusion of genciclovir 7.5mg/kg/d for 7days; (3) infusion of medication for maintaining myocardium and liver nourished; (4) PPD test.

On Day 2, she was afebrile. Laboratory test showed CRP, RF, ASO, C_3, C_4, ACCP, ANCA, ANA series, and HLA-B_{27} were negative. ANA titer was positive (1:100). MP-IgG positive. Retested EBV-DNA 1.66×10^4, the total IgE 135.8IU/ml. Retested echo showed LVED 33.8mm, LVEF 73%. The opening of the RCA dilated about 16.6mm and extended about 23.6mm, the far end width was 3.9mm. LCA was 5.8–6.4mm (Fig. 14.21a). LAD was 3.9mm and LCX was 3.5mm (Fig. 14.21b) without thrombosis in the dilated coronary artery. ASD was about 4.8mm. On Day 3, her blood glucose was normal, therefore, glycogen storage disease could be excluded. Results from examinations on related connective tissue diseases were normal. MP-IgG was slightly positive. Carotid artery ultrasound showed the common carotid artery

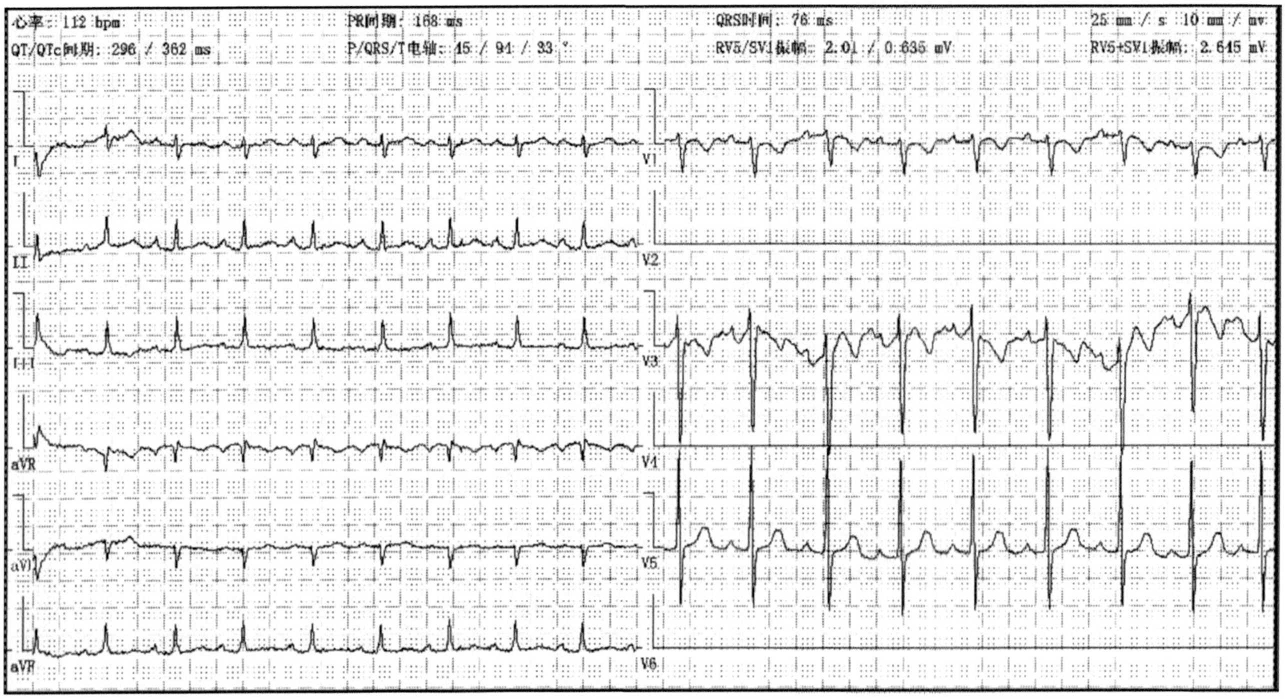

Fig. 14.17 On the day of admission, ECG showed PR interval prolonged (168ms)

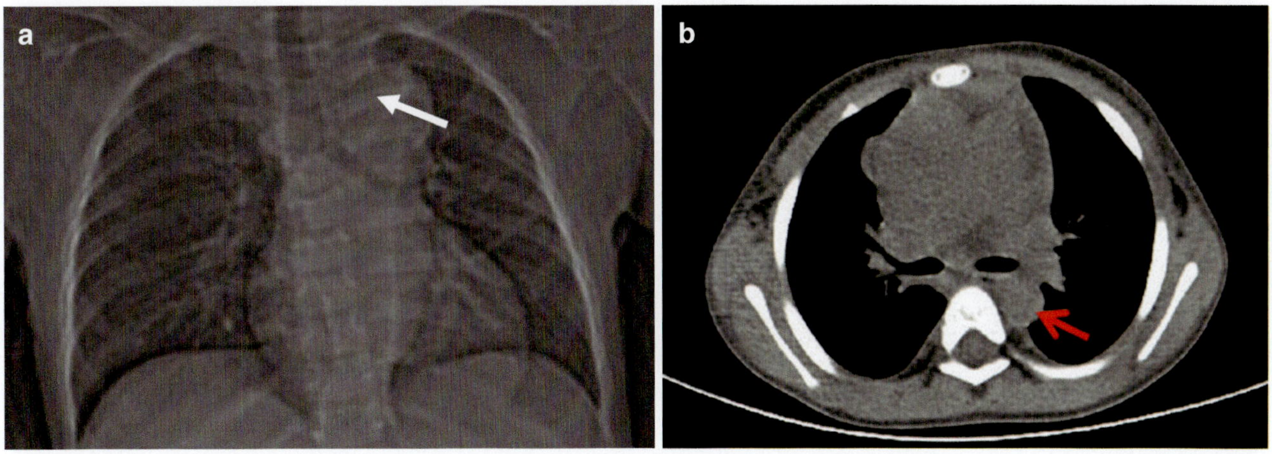

Fig. 14.18 On Day admission, chest DR image in A-P showed aortic arch dilation (**a**) transverse CT image showed thoracic aortic dilation (**b**)

was tortuous and its thickness was about 1.0–1.3 mm (Fig. 14.22a). Bone marrow test revealed they were significant proliferated, with sister nuclear and Howell-Jolly bodies (Fig. 14.22b). On Day 4, there were scattered bleeding spots around her eyelids after she cried. Left arm BP was normal. Doppler ultrasound revealed renal artery, superior vena cava and superior mesenteric artery were normal. Coronary artery CTA and three-dimensional reconstruction showed three innominate artery, left common carotid artery and left subclavian artery were dilated and tortuous (Fig. 14.23a). The proximal segments of LAD,LCX and RCA were tortuous and dilated (Fig. 14.23b). The proximal portion of RCA dilated, showing aneurysm dilatation about 22.6mm (Fig. 14.24a), and the range was about 25.7mm (Fig. 14.24b). ASD was about 4.8mm. The diameters of main branches of each coronary artery were as follows: LM 7.7mm, LAD 3.9mm (Fig. 14.25). LCX 3.5mm, distal segment of RCA was 3.9mm. She had KD with high index at recovery phase, giant CAA and superior vena cava syndrome (SVCS) could not be excluded. Therefore, treatment plans were formed as follows (1) she received warfarin in one dose 1.75mg (0.1mg/kg/d) oral, with DIC monitored every other day to maintain INR between 2 and 3,and discontinuing dipyridamole (see analysis); (2) tests for NK-cells or other immune indicators recommended by pediatric hematologist. If normal, chronic active EB virus infection was not established. Platelets were normal, macrophage activation syndrome (MAS) could be excluded. Eyelids edema, lip thick, peripheral blood vessels around the mandible and papillary level were prominent and blue, and the bleeding point around the eyelids (after crying). Anterior veins and forearm veins were prominent with cyanotic, indicating SVCS. (3) pediatric rheumatologist denied renal disease and vasculitis; (4) tuberculosis specialist told that she had tuberculosis infected but no active stage only follow-up.

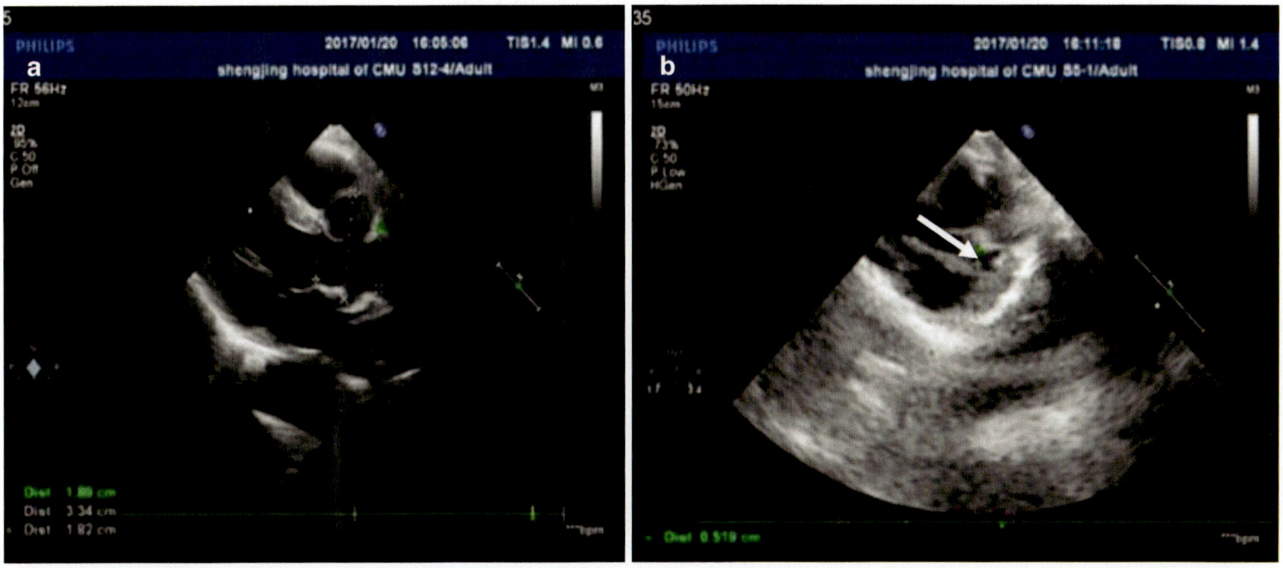

Fig. 14.19 On the 2 days before admission, echocardiography showed aortic aneurysm dilated to 33.4 mm (**a**), LCA dilated to 5.2 mm (**b**).

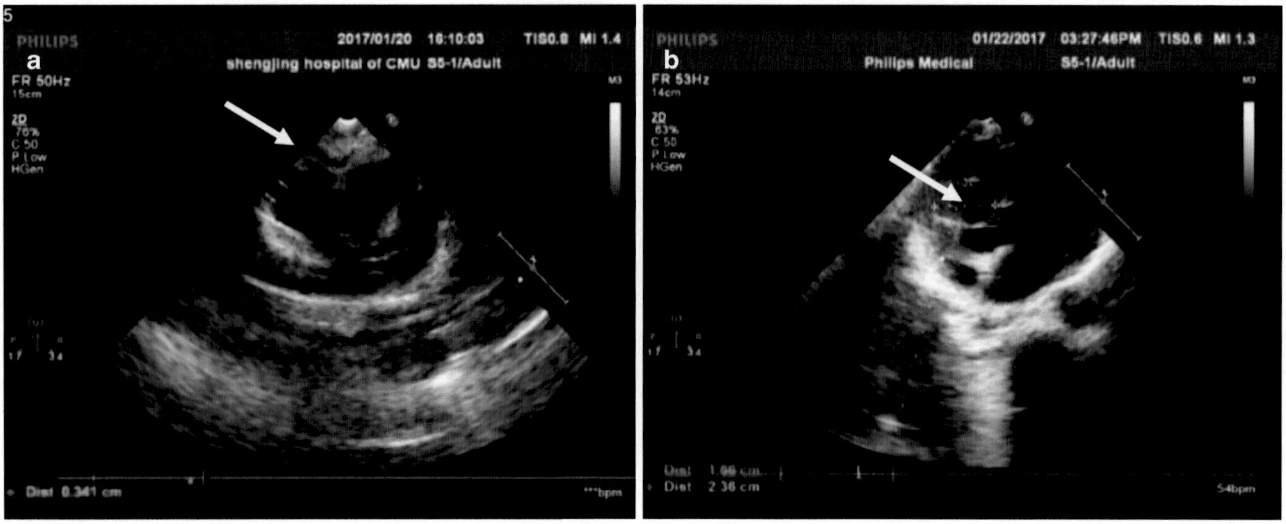

Fig. 14.20 Echocardiography showed RCA dilated to 3.4 mm on the 2 days before admission (**a**), right coronary sinus dilated to 16.6 mm × 23.6 mm on the day of admission (**b**)

On Day 10, retested INR 2.1, warfarin was reduced to 1.25mg once a day. On Day 16, she had fever with vomiting once. Retested INR was 1.3, oral warfarin 1.25mg once a day. Aortic arch ultrasound was normal. Echo showed LCA dilated about 8.8mm (Fig. 14.26a). LAD dilated about 4.8mm (Fig. 14.26b, upper arrow). LCX dilated about 5mm (Fig. 14.26b, lower arrow). The middle segment of RCA moderately dilated about 3.2mm (Fig. 14.27a). And MV mildly regurgitated (Fig. 14.27b). AV mildly regurgitated (Fig. 14.28a). In addition, there was echo reflex in the LCA (Fig. 14.28b). On the following day, she was afebrile. Test blood work showed WBC 3.1×10^9/L, NE 51.2%, HGB 107g/L, PLT 144×10^9/L, CRP 24.70mg/L. For her disease was so complex and clinical symptoms without significant improved after treatment, we advised her oral warfarin, aspirin, fructose and levocarnitine, transfer to the Beijing Children's Hospital as soon as possible.

14.3.1 Follow-up

She was diagnosed with CAA in Beijing Children's Hospital. After Oral medication we prescribed at discharge for several weeks, her general state was improved. Nine months later, she felt sick in the morning, and suddenly died in home a few minutes later.

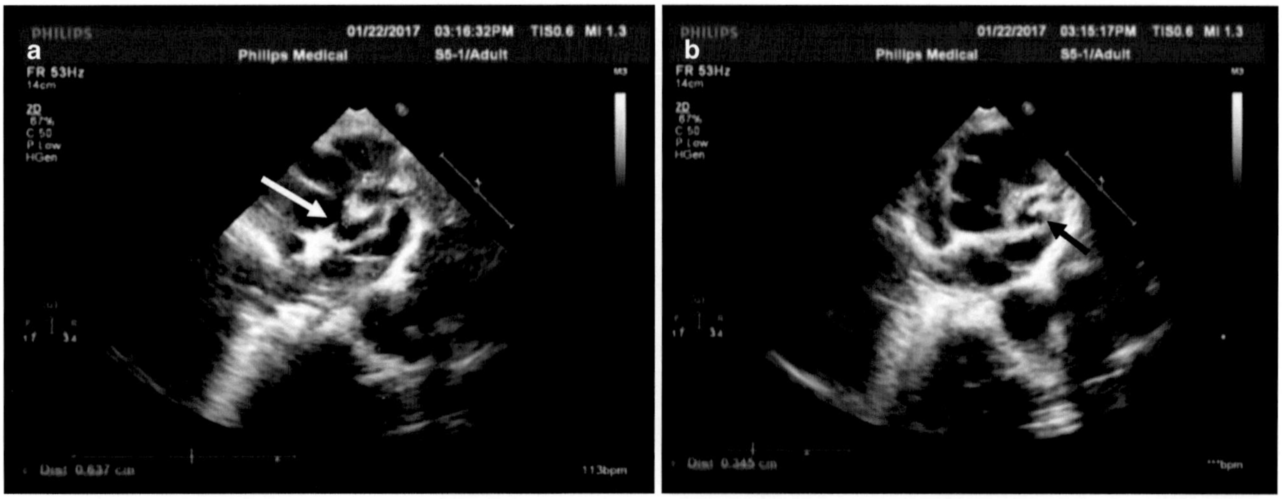

Fig. 14.21 On the day of admission, echocardiography showed LCA dilated to 5.8–6.4 mm (**a**), LCX dilated to 3.5 mm (**b**)

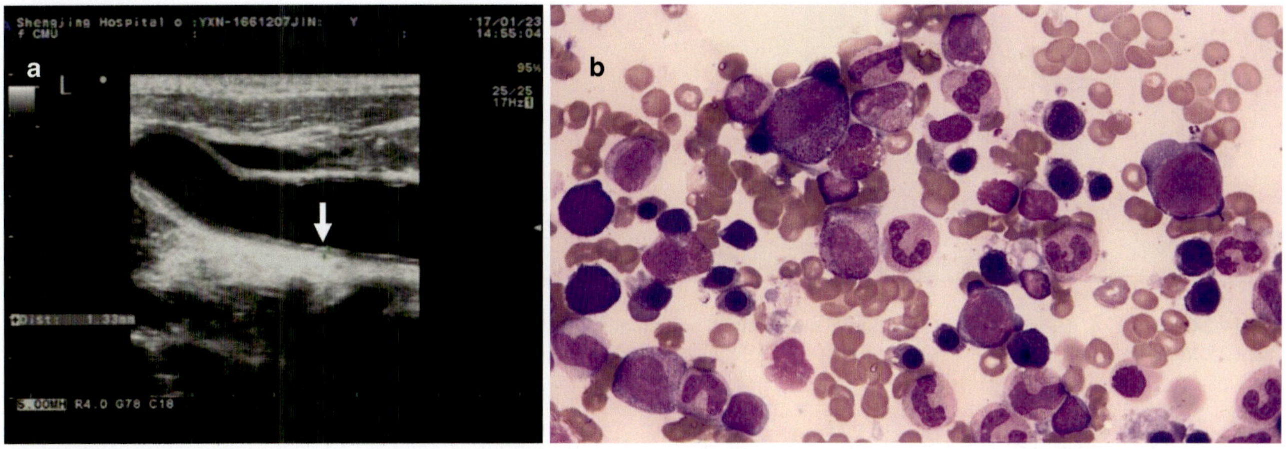

Fig. 14.22 On Day 3 of illness, ultrasound showed the intima thickness at left carotid artery reached up to 1 mm (**a**), bone marrow showed significantly proliferate (**b**)

14.3.2 Diagnosis

1. AKD, sequela period?
2. Giant CAA
3. Takayasu's Arteritis need to exclude
4. EBV infection
5. TB infection
6. ASD

14.3.3 Discussion

The diagnosis of atypical KD was not sufficient. Half year ago she had fever for more than 5 days, along with bilateral coronary artery dilatation; other symptoms were difficult to collected because it happened half a year ago and she still with different symptoms.

She didn't exclude Takayasu's Arteritis: her echo showed aortic sinus aneurysm, bilateral carotid artery wall thickened, and her legs Bp lower than arms. But she had no vascular murmur in abdominal aorta, no hypertension, and Doppler ultrasound showed the blood flow of renal artery and aortic arch were normal, Bp less than 10 mmHg and connective tissue disease antibodies were negative.

14.3.4 Case Specific Clinical Features

1. Differential diagnosis of SVCS should be considered. It has been reported that the syndrome is caused by the stenosis or occlusion of the vena cava before the blood of superior vena cava returning to the right atrium. The clinical manifestations include facial swelling, thick neck, dilate veins over neck and anterior chest. When the odd vein is blocked, dilated veins will be seen on the chest

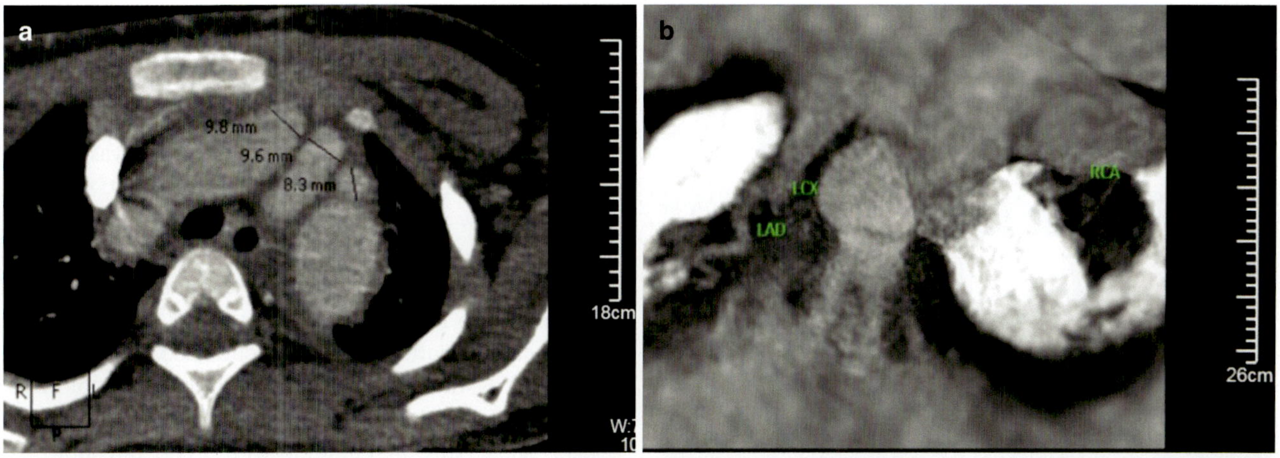

Fig. 14.23 On Day 4 of admission, innominate artery, left common carotid artery and left subclavian artery were dilated and tortuous (**a**). The proximal segments of LAD, LCX and RCA were tortuous and dilated in coronary CTA (**b**)

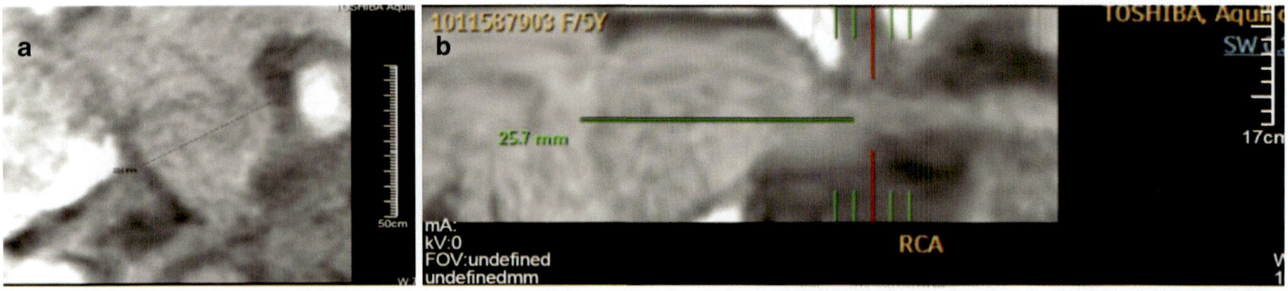

Fig. 14.24 On Day 4, coronary artery CTA showed the proximal portion of RCA aneurysm dilated about 22.6mm (**a**), long axis section of RCA about 25.7mm (**b**)

wall and the upper abdominal wall. When blocked at the end of the superior vena cava or the junction of the odd vein, dilated veins will be seen on the upper chest. When the superior vena cava is severely blocked, there will be signs of obstruction in airway (for wheezing) and even ejection of vomiting. Several causes are speculated: (1) A tumor invades or oppresses the superior vena cava; (2) Oppression of non-malignant diseases, such as post sternal thyroid tumor, thymoma, bronchus cyst, or cervical chronic fibrous tissue inflammation leading to compression around the superior vena cava, such as idiopathic sclerosis of mediastinitis, mediastinal fibrosis and so on; (3) Thrombosis of the superior vena cava, congenital heart disease and postoperative central venous catheterization or pacemaker implantation can cause thrombosis. This girl had facial edema, dilated veins on neck and anterior chest. But imaging results from pulmonary CT and superior vena cava vascular Doppler ultrasound were normal, which did not support tumor compression or superior vena cava thrombosis. Bone marrow puncture did not support tumor. Therefore diagnosis of tumor was excluded.

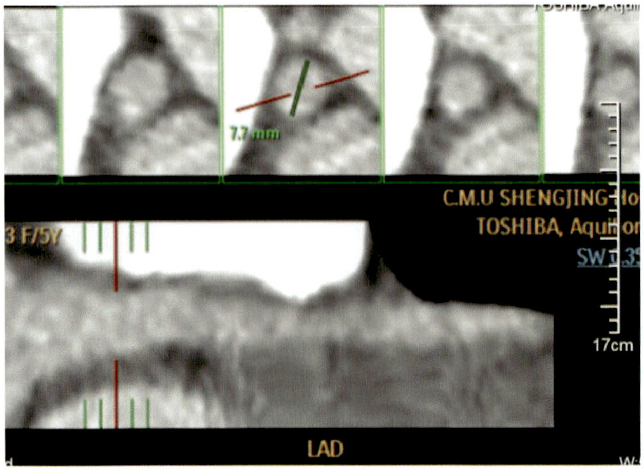

Fig. 14.25 On Day 4 of illness, coronary CTA shows LM expansion

2. Differential diagnosis of hemophagocytic syndromes (HPS) was considered. Positive EB DNA, hepatosplenomegaly, bilateral palpebral edema, and liver dysfunction together seemed likely to agree with HPS. But she didn't have persistent fever, and DIC, HGB, PLT, and bone marrow test were normal. Therefore HPS was excluded.
3. Differential diagnosis of chronic active EBV infection (CAEBV) was considered. The diagnosis criteria for CAEBV include [11]: I. the following conditions persist more than 6 months: a) symptoms persist from the initial infection of EB virus; b) abnormal titer of EB virus antibody (including EB VCA-IgG>1:5120, EA-IgG>1:640 or NA-IgG>1:2); II. Histological signs of major organ injury: a) Lymphadenitis; b) Hemophagy; c) Meningitis; d) Persistent hepatitis; e) Splenomegaly; f) Interstitial pneumonia; g) Dysplasia of bone marrow; h) Retinitis. III. EBV are confirmed from damaged tissue and peripheral blood: a) EBV-DNA, RNA or protein increases in damaged tissue; b) EBV DNA increases in peripheral blood. Attention: a diagnosis of CAEBV should meet with at least one of the above items, and any known immunodeficiency including HIV infection should be ruled out. Although the pathogenesis is not clear, severe cardiovascular damage is common in children with CAEBV. Based on the guidelines listed above, it was impossible to confirm that it has been 6 months. Hepatomegaly and liver dysfunction were not clear whether she had had before this. As a result, persistent hepatitis cannot be diagnosed. Besides, she was splenomegaly. EBV-DNA in peripheral blood was 1.05×10^5, but bone marrow was almost normal. As a result, she could not be diagnosed with CAEBV.
4. It has been reported that KD and coronary artery injury are related to EBV infection or HPS [12, 13]. However, some cases report that EBV infection and KD overlap in immune dysfunction, leading to the formation of coronary aneurysm. In China, it has been reported that coronary aneurysms in children with EBV infection are similar to those associated with KD [14], but there are other KD manifestations except fever and coronary

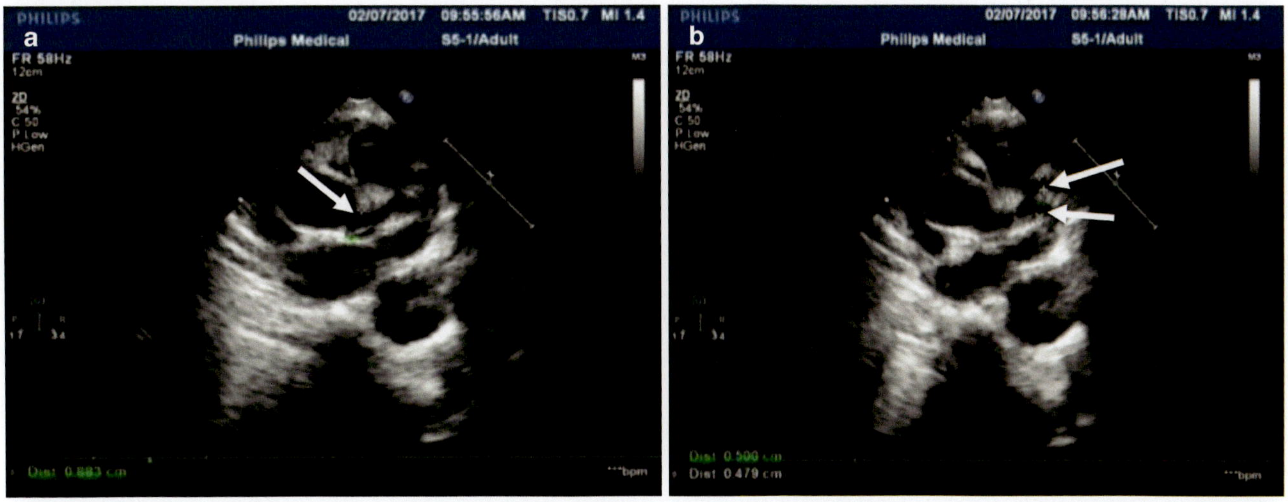

Fig. 14.26 On Day 16 of illness, echocardiography showed LCA dilated to 8.8 mm (**a**), LAD dilated to 4.8 mm (**b**) (superior arrow), LCX dilated to 5 mm (**b**) (inferior arrow)

aneurysms. EBV infection can also contribute to the formation of coronary aneurysms [15].

5. This case was characterized by atypical symptoms and no effective therapy. Echo indicated the presence of giant coronary sinus aneurysm. This change is more commonly seen in coronary arterial-pulmonary fistula, but it was not found in her echo. Laboratory test revealed positive EBV infection. When she was admitted to the hospital, examination found facial swelling, prominent veins on her neck and chest along with hepatosplenomegaly. We could not conclude whether she had EBV infection before her admission. The symptoms of KD were not incompletely, fever persisted for more than 5 days, as for the change of lymph node usually recovered less than 2 weeks. Thus, it has no significance after 6 months to the onset of illness. After receiving treatments for antiviral, liver protection and anticoagulation, her symptoms did not improve. Although her face was special, the blood glucose was at normal level, thus glycogen storage disease was excluded. Examination revealed negative connective tissue disease related antibody, therefore this one was excluded, too. The diagnosis was not very clear, perhaps the EBV infection related KD, but the dilated veins above chest cannot be explained, the patient should follow up, but she had died unfortunately, and her diagnosis kept secret forever.

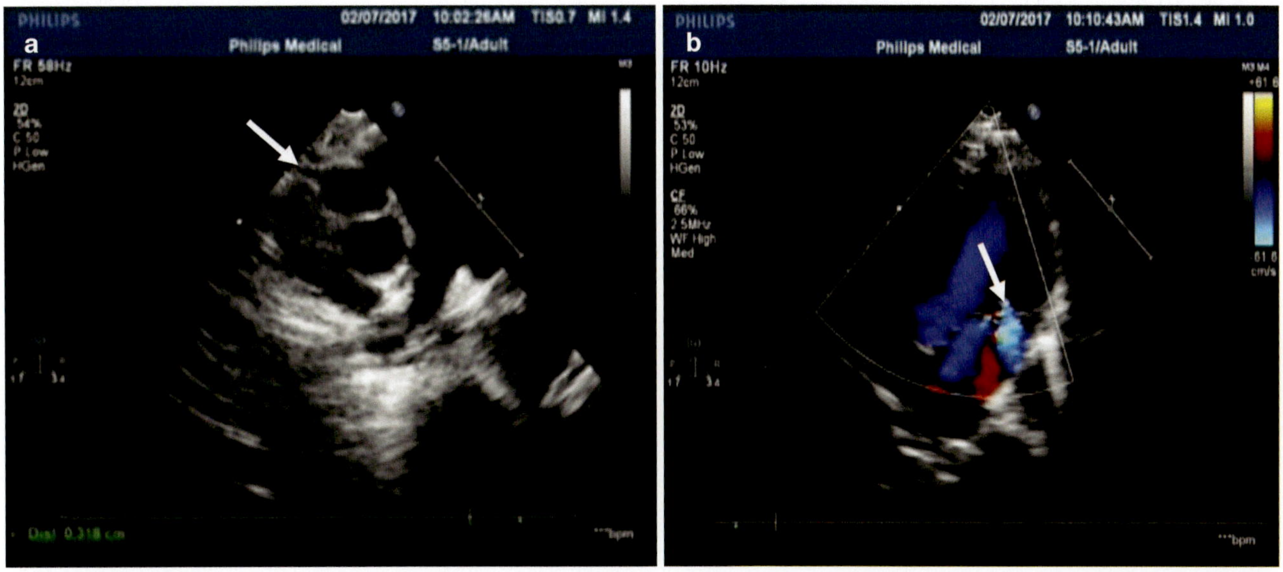

Fig. 14.27 On Day 16 of illness, echocardiography showed the middle segment of RCA slightly dilated to 3.2 mm (**a**) (white arrow), mild mitral valve regurgitation (**b**)

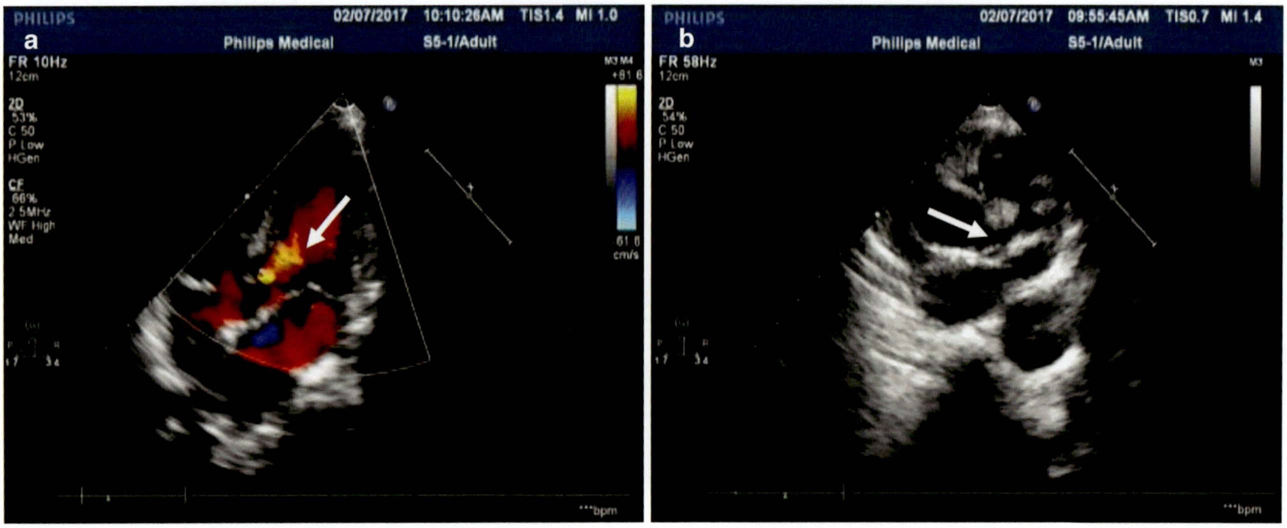

Fig. 14.28 On Day 16 of illness, echocardiography showed mild aortic valve regurgitation (**a**), additional echogenicity was found in LCA (**b**)

Xiao-zhe Cui

References

1. Newburger JW, Takahashi M, Gerber MA, et al. Diagnosis, treatment, and long-term management of Kawasaki disease: a statement for health professionals from the Committee on Rheumatic Fever, Endocarditis and Kawasaki Disease, Council on Cardiovascular Disease in the Young, American Heart Association. Circulation. 2004;110(17):2747–71.
2. Zhu FT. Practical paidonosology [M]. 6th ed. Beijing: People's Medicine Publishing House; 1996. p. 684.
3. Ristovski L, Milankov O, Vislavski M, et al. Atypical Kawasaki disease. Med Pregl. 2016;69(1-2):53–7.
4. Eleftheriou D, Levin M, Shingadia D, et al. Management of Kawasaki disease. Arch Dis Child. 2014;99(1):74–83.
5. Dionne A, Meloche-Dumas L, Desjardins L, et al. NT-pro BNP diagnostic algorithm for Kawasaki Disease compared to AHA Algorithm. Pediatr Int. 2016;59(3):265–70. https://doi.org/10.1111/ped.13154.
6. Culora GA, Moore IE. Kawasaki disease, Epstein-Barr virus and coronary artery aneurysms. J Clin Pathol. 1997 Feb;50(2):161–3.
7. Honda T, Ogata S, Ishii M. Incomplete Kawasaki disease: early findings consist of congestive heart failure due to valvular heart disease. Heart Asia. 2011;3(1):92.
8. McCrindle BW, Rowley AH, Newburger JW, et al. Diagnosis, treatment, and long-term management of Kawasaki Disease: a scientific statement for health professionals from the American Heart Association. Circulation. 2017;135(17):e927–99.
9. Printz BF, Sleeper LA, Newburger JW, et al. Noncoronary cardiac abnormalities are associated with coronary artery dilation and with laboratory inflammatory markers in acute Kawasaki disease. J Am Coll Cardiol. 2011;57(1):86–92.
10. Ebersberger U, Rieber J, Wellmann P, et al. Poly arteritis nodosa causing a vast coronary artery aneurysm. J Am Coll Cardiol. 2015;65(5):e1–2.
11. Subspecialty Group of Endocrinologic, Hereditary and Metabolic Diseases, the Society of Pediatrics, Chinese Medical Association. Consensus statement on diagnosis and treatment of congenital adrenal hyperplasia due to 21-hydroxylase deficiency. Chin J Pediatr. 2016;54(8):569–76.
12. Kawamura Y, Miura H, Matsumoto Y, et al. A case of Epstein-Barr virus-associated hemophagocytic lymphohistiocytosis with severe cardiac complications. BMC Pediatr. 2016;16(1):172.
13. Pavone P, Cocuzza S, Passaniti E, et al. Otorrhea in Kawasaki disease diagnosis complicated by an EBV infection: coincidental disease or a true association. Eur Rev Med Pharmacol Sci. 2013;17(7):989–93.
14. Kato S, Yoshimura K, Tanabe Y, et al. A child with Epstein-Barr Virus-associated hemophagocytic lymphohistiocytosis complicated by coronary artery lesion mimicking Kawasaki disease. J Pediatr Hematol Oncol. 2013;35(7):e317–9.
15. Nishimura S, Ehara S, Hanatani A, et al. Chronic active Epstein-Barr virus infection complicated with multiple artery aneurysms. Eur Heart J Cardiovasc Imaging. 2014;15(11):1255.

15 Vaccination Induced KD-Case 52-Polio Vaccine

Hong Wang and Jing Dong

Abstract

The etiology of KD is unknown, but it is currently recognized that the infection is caused by allergic vasculitis, often involving small and medium arteries. There are two types of immunization: inactivated vaccines (dead vaccines) and attenuated live vaccines. In the US, KD after vaccination happens mostly associated with Pediarix [DTaP, hep B, and intramuscular injection of polio vaccine (IPV) combined] but did not show an increase of KD [Hua et al., Pediatr Infect Dis J. 28(11):943–7, 2009; Abrams et al., Vaccine. 33(2):382–7, 2015], though there is a different opinion [Chang and Islam Pediatr Int. 2018]. The DTaP, hep B, and IPV vaccines are live attenuated vaccines. Polio vaccine comes in two forms: injections and sugar pills. IPV first was produced in 1953 by Dr. Jonas Salk, for intramuscular injection. In 1960s, Dr. Albert Sabin produced attenuated live vaccine, also called Sabin vaccination. It was for oral polio vaccine (OPV), though there was literature reporting that OPV cab resulted in acute disseminated encephalomyelitis [Shibazaki et al., Intern Med. 45(20):1143–6, 2006]. OPV was popular in China as sugar coated pills, and supposed to be taken orally three times. The disadvantage of OPV is that it will cause KD and diarrhea in patients who have innate immune deficiency. Cooling reservation are important factors to keep it effective.

Redden sign surrounding Bacille Calmette-Guérin (BCG) vaccination scar is very important in KD diagnosis [Kuniyuki and Asada, J Am Acad Dermatol. 37(2 Pt 2):303–4, 1997; Hulme, Emerg Med J. 29(7):598–9, 2012; Garrido-García et al., Pediatr Infect Dis J. 36(10):e237–41, 2017; Gamez-Gonzalez et al., Hum Vaccin Immunother. 13(5):1091–3, 2017]. It usually happened between days 31–806 after BCG inoculated [Araki et al., J Int Med Res. 46(4):1640–8, 2018].

This chapter presented an 85-day-old boy who developed KD after IVP. He had taken oral pill one month ago without any uncomfort. This time he was asked to have IPV. KD most happened in person with allergic. IPV may be easier to trigger allergic reaction and developed KD. Fortunately, his prognosis was nice.

A previous healthy 85-day-old boy had significant past medical history and family history.

He presented on Day 7 of illness. On the first day, he had polio vaccine. About six hours later, he had remitted fever >39°C. On the second day he was brought to a local hospital and was diagnosed with vaccine reaction. He took oral acetaminophen for 3 days. On Day 4, his fever did not regress and rashes developed all over the body, without itch, along with bilateral conjunctivitis (Fig. 15.1a). Red lips, strawberry tongue, edema in hands and feet were also developed. He was admitted to the local hospital and received infusion of azithromycin for one day and other antivirus medications for two days. His fever did not subside and cracked lips developed. Thus, he was transferred to our pediatric cardiology ward. He had developed significant malaise and irritability during sleep since the onset of illness. He lost appetite, but without nausea, vomit, or diarrhea. He did not cough or cry when urinating. Examination revealed the followings: his body temperature was 38.5°C, HR160 bpm, RR 28bpm, and weight 7.5 kg. His mental state was well. Lips were strikingly cracked (Fig. 15.2b). He had strawberry tongue, bilateral no-purulent conjunctivitis, and congested rashes all over the body and around BGC scar (Fig. 15.2a). Hepatomegaly was 3 cm below the right costal margin. When examined at the area, he did not cry. Edema was in hands (Fig. 15.2b) and feet. CRT<3 s, perianal was red without peeling. Others were normal. Blood work at admission revealed WBC 30.0 × 109/L, NE 67.8%,

H. Wang (✉)
Department of Pediatric Cardiology, Shengjing Hospital of China Medical University, Shenyang, China

J. Dong
Department of cardiology Function, Shengjing Hospital of China Medical University, Shenyang, China

H. Wang (ed.), *Paediatric Kawasaki Disease*, https://doi.org/10.1007/978-981-15-0038-1_15

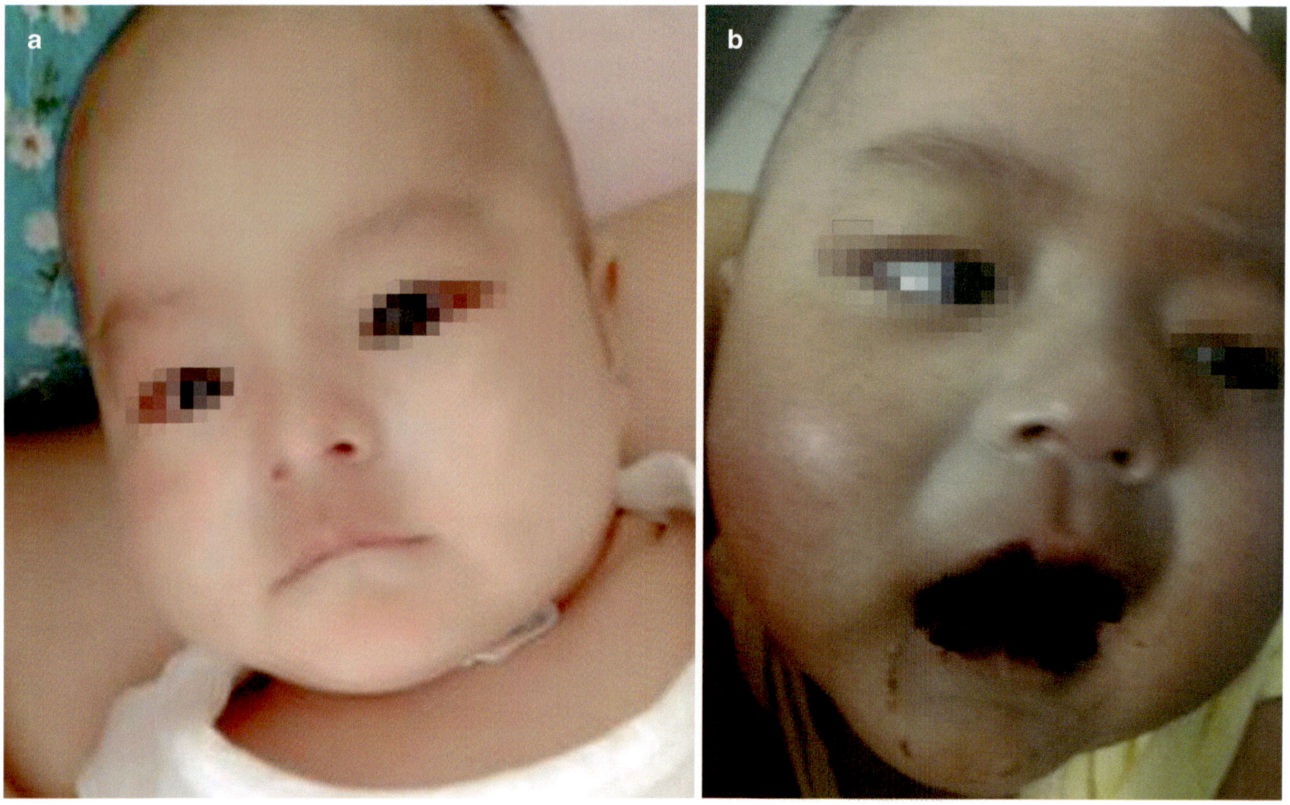

Fig. 15.1 On Day 4 of illness, he developed bilateral conjunctivitis (**a**). On Day 7 of illness, his lips were strikingly cracked (**b**)

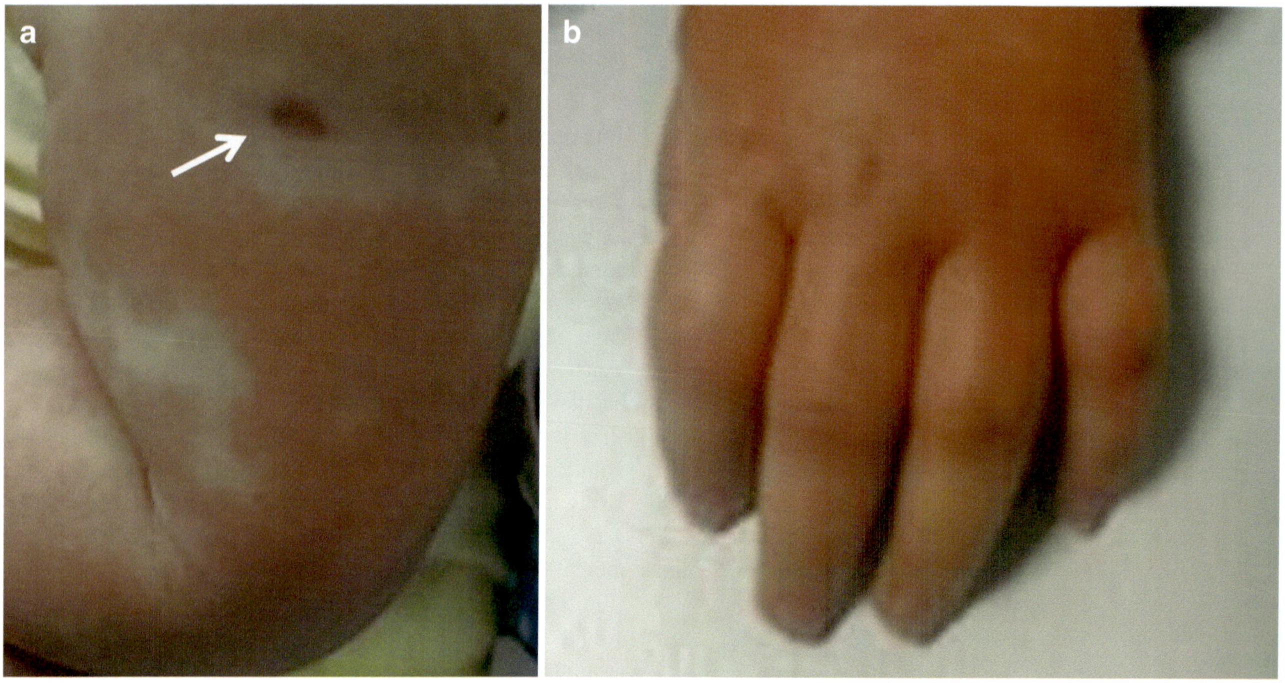

Fig. 15.2 On Day 7 of illness, skin around Bacille Calmette-Guérin (BCG) was red (**a**). Fingers were edema (**b**)

HGB 96 g/L, PLT 396 × 109/L. Urine WBC 251.67/μl, urinary cast 5.56 (0–2.25/μl), bacteria 172.10 (0–111.4/μl), RBC 1.30 (0.1–2.2/HP), WBC 45.30 (0.1–2.2/HP), CRP 161 mg/L, NT-pro BNP 823.2 pg/ml, D-Dimer 1267 μg/L. Blood and gas analysis was normal. Cervical ultrasound showed lymphadenectasis about 2.1 cm × 1.0 cm on the left (Fig. 15.3a). He had met the 5/5 criteria for KD. He was treated with: (1) blood drawn for culture; (2) IVIG 1g/kg/d for 2 days; (3) aspirin 30–50mg/kg/day and dipyridamole 3–5mg/kg/day, in three divided doses oral; (4) infusion of creatine phosphate sodium 0.5g/day.

On Day 8, his fever regressed to 37°C with running nose. His appetite got better. Physical examination did not show improvements. Laboratory test revealed: urine glucose ++++ (sample take during glucose infusion). Liver function ALB 29.1g/L, GTP 50U/L, γ-GT 439U/L. MP-IgM and CP-IgG were positive. EB-IgG NA and EB-IgG VCA were positive, PINF-IgA was positive. Liver ultrasound revealed enlarged liver (Fig. 15.3b). ECG showed I AVB (Fig. 15.4). Chest CT scan showed inflammation scattered at both lungs (Fig. 15.5a). Having hypoalbuminemia, MP infection, liver dysfunction, and PINF infection, he was treated with infusion of (1) erythromycin; (2) albumin; (3) medications to protect liver on next day.

On Day 9, he was afebrile. Bilateral conjunctivitis, rashes, edema hands and feet were improved, but lips were still red and dry (Fig. 15.5b).

On Day 10, he was afebrile for 48 hours. Bilateral conjunctivitis, rashes, edema hands and feet were settled, with only lips remaining cracked. The dose of aspirin was reduced to 3–5 mg/kg/dayqd. Retested blood work revealed WBC 11.26 × 109/L, NE 35.8%, HGB 84g/L, PLT 504 × 109/L, CRP 24.8mg/L, GPT 41U/L, AST 36U/L, γ-GT 278U/L, NT-pro BNP 987.6pg/ml, D-dimer 1051 μg/L. Urine WBC 13.80/HP, urinary cast 9.19/μl. ALB recovered to 37.7 g/L. ECG still showed I AVB (Fig. 15.6). Echo showed normal coronary artery (Fig. 15.7a–b). He was discharged.

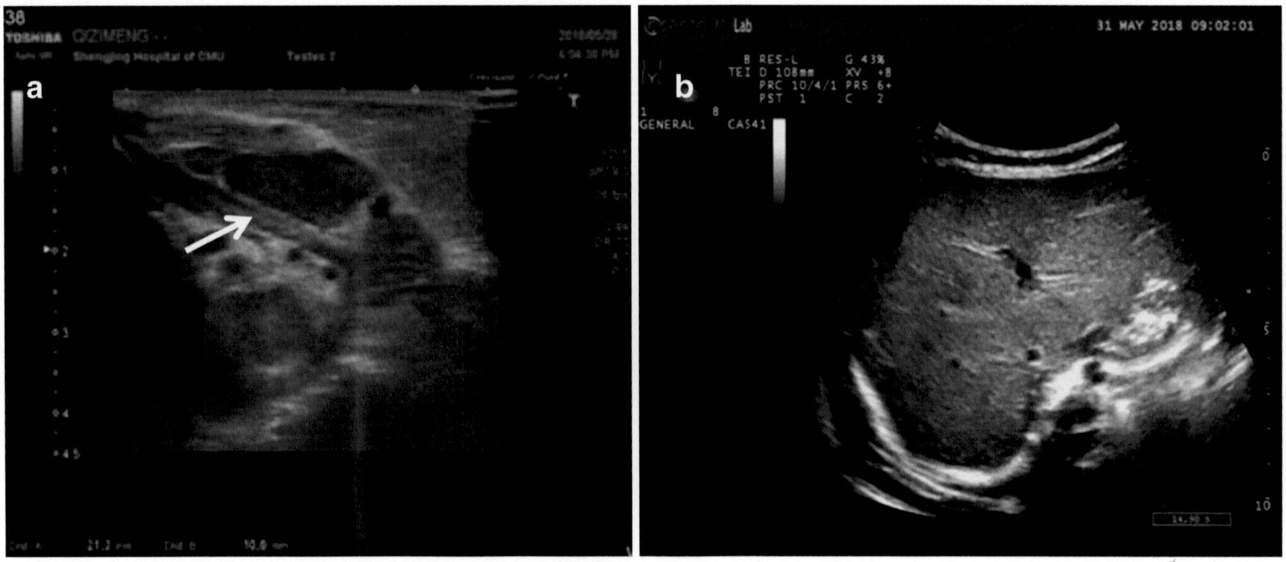

Fig. 15.3 On Day 7 of illness, ultrasound showed left cervical lymphadenopathy about 2.1 cm (**a**), on the Day 8 of illness, liver ultrasound showed the liver enlargement (**b**)

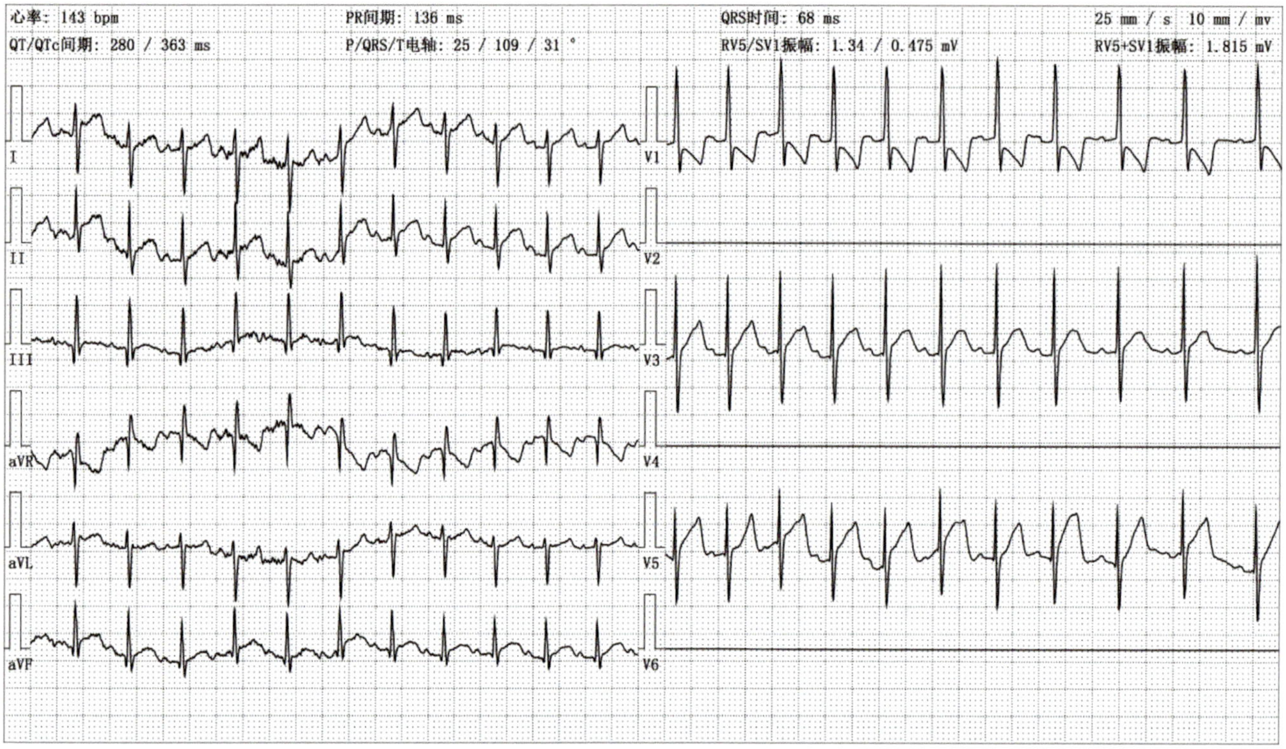

Fig. 15.4 On Day 8 of illness, ECG showed I AVB (HR143bpm, PR interval was 135 ms)

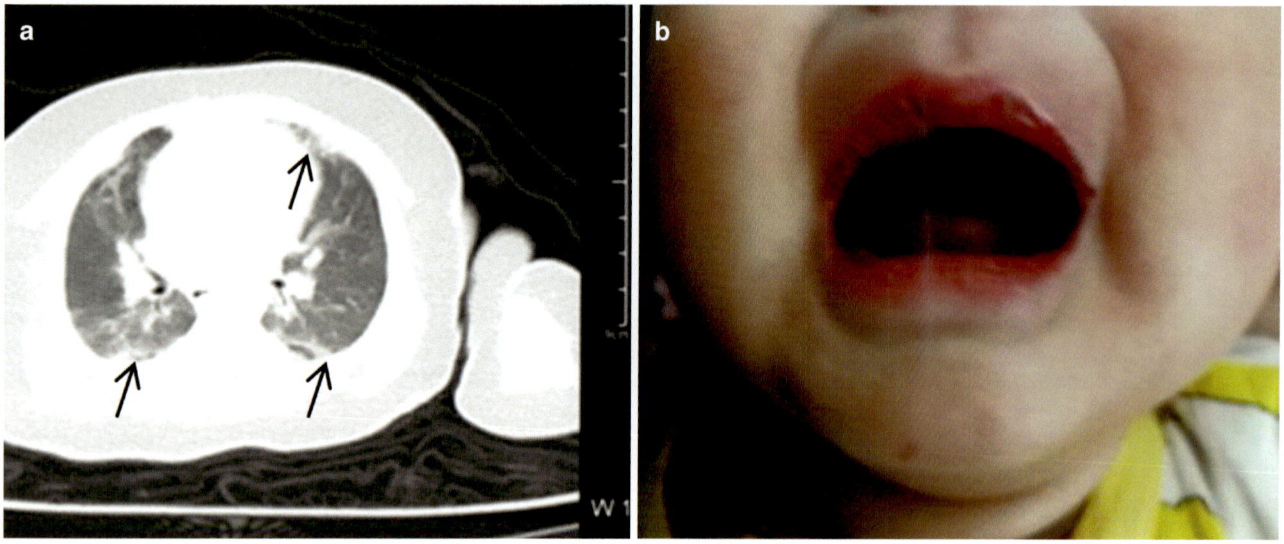

Fig. 15.5 On Day 9 of illness, chest CT showed inflammation scattered on both lungs (**a**). His lips still red and dry (**b**)

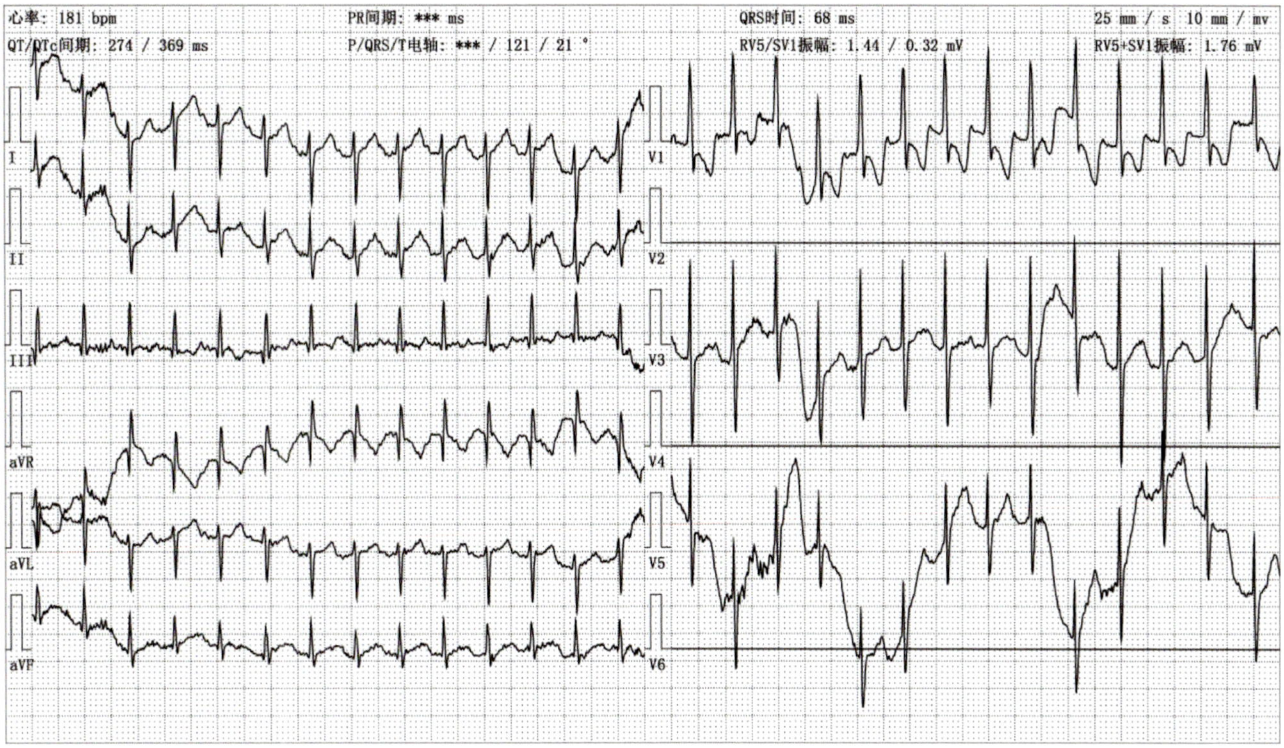

Fig. 15.6 On Day 10 of illness, his ECG was I AVB (HR 181bpm, PR interval was 155 ms)

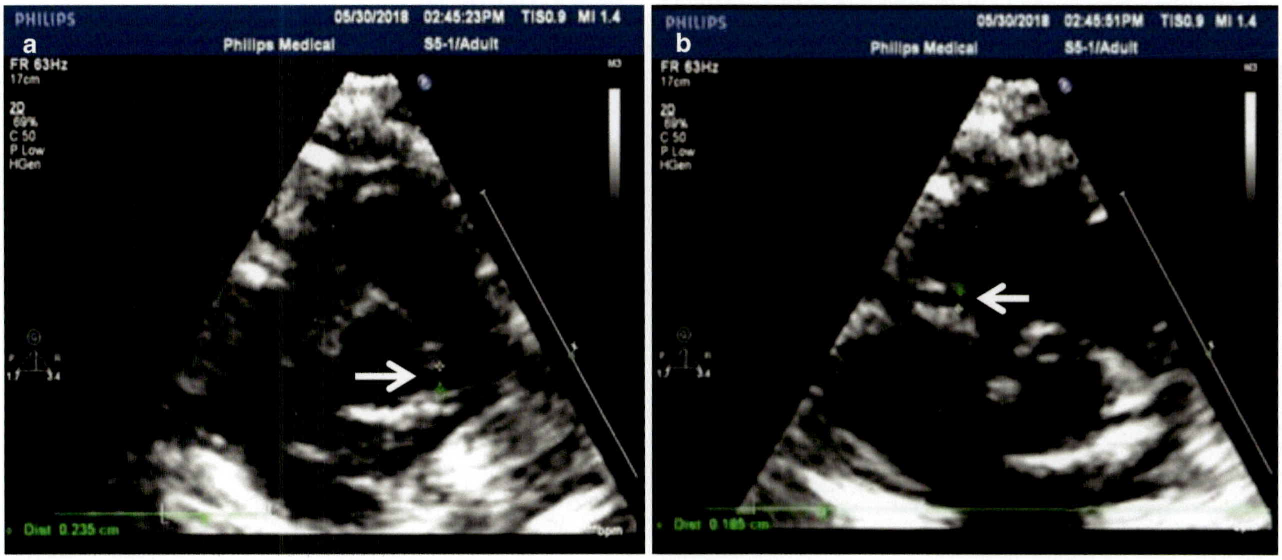

Fig. 15.7 On Day 10 of illness, echo showed normal LCA (**a**) and RCA (**b**)

15.1.1 Clinical Course of the Patient

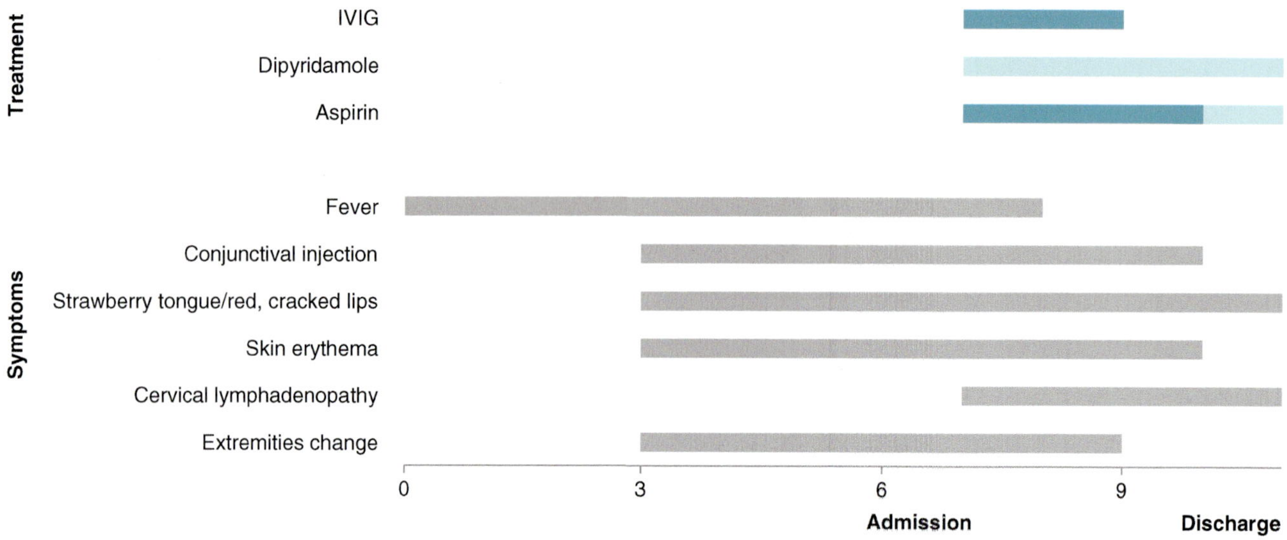

15.1.2 Follow-up

After discharge, he was prescribed to take (1) erythromycin for one week; (2) ferralia and vitamin C for one month; (3) aspirin, dipyridamole and FDP. Peeling skin occurred around fingernails at 2 weeks of illness, followed by peeling skin around toenails 5 days later (Fig. 15.8). His fingernails (Fig. 15.9a) and toenails became shriveled (Fig. 15.9b) at one month of illness. Retested blood work revealed PLT, ESR, NT-pro BNP, and DIC were normal, and tested routine urine was normal at 2 months of illness. ECG (Fig. 15.10) and echo showed normal measurements. Thus, all medication were stopped except for ferralia and vitamin C for additional one month.

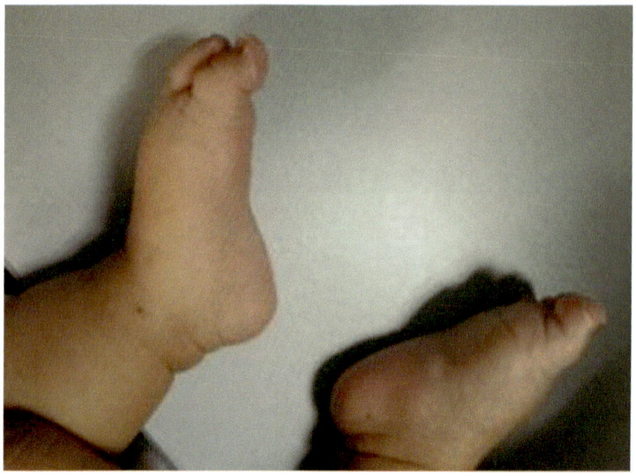

Fig. 15.8 On Day 21 of illness, peeling skin occurred around toenails

At 6 months of illness, repeated echo showed normal results (Table 15.1).

15.1.3 Diagnosis

1. KD
2. Liver dysfunction
3. Hypoalbuminemia
4. Sterile urethritis
5. Moderate anemia
6. MP infection
7. PINF infection
8. Acute pneumonia.

15.1.4 Discussion

He had met the criteria of KD for he had prolonged fever over 5 days, and antibiotics treatment had no effects, along with (1) congested rashes all over body and redden Bacille Calmette-Guérin (BCG) inoculation site; (2) bilateral no-purulent conjunctivitis; (3) strikingly red and cracked lips, and straw berry tongue; (4) edema in hands and feet; (5) cervical lymphadenectasis about 2.1 cm on the left. He had met the criteria of sterile urethritis for (1) he had KD; (2) he did not cry when urinating; test urine revealed significantly increased WBC, without/or little RBC, without positive bacteria growth in cultural test. Therefore, special antibiotics were not needed. He recovered after IVIG. Different diagnosis of sepsis should be considered.

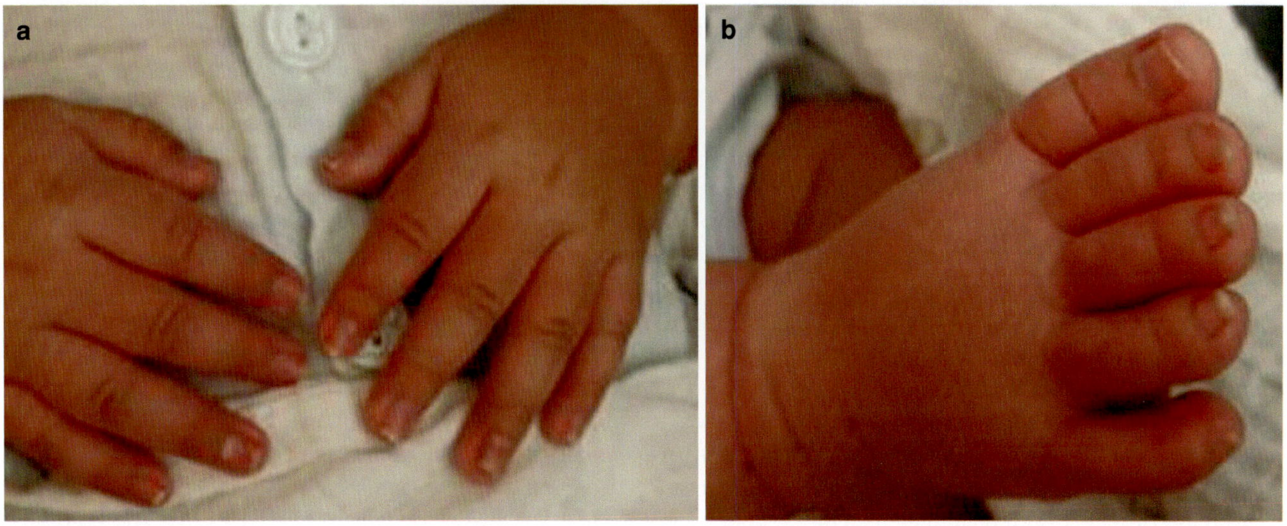

Fig. 15.9 On Day 37 of illness, fingernails (O) and toenails (P) became shriveled

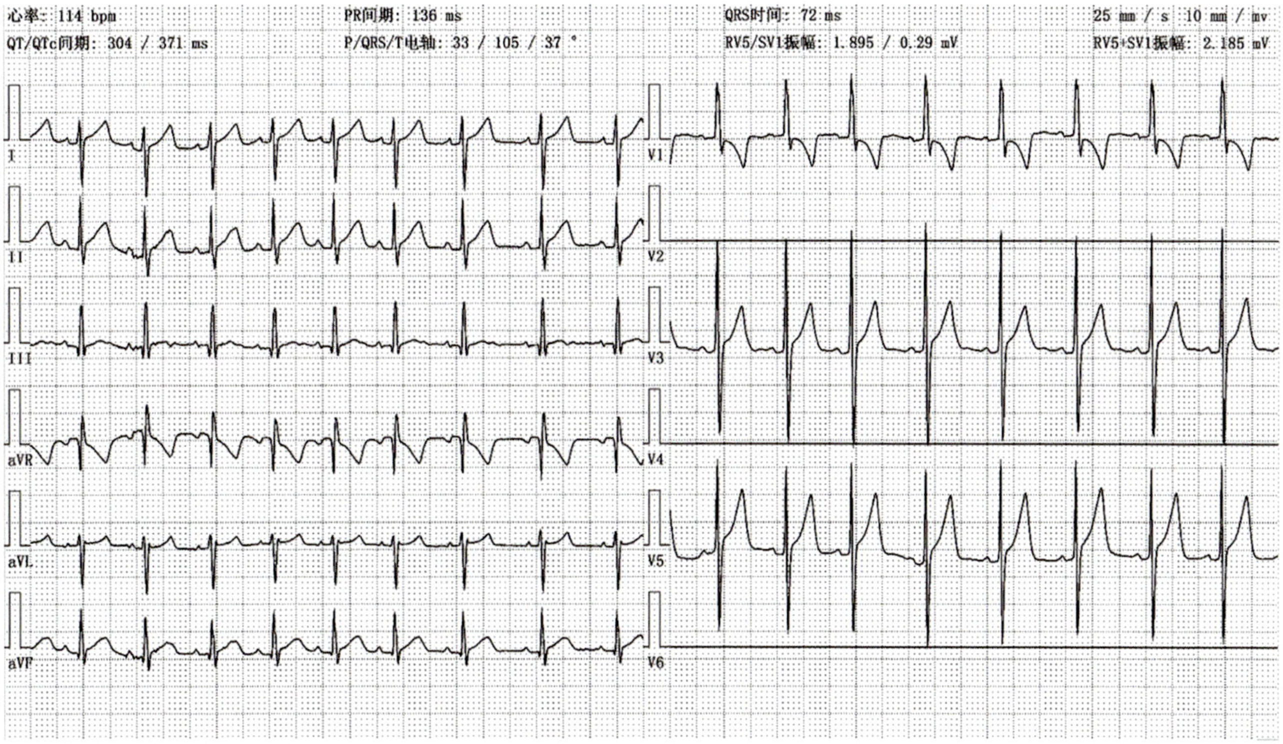

Fig. 15.10 On Day 21 of illness, ECG was normal (HR 114bpm, PR interval was 136 ms)

15.1.5 Case Specific Clinical Features

1. Less than one year old, male, CRP>100, WBC>15 × 109/L, and hypoalbuminemia were high risk factors for developing CAA. Fortunately, this patient was treated timely, and the condition rapidly evolved favorably with IVIG and he did not have coronary artery lesion.
2. Elevated NT-pro BNP in KD are usually caused by two possibilities: increased pressure of atrium/ventricular or encephalocoele. The later usually occurred with sterile meningitis. Thus, once NT-pro BNP increased, routine EEG check is followed. This boy had no neck stiffness; therefore, the first choice of examination should be a non-invasive EEG. On the day of admission, because the

sedative effect was not very well, EEG was not performed. On the following day, his fever subsided and the mental state improved. He ate and played normally. His clinic-laboratory responses were excellent, too. EEG, head CT, and MR were not performed.

3. D-dimer and FDP elevation usually indicates tissue disintegration in multiple organs, as evidenced by the involvement of the lungs, liver, blood, and urinary system. Lucky enough all were recovered quickly in this patient. As a common phenomenon often seen in clinical practice, hepatomegaly usually retested when the patient's liver was enlarged bigger than at admission.
4. In the USA, KD after vaccination most happens with Pediarix [DTaP, hep B, and intramuscular injection of polio vaccine (IPV) combined] but did not show an increase of KD [1–2] though there is a different opinion [3]. IPV was first produced by Dr. Jonas Salk for intramuscular injection in 1953. In 1960s, Dr. Albert Sabin produced attenuated live vaccine, also Sabin vaccination. It was designed for oral polio vaccine (OPV), though there was literature reporting that OPV could result in acute disseminated encephalomyelitis [4]. OPV was popular in China as sugared pills, it should be taken orally three times a day. The disadvantage of OPV is that it will result in diarrhea in a person with innate immune deficiency disease. Cooling reserves are important to keep its effect. This boy had taken a sugared pill one month ago without any adverse effects reported. This time he was vaccinated via IPV. KD mostly occurs in persons with allergies. It may be easier to trigger allergic reaction when using IPV for vaccination, thus cause recipients developing KD. Fortunately, his prognosis was good.
5. KD in infants usually are atypical. This boy developed KD step by step as classic cases stated in textbooks. Skin around BCG scar was red, similar to those happening in most babies. Of course, there was the center skin red, too. It can be recovered in 2 weeks without administrating anti-tuberculosis reagents [5]. BCG scar redden is more important in KD diagnosis [6–8]. It usually happens between days 31 and 806 after BCG inoculated [9]. Some KD developed paronychia appearance at recovery phase (Fig. 15.11). After desquamation, some KD patients have nails with knife cut/insect cut cross furrow (Fig. 15.12a) around 2 month of illness. At 3–4 months, the distal nail may be broken or fall off (Fig. 15.12b). The border of peeling skin around anus in KD is clear (Fig. 15.13a), whereas it is blurry in patients with streptococcal infection (Fig. 15.13b). Regarding to the cracked lips, most recovered, and few developed fatty streaks around lips (Fig. 15.14a–b). This may last forever. Treatment with ointment erythromycin may be beneficial for this.
6. As to when they can be re-vaccinated, AHA suggests that measles, mumps, and varicella immunizations should be deferred for 11 months after receiving high dose IVIG [10]. But children with high risk of exposure to measles may receive vaccination earlier and then be re-immunized at least 11 months after IVIG administration, if they have an inadequate serological response.

Table 15.1 The dynamic changes of lab parameters

Illness	5 day	6 day	10 day	13 day	15 day
WBC ($\times 10^9$/L)	14.5	14			
NE (%)	73.6	75			
HGB (g/L)	128	122			
PLT ($\times 10^9$/L)	256	251			
CRP (mg/L)	86		12.5		5.6
ESR (mm/h)		64			
cTnI (μg/L)	0.053		0.239	0.042	0.029
hs-cTnT (ng/ml)	0.029		0.042	0.009	
NT-pro BNP (ng/ml)	4804		233		

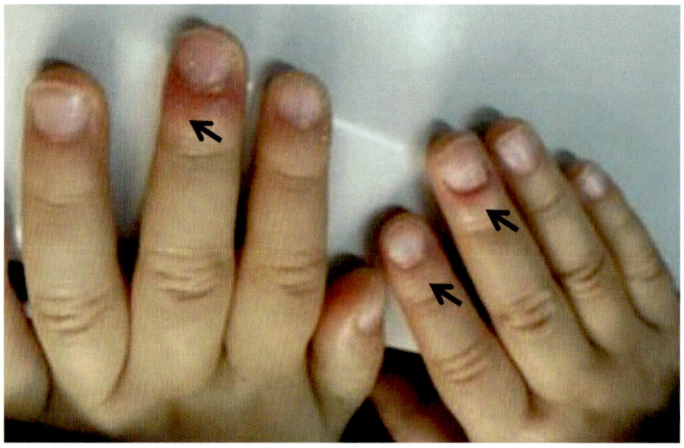

Fig. 15.11 Another KD girl was with paronychia appearance at two months of illness

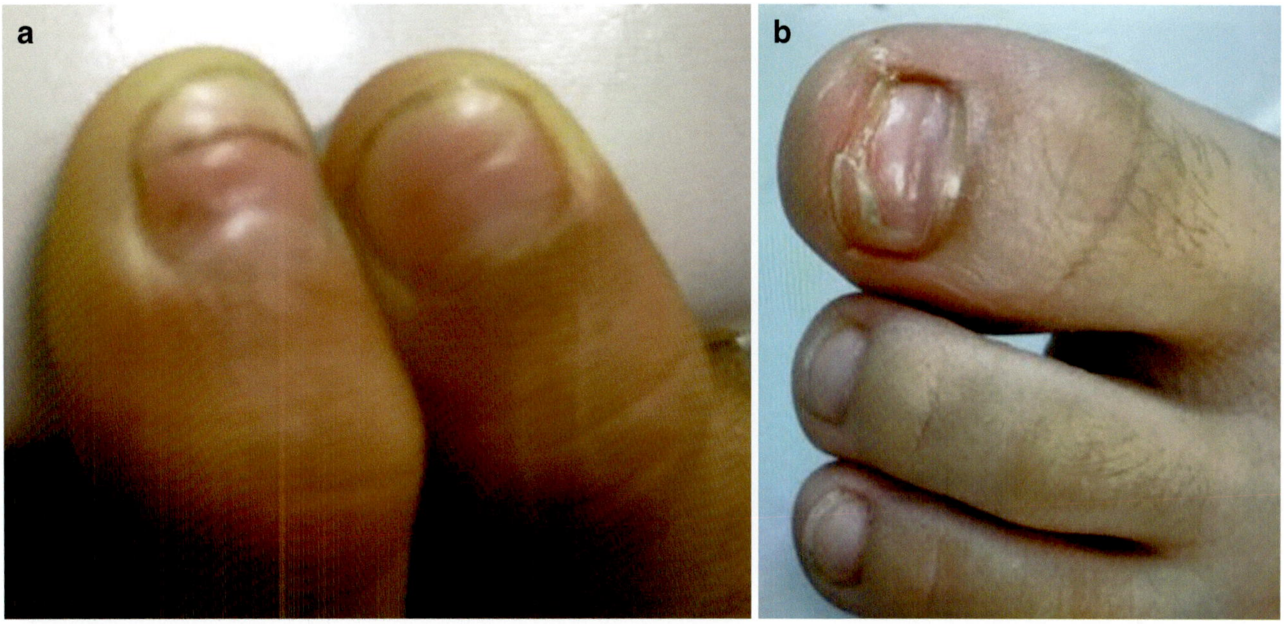

Fig. 15.12 Another KD boy, after desquamation, their nails with knife cut/insect cut cross furrow at about 1.5 months of illness (**a**) and his toe-nails broken at about 2 months of illness, the distal nail fall off (**b**)

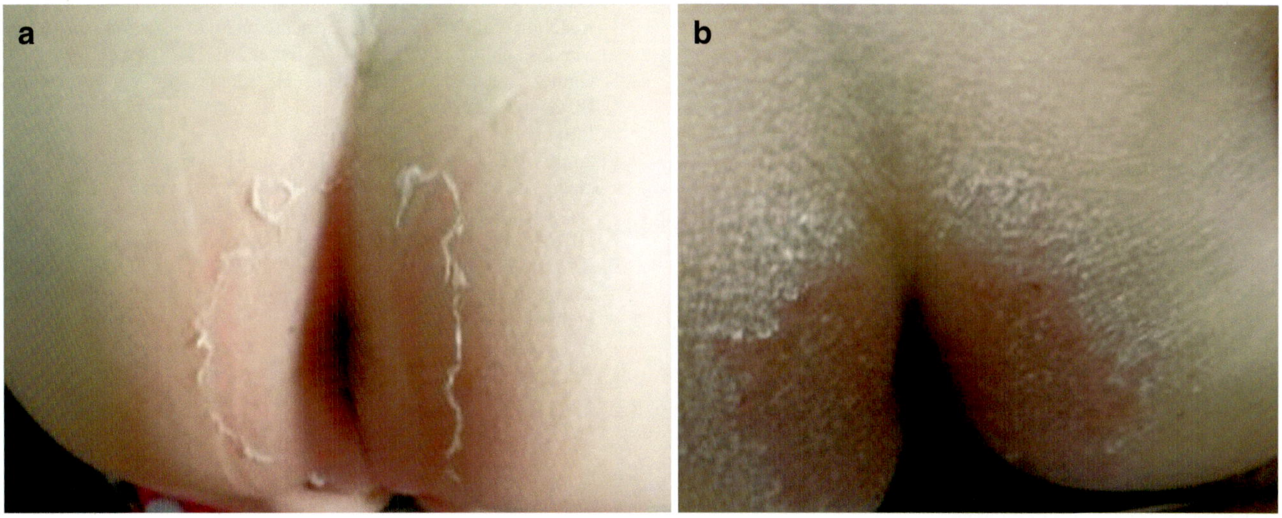

Fig. 15.13 Another KD girl, the border of peeling skin around anus was clearly (**a**), while a streptococcal infection girl the border was blurry (**b**)

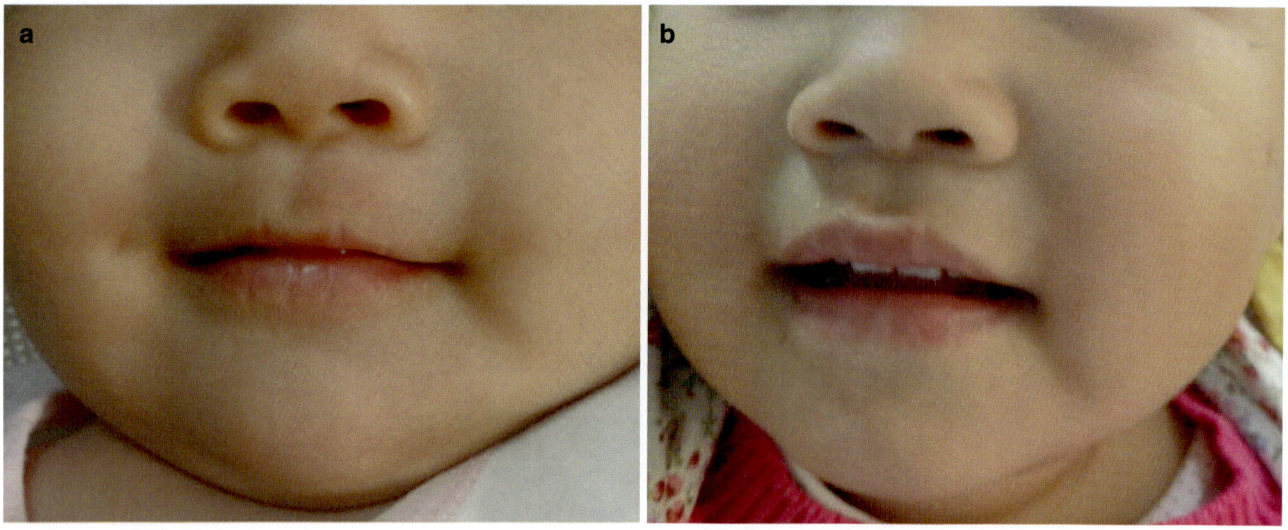

Fig. 15.14 Another KD girl with lips crack, left fatty streaks around lips at two months (**a**) and two years (**b**) of illness

References

1. Hua W, Izurieta HS, Slade B, et al. Kawasaki disease after vaccination: reports to the vaccine adverse event reporting system 1990–2007 the pediatric infectious disease journal. Pediatr Infect Dis J. 2009;28(11):943–7.
2. Abrams JY, Weintraub ES, Baggs JM, et al. Childhood vaccines and Kawasaki disease, vaccine safety datalink, 1996–2006. Vaccine. 2015;33(2):382–7.
3. Chang A, Islam S. Kawasaki disease and Vasculitis associated with immunizations. Pediatr Int. 2018; https://doi.org/10.1111/ped.13590.
4. Shibazaki K, Murakami T, Kushida R, et al. Acute disseminated encephalomyelitis associated with oral polio vaccine. Intern Med. 2006;45(20):1143–6.
5. Kuniyuki S, Asada M. An ulcerated lesion at the BCG vaccination site during the course of Kawasaki disease. J Am Acad Dermatol. 1997;37(2 Pt 2):303–4.
6. Hulme P. CT3 Emergency Medicine. Towards evidence based emergency medicine: best BETs from the Manchester Royal Infirmary. BET 1: BCG scar changes in Kawasaki's disease. Emerg Med J. 2012;29(7):598–9.
7. Garrido-García LM, Castillo-Moguel A, Vázquez-Rivera M, et al. Reaction of the BCG scar in the acute phase of Kawasaki disease in Mexican children. Pediatr Infect Dis J. 2017;36(10):e237–41.
8. Gamez-Gonzalez LB, Hamada H, Llamas-Guillen BA, et al. BCG and Kawasaki disease in Mexico and Japan. Hum Vaccin Immunother. 2017;13(5):1091–3.
9. Araki T, Kodera A, Kitada K, et al. Analysis of factors associated with development of Bacille Calmette-Guérin inoculation site change in patients with Kawasaki disease. J Int Med Res. 2018;46(4):1640–8.
10. Kawasaki disease. In: Red book. 2015 Report of the committee on infectious diseases. Elk Grove, IL: American Academy of Pediatrics; 2015:494–500.

KD with Myocardial Tumor

16

Yali Zhang, Hong Wang, Xiaona Yu, Yang Hou, Bai Gao, and Jing Dong

Abstract

To the author's knowledge, cardiac tumor combined with KD has not yet been reported. Primary cardiac neoplasm (PCN) was rare. Autopsy confirmed its morbidity between 0.17% and 0.28% (Zhong-min et al., Practical clinic cardiac surgery [M] 623–631, 2010). With echo, CT, and MR application, more and more asymptomatic patients are found by chance. PCN was divided into benign and malignant, at a ratio of 3:1. According to the morbidity, benign tumor was cardiac myxoma, cardiac fibroma, cardiac rhabdomyoma, and so on. About 66.7% of benign cardiac tumor is myxoma, which mostly come from atrial septum. Cardiac fibroma was the second common cardiac benign tumor (Toyama et al., Rep Case Kyobu Geka 70(4):317–319, 2017). Although it was called benign tumor, it is with the character of malignancy. Surgery usually cannot remove the tumor completely and they recur after operation. Furthermore, it also results in sudden death in children (Aw et al., Pediatr Cardiol 8(2):394–400, 2017). Cardiac rhabdomyoma is a rare PCN with skeletal muscle differentiation, which is the most common PCN in children, especially in newborns and infants. It may be partially or completely dissipated; so conservative treatment is generally recommended (Dinesh Kumar et al., Ann Card Anaesth. 19(4):728–732, 2016). Only when cardiac rhabdomyomas cause hemodynamic obstruction or heart rhythm disorders that affect cardiac function, medical treatment or surgical resection is necessary. The main purpose of surgery is to relieve hemodynamic blockage, protect ventricular and valve function, and prevent conduction damage. We are reporting a case of left ventricular mass presenting with KD.

16.1 Case 53 Kd with Myocardial Tumor

A 28-month-old boy had an unremarkable antenatal and family history, except that he had a hernia repair operation at the Beijing Institute of Pediatrics when he was one year old.

He presented on Day 10 of illness with a prolonged fever for 10 days, along with red lips, bilateral conjunctival congestion, rashes for 6 days. He was diagnosed with KD, systemic inflammatory response syndrome, and liver dysfunction on Day 4 of illness at a local hospital. He was given infusion of one dose IVIG 2g/kg/day, second-generation cephalosporin, and oral aspirin on Day 4 of the illness. His fever subsided, and both conjunctival congestion and rashes improved on Day 6. But his fever recurred to 38.7°C on Day 9, along with rashes and bilateral conjunctival congestion. Since the onset, his mental status, diet, and sleep were normal. Examination revealed the following results: his body temperature 37.6°C, PR 105 bpm, RR 24 bpm, weight 14kg. There were scares formed from congestive rashes on his arms, with cervical lymphadenectasis and red lips. Liver was enlarged 2cm below the right costal margin, medium texture. Others were normal. One day before admission, blood work revealed WBC 8.5×10^9/L, NE 66.5%, HGB 119g/L, PLT 436×10^9/L, CRP 16mg/L. At admission, blood test results were as follows: WBC 8.61×10^9/L, NE 67.6%, HGB 114g/L, PLT 556×10^9/L, CRP 22.40mg/L, NT pro-BNP 1257pg/ml,

Y. Zhang
Department of PICU, Zhengzhou University, Zhengzhou, China

H. Wang (✉)
Department of Pediatric Cardiology, Shengjing Hospital of China Medical University, Shenyang, China

X. Yu
Department of Ultrasound, Shengjing Hospital of China Medical University, Shenyang, China
e-mail: yuxn@sj-hospital.org

Y. Hou
Department of Radiology, Shengjing Hospital of China Medical University, Shenyang, China

B. Gao
Department of Neurology Function, Shengjing Hospital of China Medical University, Shenyang, China

J. Dong
Department of Cardiology Function, Shengjing Hospital of China Medical University, Shenyang, China
e-mail: dongj@sj-hospital.org

H. Wang (ed.), *Paediatric Kawasaki Disease*, https://doi.org/10.1007/978-981-15-0038-1_16

Na^+ 133mmol/L, PT 14.3s, APTT 29s, Fib 3.7g/L, D-dimer 307μg/L. ALB 34.0g/L, GTP 56U/L. AST, CK, CK-MB, CK-MB-mass, cTnI, and hs-cTnT were normal. Cervical ultrasound showed bilateral lymphadenectasis; the larger one was about 2.0cm×0.8 cm on the left and 1.8 cm×0.7 cm on the right. Chest DR was normal (Fig. 16.1). He had met the criteria for KD with IVIG resistance and was treated with (1) IVIG one dose 2g/kg over 10 hours; (2) aspirin 30–50mg/kg/day, dipyridamole 3–5mg/kg/day, in divided three doses oral; (3) myocardial nutrition management.

On Day 11, his fever settled down. ECG showed J point elevation (Fig. 16.2a). On Day 12, the rashes and conjunctival congestion improved. He felt sleepy and lost appetite. Examination revealed a positive left palmar reflex. Blood work revealed positive PINF virus antibody titer. ECG was normal (Fig. 16.2b). EEG showed abnormal signals; background rhythm slowed down, **θ** wave was dominant, 4–6 Hz medium amplitude (Fig. 16.3). Lumbar puncture test showed

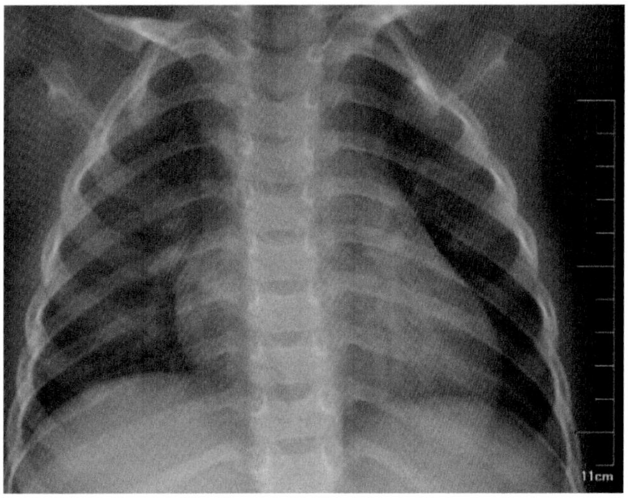

Fig. 16.1 On Day 10, chest DR was normal

CSF pressure was 60 drops/min, Pan's reaction was positive, WBC 20×10^6/L, RBC 4000×10^6/L (puncture bleeding at beginning), CSF glucose 2.73mmol/L, chlorine 124.2mmol/L, protein 0.47g/L. CSF smear and culture were normal. For he was suspected to have CNS complication, he was given infusion of deproteinized calf serum, mannitol, and furosemidum for 2 days; continued to receive infusion of second-generation cephalosporin. On Day 13, he was afebrile over 48h. His mental state was still bad. He lost appetite and vomited once but no defecation. His conjunctiva was mildly congested. Left palmar reflex was positive. Liver ultrasound showed hepatomegaly, 1.8cm below the right costal margin (Fig. 16.4a). Pediatric neurologist suggested: (1) head MRI and VBAEP; (2) continuing treatment on nourishing nerves, changing mannitol to q12h; (3) infusion of naloxone. On Day 14, without being given naloxone, his metal state and appetite improved, and his sleeping pattern was normal. Conjunctival congestion was relieved, lips were slightly red. Bilateral palmar reflex was positive, Babinski sign was negative on the left, while positive on the right. Tested blood work revealed WBC 6.43×10^9/L, NE 30.4%, HGB 103g/L, PLT 780×10^9/L, CRP 7.23mg/L, ESR 66mm/h. VBAEP was normal. Echo showed normal LVEF (Fig. 16.4b), LCA (Fig. 16.5a), and RCA (Fig. 16.5b). Aspirin was reduced to one dose 3–5 mg/kg/day.

On Day 15, he vomited several times. After receiving infusion of omeprazole, his vomiting was gradually relieved. His mental state was not improved, and he lost appetite again. Repeated CBC test revealed WBC 8.08×10^9/L, NE% 39.7%, HGB 107g/L. PLT 661×10^9/L. Serum amylase was normal. Serum lipase 65.4(<60) U/L; Abdominal CT scan showed ventosity, appendiceal fecalith (Fig. 16.6), and multiple lymphadenectasis in the mesentery. The pancreas was normal. Pancreatitis was not excluded. Without abdominal pain or vomiting, he was only permitted to take low fat liquid and liquid infusion. On Day 16, he still had no appetite, but mental

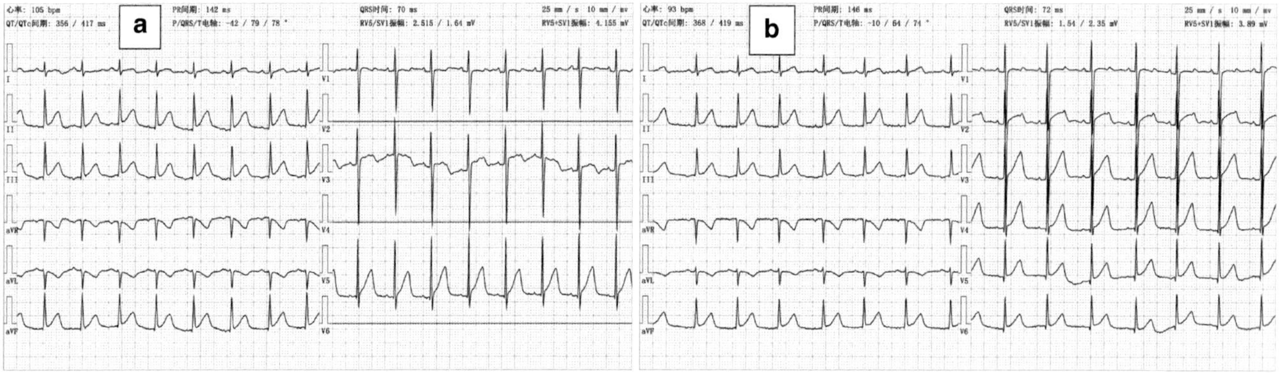

Fig. 16.2 ECG showed J point elevation on Day 11 (**a**), while normal on Day 12 (**b**)

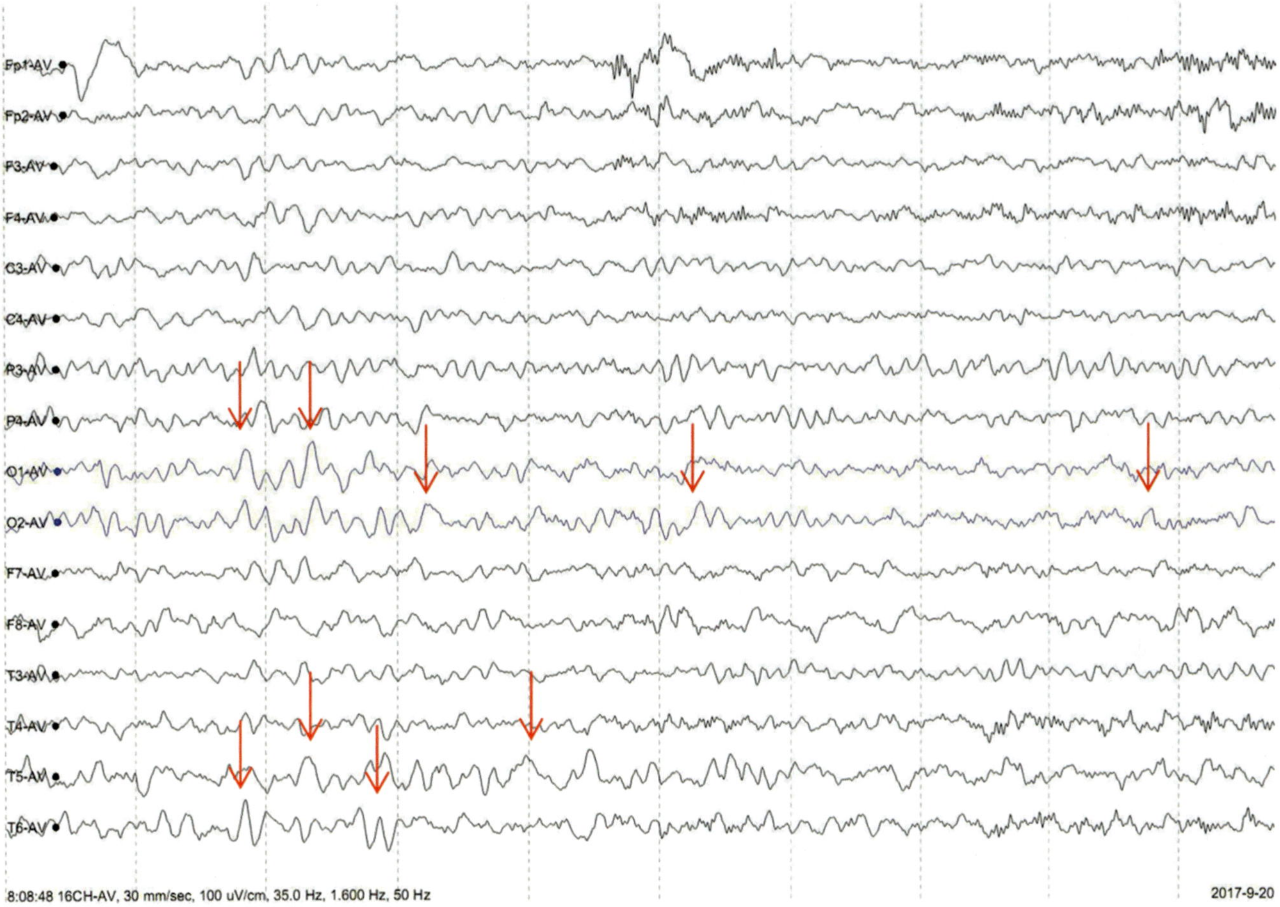

Fig. 16.3 On Day 12, EEG showed background rhythm slow down, **θ** wave was dominant, 4–6Hz medium amplitude

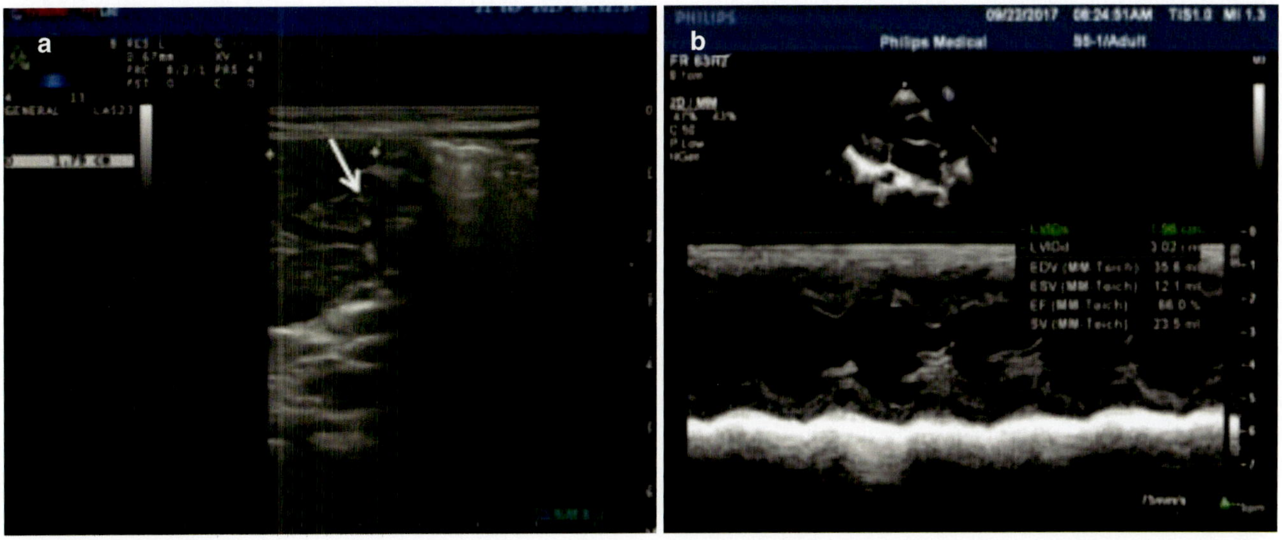

Fig. 16.4 On day 13 of illness, liver ultrasound showed hepatomegaly, 1.8cm below the arch of ribs at right midclavicular line (**a**). On day 14, echocardiography showed normal LVEF (**b**)

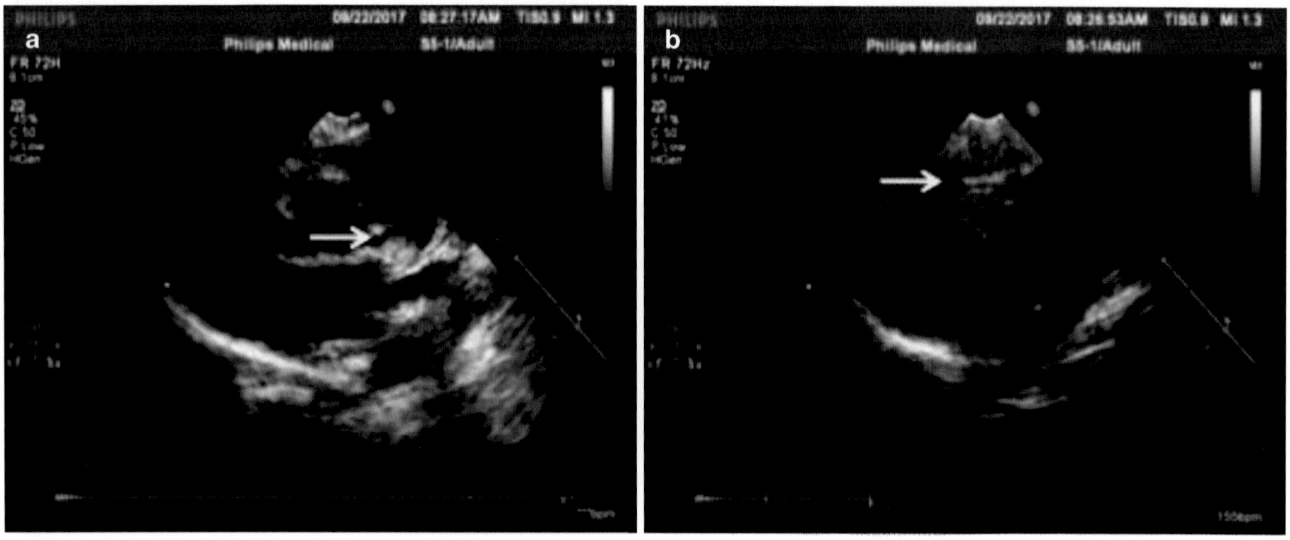

Fig. 16.5 On day 14 of illness, echocardiography showed normal LCA (**a**) and RCA (**b**)

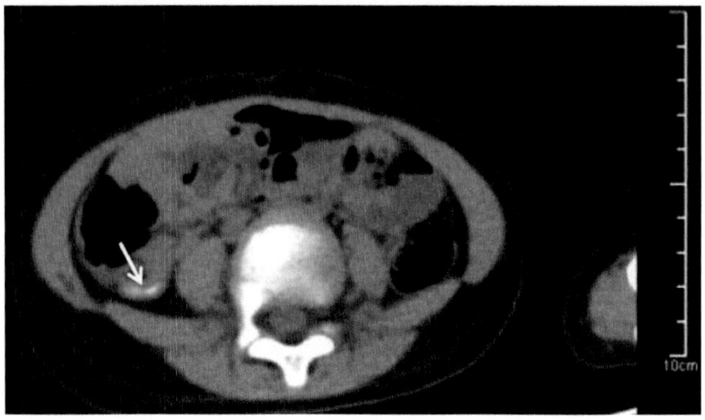

Fig. 16.6 On Day 15, abdominal CT showed appendiceal fecalith

state got better. Repeated EEG test showed slow background rhythm, the bilateral occipital region dominated by 4–6 Hz medium-high amplitude θ wave, and a little high-amplitude 3Hz δ wave (Fig. 16.7a). Head MRI and VABEP showed normal results. On Day 17, his appetite was improved. Bilateral palmar reflex was positive. Bilateral Babinski signs were negative. Low fat liquid food was permitted. On Day 18, his mental state was stable, bilateral palmar reflex was still positive. Serum amylase was normal, serum lipase was 65.4(<60) U/L, and urine amylase was 871 (<640) U/L. For he had developed pancreatitis, treatment plans were listed as the following: (1) liquid low fat food was permitted and he was given infusion of liquid; (2) he was continually given infusion of second-generation cephalosporin. On Day 19, repeated EEG showed background rhythm slowed down, mainly θ wave. The bilateral occipital region was dominated with 4–7 Hz medium-high amplitude θ wave, and a small amount of high-amplitude 3Hz δ wave (Fig. 16.7b). Echo showed normal LCA, LAD (Fig. 16.8a), RCA (Fig. 16.8b), and LVED (Fig. 16.9).

On Day 20, his body temperature reached to 38.7°C twice, without other symptoms. On Day 21, his fever regressed to 38°C. Physical examination showed his mental state was bad, he had pharyngeal congestion, and his right palmar reflex was positive. Retested CBC showed WBC 4.0×10^{9}/L, NE 0.55×10^{9}/L, HGB 122 g/L, PLT 393×10^{9}/L. It was difficult to distinguish IVIG resistance from possible infection for the reoccurred fever, and aseptic meningitis was suspected. Treatment with methylprednisolone would be beneficial for his situation. After getting consents from his parents, he was treated with (1) infusion of methylprednisolone 1.4mg/kg/day; (2) continuing oral aspirin; (3) oral lysine inositol vitamin B_{12} 5ml twice a day, oral brain protein hydrolysate tablets, 1 piece, twice a day. On Day 22, his mental state was stable and he was afebrile. The dose of methylprednisolone was reduced to 1mg/kg/day oral. On Day 23, his appetite got better, right palmar reflex was positive. MP IgG and CP IgG were positive. He took azithromycin for 3 days, and he was discharged.

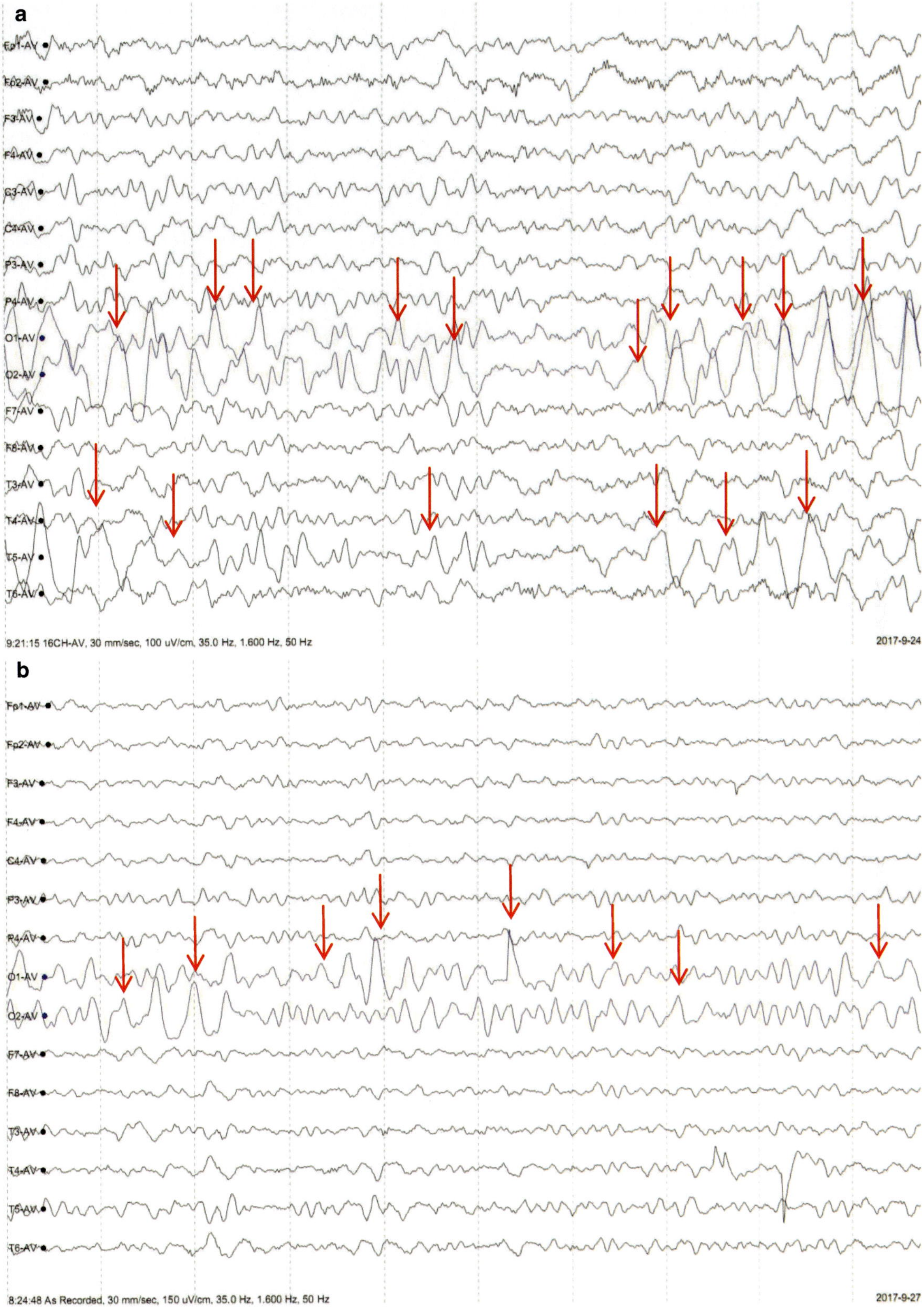

Fig. 16.7 EEG showed background rhythm slows down, more θ waves, the bilateral occipital region is dominated by 4–6 Hz medium-high amplitude θ wave, and a small amount of high-amplitude 3Hz δ wave on Day 16 (**a**) and 19 (**b**) of illness

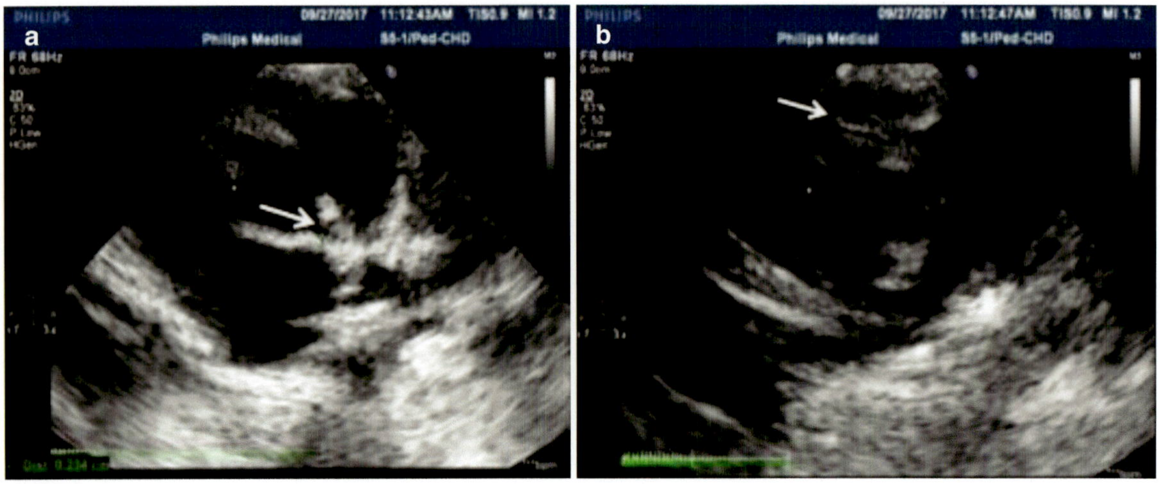

Fig. 16.8 On day 19 of illness, echocardiography showed LCA 2.3 mm (**a**), RCA 1.8 mm (**b**)

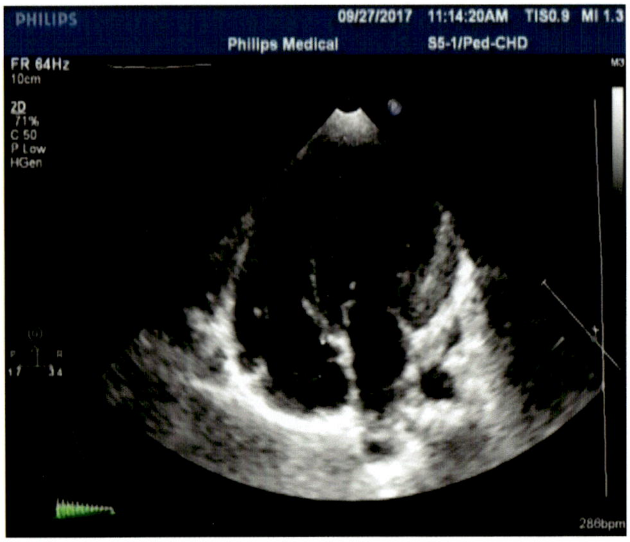

Fig. 16.9 On day 19 of illness, echocardiography showed normal LVED

16.1.1 Clinical Course of the Patient

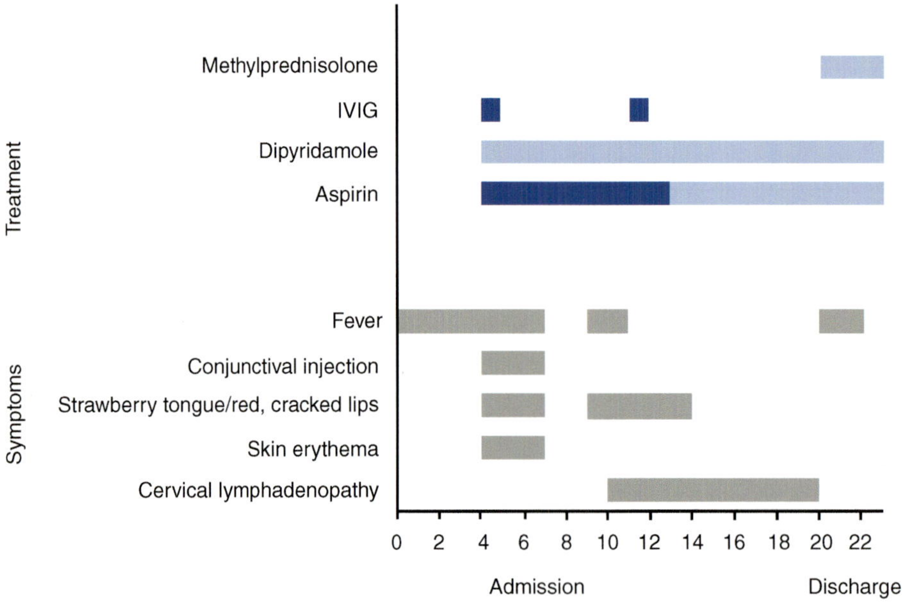

16.1.2 Follow-up

After discharge, methylprednisolone tablets were gradually reduced starting from Day 8 and withdrawn on Day 30. Repeated CBC test showed WBC 11.28×10^9/L, NE% 30.5%, NE 3.44×10^9/L, HGB 119g/L, PLT 634×10^9/L. On one month of illness, EEG showed background rhythm was slow, and the bilateral occipital region was dominated with high amplitude 3Hz δ wave, some 4–6 Hz medium-high amplitude θ wave (Fig. 16.10a). Echocardiography showed interventricular septum 5.2mm, LVD 30.5mm, LVEF 70%, a 17mm×14mm medium echo mass was identified in the left ventricular posterior wall (Fig. 16.11a). A 3.0 mm left-to-right shunt signal could be detected in the middle of the atrial septum. Coronary artery was normal.

On Day 45, retested blood work revealed WBC 7.35×10^9/L, NE 43.7%, HGB 121g/L, PLT 369×10^9/L, ESR 2mm/h (Table 16.1). E EG was normal (Fig. 16.10b). Echo showed LVD 31mm, left ventricular posterior wall thickness 4mm, EF 62%, a

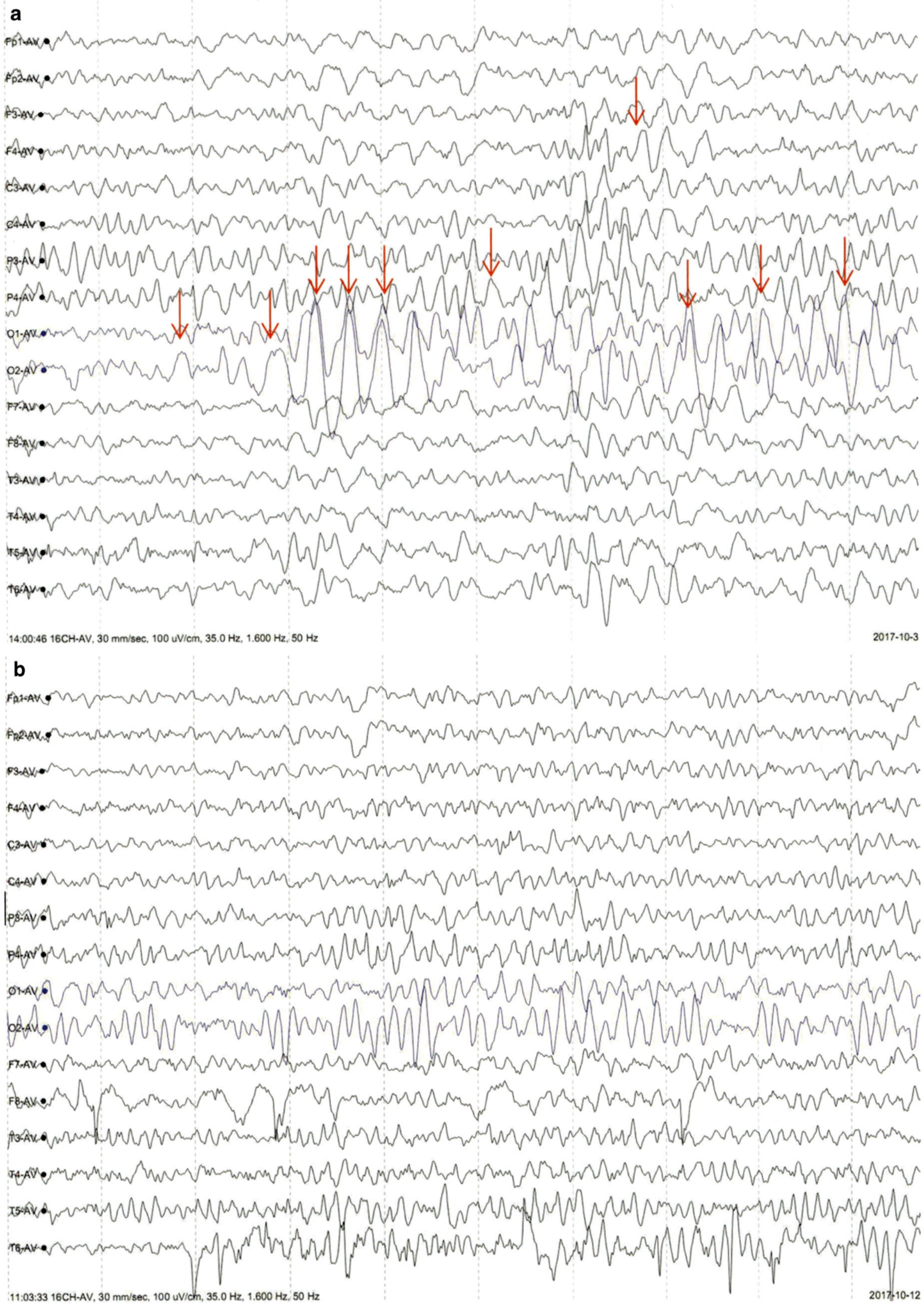

Fig. 16.10 EEG showed background rhythm was slow, the bilateral occipital region is dominated high-amplitude 3Hz δ wave, some 4–6 Hz medium-high amplitude θ wave at one month (**a**) and normal on Day 40 (**b**)

18mm×14mm medium mass in the left ventricular posterior wall (Fig. 16.11b), LCA 2.5mm, RCA 2.2mm. On Day 46, CMR was performed and showed normal left atrium and ventricle (left atrial diameter 22mm, left ventricular diastolic diameter about 35mm). There was a solid signal in the left pericardium, expansively growing (Fig. 16.12), compressed the left atrial ear, and the anterior wall of the left ventricle was unclear. The mass diameter was about 30mm×19mm×22mm (Fig. 16.13), slight deformation of left ventricular cavity in affected segment. Delayed scanning showed a significant uniform enhancement of the mass (Fig. 16.14). The remaining left ventricular wall was normal (4mm septum) and the contraction movement was normal. There was a little liquid signal in the pericardial cavity. A cardiac surgery specialist was consulted with, and he highly suspected a benign myocardial fibroid and suggested follow-up plan. We informed his parents of the child's condition, and referred him for cardiac ultrasound at Beijing Anzhen Hospital. It was still undiagnosed. At 7 months of illness, DIC was normal. PDE showed the mass of left ventricular increased to 24mm×19 (Fig. 16.15). ECG was normal (Fig. 16.16).

16.1.3 Diagnosis

1. KD, IVIG resistant
2. Cardiac tumor
3. CNS involvement
4. Hyponatremia
5. Granulocytopenia
6. Pancreatitis was not excluded

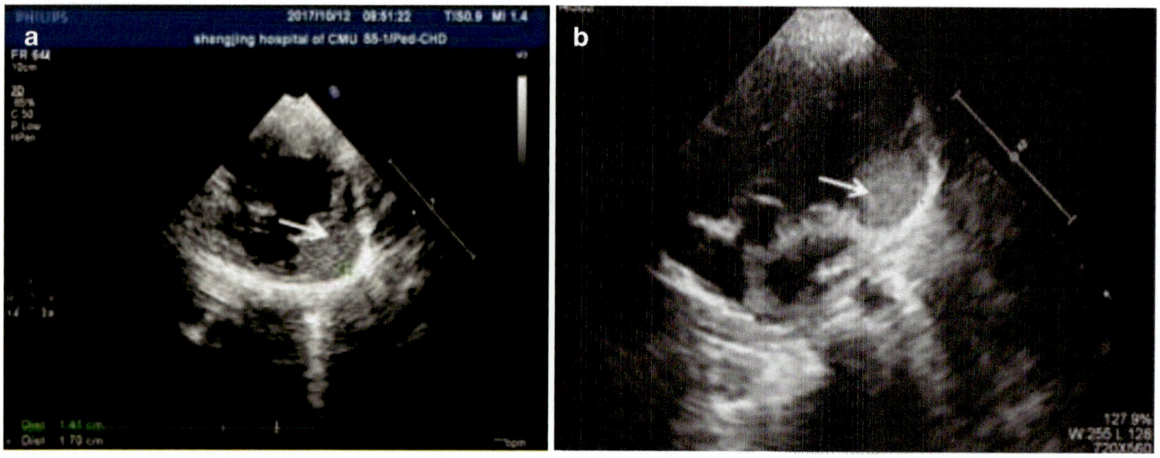

Fig. 16.11 Echo showed a 17 mm × 14 mm medium mass can be seen in the left ventricular posterior wall on Day 30 (**a**), and 18 mm × 15 mm medium echo mass on Day 45 (b)

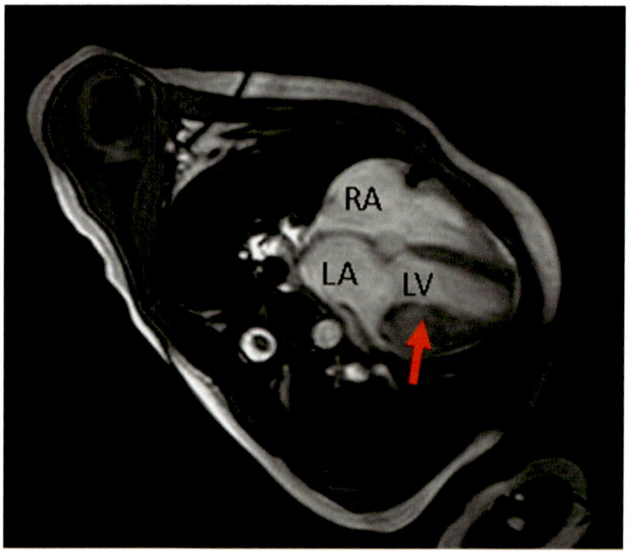

Fig. 16.12 On Day 46 of illness, CMR showed a solid signal in the left pericardium, expansively growing

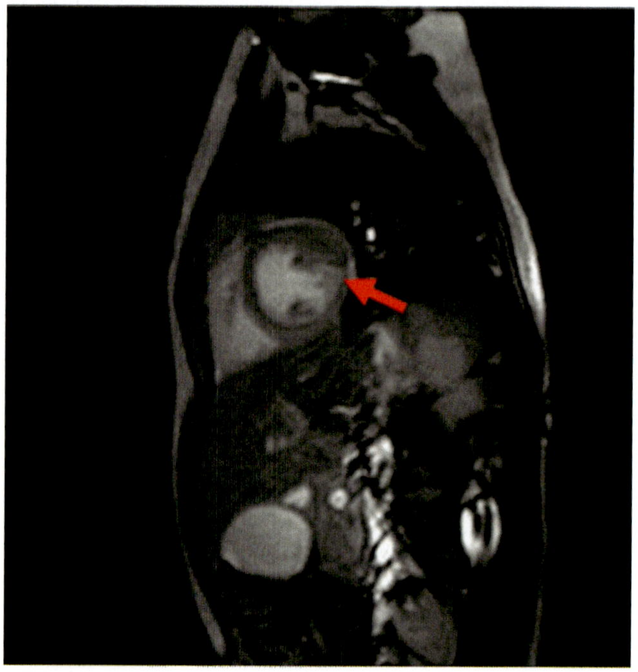

Fig. 16.13 On Day 46 of illness, CMR delayed scanning showed a significant uniform enhancement of the mass (red arrow)

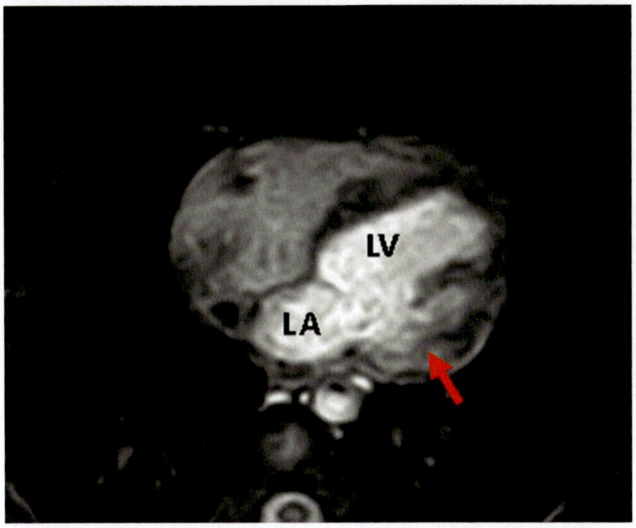

Fig. 16.14 On Day 46 of illness, CMR showed the mass diameter was about 30 mm × 19 mm × 22 mm, left ventricular cavity was slight deformation in affected segment (red arrow)

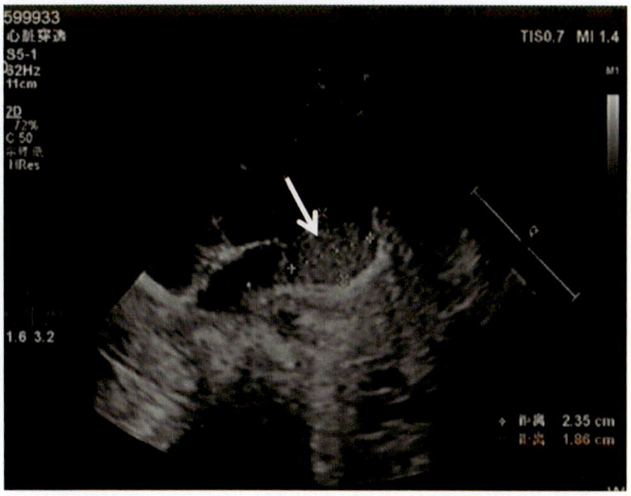

Fig. 16.15 At 7 months, echo showed a 24 mm × 19 mm medium echo mass can be seen in the left ventricular posterior wall

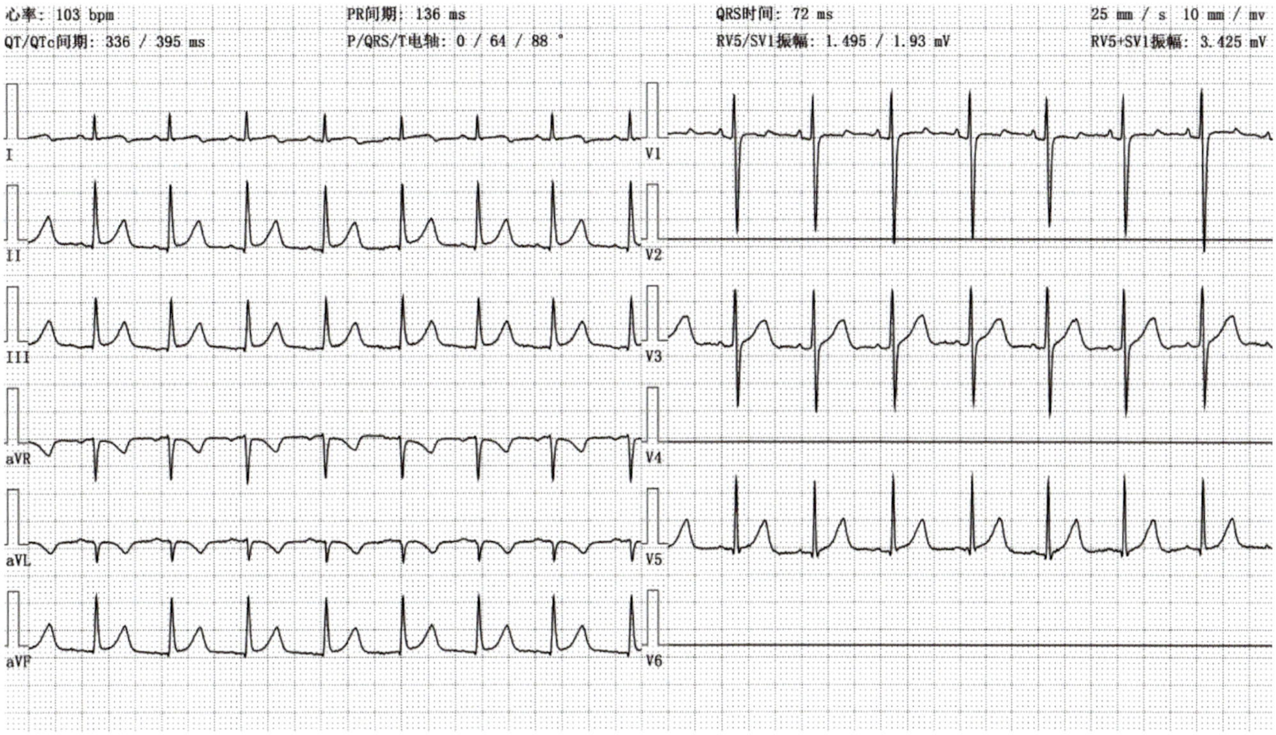

Fig. 16.16 At the 7 months, ECG was normal

Table 16.1 The summary of dynamic changes of lab parameters

Time of illness	9 days	10 days	14 days	15 days	21 days	1 months	1.5 months
WBC(×10⁹/L)	8.5	8.61	6.43	8.08	4.0	11.28	7.35
NE(%)	66.5	67.6	30.4	39.7	13.8	30.5	43.7
HGB(g/L)	119	114	103	107	122	119	121
PLT(×10⁹/L)	436	556	780	661	393	634	369
CRP(mg/L)	16	22.4	7.23				
ESR(mm)			66				2
ALB(g/L)		34					
GPT(U/L)		56					
NT pro-BNP(μg/ml)		1257					

16.1.4 Discussion

He had met the criteria of incomplete KD for he had persistent fever for more than 5 days, and (1) cervical lymphadenectasis; (2) conjunctival hyperemia without purulent discharge in both eyes; (3) red lips; (4) rashes.

He had met the criteria of KD IVIG resistance, too, based on the followings: (1) he was diagnosed as KD; (2) fever recurred >38°Cafter receiving infusion of IVIG 2g/kg 36h, along with rashes and conjunctival congestion.

Differential diagnosis of eye-bound membrane fever, scarlet fever, and Steven–Johnson syndrome should be considered.

It has been reported that a quarter of KD patients have CNS complications [1]. This child was highly suspected to have CNS involvement, because (1) he was KD patient, (2) he was sleepy and his mental state was bad, (3) his palmar reflex was positive initially at left, then developed to bilateral. Two days later it was positive at the right, while Babinski sign was negative on the left then positive on the right. These were significant signs for a 28 months boy; (4) his EEG was abnormal and persistently abnormal over 3 days. As to increased CSF cell numbers, according to ratio in blood routine, WBC at 12×10^6/L cell in CSF was almost normal, mildly increased protein in CSF could possibly come from bleeding during puncture procedure. Increased CSF pressure was associated with edema in his brain. After treatment with mannitol and furosemidum for 5 days, infusion of calf serum deproteinized and cefuroxime for one week, his mental state improved. With continuing to take vitamin B_{12} for 3 weeks, his EEG recovered at one month of illness.

The best time to apply IVIG to KD patients is 5-7 days of illness onset. Earlier (<4 days) application of IVIG causes patients prone to IVIG intolerance [1]. After receiving infusion of full dose IVIG on Day 4, he had fever again. It may be due to either serious disease or relevance to earlier IVIG applications.

16.1.5 Case Specific Clinical Features

1. A mass was found in echo since one month of illness. We do not know if this mass was primary tumor, or a mass secondary to KD. It was about 17 mm within the first month of KD onset, and the progress was a little bit fast by about 7 mm in the following 6 months. We deduced that it was an original mass occurred before KD onset. It is possible that sonographers focused on changes in coronary artery but missed those in left ventricular cavities. Whether the tumor was originated at left ventricle as suggested in ultrasound, or originated from the pericardium as suggested in MR, this mass/tumor was not in consistence with the left atrial myxoma [2]. Thus, we deduced it was a common cardiac fibroma, a benign tumor in heart muscle.
2. Left ventricular mass is a rare condition, of which the most common is thrombus [3], and this boy happened to have KD, and he was in a high coagulation stage with thrombocytopenia (PLT was 634×10^9/L). Echo is a very useful modality of investigation to evaluate the mass of left ventricle. This boy's echo showed the mass's feature was similar to ventricle rather than thrombus. Cardiac MRI also confirmed that the mass was a tumor rather than a thrombus. Thus, he was not given warfarin, and was followed up only [3, 4].
3. The tumor grew fast and its edge was not clear. Cardiac MRI showed it was connected with pericardium. The prognosis might not be good once it passes through the left ventricular wall and penetrates into the left ventricular cavity, making it difficult to be removed completely and prone to recurrence [5, 6].
4. The boy had vomit, without abdominal pain and fever. Serum lipase is slightly elevated on Day 15. Abdominal CT showed intestinal bloating, multiple mesenteric lymphadenectasis, but pancreas had no congestion and edema. Three days later, serum amylase 98U/L, serum lipase 65.4U/L, urine amylase 871U/L indicated he had developed pancreatitis. Thus, we deduced his abdominal CT maybe performed earlier and failed to identify positive signal.

References

1. Alves NR, Magalhães CM, Almeida Rde F, et al. Prospective study of Kawasaki disease complications: Review of 115 cases. Rev Assoc Med Bras. 2011;57(3):299–300.
2. Zhong-min L, Hetzer R, Yu-guo W. Practical clinic cardiac surgery [M]: People Health Publish House; 2010. p. 623–31.
3. Dinesh Kumar US, Shetty SP, Sujay KR, et al. Left ventricular mass: A tumor or a thrombus diagnostic dilemma. Ann Card Anaesth. 2016;19(4):728–32.
4. Toyama M, Abe T, Nakayama M, et al. Effective anticoagulation therapy prior to surgical excision of an aortic valve papillary fibroelastoma diagnosed after a transient cerebral ischemic attack. Rep Case Kyobu Geka. 2017;70(4):317–9.
5. Humez S, Gibier JB, Recher M, et al. Cardiac fibroma: a rare cause of sudden child death. Ann Pathol. 2015;35(5):445–8.
6. Aw F, Goyer I, Raboisson MJ, et al. Accelerated cardiac rhabdomyoma regression with everolimus in infants with tuberous sclerosis complex. Pediatr Cardiol. 2017;38(2):394–400.

Correction to: Paediatric Kawasaki Disease

Hong Wang

Correction to: H. Wang (ed.), *Paediatric Kawasaki Disease*, https://doi.org/10.1007/978-981-15-0038-1

The original version of this book was inadvertently published before updating author corrections. All the author corrections have been updated in this revised version.

The updated online version of this book can be found at https://doi.org/10.1007/978-981-15-0038-1

H. Wang (ed.), *Paediatric Kawasaki Disease*, https://doi.org/10.1007/978-981-15-0038-1_17

GPSR Compliance

The European Union's (EU) General Product Safety Regulation (GPSR) is a set of rules that requires consumer products to be safe and our obligations to ensure this.

If you have any concerns about our products, you can contact us on ProductSafety@springernature.com

In case Publisher is established outside the EU, the EU authorized representative is:

Springer Nature Customer Service Center GmbH
Europaplatz 3
69115 Heidelberg, Germany

Batch number: 10756367

Printed by Printforce, the Netherlands